Cancer Control

Cancer Control

Edited by

J. Mark Elwood, MD, DSc, FRCPC, FAFPHM
Vice-President, Family and Community Oncology,
British Columbia Cancer Agency,
Vancouver, Canada

Simon B. Sutcliffe, MD, FRCP, FRCPC, FRCR
Board Chair, Canadian Partnership Against Cancer;
Past President, British Columbia Cancer Agency,
Vancouver, Canada

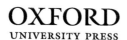
OXFORD
UNIVERSITY PRESS

OXFORD

UNIVERSITY PRESS

Great Clarendon Street, Oxford OX2 6DP

Oxford University Press is a department of the University of Oxford.
It furthers the University's objective of excellence in research, scholarship,
and education by publishing worldwide in

Oxford New York

Auckland Cape Town Dar es Salaam Hong Kong Karachi
Kuala Lumpur Madrid Melbourne Mexico City Nairobi
New Delhi Shanghai Taipei Toronto

With offices in

Argentina Austria Brazil Chile Czech Republic France Greece
Guatemala Hungary Italy Japan Poland Portugal Singapore
South Korea Switzerland Thailand Turkey Ukraine Vietnam

Oxford is a registered trade mark of Oxford University Press
in the UK and in certain other countries

Published in the United States
by Oxford University Press Inc., New York

British Library Cataloguing in Publication Data

Data available

Library of Congress Cataloging in Publication Data

Data available

Typeset in Minion
by Glyph International, Bangalore, India
Printed in UK
on acid-free paper by
CPI Antony Rowe, Chippenham, Wiltshire

ISBN 978–0–19–955017–3

10 9 8 7 6 5 4 3 2 1

To Candace, Jeremy, and Briana;
and to Margaret, Siobhan, Sian, and Katie

Preface

Cancer control is the term applied to the development of integrated population-based approaches to reduce the incidence and mortality from cancer and to minimize its impact on affected individuals. It covers a spectrum of prevention, early diagnosis, optimal treatment, and supportive and palliative care. It emphasizes the application of current best practice and new knowledge gained through research.

Cancer control has been a major initiative in several countries in recent years; in the United Kingdom, France, Australia, and Canada, for example, cancer control developments have become a political priority, in advance of any similar commitment in other diseases. This change in approach was driven by the high level of public interest and concern about cancer, and stimulated by the growing numbers of people affected; the higher public visibility of cancer, due largely to the efforts of voluntary cancer organizations; rapid scientific developments, many requiring major financial investment; and the availability of internationally comparable outcome measures such as patient survival rates.

Most countries in the developed world, at national or regional level, are at some stage in the evolution of cancer control strategic plans. These vary greatly in scope. Some plans concentrate on specific areas such as radiotherapy provision or palliative care. Some plans originate from non-government agencies and are concerned primarily with prevention, screening, or patient support. More extensive cancer plans seek to integrate and improve the whole spectrum of care. The extent to which research and evaluation is incorporated in cancer control plans varies enormously. Most variable of all is the implementation, ranging from general statements of support up to major health care reorganizations.

These developments are changing the approach used in the clinical care of cancer patients. From the traditional model of centres of excellence focusing on the patients seen in that institution, and often autonomous cancer research centres, there is a shift towards the integrated control of cancer, from prevention to palliation, and emphasis of the impact on all members of the population, and on maximizing the benefits gained from available resources.

The development and implementation of cancer control plans is a consultative process, involving public policy-makers, health care professionals (including providers, planners, and health managers), health advocacy groups and organizations, patients and those who care for them, and the informed public. As a result, most senior health care staff in oncology will be involved to some degree in cancer control developments. Advocacy groups, the informed public, and interested patients who are concerned with the 'big picture' issues, including patient choice, resource allocation, quality of care, and moving new research results into practice, will all be involved in cancer control.

This creates a need for an integrated readable overview of cancer control. No such book exists at present. This book is planned to provide interesting, relevant, topical, and we hope challenging viewpoints on key areas within cancer control, mainly from a developed country perspective, but including world-wide viewpoints. We are very grateful to the chapter authors, people with demanding positions and wide experience, representing many countries and disciplines, who have been willing to contribute their time and skills to this book. We are very aware that many important issues have not been explored fully, and that this topic is developing rapidly.

We are grateful for the insights and stimulation from a vast range of colleagues and patients over our professional lives, and the experiences we have gained in many countries. Our thanks for assistance with the editorial work goes to Ruth Grantham, Anar Dhalla, Candace Elwood, and to Georgia Pinteau, Eloise Moir-Ford, Nicola Ulyatt, and their colleagues at Oxford University Press.

Mark Elwood
Simon Sutcliffe
Vancouver, 2009

Contents

Contributors

Tara Addis, BSc
Chair,
Stakeholder Relations,
Campaign to Control Cancer (C2CC),
Toronto, Canada (Chapter 16)

Paolo Baili, PhD
Descriptive Studies and Health
Planning Unit,
Fondazione IRCCS Istituto
Nazionale dei Tumori,
Milan, Italy (Chapter 18)

Lynda Balneaves, RN, PhD
Associate Professor and CIHR
New Investigator,
University of British Columbia
School of Nursing,
Vancouver, British Columbia,
Canada (Chapter 13)

Michael Barton, OAM, MBBS, MD, FRANZCR
Professor of Radiation Oncology,
South West Sydney Clinical School,
University of New South Wales,
Sydney, New South Wales,
Australia (Chapter 9)

Courtney Beers, MPH
Alvin J. Siteman Cancer Center
and Department of Surgery,
Washington University School
of Medicine,
St. Louis, Missouri, USA (Chapter 2)

Melissa Brouwers, PhD
Associate Professor and Head of Health
Services Research,
Department of Oncology,
McMaster University;
Provincial Director, Program in
Evidence-based Care, Cancer Care Ontario,
Hamilton, Ontario (Chapter 8)

George P. Browman, MD
Clinical Professor
School of Population and Public Health
University of British Columbia, and
Department of Oncology
BC Cancer Agency,
Vancouver Island Cancer Centre,
Victoria, British Columbia,
Canada (Chapter 8)

Eduardo Bruera, MD
Department of Palliative Care and
Rehabilitation Medicine,
The University of Texas M.D. Anderson
Cancer Center,
Houston, Texas, USA (Chapter 12)

Ann N Burchell, PhD
Division of Cancer Epidemiology,
McGill University,
Montreal, Quebec, Canada (Chapter 6)

Robert Burton, MD, PhD, FAFPHM
Professor,
School of Public Health and Preventive
Medicine,
Monash University;
Melbourne, Victoria, Australia (Chapter 21)

Shirley H. Bush, MBBS, MRCGP, FAChPM
Assistant Professor,
Division of Palliative Care,
University of Ottawa;
Palliative Care Physician,
The Ottawa Hospital and Bruyère
Continuing Care,
Ottawa, Ontario, Canada (Chapter 12)

Lorraine Caron, PhD
Consulting Researcher,
Agence d'évaluation des technologies et des
modes d'intervention en santé (AETMIS),
Montréal, Québec, Canada (Chapter 17)

Harvey M.Chochinov, MD, PhD, FRSC
Distinguished Professor and
Canada Research Chair in Palliative Care,
Department of Psychiatry,
University of Manitoba;
Director,
Manitoba Palliative Care Research Unit,
CancerCare Manitoba,
Winnipeg, Manitoba, Canada (Chapter 14)

Roberta Ciampichini, PhD
Descriptive Studies and Health
Planning Unit,
Fondazione IRCCS Istituto
Nazionale dei Tumori,
Milan, Italy (Chapter 18)

Graham A. Colditz, MD, DrPH, FAFPHM
Alvin J. Siteman Cancer Center
and Department of Surgery,
Washington University School of Medicine,
St. Louis, Missouri, USA (Chapter 2)

Maximilian de Courten, MD, MPH
Associate Professor of Clinical Epidemiology,
School of Public Health and
Preventive Medicine,
Monash University,
Melbourne, Victoria, Australia (Chapter 21)

Geoff Delaney, MBBS, MD, PhD, FRANZCR
Professor and Director of Cancer Services
Sydney South West Area Health Service,
Liverpool, New South Wales,
Australia (Chapter 9)

Helen Dixon, PhD
Senior Research Fellow,
Centre for Behavioural Research in Cancer,
Cancer Council Victoria,
Carlton, Victoria, Australia (Chapter 3)

J. Mark Elwood, MD, DSc, FRCPC, FAFPHM
Vice President,
Family and Community Oncology,
BC Cancer Agency,
Vancouver, British Columbia,
Canada. (Chapters 1, 16, 23)

Carla D.L. Ens, MSc, PhD
Department of Community Health Sciences,
University of Manitoba,
Winnipeg, Manitoba, Canada (Chapter 14)

Béatrice Fervers, MD, PhD
Centre Léon Bérard, EA 4129 "Santé,
Individu, Société", Université de Lyon, Lyon,
France (Chapter 8)

Eduardo L. Franco, MD, DrPH
Professor of Epidemiology and Oncology;
Director,
Division of Cancer Epidemiology,
McGill University,
Montreal, Quebec, Canada (Chapter 6)

William Friedman, PhD
Chief Operating Officer and Director of
Public Engagement,
Public Agenda,
New York, NY, USA (Chapter 16)

Lindsay Hedden, MSc
Research Scientist,
National Centre for Health Economics,
Services, Policy and Ethics in Cancer;
Research Scientist,
British Columbia Cancer Agency,
Vancouver, British Columbia,
Canada (Chapter 19)

David J. Hill, AO, PhD
Director,
Cancer Council Victoria,
Carlton, Victoria, Australia;
President (2008–10),
International Union Against
Cancer (UICC) (Chapter 3)

**Michael Jefford, MBBS, MPH,
MHlthServMt, PhD, MRACMA, FRACP**
Clinical Consultant,
Cancer Council Victoria;
Associate Professor of Medicine,
University of Melbourne;
Consultant Medical Oncologist,
Division of Haematology and
Medical Oncology,
Peter MacCallum Cancer Centre,
Melbourne, Victoria,
Australia (Chapter 11)

Patricia Kelly, MA
Chief Executive Officer,
Campaign to Control Cancer (C2CC),
Toronto, Ontario, Canada (Chapter 16)

Jon F. Kerner, PhD
Chair, Primary Prevention Action Group,
Senior Scientific Advisor for Cancer
Control and Knowledge Translation,
Canadian Partnership Against Cancer,
One University Avenue, Suite 300,
Toronto, Ontario M5J 2P1 (Chapter 5)

Anne Leis, PhD
Professor and Dr. Louis Schulman
Cancer Research Chair,
Department of Community Health
and Epidemiology,
University of Saskatchewan,
Saskatoon, Saskatchewan,
Canada (Chapter 13)

Jerzy Leowski Jr, MD
Regional Adviser,
Non-communicable Diseases,
World Health Organization,
Regional Office for South-East Asia,
New Delhi, India (Chapter 21)

Ian T. Magrath, DSc (Med), FRCP, FRCPath
President,
International Network for Cancer
Treatment and Research (INCTR),
Brussels, Belgium (Chapter 22)

Andrea Micheli, PhD
Descriptive Studies and Health Planning Unit,
Fondazione IRCCS Istituto
Nazionale dei Tumori,
Milan, Italy (Chapter 18)

Anthony B. Miller, MD, FRCP
Associate Director, Research,
Dalla Lana School of Public Health,
University of Toronto,
Toronto, Ontario, Canada (Chapter 4)

Craig Mitton, PhD
Associate Professor,
University of British Columbia,
Vancouver, British Columbia,
Canada (Chapter 19)

Claire Neal, MPH, CHES
Director of Education and
Program Development,
Lance Armstrong Foundation,
Austin, Texas, USA (Chapter 16)

Doreen Oneschuk. MD, CCFP
Division of Palliative Care Medicine,
Palliative Care Program,
Grey Nuns Community Hospital,
Edmonton, Alberta,
Canada (Chapter 13)

Susan E. O'Reilly, MB, FRCPC
Vice President,
Cancer Care,
BC Cancer Agency,
Vancouver, British Columbia,
Canada (Chapter 10)

Stuart J. Peacock, DPhil
Co-Director,
(Canadian) National Centre for
Health Economics, Services,
Policy and Ethics in Cancer;
Senior Scientist,
British Columbia Cancer Agency;
Associate Professor, University of British
Columbia,
Vancouver, British Columbia, Canada
(Chapter 19)

Mike Richards, CBE, MD, FRCP
National Cancer Director,
England (Chapter 7)

Stephen Sagar, MBBS, MRCP, FRCR, FRCPC, DABR
Radiation Oncologist,
Juravinski Cancer Centre;
Associate Professor,
Departments of Oncology and Medicine,
McMaster University,
Hamilton, Ontario,
Canada (Chapter 13)

Mark Sarner
President/CEO,
Manifest Communications,
Toronto, Ontario,
Canada (Chapter 16)

Carol Sawka, MD
Professor of Medicine,
University of Toronto, and VP Clinical
Programs and Quality Initiatives,
Cancer Care Ontario,
Toronto, Canada (Chapter 8)

Lisa Schwartz, PhD
Arnold L. Johnson Chair in
Health Care Ethics,
Department of Clinical Epidemiology
and Biostatistics,
McMaster University,
Hamilton, Ontario, Canada (Chapter 20)

Dugald Seely, ND, MSc
Research Director,
Canadian College of Naturopathic Medicine,
Toronto, Ontario, Canada (Chapter 13)

Simon B. Sutcliffe, MD, FRCP, FRCPC, FRCR
Board Chair,
Canadian Partnership Against Cancer,
Canada;
Past President, BC Cancer Agency,
Vancouver, British Columbia,
Canada (Chapters 1, 15, 16, 23)

Genevieve N. Thompson, RN, PhD
Manitoba Palliative Care Research Unit,
CancerCare Manitoba;
Research Associate,
Faculty of Nursing,
University of Manitoba,
Winnipeg, Manitoba, Canada (Chapter 14)

Jaya Venkatesh, MHA, CMA
Director,
Business Strategy and Operations,
Provincial Systemic Therapy Program,
BC Cancer Agency,
Vancouver, British Columbia,
Canada (Chapter 10)

Arduino Verdecchia, PhD
National Centre of Epidemiology,
Health Surveillance and Promotion,
Istituto Superiore di Sanità,
Rome, Italy (Chapter 18)

Marja Verhoef, PhD
Professor and Canada Research Chair in
Complementary Medicine,
Department of Community
Health Sciences,
University of Calgary,
Alberta, Canada (Chapter 13)

Part 1

The cancer challenge

Chapter 1

Cancer control and the burden of cancer

Mark Elwood, Simon Sutcliffe[1]

An introduction to cancer control

The terms 'cancer treatment', 'cancer care', and 'cancer control' are often used interchangeably, as if their meaning implied a common understanding of purpose, action, and outcome. However, whilst they share a purpose to reduce the 'burden of cancer' at an individual or population level, they differ substantially in relation to the population served, the interventions applied, and the outcomes (end-points) achieved.

Consider the following definition of cancer control:

> Cancer control aims to reduce the incidence and mortality of cancer, and to enhance the quality of life of those affected by cancer, through an integrated and coordinated approach directed to primary prevention, early detection, treatment, rehabilitation and palliation.

The definition establishes that, if cancer control outcomes are to be improved, the population to be served is the whole population, comprised of: the healthy, the high risk, and those who harbour asymptomatic (pre-clinical) cancer; those with a cancer diagnosis who need treatment; those who are living with cancer as a chronic disease; those who are 'cured' of their cancer; and those who are dying of their cancer and require measures to bring dignity and comfort to the end of life. Cancer control is as much about health, its promotion and maintenance, as it is about managing the disease, cancer. By distinction, cancer care and cancer treatment refer to interventions in those with an established diagnosis of cancer – either as a focus on therapeutic interventions (treatment), or on the needs of cancer patients and their families for all aspects of care that confer 'living better' with cancer. To use an analogy with a communicable disease, onchocerciasis or River Blindness, treatment would imply measures to remediate blindness, care would imply optimal support for the blind or visually impaired, whilst control would encompass all measures to eradicate the cause and pathogenesis of a vector-mediated, parasitic illness.

These concepts are fully elaborated by Caron and colleagues [1], and discussed further in Chapters 15 and 17. An adaptation of their framework is shown in Table 1.1 and highlights that *treatment* is essentially a facility-based intervention according to defined or accepted protocols; *care* describes the coordination and integration of activities to enhance well-being, including treatment episodes, across the various locations and circumstances in which care is provided; and *control* refers to the system response to meet the needs of the population served, encompassing issues of awareness, communication, education, access, support, costs, etc. associated with interventions to control cancer.

[1] J. Mark Elwood, MD, DSc, FRCPC, FAFPHM, Vice-President, Family and Community Oncology, BC Cancer Agency, Vancouver, British Columbia, Canada; and Simon B. Sutcliffe, MD, FRCP, FRCPC, FRCR, Board Chair, Canadian Partnership Against Cancer, Canada, and Past President, BC Cancer Agency, Vancouver, British Columbia, Canada.

Table 1.1 Contrasts between cancer treatment, cancer care, and cancer control

Approach	Cancer treatment	Cancer care	Cancer control
Target population	Patients with cancer diagnosis requiring treatment	Patients with cancer diagnosis requiring care	Entire population from healthy to end-of-life care Risk reduction
Structural features	Facilities, centres, and hospitals	Integrated care networks	Inter-sectoral approach to health and illness
Level of integration in service delivery	Integrated treatment protocols	Clinical care 'pathways'	Public health, health care system, and community service
Management focus	Institution, service organization	Continuity of care	Health system performance

An important point about cancer control in relation to care and treatment is the breadth and nature of the interventions and to whom they are to be applied. Interventions to reduce the incidence of cancer, i.e. the number of new cases of cancer (cancer diagnoses), aim to prevent cancer arising in the population without cancer – interventions to minimize risk, remove causal factors, and address circumstances leading or contributing to adverse choices, behaviours, or exposure. Cancer control encompasses reduction in mortality, both as a consequence of reducing incidence and of improving survival in those with a diagnosis of cancer; it also encompasses all measures of care that contribute to an improved quality of life for those experiencing cancer.

The definition of cancer control implies that improvements in outcomes are expected – a *reduction* in incidence, a *reduction* in mortality, and an *improvement* in quality of life. Thus, beneficial change is inherent in the definition of cancer control. Accordingly, a plan of action is required – contextually appropriate to the circumstances of the population to be served – along with a means of implementation, a clarification of roles of engaged parties, and an evaluation that not only establishes that outcomes improve, but also describes the efficiency and effectiveness of the measures in relation to the elements of cancer control, as well as to other health states and competing choices for the allocation of resources.

In summary, if the population's needs are to be served in a manner that will reduce cancer incidence and mortality, and improve quality of life for those experiencing cancer, a plan is required that defines the population(s) to be served, the range of interventions to be applied (from prevention to end-of-life care), the level of service access, quality and safety to be applied, and the measures to be applied to define the benefit (absolute and relative). Whilst the content and implementation of activities will differ according to the national context and resources, the principles of cancer control are common to all populations. The following chapters address the elements of cancer control, the intent being to raise awareness and understanding of the state of current knowledge, whilst acknowledging that implementation at a population level will differ according to the real-life circumstances facing nations and varying levels of development and resource availability.

Measures of the burden of cancer

The burden of cancer is often expressed in terms of the most easily observable statistics, those of deaths (mortality), and newly diagnosed cases (incidence). For example, the World Cancer

Report 2008 from the World Health Organization (WHO) and the International Agency for Research in Cancer (IARC) [2], interprets cancer burden primarily in terms of incidence numbers, estimating that in 2008 there were 12.4 million incident cases of cancer in a world population of 6.7 billion, and this is estimated to rise to 26.4 million new cases in 2030. This projection, like most, is driven predominantly by growth in population numbers and aging of the population, and the incidence rate component is estimated as a one per cent annual increase. In many developed countries, however, the trend in incidence rate of all cancer has been neutral or downwards; in the United States, incidence rate fell by 0.8 per cent per year from 1999 to 2005 [3]. There is still often confusion between trends in incidence numbers and trends in rates. Whereas trends in numbers are critical in terms of service demands and costs, increases due to population growth and population aging are outside the realm of cancer control, which targets the cancer risk to the individual expressed as the age-adjusted or age-specific cancer incidence rate. Cancer organizations have not been immune from this problem, and the public is often confused by messages that cancer is an ever-increasing problem (and therefore deserving of their interest and contributions) and that cancer is being reduced or controlled (showing the value of their contributions and of research). Simple presentations showing the proportion of future trends due to population growth, due to population aging, and the residual, which is due to changes in cancer incidence rates, are useful; for example, in Canada, the numbers of new cases and deaths from cancer have risen greatly in the last 30 years, despite little change in incidence rates at different ages, and in spite of some reductions in death rates [4], Figure 1.1.

Incidence, mortality, and years of life lost

Reported cancer incidence rates depend on the recognition, diagnosis, and classification of cancer. Rapid changes in the recorded incidence of some cancers may be due to changes in classification systems or diagnostic abilities. Processes which diagnose cancers that would previously have gone undetected, and processes which diagnose cancers earlier and therefore shift the age distribution downwards, will increase age-standardized incidence rates. Many 'silent' cancers are found in pathological examinations in individuals who have died of other causes, having been unobserved in life. Such cancers may be detected with the use of further tests; but the benefits and risks of such extra diagnosis are difficult to assess. This has been particularly marked in prostate cancer, where recent incidence trends in developed countries have been greatly affected by the increasing use of a blood test for prostate specific antigen (PSA) [5]. This effect also applies to other cancers for which screening is done, such as breast and colorectal cancers; changing diagnostic methods are also thought to relate to increases in the recorded incidence of melanoma, renal, and thyroid cancers [3,6]. So, whereas one of the prime objectives of successful cancer control is to reduce the incidence of cancer through successful primary prevention, successful early detection (sometimes confusingly referred to as secondary prevention), may act to increase incidence. In developing countries, with less effective and widespread medical services, the issues of consistency of diagnoses can be even more critical.

The great majority of reports on cancer incidence omit what is in some populations the most common cancer of all, non-melanoma skin cancer. These are cancers arising in the skin, apart from melanoma, which are very common in light-skinned populations exposed to high levels of sun exposure. They are very common, often multiple in an individual, and almost always easily cured by simple surgical excision, but because of the work load needed to record them these cancers are usually not included in cancer registries. In white-skinned Australians, non-melanoma skin cancers (estimated by special surveys) are more common than all other cancers combined, and the cumulative incidence risk is over 50 per cent by age 65; that is, more people get skin cancer than avoid it [7]; however, they cause few deaths.

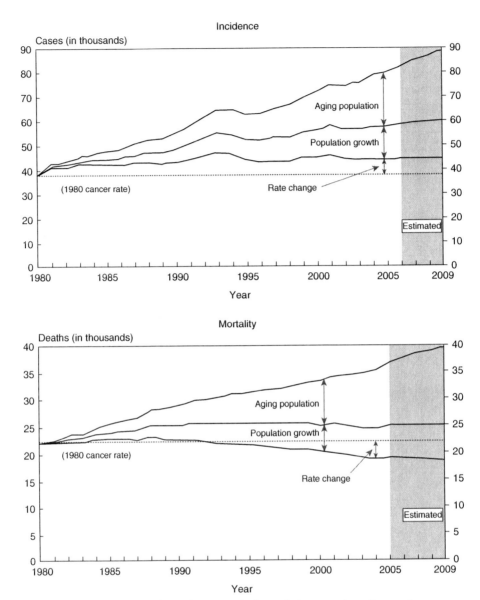

Fig. 1.1 The dominant effects of age changes and of population growth on the numbers of new cases and deaths from cancer. Data for Canada for 1980–2009, for males. For mortality, age-specific deaths rates have fallen, but numbers of deaths continue to rise.
From: Canadian Cancer Society's Steering Committee: Canadian Cancer Statistics 2009. Toronto: Canadian Cancer Society, 2009 [4]; with permission.

A more robust measure of cancer burden is cancer mortality; the prime objective of cancer control is to reduce cancer mortality. In interpreting trends, the issues of distinguishing population growth, population aging, and the underlying age-dependent mortality rates are analogous to those applying to incidence. Recorded mortality rates depend on death certification practices. While on an individual basis the recorded cause of death is often inaccurate, on a population

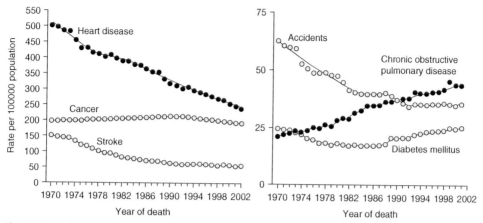

Fig. 1.2 Trends in six leading causes of death in the United States. Age-standardized rates. From: Jemal et al., JAMA 294: 1255–59, Copyright © 2005 American Medical Association. All rights reserved.

aggregate basis, mortality rates for total cancer and for the major types of cancer are quite robust, although issues of certification do need careful consideration. This is particularly the case where a cancer may be frequently diagnosed in life but is not the cause of death, with again the clearest example being prostate cancer.

Reporting the rank order of causes of death is popular with the public and the media but sometimes misleading, as it depends critically on the groupings used. In recent statistics, cancer is given as the leading cause of death in, for example, Australia and Canada, with cardiovascular disease (heart disease and stroke) coming second. This represents the success in the reductions in mortality in cardiovascular diseases [8] (Figure 1.2). In the United States, the combined total of cardiovascular diseases still exceeded that of cancer in 2005 [9], but if the cardiovascular total is split into stroke and heart disease, then cancer emerges as the leading cause of death; also, on current trends, cancer is likely to overtake cardiovascular disease by 2010. In contrast, many World Health Organization (WHO) publications, including the important 'burden of disease' work, subdivide cancer into several specific cancers, with the result that cancer appears very low in the rank order of causes of death [10].

The burden of disease can be expressed by measures which take into account both numbers of deaths and age at death, for example, by 'years of life lost' (YLL) calculations, that is, by years of expected life lost, compared to normal life expectancy, or up to an arbitrary limit, such as age 70. This is a very crude measure, as it treats each year of life up to that age as equally important, but discounts completely expected years of life after the cut-off age; although weighting systems can be used to give different weights to life years at differing ages.

Prevalence

Prevalence of cancer is quite a complex issue. The simplest definition is the number of people living in a community who have had a diagnosis of cancer; most calculations (as with incidence) exclude non-melanoma skin cancer because of its extremely good prognosis and minimum disability. A time cut-off is often used because of the difficulty of linking data over a long period; for example, using only diagnoses in the previous 5, 10, or 15 years; referred to as 'limited-duration' prevalence. Estimates of the prevalence unrestricted by date of diagnosis ('complete prevalence') can be made from such data [11]. For the United States in 2006, with a total population of

298.4 million, total cancer prevalence estimates were 4.1 million within 5 years of diagnosis, 6.8 million within 10 years, 8.9 million within 15 years, and 11.4 million estimated 'complete' prevalence [12]. This total prevalence figure is 3.8 per cent of the total population, or one person in 26. While successful primary prevention will reduce prevalence by reducing incidence, other cancer control measures, such as better and earlier diagnosis and improvements in treatment giving longer survival after diagnosis, will increase the prevalence of cancer, so rising prevalence rates usually represent successes in cancer control; Canadian estimates show a 21 per cent increase over six years up to 2004 [13]. Table 1.2 shows the inter-relationships between several measures of burden of disease, for the United States; the 15-year prevalence estimate for 2009 is 7.5 times the annual incidence rate.

People alive after a diagnosis of cancer will cover the spectrum from those whose lives are unaffected by their previous diagnosis because the disease was minor or previous treatment was successful, to people who require extensive care and have severe disabilities [14]. Estimates have been made of the prevalence of patients in such different groups, as described further in Chapter 18.

Survival after diagnosis

Cancer survival relates to the time course of disease after diagnosis, extending to death due to cancer or other causes, and is usually expressed as the proportion of patients alive at, for example, five years after diagnosis, or as the median survival, being the time point at which 50 per cent of a group of diagnosed patients are still alive. To be meaningful in terms of cancer control, cancer survival rates should be based on all patients with a particular type of cancer diagnosed in a given population, rather than being restricted to a particular hospital where selection by referral will occur. Population measures are usually expressed as the relative survival ratio, being the ratio of the observed survival for a group of cancer patients to the survival expected for people of the same age and sex in the general population, based on population mortality data (life tables). The slope of the curve of relative survival by time represents the excess death rate compared to the general population death rate, and one definition of 'cure' is the demonstration that the curve becomes horizontal, so that the mortality after that time is the same as in the non-cancer population. Cancer survival is the most direct measure of the effects of the combination of timely diagnosis and effective therapy, and as such has major importance; the comparison of cancer survival rates between European countries was the major driver of changes in cancer care services in England, as described in Chapter 7. The experience with this comparative analysis within Europe has been extended to worldwide comparisons through the Concord programme [15], which as well as providing important factual information, has further clarified the challenges of making valid comparisons between countries and between time periods. For example, in US data, the use of state- and race-specific instead of national life tables has been shown to considerably influence relative survival ratios, and differences in pathological classification, for example for gastrointestinal tumours, between Japanese and North American pathologists has given considerable differences in recorded survival [15]. More challenging is taking into account variations in diagnostic practice, not only through screening but also through differences in normal clinical diagnosis, as a chronologically earlier diagnosis will increase lead time, which will increase the survival time after diagnosis even if true natural history is unaffected.

Disparities in cancer burden and outcomes

Disparities in cancer burden and outcomes, between and within countries, show many opportunities and gaps in cancer control. Cancer incidence varies greatly between countries, over time,

Table 1.2 Key measures of the cancer burden, for the United States, 2000 and estimates for 2009

	US estimates year 2000	Ratio to incidence	US estimates year 2009	Ratio to incidence	Source
Total population	282.2 million		306.8 million		
Incidence – number of new cases	1,220,110		1,479,250		[35,36]
Deaths – number of deaths	552,200	0.45	562,340	0.38	[33,36]
Person-years life lost – person-years	8,450,000	6.9			[33]
Prevalence, diagnosis in last 15 years	8,400,000	6.9	11,100,000	7.5	[36,45]
	Costs $billions 2000	Costs per incident case $	Costs $billions 2009	Costs per incident case $	Source
Health care costs - direct/year	37.0	30,325	93.2	63,005	[36,45]
indirect morbidity costs/year	11.0	9,016	18.8	12,709	[36,45]
indirect mortality costs/year	59.0	48,356	116.1	78,486	[36,45]
Overall costs	107.0	87,697	228.1	154,200	
Value of lives lost @ $150,000 per YLL	960.6	787,306			[33]
Lifetime lost productivity	232.4	190,475			[35]

and by key demographic indicators such as age and sex; some differences may be due to differences in external risk factors which can be targeted, such as smoking; other differences may reflect intrinsic biological factors which may not be amenable to change within our present knowledge; yet others may be linked to complex factors such as socio-economic circumstances. Disparities in cancer outcomes, such as survival and mortality rate, may point to key issues that require attention. Within the countries of Europe, there are very substantial differences in cancer survival, and survival is related to several measures of total and health-related national resources, as discussed further in Chapter 18 [16,17]. Survival, adjusted for other mortality, is substantially lower in older patients, suggesting less effective health care [17].

In the United States, cancer survival is substantially lower in the black than in the white population for almost all cancers. For example, 5-year survival rates for breast cancer were 84.7 per cent in white women and 70.9 per cent in black women; for colorectal cancer they were 60.8 per cent in white women and 50.5 per cent in black women [15]. Survival is lower in those without health insurance, and in lower socio-economic groups [18–20]. This reflects both a worse stage distribution, implying lower awareness of symptoms or less access to good diagnostic and screening services, and also worse outcomes within stage categories, implying less access to treatment, lower quality of treatment, or less complete participation in treatment. It is relevant that in the United States, within the Veterans Affairs system that provides relatively standardized care for military veterans, several cancer outcomes show much less racial variation [21]; the authors of the Concord study concluded that the data 'strongly suggest that equal treatment yields equal outcome, irrespective of race' [15]. The Concord study shows that in Australia and Canada cancer survival was high, with only small regional variations, reflecting more equitable good care systems.

Indigenous people in several countries – Native Indians in the United States [22], aboriginals in Australia [23], and Māori in New Zealand [24] all show a similar pattern: compared to the majority white population, they have higher rates of lung cancer (as smoking prevention has been less effective), and of cervical cancer (as participation in screening is lower), and lower cancer survival in general (probably due to both later stage at diagnosis and issues of access to and participation in care). These populations are key examples of the failure to extend the benefits of existing cancer control systems and knowledge across the barriers of socio-economic and educational disadvantages, rural and remote locations, and cultural differences. These differences are consistent with the demographic transitions in developing countries described in Chapters 21 and 22.

Disability- and quality-adjusted life years

The concept of disability-adjusted life years (DALYs) was developed to estimate effects both on length of life (mortality) and on quality of life (morbidity), and has been the focus of the 'Burden of Disease' programme of the World Health Organization [25]. The burden of a disease is measured by the years of life lost up to normal life expectancy (YLL), plus the years lived with disability, calculated as the years lived with the disease (YL) multiplied by an assessment of disability D ranging from very severe (scores approaching 1, equivalent to death) to no disability (score 0, so there is no addition to the DALY calculation); thus the total DALYs = YLL + YL × D. The D scores are typically assessed by disease, age, and sex. The WHO uses the same normal life expectancy for all world populations, rather than the observed country-specific life expectancies. In some work, years of life at different ages are considered equal, but in others years at younger and older ages are weighted less, on both human capital and social preference grounds [26]. Since 2000, the WHO has published regular burden of disease updates for the world and 14 regions, which include mortality estimation, cause of death analysis, and measurement and evaluation of functional health status (http://www.globalburden.org/index.html).

The use of DALYs allows comparisons of the impact of different interventions to include both programmes designed to reduce mortality and those designed to reduce morbidity and increase quality of life. For example, in Australia a range of cancer control initiatives including preventive programmes, screening programmes and therapeutic and supportive interventions were compared using the gain in DALYs (that is, the extent to which the total of DALYs currently lost from the disease is reduced by the intervention) as the key outcome measure, and comparing this with the costs of each programme, to allow a rational system of priority ranking [27]; this is further discussed with results shown in Application 4 in Chapter 19.

Other work uses quality-adjusted life years (QALYs). The QALY is a 'health expectancy' measure related to life expectancy, while the DALY is a 'health burden' or 'health gap' measure related to 'years of life lost'. The familiar concept of 'life expectancy' gives the expected life years remaining to a person, irrespective of the quality of that life; to calculate QALYs a quality score Q where 1 represents full health and lower scores represent compromised quality is applied to each life-year. In contrast, as noted earlier, the DALY is a health burden measure: it is the sum of the number of person-years of life lost and the years of life lived with a disability, these assessed using a D score which increases with increasing disability from 0 to 1. So, where these scores are measured by the same methods, $D = 1 - Q$, and $Q = 1 - D$. A beneficial intervention will reduce the burden of disease assessed in DALYs, and will increase the expectancy of life assessed in QALYs. In practice there are other differences in how the measures are calculated, for example, giving different weights to years of life at different ages, and taking into account variations in health status over time [28].

Both these calculations have the weakness that the methods used to obtain the disability scores are always open to challenge, and may be based on the largely subjective views of relatively small numbers of people. They can also be challenged on their ethical basis: both methods are explicit in rating a year of life of a person with a disability less valuable than a year of life of a non-disabled person, which may be regarded as contrary to, for example, the United Nations Declaration of Human Rights [29].

Economic impacts

Extending beyond the concepts of disability- or quality-adjusted life years, the impact of cancer and the potential benefits of cancer control programmes can take into account the effects of cancer on society in economic costs. One simple example shows the importance of such issues. As noted earlier, in Australia non-melanoma skin cancers are very common; indeed, it is the cancer with the greatest burden in terms of direct health care costs, the costs being twice those of lung cancer although the DALY burden is only five per cent of that of lung cancer [27].

The economic effects of cancer include direct costs of health care services for cancer (including prevention, screening, supportive and palliative care), and indirect costs including loss of economic earning potential, reductions in the tax base, and the impact of cancer on the activity of family members and carers [30]. Indirect costs may also include the patients' costs for travel to treatment appointments, and for supportive care and non-specific medications, for example, for nausea. The impact of current or proposed cancer control methods can be assessed in these terms. Such estimates may be looked at questionably by physicians and scientists used to more precise methods of measurement, as inevitably these projections require many assumptions. But it is more relevant to compare these methods, not to the outcomes of laboratory experiments or clinical trials, but to other similar analyses which drive policy, for example, investments in roads, communication infrastructure, industry, or in other social programmes. Predictive modelling forecasting the economic burden of cancer and the economic and social benefits that could result from successful cancer control have often provided persuasive information to government policy makers, one example being the work on economic projections done by the Canadian Strategy for Cancer Control [31]. For instance, a report from the Milken Institute in the United States in 2007 [32] estimates the economic burden of chronic diseases including cancer in terms of treatment costs, productivity losses, and foregone economic growth based on estimated returns of human capital investment. This shows, for example, that while the number of people reporting chronic diseases in United States in 2003 was 10.6 million for cancer compared to 49.2 million for pulmonary conditions, the loss in productivity was $271 billion for cancer compared to $94 billion for pulmonary conditions, with additional treatment expenditures of $48 billion for cancer and $45 billion for pulmonary conditions.

Two approaches to valuing mortality losses are the *human capital* (HC) approach, in which age- and sex-specific average earnings data is added to information on years of life lost, thus giving greater weight to higher earning years of life; for example, years for men aged 55–59 would carry more weight than those for women aged 60–69, or aged 15–19; and the *willingness-to-pay* (WTP) method, in which weights are derived from surveys assessing how much people would be willing to pay for an extra year of life at different ages. Both methods have been applied in recent US analyses [33,35].

Using the WTP method, the person-years of life lost (PYLL) for cancers in the United States in 2000, and then projected to 2020, were used with a figure of $150,000 per year based on WTP research, and an annual discount rate of 3 per cent [33]. This compares to a gross domestic product (GDP) per capita in the US of $36,000; the WHO has suggested that a valuation of a year of life at three times a country's per capita GDP is appropriate in international health care assessments [34]. Some overall results are given in Table 1.3. The total value of life lost in the United States from cancer in 2000 was $960 billion, increasing to $1471 billion in 2020 (using the American billion, 1000 million). Whereas the death rates from all cancer are much higher in older people, the PYLL and value of life lost are comparable for those under 65 and those over 65. Also notable is that in 2000, although the death rates were higher in men, the PYLL and value of life lost were both higher for women. The analysis gives detailed data by cancer type, and using various scenarios for the projections; the greatest value of life lost (both sexes) was for lung cancer, followed by colorectal cancer and breast cancer.

Using the human capital approach, applied to essentially the same US epidemiological data on cancer, estimates were made of lost earnings based on the probability of employment and expected earnings (and benefits) for different age and sex groups [35]. To this base model were added estimated costs of caregiving and household activities (equal to 72 per cent of employment earnings in men, but 180 per cent in women), and again a 3 per cent discount rate to estimate present value. This method will give more importance to high-earning periods of life, whereas the WTP method described previously used the same value for any year of life. In the human capital analysis, the present value of lost earnings (PVLE) for all types of cancer in 2000 was $116 billion, projected to increase to $148 billion by 2020, with the biggest contributors being lung, colorectal, and breast cancers. Continuing the present trend of reducing mortality rates by 1 per cent per year for six major cancers would reduce productivity losses by $814 million per year.

These figures are much lower than those given by the WTP method, where the average value of a year of life lost is $133,000 (different from $150,000 because of discounting), whereas the value based on lost productivity is only $28,000. The human capital approach focuses on economic productivity, ignoring other aspects of life; however, the WTP method as used here gives the same value to a year of healthy vigorous life as to a year with severe disability. Both methods give values

Table 1.3 Results of both willingness-to-pay and human capital assessments based on cancer mortality in the United States

Willingness-to-pay method, using $150,000 per year of life (a)

| | Total, 2000 | Total, 2020 | Year 2000 in more detail | | | |
| | | | Men | | Women | |
			<65 yrs	>=65 yrs	<65 yrs	>=65 yrs
Age-adjusted mortality rate per 100,000, 1999–2003			69.6	1446.5	60.2	883.7
Person-years of life lost (millions)	8.45		2.15	1.88	2.33	2.08
Value of life lost ($ billions)	960.6	1472.5	222.4	245.8	227.9	264.5
Average value per PYLL ($ thousand)	113.7					

Human capital approach, based on estimated earnings (b)

| | Total, 2000 | Total, 2020 | Estimates for 2010 | | |
			Total	Men	Women
Person-years of life lost (excludes age under 20)	8.29				
Present value of lifetime earnings PVLE ($ billion)	115.8	147.6	124.9	81.2	43.7
Caregiving, household activity	116.6	160.4	136.8	58.5	78.3
Total including caregiving etc.	232.4	308.0	261.7	139.7	122.0
Average PVLE per year of life lost ($ thousand)	28.0				

(a) Data from Yabroff et al. 2008 [33].
(b) Data from Bradley et al. 2008 [35].

much higher than the estimated direct costs of cancer care, about $93 billion in 2009 [36]. Both methods as used here are based only on the impact of cancer deaths: loss of productivity and loss of quality of life due to cancer morbidity are not considered. These economic analyses can be influential in targeting investments in cancer control strategies and in research; for example, both methods highlight the great impact of lung cancer, which has generally been poorly supported by research and indeed in the public interest compared to some other cancers like breast cancer [37].

Direct health care costs

The direct health care costs of cancer are critical in cancer control as the balance between needs and resources is a limiting factor in cancer control in all countries, and the justification of cancer control policies includes increasing value for the investments made in health services and in research. Direct care costs in the United States were estimated in 2009 as $93.2 billion [36], equating to $63,000 per incident case (see Table 1.2); this is at least twice as high as in most other countries. The United States does show the best survival rates overall [15], although with considerable internal racial and geographic variations; but the differences in survival between the United States and Canada, Australia, and some countries in Europe are small, while all these countries have much lower health care costs. The aspect of cost which receives most attention is drug costs, and they are rising rapidly, as discussed in Chapter 10 in this book. Rational and evidence-based cancer control has a major role: in the United States in 2004 Medicare drugs for oncology totalled $5.3 billion, but of this $1.5 billion was for erythroid growth factors [38], which are of questionable value and are much less used outside the United States [39].

The wider perspective

The burden of cancer can thus be considered at a macro level in terms of its effects on mortality, on morbidity, on health services demand, and on society as a whole. Considerations at the micro level deal with the effects of cancer and its interventions on quality of life in individual patients and groups of patients, and also on their families and carers, and are discussed in several chapters in this book. The impact of cancer, as with any other disease or disability, depends not only on its biological effects on the individual, but also on the attitudes and reactions of the family and the wider community to the disease and its sufferers. Such reactions can be supportive and positive, but can also be insensitive and negative. In most developed countries there has been a major shift in individual and societal attitudes within the last few decades, with open communication about cancer and its treatments and effects, and the acceptance of people who have been diagnosed with cancer as fully functional members of their families and communities. This attitude in the best circumstances has produced a positive and supportive atmosphere around cancer 'survivors', seen most clearly in the social networks and support surrounding women with breast cancer. There are, however, considerable differences in the level of support and acceptance of breast cancer compared with some other cancers such as colorectal and lung cancer [40], and other diseases; for example, the need to achieve a similar level of societal acceptance and support for sufferers from psychiatric disease as now exists for patients with cancer has been stressed [41].

Cancer control and the burden of cancer

There is an inverse relationship between cancer control and the burden of cancer – the more effective the control of cancer, the less the burden. It is important to recognize that cancer is a process that starts in health and so is amenable to control measures exerted both in health and illness. The diagnosis of cancer is an event in the process, the growth of neoplastic cells, from which the consequences of disease and its therapy contribute to the burden of cancer, both individual and societal. This burden is a consequence of the failure to control cancer from an incidence, mortality, functionality, and quality of life perspective.

Figure 1.3 demonstrates the increasing 'burden' of cancer with increasing age in a population. The lifetime cumulative risk of developing cancer, for example in Canada, is around 42 per cent (males 45, females 40), and of dying from cancer is around 26 per cent (males 28, females 24)[4]. The areas under the two curves are a chronological expression of the population burden of cancer, relating to the mortality and incidence burdens; the area between the two curves relates to those who have experienced cancer incidence but not mortality, that is, cancer prevalence or cancer survivors. The segment of the population above the incidence curve represents the majority of the population who have not experienced cancer incidence, but have the accruing liability of the process of carcinogenesis, and includes those who will subsequently develop cancer. Cancer incidence increases rapidly and substantially after the age of 50 years; although risk of cancer

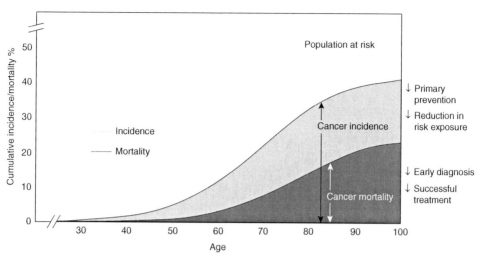

Fig. 1.3 Concept of the rising burden of cancer mortality and of incidence with age, and the role of cancer control. Cancer incidence will be reduced by successful primary prevention, altering risk and exposure profiles, although it can be increased by earlier diagnosis; cancer mortality will be reduced, in addition, by early detection and successful treatment; for cancer prevalence, represented by the area between the curves, the burden will be decreased by treatments with lower morbidity and supportive care increasing quality of life.

commences from birth, cancer will not be a major population burden if life expectancy from birth is less than about 55 years, but it will be an exponentially increasing burden as a consequence of increasing longevity.

Studies on the natural history of pre-cancerous lesions determined by early detection procedures and of benign precursor lesions in relation to the development of invasive cancer, e.g. bowel polyps, indicate that the process of carcinogenesis is initiated years or decades prior to the diagnosis of cancer. Thus the factors underlying susceptibility and risk are at play long before clinical cancer is evident. Indeed, one might say that being born, indeed being conceived, constitutes eligibility for cancer and that living involves exposure to factors that will either increase or decrease the probability of developing cancer in later life.

The risk factors for cancer and the magnitude of the attributable risks of various factors are well recognized. The choices, however, of what control can be exerted over exposure to risk vary:

♦ The risk may be truly optional, i.e. there is recognition of the risk, and the ability to mitigate the risk through exercising an applicable choice. This implies that not only is it possible to remove exposure to the risk factor, but that life circumstances (mental, physical, social, economic) are conducive and appropriate to make a sustainable change to risk exposure.

♦ It may be conditional, i.e. there may be knowledge and recognition of risk exposure, but changing exposure may be limited by, or be conditional upon, sustainable changes in life circumstances that pre-dispose to risk exposure (primordial risk factors), and may inhibit changing the exposure.

♦ It may be an unalterable exposure, a consequence of hereditary genetic predisposition (e.g. familial adenomatous polyposis, the breast cancer genes BRCA I or II, Li Fraumeni syndrome) or the presence of a risk factor that cannot be feasibly mitigated (morbid obesity, physical handicap) in the context of the individual's life circumstances.

The options available for intervention to reduce the burden of cancer, and their degree of success, will cover the natural history of the condition and include: primary prevention; early diagnosis including for a few cancers population-based screening; therapy with direct effects on the cancer; therapies to overcome or more likely ameliorate the secondary effects of the cancer; therapies to supplement the individual's physical and mental coping skills; and practical measures to reduce the effects of disability, culturally appropriate supportive and palliative care. Society's attitudes to those affected by the disease will influence both the availability and the success of these interventions. Decisions, policy, funding, or indeed lack of attention, by local communities and regional, national, and international governments influence all these approaches to the cancer burden.

The impact of the broader societal development context upon cancer control can be illustrated through the Human Development Index (HDI), an index combining normalized measures of life expectancy at birth, literacy, educational attainment, and gross domestic product per capita [42,43]. Comparing countries, cancer control outcomes correlate with the HDI, which is not of surprise given that the HDI incorporates measures of education, employment, and the economy. What is more relevant, however, is that it is difficult to enhance cancer control outcomes if there is not commensurate enhancement in measures to improve the HDI. Transposing the processes and procedures that contribute to more favourable cancer outcomes in countries with a high HDI to countries with a lower HDI, whether preventive or interventional to manage established cancer, are unlikely to have impact unless they act in concert with, and in the context of, measures to enhance human development. Given that the factors influencing human development – clean water, nutritious food, physical activity, education, employment, and personal and societal growth – are operative throughout childhood, adolescence and early adult life, the relevance of social and economic development in relation to risk factor exposure choices, behaviours, and health options to the 'accruing liability' and the future burden of cancer is apparent [44]. Not only is this relevant for health and cancer outcomes, but also for the consequences of societal inequity associated with social exclusion, marginalization, dissatisfaction and the inability to capitalize on personal and societal development and well being.

How then should we think about how best to advance cancer control from the perspectives of the nation under consideration and the potential roles of those who might offer assistance? A simple analogy is that of saving people who fall into a river and are at risk of drowning. Strategically, is it better to go 'downstream' and maximize efforts to save people before drowning, or is it better to go 'upstream' and prevent them from falling into the river? Whilst the answer might reasonably be 'do both', the answer needs to be placed in the context of the ability of the nation to commit resources to going 'upstream' or 'downstream', and the reality that for nearly all nations 'more people will continue to fall in' and it is becoming increasingly expensive to implement 'downstream' solutions.

The chapters in this book address issues of the accruing liability for cancer burden posed by risk factors and environmental exposure, as well as the burden of established cancer. The intent is to provide 'current state' knowledge about measures to reduce the burden through effective interventions, recognizing that the principles of population-based cancer control (what should be done and why?) are common to all nations. The challenge is the application of the principles within the 'real life' context of nations (how, by whom, and when?) and the ability to address the underlying inequities and disparities that militate against the opportunity to access and benefit from health interventions that precede improvement in cancer control outcomes.

References

1 Caron L, De Civita M, Law S, & Brault I (2008). Cancer control interventions in selected jurisdictions: design, governance, and implementation, monograph. *Agence d'évaluation des technologies et des modes d'intervention en santé (AETMIS)*. [cited 2009 May 26];[1–343]. Available from: http://www.aetmis. gouv.qc.ca/site/250.1043.0.0.1.0.phtml.

2 World Health Organization, International Agency for Research on Cancer (IARC) (2008). *World Cancer Report* 2008. *IARC.*[cited 2009 July 2];[1–524]. Available from: http://www.iarc.fr/en/ publications/pdfs-online/wcr/2008/index.php.

3 Jemal A, Thun MJ, Ries LA, et al (2008). Annual report to the nation on the status of cancer, 1975–2005, featuring trends in lung cancer, tobacco use, and tobacco control. *J Natl Cancer Inst.*, **100**(23):1672–1694.

4 Canadian Cancer Society's CCS Steering Committee. *Canadian Cancer Statistics 2009.*[1–124]. Available from: http://www.cancer.ca/canada-wide/about%20cancer/cancer%20statistics/~/media/ CCS/Canada%20wide/Files%20List/English%20files%20heading/pdf%20not%20in%20publications% 20section/Stats%202009E%20Cdn%20Cancer.ashx.

5 Sarma AV & Schottenfeld D (2002). Prostate cancer incidence, mortality, and survival trends in the United States: 1981–2001. *Semin Urol Oncol.*, **20**(1):3–9.

6 Black WC (2000). Overdiagnosis: An underrecognized cause of confusion and harm in cancer screening. *J Natl Cancer Inst.*, **92**(16):1280–1282.

7 Staples MP, Elwood M, Burton RC, Williams JL, Marks R, & Giles GG (2006). Non-melanoma skin cancer in Australia: the 2002 national survey and trends since 1985. *Med J Aust.*, **184**(1):6–10.

8 Jemal A, Ward E, Hao Y, & Thun M (2005). Trends in the leading causes of death in the United States, 1970–2002. *JAMA*, **294**(10):1255–1259.

9 Kung HC, Hoyert DL, Xu J, & Murphy SL (2008). Deaths: final data for 2005. *Natl Vital Stat Rep.*, **56**(10):1–120.

10 Becker R, Silvi J, Ma FD, L'Hours A, & Laurenti R (2006). A method for deriving leading causes of death. *Bull World Health Organ.*, **84**(4):297–304.

11 Capocaccia R & De Angelis R (1997). Estimating the completeness of prevalence based on cancer registry data. *Stat Med.*, **16**(4):425–440.

12 Horner MJ, Ries LAG, Krapcho M, et al (2009). Surveillance epidemiology and end results SEER cancer statistics review, 1975–2006. *National Cancer Institute (NCI)*. [cited 2009 July 3]. Available from: http://seer.cancer.gov/csr/1975_2006/index.html.

13 Canadian Cancer Society (CCS) (2008), National Cancer Institute of Canada. *Canadian Cancer Statistics 2008.* [cited 2009 July 3];[1–108]. Available from: http://www.cancer.ca/canada-wide/ about%20cancer/cancer%20statistics/canadian%20cancer%20statistics.aspx?sc_lang=en.

14 Pollack LA, Greer GE, Rowland JH, et al (2005). Cancer survivorship: a new challenge in comprehensive cancer control. *Cancer Causes Control*, **16**(Suppl 1):51–59.

15 Coleman MP, Quaresma M, Berrino F, et al (2008). Cancer survival in five continents: a worldwide population-based study CONCORD. *Lancet Oncol.*, **9**(8):730–756.

16 Berrino F, De Angelis R, Sant M, et al (2007). Survival for eight major cancers and all cancers combined for European adults diagnosed in 1995 – 99: Results of the EUROCARE-4 study. *Lancet Oncol.*, **8**(9):773–783.

17 Sant M, Allemani C, Santaquilani M, Knijn A, Marchesi F, & Capocaccia R (2009). EUROCARE-4. Survival of cancer patients diagnosed in 1995 – 1999. Results and commentary. *Eur J Cancer*, **45**(6):931–991.

18 Bradley CJ, Given CW, & Roberts C (2001). Disparities in cancer diagnosis and survival. *Cancer*, **91**(1):178–188.

19 Halpern MT, Ward EM, Pavluck AL, Schrag NM, Bian J, & Chen AY (2008). Association of insurance status and ethnicity with cancer stage at diagnosis for 12 cancer sites: a retrospective analysis. *Lancet Oncol.*, 2008; **9**(3):222–231.

20 Ward E, Jemal A, Cokkinides V, et al (2004). Cancer disparities by race/ethnicity and socioeconomic status. *CA Cancer J Clin.*, **54**(2):78–93.

21 Rabeneck L, Souchek J, & El-Serag HB (2003). Survival of colorectal cancer patients hospitalized in the Veterans Affairs Health Care System. *Am J Gastroenterol.*, **98**(5):1186–1192.

22 Espey DK, Wu XC, Swan J, et al 2007. Annual report to the nation on the status of cancer, 1975–2004, featuring cancer in American Indians and Alaska Natives. *Cancer,* **110**(10):2119–2152.

23 Condon JR, Barnes T, Armstrong BK, Selva-Nayagam S, & Elwood M (2005). Stage at diagnosis and cancer survival for Indigenous Australians in the Northern Territory. *Med J Aust.*, **182**(6):277–280.

24 Jeffreys M, Stevanovic V, Tobias M, et al (2005). Ethnic inequalities in cancer survival in New Zealand: linkage study. *Am J Public Health,* **95**(5):834–837.

25 Lopez AD & Mathers CD (2006). Measuring the global burden of disease and epidemiological transitions: 2002–2030. *Ann Trop Med Parasitol,* **100**(5–6):481–499.

26 Mathers CD, Lopez AD, & Murray CJL (2006). The Burden of disease and mortality by condition: data, methods, and results for 2001. In Lopez AD, Mathers CD, Ezzati M, Jamison DT, & Murray CJL eds. *Global Burden of Disease and Risk Factors,* pp. 45–240. Oxford University Press, New York

27 Cancer Strategies Group (2001). *Priorities for action in cancer control* 2001–2003. 1–112. Commonwealth Department of Health and Ageing, Canberra.

28 Sassi F (2006). Calculating QALYs, comparing QALY and DALY calculations. *Health Policy Plan,* **21**(5):402–408.

29 Arnesen T & Nord E (1999). The value of DALY life: problems with ethics and validity of disability adjusted life years. *BMJ,* **319**(7222):1423–1425.

30 Brown ML, Lipscomb J, & Snyder C (2001). The burden of illness of cancer: economic cost and quality of life. *Annu Rev Public Health,* **22**:91–113.

31 Canadian Strategy for Cancer Control (2005). Establishing the strategic framework for the Canadian Strategy for Cancer Control. 1–34. *Canadian Strategy for Cancer Control, Ottawa.*

32 DeVol R, Bedroussian A, Charuworn A, et al (2007). An unhealthy America: the economic burden of chronic disease—charting a new course to save lives and increase productivity and economic growth. *Milken Institute.* [cited 2009 Apr. 8];[1–186]. Available from: http://www.milkeninstitute.org/publications/publications.taf?function=detail&ID=38801018&cat=ResRep.

33 Yabroff KR, Bradley CJ, Mariotto AB, Brown ML, & Feuer EJ (2008). Estimates and projections of value of life lost from cancer deaths in the United States. *J Natl Cancer Inst.*, **100**(24):1755–1762.

34 World Health Organization (WHO) Commission on Macroeconomics and Health (2001). Macroeconomics and health: investing in health for economic development. *WHO,*[cited 2009 July 3];[1–202]. Available from: http://www.emro.who.int/cbi/pdf/CMHReportHQ.pdf.

35 Bradley CJ, Yabroff KR, Dahman B, Feuer EJ, Mariotto A, & Brown ML (2008). Productivity costs of cancer mortality in the United States: 2000–2020. *J Natl Cancer Inst.*, **100**(24):1763–1770.

36 American Cancer Society. Cancer facts & figures 2009. 1–68. 2009. Atlanta, American Cancer Society. 24-4-2009. [cited 2009 Jun 23]. Available from: http://www.cancer.org/docroot/STT/content/STT_1x_Cancer_Facts__Figures_2009.asp?from=fast.

37 Cassidy J (2007). Is breast cancer advocacy distorting the cancer budget to the disadvantage of other tumours? *Breast Cancer Research* 9(Suppl 2):S6.

38 Meropol NJ & Schulman KA (2007). Cost of cancer care: issues and implications. *J Clin Oncol.*, **25**(2):180–186.

39 Steinbrook R (2007). Erythropoietin, the FDA, and oncology. *N Engl J Med.*, **356**(24):2448–2451.

40 Chapple A, Ziebland S, & McPherson A (2004). Stigma, shame, and blame experienced by patients with lung cancer: qualitative study. *BMJ.*, **328**(7454):1470.

41 Hanne M & Hawken SJ (2007). Metaphors for illness in contemporary media. *Medical Humanities* 33(2):93–99.

42 Bhanojirao VV (1991). Human development report 1990: review and assessment. *World Development*, **19**(10):1451–1460.

43 Noorbakhsh F (1998). A modified human development index. *World Development*, **26**(3):517–528.

44 Halfon N & Hochstein M (2002). Life course health development: an integrated framework for developing health, policy, and research. *Milbank Q.*, **80**(3):433–479.

45 American Cancer Society (ACS) (2000). Cancer facts & figures 2000. *ACS.* [cited 2009 Apr. 24];[1–39]. Available from: http://www.cancer.org/downloads/STT/F&F00.pdf

Part 2

Prevention and screening

Chapter 2

Active cancer prevention

Graham Colditz, Courtney Beers[1]

The success and further potential of prevention

Fifty to sixty per cent of cancer deaths can be prevented [1]. Such estimates traditionally draw largely on international variation in cancer incidence and mortality, as well as the changes in risk observed in studies of migrants and reduction in risk of smoking-related cancers after stopping smoking. Recently a small number of randomized trials of prevention strategies including vaccination have added to the evidence base. Given that the majority of cancer can be prevented with what we already know, public health authorities, health care providers, and individuals have responded with the adoption of prevention targets and strategies that include implementation of regulations to enforce health-related protections, global public health campaigns to impact personal, community, and corporate decisions that improve lifestyle, and decrease environmental and occupational exposures to carcinogens. Active strategies to prevent cancer are the focus of this chapter. Other strategies such as early detection and effective treatment of diagnosed cancer cases are also clearly critical in improving quality of life for individuals with cancer and for decreasing cancer-related deaths, and are addressed elsewhere in this book.

There is still much work to be done as the number of cancer deaths is expected to grow from 12 million new cases and 7 million deaths from cancer in 2008 to a projected 26 million new cases and 11.4 million deaths in 2030 [2]. The leading causes of cancer mortality in the world are lung (1.4 million deaths per year), stomach (866,000), colon (677,000), and breast (548,000). Approximately 72 per cent of cancer deaths occurred in low and middle income countries in 2007, where the leading causes of cancer mortality are: lung, stomach, liver, colon and rectum, and cervix. Increasing cancer death rates can be attributed, in part, to the aging population and also the epidemic of tobacco use in the developing world [3], with additional increases in female cancers due to changing reproductive patterns [4].

One important omission from such estimates of the proportion of cancer that can be prevented is detailed understanding of the time course of risk reduction for many of the behaviours that cause cancer and consideration of achievable or sustainable change in exposure to the causes. Except in rare settings, such as cessation from smoking cigarettes, the time course to achieve reduction in the cancer burden is not quantified. Cigarette smoking does, however, offer strong evidence on the change in cancer risk after stopping smoking at the individual level. Peto has demonstrated that by 1990 in the United Kingdom smoking cessation had almost halved the number of lung cancers that would have been expected if the former smokers had continued smoking [5]. Furthermore, he showed substantial benefit of stopping at an earlier age for men in the United Kingdom compared to continuing to smoke to age 75. For example, a man who stops smoking at age 40 has a cumulative risk to age 75 of 3 per cent compared to 6 per cent if he

[1] Graham A. Colditz, MD, DrPH, FAFPHM; and Courtney Beers, MPH, Alvin J. Siteman Cancer Center and Department of Surgery, Washington University School of Medicine, St. Louis, Missouri, USA.

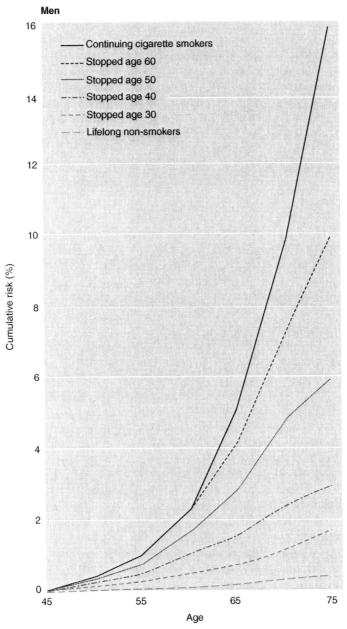

Fig. 2.1 Cumulative risk of lung cancer and age at stopping smoking, UK, men.
From Peto et al. 2000 [93], with permission from the BMJ.

stopped at 50, 10 per cent if he stopped at 60, and 16 per cent for the continuing smoker (see Figure 2.1).

The benefit of reduced risk has also been addressed in the United States with detailed data on individual smoking behaviours updated every two years among women in the Nurses' Health Study [6]. Kenfield and colleagues showed that risk of death due to lung cancer was reduced by

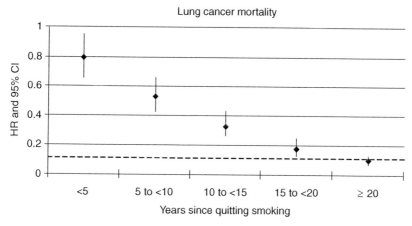

Hazard 1 = current smoker   Dashed line – never smoker

Fig. 2.2 Reduction in mortality from lung cancer compared to continuing to smoke, by time since quitting smoking, Nurses' Health Study, 1980 to 2004. The y-axis is a log scale. The error bars denote 95 per cent confidence intervals. The reference category consists of current smokers. The horizontal dashed line indicates a never-smoker's risk. Adjusted for age (months), follow-up period, history of hypertension, diabetes, high cholesterol levels, body mass index, change in weight from age 18 years to baseline (1980), alcohol intake, physical activity, previous use of oral contraceptives, postmenopausal oestrogen therapy use and menopausal status, parental history of myocardial infarction at age 65 years or younger, cigarettes smoked per day during the period prior to quitting, and age at starting smoking.
From Kenfield et al. 2008 [6], p. 2046, with permission from the *JAMA*.

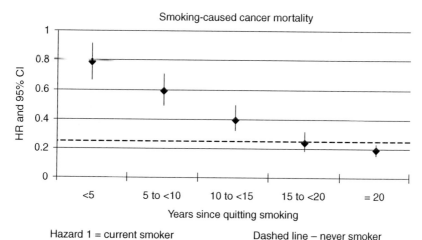

Hazard 1 = current smoker   Dashed line – never smoker

Fig. 2.3 Reduction in mortality for all smoking related cancers compared to continuing to smoke, by time since quitting smoking, Nurses' Health Study, 1980 to 2004. Details as described in Figure 2.2.
From Kenfield et al. 2008 [6], p.2046, with permission from the *JAMA*.

50 per cent within 10 years of stopping, and a similar reduction in mortality was observed for all smoking-related cancers [6] (see Figures 2.2, 2.3).

In contrast with data on individuals, Barnoya and Glantz evaluated the population changes in cancer mortality after the introduction of the California Comprehensive Tobacco Control Program in 1988. They observed a significant reduction in lung cancer in San Francisco compared to other US SEER registries corresponding to a 6 per cent reduction in lung cancer incidence over the 10 years after the programme was introduced [7]. Reductions were also observed for bladder cancer, but not for cancers known not to be related to smoking. The California Comprehensive Tobacco Control Program is a population-wide effort to reduce tobacco consumption in the state. This programme stressed clean indoor air and policies to create smoke-free environments [8] and increased taxation resulting in an accelerated decline in smoking prevalence [9]. Evidence clearly supports population-level prevention strategies for tobacco control and reduction in smoking-related cancers. Though not immediate, the trend to reduced cancer burden is well documented.

The impact of change in level of exposure to other causes of cancer, or following the implementation of prevention strategies, is less well supported by rigorous evaluation. Several important aspects of the time course of prevention interventions must be considered. These are (1) the ability of interventions to sufficiently change the exposure, (2) the timing in the process of carcinogenesis, or the development of cancer, and (3) how sustained the behaviour change is over time [10]. This last issue, in particular, plagues randomized trials of screening and lifestyle change (e.g. with diet or vitamins) in that adherence to the experimental and control interventions has not been high [11–13]. For example, approximately 40 per cent of women stopped the intervention in the Women's Health Initiative and many of the control women 'dropped in', or began using the intervention agents. For interventions of calcium and vitamin D, the magnitude of the intervention was not sufficiently large (vitamin D) nor did the calcium supplementation adequately address low-intake women to achieve the reductions in colon cancer incidence observed in epidemiologic studies and polyp prevention trials [14].

Vaccination programmes offer yet another insight to the time frame of intervention and the ultimate reduction in cancer incidence. For cervical cancer prevention with human papilloma virus (HPV) vaccine, the current US Center for Disease Control (CDC) recommends vaccination for women between ages 13 and 26; the benefit of this prevention will be observed many years hence. Hepatitis vaccination programmes in Africa and Asia offer further illustration of these points. In the Gambia a programme launched in 1986 aims to evaluate the effectiveness of childhood vaccination with hepatitis B and current estimates are that the final outcome of reduced hepatocellular carcinoma in adults should be measurable from 2017 onwards [15]. In Asia with nationwide hepatitis B vaccination implemented in Taiwan in 1984, results at 10 years show significant reduction in hepatocellular carcinoma in children [16]. Clearly many years of follow-up are required to demonstrate protection of adults, though this outcome is implied by results to date.

In sum, the time course to achieve reduction in cancer incidence through active prevention programmes may vary substantially. The timing of the intervention in the time course of carcinogenesis, and the ability of individuals or populations to maintain the lifestyle changes necessary to reduce the cancer burden, both contribute to the ultimate benefit of the active prevention intervention. One population that shows how much reduction can be achieved through long-term adherence to a cancer reducing lifestyle is the members of the Seventh Day Adventist Church in the United States. This population avoids smoking, alcohol, and consumption of meat, being largely lacto-ovo-vegetarian, and shows an overall 27 per cent lower cancer mortality among men than the US population at large [17]. Reductions in cancer mortality among women were lesser, in part because of the burden of breast and other reproductive cancers that may not respond to changes in diet and smoking.

Given the potential impact on disease burden, cancer prevention is an international health priority. However, there is wide variation in the resources allocated to prevention and in the approaches and effectiveness of programmes. Success is often dependent upon political commitment, regulatory/legislative backing, funding, and involvement of stakeholders in the programme development and implementation phases. Strategies range from regulation and taxation of cigarettes to health-service coverage of counselling or pharmaceuticals to support cessation. A determinant of successful prevention programmes is identified in Richmond and Kotelchuck's health policy model as the interplay between the three critical components of prevention: scientific knowledge base, political will, and a social strategy [18]. These components are evident in the following descriptions of international prevention programmes focused on individual, health care providers, community, and/or regulatory approaches in nine key areas.

Nine focus areas for active prevention

We focus on nine key areas where prevention efforts have the potential to significantly impact cancer incidence, quality of life, and mortality in developed countries and worldwide: tobacco, alcohol, physical activity, weight control, diet and dietary supplementation, sun exposure, infections, environmental and occupational exposures, and medications.

In Table 2.1, we summarize the relative contribution of these causes, based partly on a quantitative review of risk factors for specific cancers by Danaei and colleagues [19]. This approach is more conservative than the earlier approach of Doll and Peto who estimated the overall proportion of cancer that could be avoided mainly by comparing high and low risk populations [20]. Danaei and colleagues limit their prevention estimates to lifestyle changes that could reasonably be achieved, and base these estimates on a limited number of cancers for which a consensus approach leads to a causal inference. Estimates for smoking are comparable in both reports because Doll and Peto used the American Cancer Society (ACS) Cancer Prevention Study 1 mortality data (for cancers of the lung, mouth, larynx, oesophagus, bladder, and pancreas) and estimates for other cancers (such as kidney and liver) to derive their estimate of 30 per cent of cancer mortality [20].

However for obesity, for example, the ACS data indicate that 14 to 20 per cent of cancer mortality is attributable to obesity [21], whereas the Danaei estimate is limited to only breast, colon, and uterus [19], omitting causal evidence for oesophagus (as classified by the IARC report [22]) and for other cancers (liver, pancreas, multiple myeloma, and non-Hodgkin lymphoma) identified as having significant excess mortality among overweight and obese participants in the ACS cohort. Thus, in contrast with the ACS mortality data, Danaei and colleagues use more conservative consensus approaches to causal inference and attribute only 3 per cent of cancer in high-income countries to overweight and obesity. Further, Danaei and colleagues omit drugs such as postmenopausal hormones for breast and endometrial cancers, chemoprevention, and vaccination programmes against infectious agents. We have included these. For each area, we will discuss the contribution of the factor to cancer incidence and prevention; effective policy and/or programmatic approaches that have been successfully implemented to achieve sustained changes in behaviour; and the likely time course for prevention, if it is known.

Tobacco

Established as the primary cause of cancer-related deaths and considered the single largest preventable cause of cancer in the world [23], the impact of tobacco on international health is hugely detrimental. Tobacco smoking causes bladder, cervical, oesophageal, kidney, laryngeal,

Table 2.1 Proportion of cancer (per cent) that could be prevented through modification of lifestyle factors, drugs, chemopreventive agents, and vaccines

	High-income countries	Worldwide
Lifestyle factors[1]		
Smoking	29	21
Alcohol	4	5
Overweight and obesity	3	2
Physical inactivity	2	2
Diet: low fruit and vegetable intake	3	5
Sun exposure	2 (ignored by Danaei)	1 (ignored by Danaei)
Environment and occupation	1–4	? Unknown
Medical interventions[2]		
Medications		
Postmenopausal oestrogen plus progestin therapy[a]	6–10	Currently minimal
SERMs (Tamoxifen and Raloxifene)[b]	10	Currently minimal
Aspirin (colon cancer)[c]	3	Currently minimal
Vaccines		
HPV and Hepatitis B vaccines[d]	Minor impact	8–16

1. Lifestyle estimates from Danaei et al. [19]

    Risk factors were selected for consideration if they were likely to be a leading cause of worldwide or regional disease burden. An expert work group completed a systematic review to obtain a relative risk estimate. Population attributable fraction was then estimated for the selected cancers.

2. Medication estimates derived as follows:

    a. Colditz 2007; using US prevalence of use and relative risks [71].

    b. Chen et al 2007; using results from randomized trials and US population estimates [82].

    c. Aspirin: 20% reduction in risk among those using aspirin for more than 10 years is plausible but risk benefit considerations limit widespread use for colon cancer prevention. Current user estimate of 3% is based on prevalence of long term uses in Chan et al [94].

    d. Vaccines: Cervix, stomach, and liver cancer account for over 33% of cancer mortality in low and middle income countries; 18% worldwide [64]. Vaccines have been shown to be effective. Preventive benefit is determined by delivery of vaccine to population to reduce cancer by 50 to 100%.

lung, oral, pancreatic, and stomach cancers and acute myeloid leukaemia (AML) [24]. In the United States alone, smoking causes at least 30 per cent of cancer deaths annually; globally tobacco will kill more than five million people. Risk increases with daily consumption as well as duration of smoking. Second hand smoke poses significant risk as well, which makes tobacco the only legal consumer product that can harm everyone exposed to it. Furthermore the reduction in mortality from tobacco-related cancer after cessation from smoking is substantial, attaining mortality rates of never-smokers in 20 to 30 years [6].

The World Health Organization promotes population-wide anti-tobacco policies and programming as evidenced in its MPOWER [25] strategy:

Monitor tobacco use and prevention policies

Protect people from tobacco smoke

Offer help to quit tobacco use

Warn about the dangers of tobacco

Enforce bans on tobacco advertising, promotion, and sponsorship

Raise taxes on tobacco

Approaches to tobacco control include restriction on who can purchase tobacco products and where individuals can smoke, advertising bans, clear warnings and health information on labels (including pictorial representations of the detrimental effects of smoking), and price increases through taxation.

The effectiveness of strict restrictions on advertisements and health labels has been demonstrated in Brazil, where the prevalence of smoking declined from 35 per cent of adults in 1989 to 22 per cent in 2003 after legislative action related to tobacco promotion [26]. Though tobacco is critical to Brazil's industry, the Ministry of Health has taken multiple approaches to reducing tobacco use. In 2000, law was enacted that restricted advertisement of tobacco products and forbid merchandising at and sponsorship of cultural and sports events (Federal Law 10.67). Additionally, Brazil requires poignant health warnings and images on all tobacco products.

Approaches at the provider and individual levels have also proven to be effective when implemented as part of large-scale state-driven programmes such as those in California and Massachusetts. Funded by the California Tobacco Tax and Health Promotion Act in 1988, the California Tobacco Control Program (CTCP) was the first of its kind with a comprehensive, social-norm approach to reducing tobacco use state-wide. Despite tobacco industry spending in California being more than 5 times greater than the tobacco control programme funding, focused programmatic attention on countering pro-tobacco influences in the community, reducing second hand smoke exposure, and reducing tobacco availability, were effective as demonstrated by decreasing smoking-attributable cancer mortality rates in adults 35 years and older to a point where they are significantly lower than comparable US rates [27]. Efficacy of this comprehensive state programme is also evidenced by results of random surveys employed to assess smoking prevalence (13.7 per cent in adults in 2005 – a 28 per cent decline since 1990), smoking cessation (quit attempts in the past year were reported for 52.9 per cent of smokers in 1990 and 58.5 per cent in 1999–2005), sustained quit attempts of 90 days or longer (10.9 per cent of smokers in 1999 as compared to 13.7 per cent in 1999–2005), increased use of nicotine replacement therapy to facilitate quit efforts (13.7 per cent in 1996 versus 18.8 per cent in 2005), and other factors, not all of which produced positive results [28].

In sum, comprehensive tobacco control programmes are necessary to achieve reductions in cigarette smoking – furthermore these must be sustained over time to achieve long term health benefits and reductions in the burden of cancer. The reduction in risk of lung cancer is rapid with 50 per cent risk reduction in less than 10 years [6]. Complementing population strategies a range of individual cessation approaches is now widely used. A remaining challenge for tobacco control policies and priorities is the trade-off between focusing on children and youth to prevent initiation or focusing on adults to achieve cessation and faster returns of a reduced cancer burden. The 1994 report of the US Surgeon General highlights the importance of balancing the priorities and maintaining a focus on youth to avoid industry dominance and recruitment of a new generation of smokers [29].

Alcohol consumption

Alcohol is estimated to cause 4 per cent of all cancers in high income countries [19], with a higher burden in men than women reflecting overall intake. Health risks increase with heavier drinking leading to oral cavity, pharynx, larynx, oesophagus, liver, breast, and colorectal cancers [30]. Risks increase further when heavy alcohol use is combined with smoking.

The public health message regarding alcohol can easily be confused since research has demonstrated protective effects of alcohol on cardiovascular disease [31]. Data from the American Cancer Society study of 46,000 deaths among 490,000 men and women highlight the trade-off of protection against cardiovascular disease and the increase in cancer. The J-shaped curve for alcohol consumption and all-cause mortality has its lowest point at 1 drink per day for both men and women [31]. From a cancer perspective and for public health benefits, programmatic approaches should focus on decreasing consumption through laws and regulation, sale and driving restrictions, and/or pricing and taxation, for example; in general, including both a population-based and individual-level approach. The time course for change in risk following reduction in alcohol intake is not well quantified.

Physical activity

Globally, inactivity causes close to 2 million deaths each year [32]. Lack of activity is linked to most major chronic diseases, including type II diabetes, osteoporosis, stroke, cardiovascular disease, and cancer. Based on a rigorous systematic review of published evidence, the World Cancer Research Fund reports there is convincing evidence that physical activity decreases risk for colon cancer, probable evidence of a decrease in post-menopausal breast cancer and endometrial cancer, and suggestive evidence of an impact on lung, pancreas, and pre-menopausal breast cancer [30]. Growing evidence points to physical activity substantially reducing pre-menopausal breast cancer [33,34] as well as other chronic diseases.

Physical activity recommendations have varied but largely aim to achieve the equivalent of 30 minutes of moderate activity per day, such as brisk walking [35]. Methods for initiating and sustaining this level of physical activity have been studied extensively. Among the approaches that are effective in increasing physical activity are informational interventions ('point of decision' prompts to encourage stair use and community-wide campaigns); behavioural and social interventions (school-based physical education, social support in community settings, and individually-adapted health behaviour change); and environmental and policy intervention (creation of or enhanced access to places for physical activity combined with informational outreach activities) [36].

Providing general health recommendations alone does not ensure uptake. Studies indicate that the use of primary care based programmes employing exercise 'on prescription' can be beneficial. One New Zealand study in general practice indicated that the proportion of middle-aged women attaining 150 minutes of moderate activity per week increased from 10 per cent at baseline to 39 per cent at 24 months, quality of life improved, although no significant differences in clinical outcomes were observed [37].

Overall, the metabolic effects of increasing physical activity are well documented both for the insulin-glucose pathways and other endogenous hormones, but the time course for change in risk of cancer remains largely undocumented.

Weight control

Obesity is increasing at epidemic rates around the world [22]. US data from 2003 to 2004, report that 66 per cent of adults are overweight or obese (BMI ≥25) and 32 per cent of adults are obese (BMI ≥30) with a rising trend since 1988 [38]. Overweight and obesity cause a substantial proportion of several cancers, including oesophageal, colorectal, endometrial, kidney and post-menopausal breast cancers [22] Public health recommendations call for adults to stay within the recommended BMI range (18.5–24.9) and avoid weight gain. Accordingly, in its Global Strategy on Diet, Physical Activity, and Health, the WHO identifies energy balance and maintenance of a healthy weight as a public health priority and charges member states to develop and support multi-sectoral programmes to address weight, diet, and physical activity; thereby decreasing non-communicable disease worldwide [39].

Programmatic recommendations include interventions that integrate physical activity and diet for more sustained behaviour change. At the grade school level, Gortmaker and colleagues have successfully integrated approaches to diet, activity, and TV viewing into the school curriculum, achieving a sustained intervention and significant increases in fruit and vegetable consumption, reduction in TV viewing [40], and in a second study also reducing obesity [41]. In adult populations, a randomized trial achieved sustained weight reduction over two years through diet and activity interventions by health care providers, and resulted in reduced progression to diabetes among men and women at elevated risk [42]. Whole community interventions are exemplified by one in Belgium that included multiple strategies (media campaign, environmental approaches, use of pedometers, and local projects) and resulted in a significant increase in the proportion of the population achieving a target of 10,000 steps per day [43].

Given the preponderance of evidence that sugar-sweetened beverages increase the risk of obesity and diabetes, a growing number of interventions are now focused on strategies to reduce intake through substitution of other beverages that do not contribute to the excess energy intake. In addition to individual behaviour change, strategies that alter access through limiting on-school campus sale and increasing taxation or removing tax protection may further reinforce behaviour change.

Because of limited success in achieving sustained weight loss, cancer outcomes have been rarely studied. One important finding from the Nurses' Health Study shows that weight loss after menopause that is sustained results in a significant reduction in incidence of breast cancer in the short term [44]. This is consistent with changes in hormone levels with weight loss. The time course of risk reduction for other cancers or precursor lesions remains to be clarified.

Diet and dietary supplementation

Related to physical inactivity and weight control, though having an effect on cancer prevention that is independent from weight, diet is now estimated to account for considerably less than 35 per cent of cancers as estimated by Doll and Peto [20], though the evidence was limited and they gave an acceptable range from 10 to 70 per cent. Most estimates for the contribution of diet have included overweight/obesity in the effect of diet, yet only total energy intake exceeding energy expenditure is convincingly related to weight gain. Specific components of diet increase cancer risk at specific sites, such as red and processed meat and colon cancer, contaminants such as aflatoxin and liver cancer, while non-starchy vegetables reduce risk of cancers of the mouth, oesophagus, and stomach [30]. Because of benefits in preventing other major chronic diseases such as cardiovascular disease and diabetes, it is estimated that a global increase in fruit and vegetable consumption would save 2.7 million lives annually [32].

International recommendations prescribe a diet high in fruits and vegetables (at least 4–13 servings per day) with emphasis placed on nutrient-rich green leafy vegetables, orange vegetables, and legumes. Avoiding certain foods potentially decreases cancer risk, such as salt-preserved meats or other foods, red meat, and very hot food or drinks. The US National Cancer Institute (NCI) recommends that only 20 to 35 per cent of daily calories be from fat; comprised of primarily polyunsaturated or monounsaturated fats in fish, nuts, and vegetable oils, 10 per cent saturated fats, and as little trans fat as possible [45].

Randomized trials of fibre, fruit and vegetables, and risk of colon polyp recurrence have not shown any benefit from increased intake [46,47], and the Women's Health Initiative trial of reduced fat intake (along with increased fruit and vegetable intake) to prevent breast cancer did not show a significant reduction in risk over 8.1 years [48]. The level of adherence to diet in this long-term study limited the likelihood of the trial showing benefit.

The California State Department of Public Health has promoted '5-a-day' consumption of fruit and vegetables, using a number of strategies including worksites. This and similar approaches have been promoted in many countries. Research projects modelled on this strategy were implemented in nine NCI funded projects to evaluate its effectiveness. For example, Sorensen and colleagues showed that a multi-component intervention that included media exposure to 5-a-day messages, programmes aimed at individual behaviour change, and worksite environment changes could significantly increase fruit and vegetable consumption [49]. Multi-component interventions to achieve sustained dietary changes are supported by studies such as this. Barriers to achieving a maximally healthy diet include higher costs and lack of ready access to fresh fruit and vegetables.

Strategies to improve diet and lower disease risk include counselling and regulatory approaches as well as farm-based interventions. Rather than focus on whole food consumption, much research has focused on specific nutrients leading to chemoprevention strategies that modify exposure to bioactive agents. For example in Finland, to overcome low selenium levels in the soil and because trials indicated that higher selenium may reduce cancers of the lung, colon, and prostate [50], a fortification intervention was introduced. Selenium was applied with fertilizer, and blood selenium levels rose rapidly following the ecologic intervention, though there has been no apparent decline in incidence of prostate or colon cancers [51]; and a subsequent randomized controlled trial in the United States (the SELECT trial) showed no overall benefit of increased selenium, nor a reduction in prostate or colon cancers [52]. Thus it is highly unlikely that increasing selenium intake will be beneficial for cancer prevention.

Other nutritional agents have also been tested in chemoprevention trials in the developed world and in China [53]. Based on evidence that people in Linxian, China, had low intakes of several nutrients, a randomized trial comparing combinations of retinol, zinc, riboflavin, niacin, vitamin C and molybdenum, beta-carotene, vitamin E, and selenium was undertaken [54]. Significant reductions in mortality were observed for those who received the combination of beta-carotene, vitamin E, and selenium – and the reduction was greater for those who began the therapy at a younger age. In contrast, studies have shown no benefit of beta-carotene in high risk smokers (The Alpha-Tocopherol Beta-Carotene trial was stopped early because of excess lung cancer in men randomized to beta-carotene) [55], or in men at high risk due to smoking or asbestos exposure [56]. Similarly among average risk populations [57] no benefit was observed. Together these trials show strong evidence against the hypothesis that beta-carotene can substantially reduce risk of lung cancer. However, if dietary antioxidants such as beta-carotene act early in the carcinogenic process, trials such as these would not have detected any benefit. Further study of diet across the full time course of carcinogenesis is clearly necessary.

Substantial evidence supports a link between vitamin D and reduced incidence of colon cancer – the third most common cancer among both men and women in the United States. Studies show that people with higher circulating vitamin D levels can have as little as half the risk of developing colon cancer as those with lower vitamin D levels [58]. This and other possible benefits were reviewed systematically by the International Agency for Research on Cancer (IARC) [58], and led to the recommendation that better understanding of possible adverse health effects of population supplementation, and the possible variation in benefits depending on the baseline serum 25-hydroxyvitamin D level, are necessary before recommending routine vitamin D supplementation for cancer prevention. Further research is needed to define the optimal dose or level of vitamin D, its efficacy in reducing cancer incidence, and the time course for change in risk of cancer after increasing levels.

Sun exposure

The sun, as the primary source of ultraviolet radiation, poses a significant risk of skin cancer particularly in fair-skinned Caucasians. Internationally, nearly 60,000 deaths are attributed to over-exposure leading to malignant melanomas and skin cancer annually [59]. Observing trends of increasing rates of skin cancer, the US National Cancer Institute reports 60,000 new cases in 2007 in the United States alone [45]. Prevention recommendations as simple as avoiding the sun in peak hours (approximately 10 a.m. to 3 p.m.), covering skin whenever possible, protecting exposed skin with sunscreen, and avoiding tanning booths are effective in reducing skin cancer incidence if these lifestyle changes are adopted, particularly, at an early age.

The Center for Disease Control Task Force on Community Preventive Services concluded that school-based educational/policy interventions (for children) and recreational-based educational/policy interventions (for adults) were effective in reducing sun exposure [60]. Both types of interventions are well represented by the Australian SunSmart programme, ongoing since 1982, (formerly Slip! Slop! Slap!) which aims at reducing UV exposure through access to shade and consistent use of protective clothing, hats, sunglasses, and sunscreen. Examples of SunSmart programming include accreditation of schools that adhere to its policy and practice requirements and collaboration with governmental agencies to protect outdoor workers. Montague et al. credit the programme with changing attitudes regarding sun tanning, increases in protective behaviour, decreased costs of sun protection gear, societal acceptance of more protective attire (including hats, sunglasses, and 'neck to knee' swimsuits for children) and, most importantly, decreasing incidence rates of skin cancer [61]. Dobbinson et al. concluded that sun-protective behaviour had increased from 1987 to 2002 during which time the SunSmart programme was active [62]. The evidence from Australia indicates that active prevention efforts including television advertising campaigns can be highly effective in improving the population-wide sun-protective behaviours, resulting in falling age-specific incidence rates for melanoma, in younger birth cohorts [63].

Infections

The aetiology of some 18 per cent of cancers worldwide can be linked to chronic infections due to agents such as Helicobacter pylori, human papillomaviruses (HPV), Hepatitis B, Hepatitis C, Epstein-Barr virus (EBV), human immunodeficiency virus (HIV), human herpes virus 8 (HHV-8), and Schistosoma haematobium [64], with the proportion of all cancer due to infections being much higher in developing countries (26 per cent, compared to 7.7 per cent in developed countries). The current burden of cancer in the developing world is dominated by infection, once smoking is accounted for. Of 10.8 million new cases of cancer worldwide (2002 figures), those caused by infectious agents are estimated as: H. pylori 5.5 per cent (mainly stomach, and lymphoma); HPV 5.2 per cent (mainly cervix, and ano-genital, mouth, pharynx); HBV and HBC 4.9 per cent (liver); EBV 1.0 per cent (nasopharynx, Hodgkin lymphoma, and Burkitt lymphoma), HIV and HHV 80.9 per cent (Kaposi sarcoma, non-Hodgkin lymphoma) and other less common agents including schistosomes, HTLV 1 per cent, and liver flukes less than 0.5 per cent. More than 25 per cent of cancer incidence in developing countries could be avoided if infectious causes of cancer were prevented [64]. Successful vaccination programmes have the potential to reduce cancer incidence and mortality; for example, Taiwan's HBV vaccination programme was initiated in 1984, and impressively high coverage rates (up to 97 per cent in 2004) have led to a consistent decline in hepatocellular cancer rates [16]. However, a recent study by Chang et al. underscores the importance of a multi-pronged approach. Though Taiwan has seen a decrease in the incidence of hepatocellular cancer in children since initiation of the vaccination programme (from 0.54 to 0.20 per 100,000 before and after the programme), vertical transmission, vaccine failure, and the lack of hepatitis B immunoglobulin injection has affected programme effectiveness and public health impact [65].

Environmental and occupational exposures

Environmental exposures account for 1 to 4 per cent of cancers. Occupational exposures such as asbestos, arsenic in drinking water, food contaminants such as aflatoxins and pesticides, and radiation exposure are classified as environmental carcinogens, but in countries with established market economies, exposure is now largely limited by regulation to reduce harm. International agencies have responded by identifying carcinogens (e.g. IARC classification of carcinogenic compounds) and regulating use, exposure, and protection for employees in the case of occupational hazards.

The WHO has identified legislative enforcement of identification and elimination/reduction approaches, government-driven dissemination of information and awareness-raising activities, and increased access to information as effective strategies to combat carcinogenic environmental exposures [66]. An end result is that, in some cases, production has been exported to countries with more lenient requirements for environmental exposure and contaminants thereby not eliminating, but shifting, the cancer risk from an international scope. Despite regulatory changes in many countries, exposure to asbestos, for example, continues through occupations such as construction, ship work, and asbestos mining. Given the long lag between exposure and lung and pleural cancers, mortality from asbestos-related disease is estimated to remain at 90,000 per year [67].

Regulation and oversight of non-occupational hazards can be more difficult; for example, indoor air pollution primarily from burning coal and cooking oil. A recent meta-analysis conducted by Zhao et al. confirmed an association in China between indoor air pollution and lung cancer [68]. In a separate study, the impact of solid fuel-related air pollution on the Chinese population was implicated in causation of approximately 420,000 premature deaths each year [69]. In the 1980s and 90s, China's Ministry of Health implemented the National Improved Stove Program that intended to improve fuel-efficiency by providing biomass stoves with chimneys. The programme was '. . . the largest and most successful improved stove programme ever implemented anywhere in the world' [70]. While the programme was successful in improving pre-programme indoor air quality levels, subsequent testing in a random sample of houses indicated the need for continued improvement, as the indoor air quality was still not compliant with Chinese indoor air pollution standards. Successful enforcement of approaches to reduce exposure to known carcinogens in both the work place and the home is necessary to achieve successful cancer prevention.

Medications

Medication use is widespread in the high income countries and limited in low and middle income countries. Strong evidence supports several medications as either causing cancer, e.g. postmenopausal hormone therapy with oestrogen plus progestin [71], or reducing cancer, e.g. oral contraceptives and ovarian cancer [72], aspirin and colon cancer [73]. For combination oestrogen plus progestin, the IARC has now classified this combination therapy as carcinogenic in humans [74] and estimates indicate that the reduction in use of hormones after the widespread publicity of the results of the Women's Health Initiative (stopped early due to excess breast cancer) accounts for approximately a 10 per cent decline in incidence among women 40 to 70 years of age [71]. Thus for this combination therapy evidence shows that risk rises with duration of use and that acting as a late promoter, removal of the drug leads to a rapid decline in incidence [71], though among women with longer durations of use risk may not return to that of women who have never used combination therapy [75]. Other less widespread drugs may also contribute to cancer risk (e.g. DES), but the population impact will be substantially smaller than the examples based on much more widespread use described in earlier sections.

For some medications that reduce risk, the benefits have been limited to date to those who have had specific indications for use of the medication. Broader population strategies may be developed for more widespread protection, such as could be achieved if all women took oral contraceptives as a chemopreventive for a minimum of 5 years (see 'Chemoprevention' herein).

Chemoprevention

Oral contraceptives As noted earlier, use of oral contraceptives (OCs) for 5 years halves a woman's risk of ovarian cancer and substantially reduces risk of endometrial cancer. The protection is long lasting and in high income countries rates of use approach 80 per cent. Adverse effects are largely limited to increased risk of breast cancer and stroke while currently using OCs. As these side-effects are strongly age-dependent, use of OCs during late teens and early 20s could be widened for greater reduction in ovarian and endometrial cancers and overall net health benefit [76].

Aspirin The use of aspirin has been extensively studied in observational epidemiologic settings that address duration of use, dose, and magnitude of risk reduction. The observational evidence is consistent with evidence from randomized primary prevention trials showing that use of 300 mg or more of aspirin a day for 5 years or more is effective in preventing colon cancer; reducing risk by approximately 25 per cent [77]. A latency of about 10 years is observed. Like all chemoprevention strategies, risks and benefits must be balanced [78]. To date, the risk-benefit considerations of cardiovascular disease, bleeding complications, stomach pain, and heart burn have precluded recommendations for aspirin use as a widespread prevention strategy [79].

Selective oestrogen receptor modulators (SERMs) Drugs such as Tamoxifen and Raloxifene have been shown in randomized controlled prevention trials to reduce risk of pre-invasive and invasive breast cancer [80,81]. While Tamoxifen increases risk of uterine cancer, this is not so for Raloxifene and the risk profile for Raloxifene looks considerably safer [82]. Based on this, we have estimated the potential for risk reduction among women over age 50 who are postmenopausal. Our estimates indicate that if the trade-off of excess adverse events versus cases of breast cancer prevented must be less than 1, then approximately 30 per cent of the 27 million women between ages 50 and 69 in the United States have benefits exceeding risks, and would achieve a 50 per cent reduction in the burden of breast cancer by taking a SERM. This is a population benefit of 42,900 fewer cases of invasive breast cancer among the more than 7 million women with sufficiently high risk to justify chemoprevention [82]. The reduction in risk observed in the chemoprevention randomized trials is rapid; within 2 years of beginning therapy, incidence curves have clearly separated. This is consistent with the pharmacologic action of the agents inhibiting oestrogen receptors. Importantly these agents show protection against oestrogen receptor (ER) positive breast cancers (risk reduction up to 76 per cent) and no protection against receptor negative cancers [81]. While models to classify risk of breast cancer have been developed and validated, to date prediction of receptor positive tumours is no more accurate than prediction of risk overall [83]. Refining risk stratification and developing tools to aid women in considering trade-offs of risks and benefits of chemoprevention therapy are necessary next steps to wide-spread use of these promising strategies for women at elevated risk of breast cancer.

Balancing priorities: high risk versus individual or tailored prevention strategies

A major challenge for active prevention programmes is to balance the components of a social strategy, actions through health care providers, those through regulatory changes and those focused on individual behaviour changes [18]. Are we to focus on provider delivered strategies tailored to the risk level of the individual or embark on active population-wide efforts? We note that in the case of colon cancer, estimates from the Health Professionals Follow-up Study indicate that the majority of men have multiple modifiable risk factors [84]. Only 3 per cent of this population of middle-aged and older men had no modifiable risk factors for colon cancer. Similar results were observed for women in the Nurses' Health Study when considering prevention of heart disease and diabetes. With population-wide changes increasing the level of physical activity, reducing intake of alcohol, increasing folate intake, reducing adult weight gain and obesity, and reducing red meat intake, up to 70 per cent of colon cancer could be avoided. Of course, screening offers additional cost-effective strategies for early detection of cancers and removal of precursor polyps [85,86]. For example, if the entire US population increased their level of physical activity through walking for an additional 30 minutes per week we would reduce the burden of colon cancer by 15 per cent [87]. This then is a highly preventable malignancy for which numerous population-wide strategies are already available to reduce the incidence of the second leading cause of cancer mortality.

The fundamental premise of epidemiology is to estimate the population average risk of disease. Risk is a population measure, not an individual measure. Epidemiology does not estimate individual risk, nor does it perfectly predict individual likelihood of disease. As noted by Rose, epidemiology does not describe why an individual case of cancer arises in the population, but rather what the causes of incidence in the population are [88].

The high-risk approach to prevention aims to identify those most at risk of disease and avoid the apparent wastefulness of mass prevention strategies, which are characterized by large societal benefits though little individual gain. However, population-level changes shift the underlying risk. The melanoma prevention efforts in Australia discussed previously illustrate the benefits of population-wide strategies. Exposure to solar radiation is accepted as the major environmental cause of melanoma. Population-wide strategies to reduce sun exposure have been implemented in Australia, the country with the highest incidence of melanoma in the world.

Does knowledge of phenotypic risk factors change the prevention messages? For melanoma, can we recommend that only a subset of the population avoid excess sun exposure? Estimates by English and Armstrong based on Australian data suggest that 54 per cent of melanoma occurs in 16 per cent of the population, who might therefore be suitable for more intensive surveillance. However, to exclude the 'low risk' segment of the population from prevention messages or strategies would eliminate the potential for prevention of 46 per cent of cases. These estimates of the proportion of disease arising from those with epidemiologic risk factors is consistent with seminal writing by Wald et al. showing that risk factors are poor markers for identification of sub-populations for prevention [89]. Hence as Rose noted, prevention strategies must be widespread.

In contrast with the high-risk approach that will be tailored to each malignancy one at a time, population-wide strategies that have benefits across multiple chronic conditions, such as smoking cessation, increase in physical activity, avoiding weight gain and improving diet, will have far greater public health benefit. For example increasing physical activity will also reduce the burden of type II diabetes, coronary heart disease, and stroke.

To eliminate large portions of the burden of cancer we typically do not need refined understanding of molecular pathways. Recommendations to stop smoking were made long before the molecular pathways from tobacco to lung cancer were described. Based on the evidence from seven prospective studies available in 1964, the Report of Surgeon General Luther Terry concluded that smoking causes lung cancer in men and recommended that men stop smoking. Subsequent to the 1964 report of the Surgeon General there have been widespread changes in patterns of smoking and ultimately changes in lung cancer incidence. The incidence of lung cancer is now falling [90].

One might well ask, 'How will refined understanding of molecular pathways to malignancy help reduce the population burden of lung cancer'? Perhaps they won't, but rather they may identify strategies for chemoprevention among former smokers, or treatment options. Perhaps greater effort should be made for understanding and interrupting the pathway from marketing, uptake of smoking and addiction, or modifying social norms related to supersizing sugar sweetened beverages?

Broad campaigns can be effective, as the melanoma prevention programme in Australia has demonstrated, and data from California noted earlier in this chapter attest to the impact of the increases in tobacco tax and anti-tobacco education campaigns to prevent smoking. Since smoking causes cancer at many organ sites, shifting the whole population distribution will have a greater impact on cancer burden than trying to identify a subset of susceptible individuals that is at sufficiently high risk (yet are a large enough subset of the population) to account for a substantial portion of the disease burden.

Balancing strategies across provider services and actions, regulatory changes that will reduce exposures and reinforce cancer reducing behaviour changes, and strategies targeted to communities and individuals remains a high priority as we plan and implement active prevention programmes to reduce the burden of cancer.

Cancer prevention: future directions

While for non-smokers population-wide approaches to increase physical activity and prevent weight gain (or achieve weight loss) offer the greatest benefits and major challenges for cancer prevention going forward, advancing technology must also be considered. As vaccines such as the HPV vaccine are developed can they be effectively delivered to the women (or adolescents) at highest risk for cervical cancer, i.e. in countries with limited health resources?

Can physical activity and weight control compete with the drive for development, fast food, and a Western lifestyle? Can tobacco control compete effectively with these same marketing forces? Evidence shows that tobacco control can be successful, with sufficient political will to allocate adequate resources and establish necessary regulatory changes to complement health care provider and individual level changes.

These are challenges in the field that the recently launched World Cancer Declaration (WCD) (www.uicc.org/wcd) sets forth as priorities for the global cancer community. Priorities for the WCD include health policy placing cancer on the agenda; cancer prevention and early detection priorities that address tobacco, reduction in exposure to environmental carcinogens, and increased access to vaccines. In the research setting, better defining the achievable changes in exposure will lead to more realistic estimates of the proportion of cancer that is preventable through active cancer prevention programmes. A refined understanding of natural history of cancers and the carcinogenic process for each cancer site will improve our ability to target prevention strategies appropriately during the life course.

Advances that refine classification of cancer and perhaps offer new prevention pathways may offer new prevention strategies for specific subsets of cancer. If such an approach is successful for say oestrogen receptor negative breast cancer that impacts a relatively small number of women, how will we identify those at high risk? How will this risk reduction strategy that is more focused on prevention of subsets of cancer be communicated to the population, to health care providers, and to policy setting bodies? Already the potential for selective oestrogen receptor modulators (such as Tamoxifen and Raloxifene) to prevent a substantial portion of postmenopausal breast cancer is exciting, particularly as the global burden will continue to rise with changing reproductive patterns in Asia [4]. Such chemopreventive agents have risks in addition to the benefits of reduced cancer incidence. Quantifying risks of therapies is always somewhat limited as studies are powered to quantify benefits, not risks. New and improved approaches to identifying and quantifying risks, and subsets of the population who may be at particular risk, will help refine approaches to balancing risk benefit trade-offs.

The use of genome-wide scans for common cancers to identify polymorphisms that may contribute to the aetiology of cancers may be added to lifestyle factors to improve risk classification [91], and targeting of prevention strategies. However, this is far from simple as the genetic markers do not yet discriminate between those who do and do not get cancer [92].

Conclusion

More than half of the seven million deaths from cancer worldwide are caused by one of the key potentially modifiable risk factors described in this Chapter. Using evidence-based strategies to impact individual and population behaviour changes, public health efforts driven by sound knowledge, legislative support/backing, and social commitment have the potential to rapidly reduce the cancer incidence and mortality in the twenty-first century. Our aging population and the burden of cancer that comes due to aging demands we act now to achieve this global benefit.

References

1 Colditz GA, Sellers TA, Trapido E (2006). Epidemiology–identifying the causes and preventability of cancer? *Nat Rev Cancer*, **6**:75–83.

2 International Agency for Research on Cancer (2008). *World Cancer Report*. International Agency for Research on Cancer, Lyon.

3 Peto R, Chen ZM, Boreham J (1999). Tobacco–the growing epidemic. *Nat Med*, **5**:15–17.

4 Linos E, Spanos D, Rosner BA, et al (2008). Effects of reproductive and demographic changes on breast cancer incidence in China: a modeling analysis. *J Natl Cancer Inst*, **100**:1352–60.

5 Peto R, Darby S, Deo H, Silcocks P, Whitley E, & Doll R (2000). Smoking, smoking cessation, and lung cancer in the UK since 1950: combination of national statistics with two case-control studies. *BMJ*, **321**:323–29.

6 Kenfield SA, Stampfer MJ, Rosner BA, & Colditz GA (2008). Smoking and smoking cessation in relation to mortality in women. *JAMA*, **299**:2037–47.

7 Barnoya J & Glantz S (2004). Association of the California tobacco control program with declines in lung cancer incidence. *Cancer Causes Control*, **15**:689–95.

8 Bal DG, Kizer KW, Felten PG, Mozar HN, & Niemeyer D (1990). Reducing tobacco consumption in California. Development of a statewide anti-tobacco use campaign. *JAMA*, **264**:1570–74.

9 Pierce JP, Gilpin EA, Emery SL, et al (1998). Has the California tobacco control program reduced smoking? *JAMA*, **280**:893–99.

10 Zelen M (1988). Are primary cancer prevention trials feasible? *J Natl Cancer Inst*, **80**:1442–44.

11 Chlebowski RT, Hendrix SL, Langer RD, et al (2003). Influence of oestrogen plus progestin on breast cancer and mammography in healthy postmenopausal women: the Women's Health Initiative Randomized Trial. *JAMA*, **289**:3243–53.

12 Demissie K, Mills OF, & Rhoads GG (1998). Empirical comparison of the results of randomized controlled trials and case-control studies in evaluating the effectiveness of screening mammography. *J Clin Epidemiol*, **51**:81–91.

13 Wactawski-Wende J, Kotchen JM, Anderson GL, et al (2006). Calcium plus vitamin D supplementation and the risk of colorectal cancer. *N Engl J Med*, **354**:684–96.

14 Martinez ME, Marshall JR, & Giovannucci E (2008). Diet and cancer prevention: the roles of observation and experimentation. *Nat Rev Cancer*, **8**:694–703.

15 Viviani S, Carrieri P, Bah E, et al (2008). 20 years into the Gambia Hepatitis Intervention Study: assessment of initial hypotheses and prospects for evaluation of protective effectiveness against liver cancer. *Cancer Epidemiol Biomarkers Prev*, **17**:3216–23.

16 Chang MH, Chen CJ, Lai MS, et al (1997). Universal hepatitis B vaccination in Taiwan and the incidence of hepatocellular carcinoma in children. Taiwan Childhood Hepatoma Study Group. *N Engl J Med*, **336**:1855–59.

17 Mills PK, Beeson WL, Phillips RL, & Fraser GE (1994). Cancer incidence among California Seventh-Day Adventists, 1976–1982. *Am J Clin Nutr*, **59**:1136S–42S.

18 Atwood K, Colditz G, & Kawachi I. Implementing prevention policies: relevance of the Richmond model to health policy judgments (1997). *Am J Public Health*, **87**:1603–6.

19 Danaei G, Vander Hoorn S, Lopez AD, Murray CJ, & Ezzati M (2005). Causes of cancer in the world: comparative risk assessment of nine behavioural and environmental risk factors. *Lancet*, **366**:1784–93.

20 Doll R & Peto R (1981). *The Causes of Cancer: Quantitative Estimates of Avoidable Risks of Cancer in the United States Today*. Oxford University Press, New York.

21 Calle EE, Rodriguez C, Walker-Thurmond K, & Thun MJ (2003). Overweight, obesity, and mortality from cancer in a prospectively studied cohort of US adults. *N Engl J Med*, **348**:1625–38.

22 International Agency for Research on Cancer (2002). Weight Control and Physical Activity. International Agency for Research on Cancer, Lyon.

23 Peto R, Lopez AD, Boreham J, Thun M, Heath C, Jr., & Doll R (1996). Mortality from smoking worldwide. *Br Med Bull*, **52**:12–21.

24 US Department of Health and Human Services (2004). The health consequences of smoking: a report of the Surgeon General. Washington, DC.

25 World Health Organization (2008). WHO Report on the Global Tobacco Epidemic. World Health Organization, Geneva.

26 Monteiro CA, Cavalcante TM, Moura EC, Claro RM, & Szwarcwald CL (2007). Population-based evidence of a strong decline in the prevalence of smokers in Brazil (1989–2003). Bulletin of the World Health Organization, **85**:527–34.

27 California Department of Health Services TCS (2006). California tobacco control update. Sacremento, CA: CDHS/TCS.

28 Al-Delaimy W, White M, T G, Zhu S-H, & Pierce J (2008). *The California Tobacco Control Program: Can We Maintain the Progress? Results from the California Tobacco Survey, 1990–2005*. La Jolla, CA: University of California, San Diego.

29 US Department of Health and Human Services (1994). Preventing Tobacco Use among Young People. A Report of the Surgeon General. Atlanta, Georgia: US Department of Health and Human Services, Public Health Service, Centers for Disease Control, National Center for Chronic Disease Prevention and Health Promotion, Office on Smoking and Health.

30 World Cancer Research Fund (2007). *Food, Nutrition, Physical Activity, and the Prevention of Cancer: A Global Perspective*. Washington, DC: AICR.

31 Thun MJ, Peto R, Lopez AD, et al (1997). Alcohol consumption and mortality among middle-aged and elderly US adults. *N Engl J Med*, **337**:1705–14.

32 Ezzati M, Lopez AD, Rodgers A, Vander Hoorn S, & Murray CJ (2002). Selected major risk factors and global and regional burden of disease. *Lancet*, **360**:1347–60.

33 Bernstein L, Henderson BE, Hanisch R, Sullivan-Halley J, & Ross RK (1994). Physical exercise and reduced risk of breast cancer in young women. *J Natl Cancer Inst*, **86**:1403–8.

34 Maruti SS, Willett WC, Feskanich D, Rosner B, & Colditz GA (2008). A prospective study of age-specific physical activity and premenopausal breast cancer. *J Natl Cancer Inst*, **100**:728–37.

35 Pate RR, Pratt M, Blair SN, et al (1995). Physical activity and public health. A recommendation from the Centers for Disease Control and Prevention and the American College of Sports Medicine. *JAMA*, **273**:402–7.

36 Kahn EB, Ramsey LT, Brownson RC, et al (2002). The effectiveness of interventions to increase physical activity. A systematic review. *Am J Prev Med*, **22**:73–107.

37 Lawton BA, Rose SB, Elley CR, Dowell AC, Fenton A, & Moyes SA (2008). Exercise on prescription for women aged 40–74 recruited through primary care: two year randomised controlled trial. *BMJ*, **337**:a2509.

38 Ogden CL, Carroll MD, Curtin LR, McDowell MA, Tabak CJ, & Flegal KM (2006). Prevalence of overweight and obesity in the United States, 1999–2004. *JAMA*, **295**:1549–55.

39 World Health Organization (2004). Global Strategy on Diet, Physical Activity, and Health. World Health Organization, Geneva.

40 Gortmaker SL, Cheung LW, Peterson KE, et al (1999). Impact of a school-based interdisciplinary intervention on diet and physical activity among urban primary school children: eat well and keep moving. *Arch Pediatr Adolesc Med*, **153**:975–83.

41 Gortmaker SL, Peterson K, Wiecha J, et al (1999). Reducing obesity via a school-based interdisciplinary intervention among youth: Planet Health. *Arch Pediatr Adolesc Med*, **153**:409–18.

42 Knowler WC, Barrett-Connor E, Fowler SE, et al (2002). Reduction in the incidence of type 2 diabetes with lifestyle intervention or metformin. *N Engl J Med*, **346**:393–403.

43 De Cocker KA, De Bourdeaudhuij IM, Brown WJ, & Cardon GM (2007). Effects of '10,000 steps Ghent': a whole-community intervention. *Am J Prev Med*, **33**:455–63.

44 Eliassen AH, Colditz GA, Rosner B, Willett WC, & Hankinson SE (2006). Adult weight change and risk of postmenopausal breast cancer. *JAMA*, **296**:193–201.

45 National Cancer Institute (2007). Cancer Trends Progress Report – 2007 Update. Bethesda, MD: NIH, DHHS.

46 Alberts DS, Martinez ME, Roe DJ, et al (2000). Lack of effect of a high-fiber cereal supplement on the recurrence of colorectal adenomas. Phoenix Colon Cancer Prevention Physicians' Network. *N Engl J Med*, **342**:1156–62.

47 Schatzkin A, Lanza E, Corle D, et al (2000). Lack of effect of a low-fat, high-fiber diet on the recurrence of colorectal adenomas. Polyp Prevention Trial Study Group. *N Engl J Med*, **342**:1149–55.

48 Prentice RL, Caan B, Chlebowski RT, et al (2006). Low-fat dietary pattern and risk of invasive breast cancer: the Women's Health Initiative Randomized Controlled Dietary Modification Trial. *JAMA*, **295**:629–42.

49 Sorensen G, Stoddard A, Peterson K, et al (1999). Increasing fruit and vegetable consumption through worksites and families in the treatwell 5-a-day study. *Am J Public Health*, **89**:54–60.

50 Clark LC, Combs GF, Jr., Turnbull BW, et al (1996). Effects of selenium supplementation for cancer prevention in patients with carcinoma of the skin. A randomized controlled trial. Nutritional Prevention of Cancer Study Group. *JAMA*, **276**:1957–63.

51 Willett WC (1999). Goals for nutrition in the year 2000. *CA Cancer J Clin*, **49**:331–52.

52 Lippman SM, Klein EA, Goodman PJ, et al (2009). Effect of selenium and vitamin E on risk of prostate cancer and other cancers: the Selenium and Vitamin E Cancer Prevention Trial (SELECT). *JAMA*, **301**:39–51.

53 Greenwald P, Anderson D, Nelson SA, & Taylor PR (2007). Clinical trials of vitamin and mineral supplements for cancer prevention. *Am J Clin Nutr*, **85**:314S–17S.

54 Blot WJ, Li JY, Taylor PR, et al (1993). Nutrition intervention trials in Linxian, China: supplementation with specific vitamin/mineral combinations, cancer incidence, and disease-specific mortality in the general population. *J Natl Cancer Inst*, **85**:1483–92.

55 The Alpha-Tocopherol BCCPSG (1994). The effect of vitamin E and beta carotene on the incidence of lung cancer and other cancers in male smokers. *N Engl J Med*, 330:1029–35.

56 Omenn GS, Goodman GE, Thornquist MD, et al (1996). Effects of a combination of beta carotene and vitamin A on lung cancer and cardiovascular disease. *N Engl J Med*, **334**:1150–5.

57 Hennekens CH, Buring JE, Manson JE, et al (1996). Lack of effect of long-term supplementation with beta carotene on the incidence of malignant neoplasms and cardiovascular disease. *N Engl J Med*, **334**:1145–9.

58 International Agency for Research on Cancer (2008). Vitamin D and Cancer. International Agency for Research on Cancer; Lyon.

59 World Health Organization (2007). The World Health Organization's Fight Against Cancer: Strategies that prevent, cure, and care. World Health Organization, Geneva.

60 Saraiya M, Glanz K, Briss P, Nichols P, White C, & Das D (2003). Preventing skin cancer: findings of the task force on community preventive services on reducing exposure to ultraviolet light. *MMWR Recomm Rep*, **52**:1–12.

61 Montague M, Borland R, & Sinclair C (2001). Slip! Slop! Slap! and SunSmart, 1980–2000: Skin cancer control and 20 years of population-based campaigning. *Health Educ Behav*, **28**:290–305.

62 Dobbinson SJ, Wakefield MA, Jamsen KM, et al (2008). Weekend sun protection and sunburn in Australia trends (1987–2002) and association with SunSmart television advertising. *Am J Prev Med*, **34**:94–101.

63 Hill D & Marks R (2008). Health promotion programs for melanoma prevention: screw or spring? *Arch Dermatol*, **144**:538–40.

64 Parkin DM (2006). The global health burden of infection-associated cancers in the year 2002. *Int J Cancer*, **118**:3030–44.

65 Chang MH, Chen TH, Hsu HM, et al (2005). Prevention of hepatocellular carcinoma by universal vaccination against hepatitis B virus: the effect and problems. *Clin Cancer Res*, **11**:7953–57.

66 World Health Organization (2007). Cancer Control: Knowledge into Action (Prevention Module). World Health Organization, Geneva.

67 World Health Organization (2006). Elimination of Asbestos-related Disease. World Health Organization, Geneva.

68 Zhao Y, Wang S, Aunan K, Seip HM, & Hao J (2006). Air pollution and lung cancer risks in China–a meta-analysis. *The Science of the Total Environment*, **366**:500–13.

69 Zhang JJ & Smith KR (2007). Household air pollution from coal and biomass fuels in China: measurements, health impacts, and interventions. *Environ Health Perspect*, **115**:848–55.

70 Edwards RD, Liu Y, He G, et al (2007). Household CO and PM measured as part of a review of China's National Improved Stove Program. *Indoor air*, **17**:189–203.

71 Colditz GA (2007). Decline in breast cancer incidence due to removal of promoter: combination oestrogen plus progestin. *Breast Cancer Res*, **9**:108.

72 Collaborative Group on Epidemiological Studies of Ovarian C, Beral V, Doll R, Hermon C, Peto R, & Reeves G (2008). Ovarian cancer and oral contraceptives: collaborative reanalysis of data from 45 epidemiological studies including 23,257 women with ovarian cancer and 87,303 controls. *Lancet*, **371**:303–14.

73 Chan AT, Giovannucci EL, Meyerhardt JA, Schernhammer ES, Curhan GC, & Fuchs CS (2005). Long-term use of aspirin and nonsteroidal anti-inflammatory drugs and risk of colorectal cancer. *JAMA*, **294**:914–23.

74 International Agency for Research on Cancer (2007). Combined estrogen-progestogen contraceptives and combined estrogen-progestogen menopausal therapy. *IARC Monogr Eval Carcinog Risks Hum*, **91**:1–528.

75 Colditz GA & Rosner B (2000). Cumulative risk of breast cancer to age 70 years according to risk factor status: data from the Nurses' Health Study. *Am J Epidemiol*, **152**:950–64.

76 Kawachi I, Colditz GA, & Hankinson S (1994). Long-term benefits and risks of alternative methods of fertility control in the United States. *Contraception*, **50**:1–16.

77 Flossmann E & Rothwell PM (2007). Effect of aspirin on long-term risk of colorectal cancer: consistent evidence from randomised and observational studies. *Lancet*, **369**:1603–13.

78 Glasziou PP & Irwig LM (1995). An evidence based approach to individualising treatment. *BMJ*, **311**:1356–59.

79 Gralow J, Ozols RF, Bajorin DF, et al (2008). Clinical cancer advances 2007: major research advances in cancer treatment, prevention, and screening–a report from the American Society of Clinical Oncology. *J Clin Oncol*, **26**:313–25.

80 Fisher B, Costantino JP, Wickerham DL, et al (1998). Tamoxifen for prevention of breast cancer: report of the National Surgical Adjuvant Breast and Bowel Project P-1 Study. *J Natl Cancer Inst*, **90**:1371–88.

81 Martino S, Cauley JA, Barrett-Connor E, et al (2004). Continuing outcomes relevant to Evista: breast cancer incidence in postmenopausal osteoporotic women in a randomized trial of raloxifene. *J Natl Cancer Inst*, **96**:1751–61.

82 Chen WY, Rosner B, & Colditz GA (2007). Moving forward with breast cancer prevention. *Cancer*, **109**:2387–91.

83 Colditz GA, Rosner BA, Chen WY, Holmes MD, & Hankinson SE (2004). Risk factors for breast cancer according to oestrogen and progesterone receptor status. *J Natl Cancer Inst*, **96**:218–28.

84 Platz EA, Willett WC, Colditz GA, Rimm EB, Spiegelman D, & Giovannucci E (2000). Proportion of colon cancer risk that might be preventable in a cohort of middle-aged US men. *Cancer Causes Control*, **11**:579–88.

85 Frazier AL, Colditz GA, Fuchs CS, & Kuntz KM (2000). Cost-effectiveness of screening for colorectal cancer in the general population. *JAMA*, **284**:1954–61.

86 Winawer SJ, Zauber AG, Ho MN, et al (1993). Prevention of colorectal cancer by colonoscopic polypectomy. The National Polyp Study Workgroup. *N Engl J Med*, **329**:1977–81.

87 Colditz G, Frazier AL, & Sorensen G (2000). Population-level change in risk factors for cancer. In: Colditz G, Hunter DJ, (eds) *Cancer Prevention: The Causes and Prevention of Cancer*, pp. 313–23. Kluwer Academic Publishers, Dordrecht.

88 Rose GA (1992). *The Strategy of Preventive Medicine*. Oxford University Press, Oxford (England), New York.

89 Wald NJ, Hackshaw AK, & Frost CD (1999). When can a risk factor be used as a worthwhile screening test? *BMJ*, **319**:1562–65.

90 Wingo PA, Ries LA, Giovino GA, et al (1999). Annual report to the nation on the status of cancer, 1973–1996, with a special section on lung cancer and tobacco smoking. *J Natl Cancer Inst*, **91**:675–90.

91 Pharoah PD, Antoniou AC, Easton DF, & Ponder BA (2008). Polygenes, risk prediction, and targeted prevention of breast cancer. *N Engl J Med*, **358**:2796–2803.

92 Pharoah PD (2008). Shedding light on skin cancer. *Nat Genet*, **40**:817–18.

93 Peto R, Darby S, Deo H, Silcocks P, Whitley E, & Doll R (2000). Smoking, smoking cessation, and lung cancer in the UK since 1950: combination of national statistics with two case-control studies. *BMJ*, **321**:323–29.

94 Chan AT, Giovannucci EL, Meyerhardt JA, Schernhammer ES, Wu K, & Fuchs CS (2008). Aspirin dose and duration of use and risk of colorectal cancer in men. *Gastroenterology*, **134**:21–28.

Chapter 3

Achieving behavioural changes in individuals and populations

David Hill, Helen Dixon[1]

In this chapter, we consider how behavioural theory and research can be translated into successful cancer prevention programmes. Such programmes may be applied at the individual, group, community or national level. The agenda for behavioural interventions in cancer prevention is set by rigorous epidemiological analysis. The ultimate goal of behavioural interventions is to enable individuals to reduce their cancer risk by engaging in recommended preventive behaviours. To reach this goal, a thorough analysis of factors underpinning the behaviour in question is needed to identify possible targets for intervention. This foundation can be strengthened by consideration of key psychological principles known to be important drivers of health-related behaviour. In this chapter, we present the *Big Five Principles of Behaviour Change* and suggest how they may be applied to promoting and evaluating change in cancer preventive behaviour. These principles draw upon a wide spectrum of behavioural research and theory, not just in the health field. They could be used to guide culture-specific programmes in any country. The principles considered are listed in Table 3.1. Research applications of these principles are reviewed together with overarching strategies for successful implementation of cancer prevention programmes. The Big Five Principles are a convenient shorthand, and could be used by cancer prevention planners as a checklist to assist in developing strategies that *all at once* push as many as possible of the effective levers for behaviour change.

Introduction

The scope of this chapter is 'cancer-related behaviour', by which we mean any behaviour, which increases or decreases the probability of occurrence, or effects of, cancer in oneself or in those for whom one has responsibility such as patients, pupils, employees, family, or electors. Hence, cancer-related behaviours include smoking, sunbathing, drinking alcohol, exercise, dietary behaviour, having a mammogram, Pap test or faecal occult blood test (FOBT), being vaccinated for hepatitis or human papillomavirus (HPV), seeking treatment or advice (including for palliation). Cancer-related behaviours also include all those professional behaviours that impact upon the above – teaching, advising, referring, recruiting, as well as examining, prescribing, inserting, cutting, irradiating, injecting, and so on.

There is quite bewildering literature covering attempts by 'authorities' such as public health departments, non-government organizations, and cancer centres to get people to change their

[1] David J. Hill, AO, PhD, Director, Cancer Council Victoria, Carlton, Victoria, Australia; President (2008–2010) International Union Against Cancer (UICC); and Helen Dixon, PhD, Senior Research Fellow, Centre for Behavioural Research in Cancer, Cancer Council Victoria, Carlton, Victoria, Australia.

Table 3.1 The Big Five Principles of Behaviour Change: MMCRR

Motivation
Modelling
Capacity (resources available and self-efficacy)
Remembering
Reinforcement

cancer-related behaviour, i.e. behaviour to reduce their own or someone else's risk of developing or succumbing to cancer. This literature is part of a broader literature on health promotion covering a host of diseases.

The evidence base to guide cancer prevention practitioners is far less definitive than it is, for instance, for the practitioner managing hypertension in a patient. Systematic reviews are relatively few, and those to be found may be of little use to a practitioner charged with designing a prevention programme for a local population.

Meta-analyses of research data have validity only when the measures aggregated across different studies are sufficiently comparable; the intervention is the same (or similar enough); measures of effect are the same; and the host organism is functionally equivalent. Usually none of these conditions apply when health behaviour interventions are combined in systematic reviews/meta-analyses. To make matters worse, the applicability for health behaviour interventions of the presumed 'gold standard' of scientific evidence, the randomized controlled trial has now been seriously questioned [1].

Health behaviour interventions are designed to affect Homo sapiens, a species which thinks, feels, and acts in ways that are largely determined by learning histories that are individual- and culture-specific. To achieve the same results as found in a researched population requires that the population in which those results are applied be functionally equivalent. This is often not the case in the way that, for instance, the respiratory systems of Asians, Africans, and Caucasians are functionally equivalent.

Accessible standard resources are of less value to the prevention practitioner than they are to the clinician dealing with specific clinical problems. In this chapter we therefore offer a set of working principles upon which to base interventions. The approach is thus principle-based rather than evidence-based in the usual sense. However, we assert that these principles are underpinned by more than a century of behavioural science research and theory, and that the literature on cancer-related behaviour change includes many examples of their successful application. The prevention practitioner should be as committed to using an evidence base as should the clinical practitioner. The difference is that the prevention practitioner needs to be involved in building, as well as applying the evidence base for their programmes, in order to achieve continuous improvement in outcomes. This has significant implications for establishing the skill sets required to implement the most effective behaviour change programmes, as we discuss later in this chapter.

In identifying the Big Five Principles of Behaviour Change we acknowledge that there may be additional principles that would add value. That is for others to argue. In the meantime, we offer the principles in the belief that they cover a very large part of the field of opportunity for catalysing benign behaviour change in others. We believe that the brevity of the list and the simplicity of the principles give them a utility for the practitioner that might be compromised by a more extended or elaborate articulation. They can be easily brought to mind by the acronym *MMCRR* (Motivation, Modelling, Capacity, Remembering, Reinforcement).

Where to focus

In focussing on the individual, we do not mean to imply that underlying ('upstream', 'primordial') factors are irrelevant. Indeed, there is ample evidence that educational, economic, and social disadvantage are strongly associated with risk factors for cancer [2,3] (see Chapter 2 also). There is also good reason to believe that making an impact on disadvantage would reduce cancer risk in affected populations [4]. We do not see that 'individual' and 'societal' explanations are at odds with each other. We do not see any necessary contest between the sociological and the psychological perspectives. On the contrary, we contend that upstream factors ultimately find expression in the behaviour of individuals, and that trends among populations and sub-populations are, after all, the aggregation of many individuals' actions. Hence, we believe that opportunities to understand and improve the health of populations are foregone when analysis and intervention at the individual level is neglected. As we discuss later, upstream factors are more complex, distant in time, and difficult for the health sector to influence but they do involve broad social agendas that extend beyond health. There are consequently opportunities to develop alliances in which changing cancer-related behaviour is one among several societal benefits of upstream interventions.

Shaping behaviour: Big Five Principles of Behaviour Change

Our articulation of the Big Five was stimulated by requests from practitioners and research colleagues for a succinct statement of what is 'really known' about health behaviour change. They wanted an answer that did not lose them in detail, but one which would provide a sound and reliable guide. These principles draw upon a wide spectrum of behavioural research and theory, not just in the health field. They represent a distillation of key concepts derived from social cognitive theory [5], the theory of planned behaviour [6], the precede-proceed model [7], the health belief model [8], basic learning theory [9], and our own practical experience. Readers will recognize them all.

The basic proposition of this model is that repeated or habitual voluntary behaviours are determined by the extent to which a person:

♦ wants to do it (conscious motivation)
♦ sees others doing it (modelling)
♦ has the required capacity to do it (resources, comprehension, training, and self-efficacy)
♦ remembers to do it (memory and prompting)
♦ is rewarded for doing it, or suffers for not doing it (positive and negative reinforcement)

Any programme to change a cancer-related behaviour would be highly successful if it could maximize the operation of all the Big Five Principles simultaneously. In the next section we articulate these principles and present examples of their application in a variety of cancer prevention settings. In practice, cancer prevention efforts have tended to utilize only a subset of these principles within particular programmes, often because in certain settings some of the principles that would be effective are judged to be impractical, unacceptable, or too expensive.

1. Motivation

Motivation is the most elusive concept in psychology and it has to do with *why* we do the things we do. Reasons for self-initiated behaviour do not have to be logical in any objective sense, so the fact that a person continues smoking in the knowledge of the dangers of smoking does not invalidate this principle. People may experience motivation as wanting, needing, or desiring to put their energy into doing things or pursuing goals. The origins of a motive may lie in physiology (e.g. satiation), learning (e.g. success), or perhaps genetics (inherited motives are more clearly evident in other species, for instance, the true-to-breed behaviour of an untrained beagle when it first encounters the scent of a hare). For our purposes it is enough to recognize that motivation is a force, an 'engine' that can initiate and maintain behaviour.

Health behaviour change strategies nearly always acknowledge motivation by communicating *arguments* and *evidence* that are intended to provide personally relevant reasons, and thereby the motivation, to do the things we cancer prevention advocates contend will prevent cancer.

There are two main points to make about motivation as a principle to use in changing cancer-related behaviour. First, motivation is a necessary condition of volitional behaviour. However it is often an insufficient cause of behaviour change on its own. Yet attempts to inform and reason with our target populations dominate cancer prevention efforts, often to the neglect of other arguably more effective principles. Second, we can do a much better job motivating our target groups by getting 'inside' the way they view the world. Sophisticated qualitative research techniques [10] are being applied increasingly in cancer prevention to provide insights into the arguments and evidence most likely to motivate culturally diverse sub-groups in society.

A group of theories known as expectancy-value theories has been found useful in creating motivational communications for cancer prevention. Their proposition is that people anticipate (i.e. can think ahead to) various outcomes of behaviours they contemplate engaging in, and that such outcomes have positive or negative values for people. People are predicted to choose behaviours that they expect will reap the most success and value, and minimize negative outcomes. Outcome expectations may take the form of physical outcomes such as the pleasurable or aversive effects of the behaviour (e.g. if I limit my food intake, I'll feel really hungry), social reactions evoked (e.g. if my diet helps me achieve a healthy weight, my partner will find me more attractive), and self-evaluative reactions (e.g. if I lose weight I'd be healthier). Helping people see how habit changes are in their self-interest and in line with broader goals they value highly should enhance motivation [5]. Short-term, attainable goals help people succeed in pursuing longer-term goals by mustering and guiding current effort.

Applied to cancer prevention, influencing outcome expectancies means promoting the benefits of performing recommended 'new' health actions, as well as the negative consequences of persisting with the current potentially harmful health actions.

Example

We often assume that knowledge of the cancer risks associated with a given behaviour will provide ample motivation for people to modify that behaviour. However, consideration of other possible motives for that behaviour can yield fruitful opportunities for intervention. For example, public education campaigns have been successful in generating awareness of the risk of skin cancer as a consequence of excessive exposure to solar UV radiation [11,12]. However, many young people continue to deliberately or inadvertently expose themselves to excessive UV radiation [13,14]. Clearly knowledge of health risks has not provided sufficient motivation to this group to change their behaviour. What then might be the competing motives for their risky sun exposure behaviour? It seems that beliefs that a tan enhances physical appearance provide an important motive for sun exposure [15]. Based on this reasoning, Mahler, Kulik, Gerrard, and Gibbons (2007) conducted an innovative, appearance-based intervention where they exposed young adults to UV photographs of sun-related skin damage to their own skin and a video of photoaging information (e.g. wrinkles and age spots). Both interventions showed evidence of less skin darkening at post-summer follow up, and those in the photoaging information condition also reported more sun protective behaviour and still showed less skin darkening one year after the intervention [16]. This study illustrates the importance of carefully considering a target population's motives for cancer-related behaviour, without assuming their primary motives centre around health concerns.

2. Modelling

Every parent knows that children can learn a particular behaviour by watching someone doing it and imitating. We learn how to do things by observation and, when we see that the behaviour is engaged in by someone we admire and/or the modelled behaviour leads to some desired outcome, we want to do it too. The concept of modelling is central to Social Cognitive Theory [5].

Applied to cancer prevention, this means providing target audiences with perceptions of models performing recommended behaviours. This should help the audience to acquire recommended behaviours and ultimately perform them in relevant situations. Using models who are admired and trusted and illustrating positive outcomes of the behaviour should be most effective. Modelling may occur face-to-face by observing others in the immediate social environment (e.g. a teacher) or 'symbolically' via mass media (e.g. television) [17].

An advantage of modelling health behaviour through mass media is that larger audiences can be reached with carefully selected and portrayed models at less cost per capita than using face-to-face methods of communication. The drawback is that mass media is by definition a shotgun approach, such that individual tailoring of the modelling situation is not possible as with other more direct methods of communication. Nonetheless, skilful media placement helps reach certain target groups relatively efficiently. As discussed later in this chapter, mass media, especially television, provide scope to utilize all of the Big Five Principles in promoting cancer-preventive behaviour.

Example

In a study to increase sun protection behaviour at community swimming pools in Virginia, USA, lifeguards were trained to model sun protection by wearing hats, protective clothing and sunscreen, and by using shaded areas at the pool site throughout the study [18]. Lifeguards received three hours' training and practice in sun protection, including how to initiate conversations supporting sun protection and how to help others engage in these behaviours. Although it was not possible to isolate the specific effects of modelling from other intervention components such as information and resource provision, the intervention produced objective improvements in child and adult sun-protection behaviours.

3. Capacity – objective and subjective resourcing

It is self-evident that no behaviour can occur without the capacity to enact it. Capacity has two components, one of which is objective, the other subjective. Both are necessary and neither alone is sufficient for behaviour change.

Objective capacity

The objective component of capacity refers to the availability of physical resources to enable health behaviour, such as fruit and vegetables for healthy eating, or shade structures for sun protection. It is no use promoting a particular health-related behaviour, if people do not have the necessary resources and environmental supports to enable action. Ecological models emphasize how the physical and social environment can influence health [19]. Models of individual health behaviour also consider how access to physical resources can help or hinder people's health actions [e.g. 5,7]. If ecological factors play a role in a health problem, then ecology-based solutions are needed within health programme efforts. Methods for achieving environmental change to support health behavioural targets include legislation, policy changes, design of neighbourhoods, and provision of physical resources.

Subjective capacity

The second, subjective component of capacity is our belief that we are actually able to carry out the required behaviour. Social Cognitive Theory [5] and the Theory of Planned Behaviour [6] cite such 'self-efficacy' beliefs as important determinants of health behaviour, and a vast body of research attests to this notion [e.g. 20,21]. We form self-efficacy beliefs on the basis of our own personal history of successful and failed attempts. To have sufficient self-efficacy for a given health behaviour people need not only objective capacity to carry out the behaviour but also a self-perception that they have the skills to do so. Thus, efforts to promote self-efficacy may seek to overcome deficits in skills and confidence in performing cancer-related behaviour. If self-efficacy beliefs can be changed by education and training, the probability of sustained behaviour change is greatly increased.

Examples–objective capacity

The importance of resourcing, as well as educating and modelling, was borne out in an intervention to increase sun protection of patrons of a public swimming pool where sun protection items such as sunscreen were provided to pool patrons [18, also cited in modelling example]. A recent sun protection intervention that employed the principle of objective capacity was a cluster randomized controlled trial that examined adolescents' use of purpose-built shade in secondary schools [22]. Observational data revealed greater student use of the newly shaded areas at intervention schools compared to full-sun areas at control schools. The finding that provision of shade proved to be an effective, practical means of reducing adolescents' exposure to solar UV radiation was especially encouraging, since adolescents have proved to be an important yet challenging target group to effect with educational strategies promoting sun protection.

Another example of applying the objective capacity principle to supporting health protective behaviour comes from Reuben and colleagues (2002) cluster randomized clinical trial, which compared the benefit of offering on-site mobile mammography in addition to an outreach programme designed to increase mammography use by educating patients. Women offered access to on-site mammography in addition to health education were almost twice as likely to undergo mammography within 3 months compared to the health education only group. Offering on-site mammography at community-based sites where older women meet proved an especially effective method for increasing screening rates among certain ethnic and sociodemographic subgroups of women who traditionally have low screening rates [23]. As can be seen, resourcing was not the only principle employed by these investigators.

Example – subjective capacity

A good example of applying the subjective capacity principle is a study conducted in Maryland, USA [24]. The target group were low-income women served by the Special Supplemental Nutrition Program for Women, Infants and Children (WIC), a group who were known to have poor nutrition. Behaviour change principles were applied within the Transtheoretical model [25] (which, incidentally, provides the important insight that behaviour change is a process not an event, and is characterized by a series of stages which call for different, tailored forms of information, training, and assistance). The researchers hired women on the WIC programme as peer leaders (which incidentally also exemplifies modelling). The peer leader's role was to raise the self-efficacy of participants to increase fruit and vegetable consumption in their families. These peer leaders conducted three 45-minute education sessions in small groups over six months.

Childcare was provided so women became fully involved in discussions of how to overcome barriers to increasing fruit and vegetable consumption and to engage them in hands-on practice in food preparation. As well as this self-efficacy-raising strategy, a number of other principles were applied, including motivation, prompting and reinforcement. Consistent with the importance of the capacity principle, women who attended the largest number of efficacy-raising sessions increased their servings most, and there was a significantly greater increase on the scale to measure self-efficacy in the intervention group compared to the control group. Overall, the intervention increased by half a serve a day, women's mean daily consumption of fruit and vegetables.

4. Remembering

Memory refers to the storing and retention of information. Sometimes in cancer prevention practice we have erred by overcomplicating matters and overlooking the obvious. People simply forget to do things, particularly behaviours that are intermittent, such as screening. Prompts are a simple solution to memory lapses and procrastination. They help bring cancer prevention recommendations to the fore, such that target issues or behaviours to be changed are given personal priority alongside the other demands of people's everyday lives. The health belief model [8] argues that such 'cues to action' remind or alert people to a potential health problem making them more likely to take preventive action. Examples of cues to action are mass media campaigns, a reminder postcard from a doctor, advice from others, illness of a friend or relative, newspaper or magazine article, SMS, or email message.

Example

In an Australian study of recruitment to a publicly funded (free) mammographic screening service, it was found that the effectiveness (and cost-effectiveness) of personal letters of invitation, followed by a second letter to non-attenders was far greater than public recruitment strategies such as local newspaper articles, community promotion, and promotion to physicians. Most effective, though not most cost-effective, were letters of invitation that specified an appointment time, followed by a second letter to initial non-attenders [26]. This suggests that the public health potential of proactive use of population and sub-population lists is considerable.

These days, with vast numbers of people who use personal computers and have access to the Internet or who carry mobile phones with them, there are almost limitless opportunities for timely prompts and advice that are not location dependent. For example, a recent randomized controlled trial used mobile phone text messaging for a smoking cessation programme [27]. Approximately 2,000 teen and adult smokers from throughout New Zealand who wanted to quit, and owned a mobile phone, were randomized to an intervention group that received regular, personalized text messages providing smoking cessation advice, and support, or a control group that received periodic distraction messages. At six weeks, more participants in the intervention had quit compared to the control group: 239 (28 per cent) versus 109 (13 per cent), relative risk 2.20. This treatment effect was consistent across subgroups defined by age, sex, income level, or geographic location. Thus phone text messaging that is affordable, personalized, age appropriate, and not location dependent appears to be a potentially useful method to help young smokers to quit.

5. Reinforcement – positive and negative

Reinforcement operates on the principle that behaviour is more likely to be repeated if it is positively reinforced or rewarded, and less likely to be repeated if it is unrewarded or punished.

Reinforcing factors may act as important incentives for the persistence or repetition of cancer-preventive as well as cancer-risk behaviours. For example, use of solariums for tanning may result in positive reinforcement at an intrinsic level (endorphin release; see [11]) and extrinsic level (social approval of tan by peers). These positive reinforcements make the behaviour more appealing than if they were absent. Conversely, negative reinforcement at an intrinsic level (e.g. painful sunburn) or extrinsic level (e.g. doctor tells you it will increase skin cancer risk) may discourage the behaviour. Negative reinforcement may also increase the likelihood of a behaviour by removing a negative stimulus when the behaviour is performed. For example, nicotine craving may be removed by smoking.

According to social cognitive theory [5] reinforcement may be direct, vicarious or self-directed. Take for example a cancer-preventive behaviour such as exercise. A jogger who experiences 'runner's high' (endorphin release) is receiving direct, intrinsic, positive reinforcement. If her coach praises her running performance, this is direct, extrinsic, positive reinforcement. If she observes high profile athletes receiving awards and recognition for their running this may provide vicarious positive reinforcement for her running in future. She may also engage in self-directed reinforcement contingent on her accomplishments; for example, if she jogs 10 km per day for one month, she will reward herself with a new pair of running shoes.

Successfully applying the principle of reinforcement to cancer prevention could involve positively reinforcing recommended behaviours and/or negatively reinforcing cancer risk behaviours. However, in the benign business of cancer control we neither have available nor would choose to use many of the draconian reinforcement contingencies that could change the cancer-related behaviour of populations. Yet we may still err in not giving enough attention to systematic canvassing of the opportunities to build positive reinforcement into our interventions and, just as important, how to avoid inadvertently building in negative reinforcement.

Example

One of us once attended a workshop to devise a strategy to increase participation in cervical screening programmes by women in at-risk categories. Workshop attendees were told that only a quarter of women on a register of those who had already had at least one Pap test returned for another after being reminded at three years that they were overdue for their next test. It would seem at least three of the Big Five Principles should have been operating here. After all, women were prompted by a letter; they knew how to engage in the behaviour because they had done it at least once before; and their previous behaviour had presumably been positively reinforced by getting an 'all clear' test result. But was it? Further discussion by the group revealed that the screened women were rarely notified of their 'all clear' result unless they took the trouble to telephone their doctor for it – which relatively few did. So the explanation for the disappointing response to recall for the Pap test may simply be the failure to systematically apply positive reinforcement of the desired behaviour (receiving as a reward for their behaviour an 'all clear' letter) when a golden opportunity existed to do so.

Heil and colleagues [28] applied the principle of positive reinforcement in a randomized controlled trial where smokers entering prenatal care were assigned to either a contingent or non-contingent voucher condition. The vouchers could be exchanged for retail items during pregnancy and for 12 weeks postpartum. Women in the contingent condition earned vouchers for biochemically verified smoking abstinence; in the non-contingent condition, women earned vouchers independent of smoking status. The results revealed that 'voucher-based reinforcement therapy' contingent on smoking abstinence during pregnancy significantly increased smoking abstinence at end-of-pregnancy (41 per cent compared to 10 per cent) and at twelve weeks postpartum (24 per cent compared to 3 per cent). Evidence from serial ultrasound examinations indicated significantly greater estimated foetal growth in the contingent condition compared to the non-contingent condition. As applied in this innovative intervention, the principle of positive reinforcement yielded positive health benefits for both mothers and their unborn infants.

A good example of reinforcement delivered en masse in cancer prevention is the use of tax increases to reduce tobacco consumption. A study on the economics of tobacco control conducted by the World Bank, in partnership with the World Health Organization, concluded that tax increases that raise the real price of cigarettes by 10 per cent would reduce smoking by about 4 per cent in high income countries and by about 8 per cent in low income or middle income countries [29]. The continuing smoker is negatively reinforced by costs; the quitter is positively reinforced by savings. For example, data from smokers between 17 and 69 years old interviewed during an annual face-to-face survey conducted by Taiwan National Health Research Institutes between 2000 to 2003, revealed that a new tobacco tax scheme introduced in 2002, brought about an average annual reduction in cigarette consumption of 13.27 packs/person (10.5 per cent) [30]. Recently Carpenter and Cook (2008) used data from over 800,000 youths from national, state, and local Youth Risk Behavior Surveys to examine the effect of tobacco taxation on youth smoking in the United States. They found that the large state tobacco tax increases of the past 15 years were associated with significant reductions in both smoking participation and frequent smoking by youths [31].

Putting it all together: implications of Big Five Principles for interventions

In this section, we illustrate how the Big Five Principles may be translated into the design of interventions. We believe that the most promising approaches to behavioural change would include as many of the Big Five Principles as possible.

Once epidemiological data has been used to identify behavioural and environmental risk factors linked to the cancer outcomes to be addressed, the next step is to consider the attitudes, knowledge, social norms and patterns of social and community organization that contribute to the behavioural risk factors. This assessment will highlight possible levers for change that may be targeted in an intervention. Where possible, draw on previous research to identify the most likely routes to improvement. A huge amount of information about what works in interventions can be gleaned from authoritative reviews and summaries. Learn from what has worked elsewhere as a starting point in choosing intervention strategies.

Where this information is not available from existing sources, it may be necessary to collect additional data pertaining to your specific target population. The 'Big Five' will provide pointers on what data to collect. For example, what *motivates* people to engage in the behaviour of interest? Do they have *capacity* to perform the desired alternative behaviour (both in terms of resources and self-efficacy)? Who would the target audience perceive to be a credible role *model* concerning recommended behaviours? What factors might *reinforce* the risk behaviour and the recommended alternative behaviour? What do the target audience know and feel about the cancer outcome and associated risk factors? What would be the best messages and channels through which to *prompt and remind* our target audience of recommended actions? Once we have a good understanding of our target audience and how their environment shapes their behaviour, we are better positioned to promote changes in cancer-related behaviour.

Carcinogenic effects are usually dependent upon the cumulative frequency and amount of exposure received in 'doses' that in themselves are only trivially toxic or aversive (such as the single cigarette). Therefore, it is hardly surprising that the cancer-related behaviours of most interest in prevention are repeated or habitual ones. When we use the term behaviour change, we really mean the reversal or redirection of a pattern of behaviour that is the end product of an individual's 'learning history'.

When people use the term 'behaviour', closer reflection usually reveals that the behaviour they have in mind is actually a chain of behaviours. Consider the complexity of the steps that need to be taken between awareness of a recommendation to take a screening test and having the test done, or purchasing and smoking a packet of cigarettes. We therefore advise doing a searching and reflective analysis of the target cancer-related behaviour it is intended to influence.

When analysing a given cancer-related behaviour, it is nearly always helpful to ask the questions; is this a habitual, contingent, or one-off behaviour? What is preventing the person who is our target from doing what we recommend? Why exactly did or would the person act this way? Can the behaviour be broken down into parts, i.e. is the behaviour actually a chain of behaviours? Are there links in the chain that lend themselves to intervention? Can any of the Big Five Principles be introduced at critical links in the chain? Can unfavourable upstream factors be offset through targeted interventions at an individual level (e.g. are there ways to neutralize educational or social disadvantage for the particular behaviour)?

Creating a problem-specific conceptual model

Kurt Lewin (1952, p. 169) famously wrote, 'There is nothing more practical than a good theory' [32]. A theory lays out the causal pathways to explain and predict phenomena in nature. In our work, we have found it useful to articulate during the planning process our own 'theories' to explain the cancer-related behaviours of interest. Doing so will test your assumptions and logic. Any such theory gives pointers to where to intervene to change the behaviour. Your theory can draw upon extant formal theories, such as those introduced above – but it should not be overwhelmed by them. It will be more fine-grained, but more likely to be of use to you. The importance of this exercise is to force you to articulate what leads to what, and why. This will guide the crafting of the intervention and help structure the evaluation of it in the field.

For example, early in the development of a skin cancer prevention programme in Australia, we developed a conceptual model illustrating factors known to influence individual risk of skin cancer (Figure 3.1) [33]. It provides a useful framework for measurement and explanation of sun-related behaviour, as it accounts for intra-personal factors as well as variations in the physical environment in which the behaviour of interest occurs.

The model also draws attention to which factors may be amenable to intervention or not. For instance, if seeking to change the environment to reduce people's risk of solar UV exposure, the physical environment (e.g. availability of shade) can be readily modified, but the solar UV levels in a particular climate cannot. At the level of individual risk factors, physical characteristics such as having a skin type that sunburns easily may not be alterable, but personal sun protection behaviours provide a more achievable means for people to reduce their risk of exposure. This in turn highlights the importance of considering which predispositions drive sun protection behaviour and whether these also provide suitable targets for intervention. For instance, a number of studies have found that pro-tan attitudes are associated with poor sun protection behaviour [15].

Once factors that are potentially amenable to intervention are identified, the relative importance of each of these factors in influencing cancer risk should be considered, to determine where intervention efforts are best concentrated. For example, multivariate analysis of predictors of sun protection behaviour for a given population might suggest that tanning norms and activity demands are much more strongly associated with sun protection behaviour than knowledge of skin cancer risk (which was found to be universally high), such that the former are more promising targets for health promotion intervention. In many cases, it will be necessary to collect

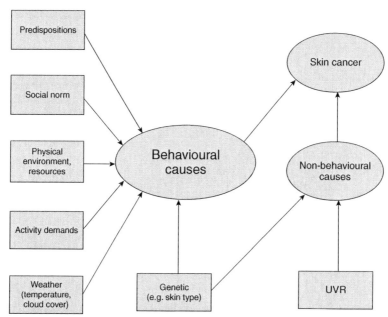

Fig. 3.1 Behavioural factors in causation of skin cancer.
From: Hill et al. 1998, p.63 [33], with permission.

and analyse local data from the specific target population to inform this process. While drawing on prior research with different populations is usually helpful, it may not necessarily be generalizable. Subjecting your model to real-world testing will also help determine whether your model includes unimportant factors, or whether there are further factors that need to be added to the model. In this formative stage of research, qualitative methods (see [10]) such as focus groups may complement quantitative, population-based surveys.

Developing and testing a problem-specific model can also provide insight into the most promising settings through which to reach target groups for intervention. For example, Hill and colleagues' (1992) assessment of behavioural and non-behavioural factors in sunburn found that people who engage in water sports are a high-risk group for excessive sun exposure [34]. This finding suggested that targeting people in these sports settings would be useful for skin cancer prevention.

Developing interventions that fit the target population

Carefully establishing an evidence base for explaining behavioural risk factors for a given cancer provides a firm foundation on which to build intervention efforts. From this foundation, health promotion planners are in a position to creatively consider how the Big Five Principles can be used as a 'toolbox' to bring about the change they seek.

Table 3.2 illustrates application of the Big Five Principles in various cancer prevention contexts. The Table exemplifies the manner in which the Big Five Principles may be applied to promoting change in a diverse range of cancer-related behaviours. This includes the potential to influence people's behaviour through law, education, and social marketing. The Big Five Principles operate

Table 3.2 Examples of application of the Big Five Principles to cancer prevention programmes

Principles	Prevention e.g. solar protection, smoking cessation	Screening e.g. cervical cancer screening, bowel cancer screening
Motivation *Provide rationale for the target behaviour.*	*Present target group with arguments & evidence to support cancer-preventive behaviour.* For example, graphic television commercial (TVC) illustrating importance of cumulative solar UV exposure to skin cancer risk; ad campaign promoting smoke free environments presents health risks to smokers & to children exposed to passive smoking. *Use arguments & evidence that resonate with target audience's view of the world.* For example, anti-smoking TVC that presents emotional as well as physical risks of smoking, such as what a child who loses a parent to tobacco-related cancer will miss out on.	*Present target group with arguments & evidence to support screening practice.* For example, letter of invitation for free FOBT presents national incidence & mortality from bowel cancer, e.g. TVC aimed to encourage under-screened women to have a Pap test conveyed that whilst a Pap test can cause discomfort & embarrassment, the consequences of not having one could be far worse.
Modelling *Provide perceptions of role models demonstrating recommended behaviours.*	*Encourage prominent & admired role models to demonstrate recommended behaviours in relevant settings.* For example, solar protection programme sponsorship of lifeguard's association ensured that lifeguards modelled sun protective behaviour at pools/beaches where both participants & spectators risk skin damage from excessive sun exposure. *Symbolically model recommended behaviours via mass media.* For example, TVC and brochure photographs modelling a smoker telephoning a smoking cessation hotline & engaging in discussion with smoking cessation counsellor.	*Provide target group with perceptions of role models initiating & participating in recommended screening behaviour.* For example, mass media campaign modelled women making & attending an appointment for a Pap test (did not show test being undertaken).
Capacity ~ Objective *Provide opportunities & support for recommended behaviours.*	*Legislation to support cancer-preventive behaviour.* For example, tax rebates allowing outdoor workers to claim expenses for sun protective clothing. *Legislation to inhibit cancer-risk behaviour.* For example, legislation to prohibit tobacco & cigarette advertising; bans on smoking in public settings such as restaurants & workplaces. *Policies in organizations such as schools, workplaces, & sports clubs that support recommended behaviours.* For example, encourage schools to develop & implement a sun protection policy that includes compulsory hat wearing for	*Government establishment of cancer screening registry.* For example, Pap test register enables women's participation in cervical screening to be centrally recorded & reminder letters to be sent out to women whose Pap tests are overdue. *Policy that provides consensus guidelines on who should be screened & how often.* For example, policy specifying that routine cervical screening with Pap smears should be carried out every two years for women with no symptoms or history suggestive of cervical pathology.

Table 3.2 (Continued) Examples of application of the Big Five Principles to cancer prevention programmes

Principles	Prevention e.g. solar protection, smoking cessation	Screening e.g. cervical cancer screening, bowel cancer screening
	children playing outside during peak UV seasons, scheduling outdoor activity to times furthest from solar noon, & inclusion of sun protection in the curriculum. *Resources that promote or enable recommended behaviours made available & accessible.* For example, standards set for protection level of sunscreen, tax on sunscreen lowered & restrictions on sales outside pharmacies removed; e.g. provision of smoking cessation phone counselling service for the cost of a local phone call.	*Subsidize cost of eligible people participating in screening.* For example, provision of FOBT test kit via mail-out to consumers. *Provide financial support to health service providers who perform tests.* For example, rebates to GPs & nurses for Pap tests; financial support for attending training.
Capacity ~ Subjective *Promote mastery learning through skills training.*	*Educate target group about recommended behaviours.* For example, Slip!Slop!Slap! ads demonstrated sun protection behaviours in a fun & empowering way. *Build skills training into interventions.* For example, smoking cessation phone counsellors provide personalized advice & support to enable smokers seeking to quit to realize their goal & deal with setbacks. *Break skills training into manageable steps.* For example, smoking cessation counsellors teach people stage-based tactics to enable them to do well in a quit attempt, such as setting a quit date, putting plans in place to make a quit attempt more successful.	*Provide & support training for health/ medical undergraduates & professionals who will be performing screening tests.* For example, workshops & on-line learning for GPs to promote competence in identifying patients eligible for bowel screening, understanding FOBT efficacy & procedure, following up patients with positive results. *Establish & monitor professional standards for performing, analysing & reporting on screening test results.* For example, college of nursing requiring Pap test nurses to gain professional credentials in Pap testing & re-establishing those credentials every 3 years. *In communication campaigns, seek to build skills & confidence of target group in initiating, attending & undertaking screening test.* For example, instruction booklet illustrating steps to collecting a faecal sample sent to consumers with free FOBT test kit. For example, cervical cancer screening programme advertisements (newspapers, cinema, outdoor, health promotion within health services) aimed to provide reassurance to women: although test uncomfortable, it should be quick; taking test won't compromise privacy.

(Continued)

Table 3.2 (Continued) Examples of application of the Big Five Principles to cancer prevention programmes

Principles	Prevention e.g. solar protection, smoking cessation	Screening e.g. cervical cancer screening, bowel cancer screening
Remembering Make people aware or conscious of the need to act – remind & prompt them.	*Help target audience keep recommended behaviour top of mind, especially at relevant settings and times.* For example, signs with sun protection symbols at outdoor pools. For example, PR activity on New Year's Eve, encouraging those considering quitting to make it a New Year's Resolution. *Disseminate prompts to reach target groups en masse using communication channels they already access.* For example, SMS or e-mail prompts with smoking cessation advice to striving quitters; TV, radio, print & outdoor smoking cessation advertising.	*Reach target audience with calls to screening action using communication channels that will reach unaware as well as aware consumers.* For example, invitation letters to undertake free FOBT sent to older adults in specified age groups. *Help target audience keep recommended screening behaviour top of mind, especially in relevant settings.* For example, work with GPs to encourage them to remind & alert under-screened women to have Pap test.
Reinforcement Positively reinforce (reward) cancer-preventive behaviour; negatively reinforce cancer-risk behaviour.	*Communicate positive consequences of preventive action, or negative consequences of failing to act.* For example, advertisement showing celebrity smoker in their heyday, then later in life bearing severe negative health effects of smoking. *Promote self-initiated rewards & incentives.* For example, printed resource highlighting financial savings of becoming a non-smoker, & illustrating appealing entertainment & leisure items (holidays, CDs etc.) that ex-smokers can buy with money instead of cigarettes. *Expectancies – present outcomes of change that have functional meaning to the target group.* For example, 'No hat, no play' rule for children in outdoor education or childcare settings. *Cultivate physical and social environments that act as incentives for cancer-preventive behaviour.* For example, smoke free areas such as prominent sporting venues, or restaurants mean smoking is negatively reinforced, in that you can't participate in those settings if you smoke; non-smoking is positively reinforced, by being able to participate in the setting.	*Communicate positive consequences of undertaking screening, or negative consequences of failing to screen.* For example, letter advising people their bowel screening test result is 'all clear' (positive reinforcement). For example, advertisement featuring a case study of a woman who didn't screen & had cervical cancer & infertility (negative reinforcement). *Build incentives into programmes.* For example, incentive payments for GPs who administer Pap tests to previously un/under-screened women.

to varying extents within each of these approaches, but are probably best captured by social marketing methods. Social marketing focuses on consumer's needs and desires, and thus calls for research with target groups to inform and evaluate programme efforts. It attempts to change and maintain voluntary behaviour of target market members by offering them benefits from and minimization of barriers to performing desired health behaviour [35]. Social marketing offers a set of procedures for promoting change in cancer-related behaviours that incorporates many of the Big Five Principles. Its concepts and practices can be used to improve local and national cancer-prevention programmes, and programmes with varying resources. (For details on applying social marketing to health behaviour and health education, see [36,37]).

Key elements of social marketing practice applied to cancer prevention are to:

◆ Sell the *product* (i.e. promote the benefits to consumers of engaging in cancer preventive behaviours, and of reduced cancer risk (consider benefits beyond health benefits too); tailor cancer-related products and services to maximize delivery of desired benefits to the target group)

◆ Use *price* to effect behaviour (reduce barriers or economic, psychological, social, or environmental costs of carrying out prescribed behaviours)

◆ *Place* marketing efforts effectively (i.e. use limited resources to reach target audiences with cancer-prevention efforts as frequently as possible and in as close proximity as possible to when the prescribed behaviour will occur)

◆ *Promote* costs and benefits to consumer (i.e. inform and persuade target audience about the costs of cancer-risk behaviour and the personal benefits of cancer-preventive behaviour using a range of promotional elements, such as advertising, public relations, direct mail, and point-of-sale promotions).

Mass media

A noticeable feature of Table 3.2 is that mass media, in particular television, have the capacity to cut across most if not all of the Big Five Principles, rendering mass media campaigns a useful centrepiece to cancer prevention efforts. In terms of capacity, the media environment can be structured to support cancer-preventive behaviour (e.g. prohibiting mass media tobacco advertising). Mass media advertising can promote access points where people can obtain resources and skills, it can model cancer-preventive behaviour, it can motivate by presenting arguments and evidence, it can remind and prompt, and it can vicariously reinforce recommended behaviours. At the individual level, measured by percentage change in target behaviour, mass media cannot compete with interventions that build on one-to-one contact with well-resourced professionals. But it has been shown to be an efficient means of changing smoking, diet, and sun-related behaviour at the whole of population level [12,38,39,40]. In Australia for instance, sophisticated multivariate analysis showed the independent significant contributions of mass media to reductions in smoking [38]. The authors concluded that increases in the real price of cigarettes and tobacco control mass media campaigns, broadcast at sufficient exposure levels and at regular intervals, are critical for reducing population smoking prevalence.

Evaluation/monitoring methods

Evaluation enables determination of the extent to which a cancer prevention or patient support programme has been successful in promoting the desired cancer-related behaviour change within the target population. Carefully articulating and documenting programme objectives in measurable terms before embarking on interventions will guide programme activities and inform evaluation efforts. Adapt the Big Five Principles to practice, by incorporating them into specific programme objectives. Through careful appraisal and study, evaluation researchers compare a programme's actual progress to prior plans, and direct interpretation of findings toward improving plans for future programme implementation. Programme activities should be evaluated at various stages of development and implementation. Ideally there will be a continuous cycle of planning, implementation, and evaluation of programmes.

Green and Kreuter (2005) distinguish between Formative, Process, and Impact evaluation [7]. Formative evaluation is carried out in the early stages of programme development. Qualitative and quantitative research methods are useful at this point. Quantitative surveys may be used to assess whether a particular demographic group would benefit from a programme, e.g. survey results may reveal that cervical cancer screening rates are especially low among certain ethnic groups within a community; the same survey may indicate that women across the community have poor knowledge of the benefits of Pap testing. Focus groups might be conducted to explore issues in depth for the target group, e.g. discussion with women in those ethnic groups might reveal that these women are uncomfortable with the idea of visiting a male medical practitioner for a Pap test as their community would frown on it, but that they do not have local access to female practitioners. Based on these findings, the programme planner may decide to target cervical cancer prevention efforts at specific sub-groups of women, train and fund female practitioners to provide screening in target communities (i.e. improve external capacity; indirectly eliminate negative social reinforcement for seeing male doctor), and educate the target community about the benefits of Pap screening (i.e. improve motivation). To maximize support for the programme within the target community, intervention efforts should be tailored to meet their needs and values. Formative research may also include pre-testing resources, messages, and concepts with the target audience, before disseminating them. For example, the programme planner may decide to use media to promote the programme in the target community and use focus groups to pre-test some communication concepts that show a woman in the target community making an appointment for a Pap test (i.e. principles of modelling and remembering).

Process evaluation research assesses whether particular intervention components are operating as intended. At a minimum this includes collecting details on the number of groups and individuals receiving programme resources or participating in programme activities. Other processes that may be evaluated are whether programme activities conform to any regulatory requirements, to the initial programme design, to relevant professional standards, or the expectations of the target group. Based on the findings of process evaluation, current programme operations may be modified to address identified shortcomings. It is obvious, but sometimes forgotten, that if outcome measures show no effect and process has not been adequately measured, there is no way to know whether the intervention does not 'work' or whether it was simply not delivered.

Programme outcomes are monitored through impact evaluation research. For cancer-related behavioural interventions, this includes monitoring population trends in the psychological or behavioural domains where change is being sought, or testing outcomes for groups known to have received certain programme strategies. More distal cancer outcomes such as patterns of disease within the population can be monitored through epidemiological studies and cancer registry surveillance. As tightly designed randomized controlled trials are not always feasible in practice, study designs for impact evaluation often include cross-sectional surveys, experimental/quasi-experimental studies, pre-post designs, and time trend analysis. Ideally studies should be designed to enable determination of whether outcomes assessed are the result of the programme's effects and not other forces.

Table 3.3 Cancer behaviour research centre examples

Centre	Website
Co-location models	
Behavioral Research Center, American Cancer Society, Atlanta, Georgia, USA	http://www.cancer.org/docroot/RES/RES_9.asp
Centre for Behavioural Research in Cancer, The Cancer Council Victoria, Australia	http://www.cancervic.org.au/about-our-research/our-research-centres/centre_behavioural_research_cancer
Viertel Centre for Research in Cancer Control, Cancer Council Queensland, Australia	http://www.cancerqld.org.au/research/vcrcc/vcrcc.asp
University-based models	
Centre for Behavioural Research and Program Evaluation, University of Waterloo, Canada	http://www.cbrpe.uwaterloo.ca/eng/index.html
Centre for Health Research & Psycho-oncology, The University of Newcastle, Australia	http://www.newcastle.edu.au/centre/cherp/
Department of Health Promotion and Health Education, Maastricht University, The Netherlands	http://www.gvo.unimaas.nl/index_uk.htm
Health Behaviour Unit, University College London, England	http://science.cancerresearchuk.org/research/loc/london/university_coll/wardlej/wardlejproj?version=1

Organizational model

As in clinical cancer medicine, there is a wasteful disconnect between the availability of evidence for effective population approaches and its widespread implementation in practice [41]. Organizational structures that co-locate prevention researchers and prevention practitioners can be successful in addressing this problem. An early co-location model was the Centre for Behavioural Research in Cancer at The Cancer Council Victoria [42]. Other co-location models and university-based models have been successful in forging close connections between research and practice; see Table 3.3. In each of these examples, the initiative and funding has come from a major organization with a remit to deliver behaviour change programmes to the population. In each case, the initiative has built significant new capacity through the development and support of a behavioural research workforce. It is our view that such capacity is essential to maximize the ongoing effectiveness of any programme to reduce cancer through behaviour change. Putting practice into research as well as putting the research into practice necessitates close interaction between practitioners and researchers. It is hard to apply science when there are no scientists.

Conclusion

The ultimate goal of modifying cancer-related behaviour is to help prevent cancer occurring or preventing it from spreading if it occurs. There is no magic bullet, as the problem is complex and people are complicated. Our purpose in this chapter has been to present a practical approach to the identification, building, and dissemination of evidence to control cancer through behaviour change. The Big Five Principles are levers for behavioural change that may be applied to all aspects of cancer control from primary prevention, through to clinical practice, patient support, and end-of-life issues.

References

1 Glasgow RE, Marcus AC, Bull SS, & Wilson KM (2004). Disseminating effective cancer screening interventions. *Cancer*, **101**(5 Suppl):1239–50

2 Ward E, Jemal A, Cokkinides V, et al (2004). Cancer disparities by race/ethnicity and socioeconomic status. *CA Cancer J Clin*, **54**(2):78–93.

3 Strong K, Mathers C, Epping-Jordan J, Resnikoff S, & Ullrich A (2008). Preventing cancer through tobacco and infection control: how many lives can we save in the next 10 years? *Eur J Cancer Prev*, **17**(2):153–61.

4 Sorensen G, Emmons K, Hunt MK, et al (2003). Model for incorporating social context in health behavior interventions: applications for cancer prevention for working-class, multiethnic populations. *Prev Med*, **37**(3):188–97.

5 Bandura A (2004). Health promotion by social cognitive means. *Health Educ Behav*, **31**(2):143–64.

6 Ajzen I & Fishbein M (1980). *Understanding attitudes and predicting social behaviour*. Prentice Hall, NJ.

7 Green LW & Kreuter MW (2005). *Health Program Planning: An Educational and Ecological Approach*, 4th edn. McGraw Hill, Boston, MA.

8 Janz NK & Becker MH (1984). The Health Belief Model: a decade later. *Health Educ Q*, **11**(1):1–47.

9 Skinner BF (1950). Are theories of learning necessary? *Psychol Rev*, **57**(4):193–216.

10 Windsor R, Baranowski T, Clark N, & Cutter G (1994). *Evaluation of Health Promotion Health Education & Disease Prevention Programs*, pp. 175–214. Mayfield Publishing Company, Mountain View.

11 Robinson JK, Rigel DS, & Amonette RA (1997). Trends in sun exposure knowledge, attitudes, and behaviors: 1986 to 1996. *J Am Acad Dermatol*, **37**(2 Pt 1):179–86.

12 Dobbinson SJ, Wakefield MA, Jamsen KM, et al (2008). Weekend sun protection and sunburn in Australia trends (1987–2002) and association with SunSmart television advertising. *Am J Prev Med*, **34**(2):94–101.

13 Livingston PM, White V, Hayman J, & Dobbinson S (2007). Australian adolescents' sun protection behavior: who are we kidding? *Prev Med*, **44**(6):508–12.

14 Jerkegren E, Sandrieser L, Brandberg Y, & Rosdahl I (1999). Sun-related behaviour and melanoma awareness among Swedish university students. *Eur J Cancer Prev*, **8**(1):27–34.

15 Arthey S & Clarke V (1995). Suntanning and sun protection: a review of the psychological literature. *Soc Sci Med*, **40**(2):265–74.

16 Mahler HI, Kulik JA, Gerrard M, & Gibbons FX (2007). Long-term effects of appearance-based interventions on sun protection behaviors. *Health Psychol*, **26**(3):350–60.

17 Bandura A. (1994). Social cognitive theory of mass communication. In Bryant J, Zillman D (eds) *Media Effects: Advances in Theory and Research*, pp. 61–90. Lawrence Erlbaum Associates, Hillsdale, NJ.

18 Lombard D, Neubauer TE, Canfield D, & Winett RA (1991). Behavioral community intervention to reduce the risk of skin cancer. *J Appl Behav Anal*, **24**(4):677–86.

19 Sallis JF & Owen NG (2002). Ecological models of health behaviour. In Glanz K, Rimer BK, Lewis FM (eds) *Health Behavior and Health Education: Theory, Research, and Practice*. 3rd edn. pp. 462–84. Jossey-Bass, San Francisco, CA.

20 Rimal RN (2000). Closing the knowledge-behavior gap in health promotion: the mediating role of self-efficacy. *Health Commun*, **12**(3):219–37.

21 Yarcheski A, Mahon NE, Yarcheski TJ, & Cannella BL (2004). A meta-analysis of predictors of positive health practices. *J Nurs Scholarsh*, **36**(2):102–8.

22 Dobbinson SJ, White V, Wakefield MA, et al (2009). Adolescents' use of purpose-built shade in secondary schools: a cluster randomised controlled trial. *BMJ*, **338**, b95; doi:10.1136/bmj.b95.

23 Reuben DB, Bassett LW, Hirsch SH, Jackson CA, & Bastani R (2002). A randomized clinical trial to assess the benefit of offering on-site mobile mammography in addition to health education for older women. *Am J Roentgenol*, **179**(6):1509–14.

24 Havas S, Anliker J, Greenberg D, et al (2003). Final results of the Maryland WIC Food for Life Program. *Prev Med*, **37**(5):406–16.

25 Prochaska JO, Redding CA, & Evers KE (2002). The transtheoretical model and stages of change. In Glanz K, Rimer BK, Lewis FM (eds) *Health Behavior and Health Education: Theory, Research, and Practice*, 3rd edn. pp. 99–120. Jossey-Bass, San Francisco, CA.

26 Hurley SF, Jolley DJ, Livingston PM, Reading D, Cockburn J, & Flint-Richter D (1992). Effectiveness, costs, and cost-effectiveness of recruitment strategies for a mammographic screening program to detect breast cancer. *J Natl Cancer Inst*, **84**(11):855–63.

27 Rodgers A, Corbett T, Bramley D, et al (2005). Do u smoke after txt? Results of a randomised trial of smoking cessation using mobile phone text messaging. *Tob Control*, **14**(4):255–61.

28 Heil SH, Higgins ST, Bernstein IM, et al (2008). Effects of voucher-based incentives on abstinence from cigarette smoking and fetal growth among pregnant women. *Addiction*, **103**(6):1009–18.

29 Jha P & Chaloupka FJ (2000). The economics of global tobacco control. *BMJ*, **321**(7257):358–61.

30 Lee JM, Hwang TC, Ye CY, & Chen SH (2004). The effect of cigarette price increase on the cigarette consumption in Taiwan: evidence from the National Health Interview Surveys on cigarette consumption. *BMC Public Health*, **4**:61.

31 Carpenter C & Cook PJ (2008). Cigarette taxes and youth smoking: New evidence from national, state, and local Youth Risk Behavior Surveys. *J Health Econ*, **27**(2):287–99.

32 Lewin K (1951). Problems of research in social psychology. In Cartwright D (ed), *Field Theory In Social Science: Selected Theoretical Papers*. pp. 155–169. New York, Harper & Row.

33 Hill D, Boulter J, & Dixon H (1998). Sun related behaviour of populations: determinants, trends, and measurement. *The Royal Society of New Zealand. Miscellaneous Series*, **49**:63–4.

34 Hill D, White V, Marks R, Theobald T, Borland R, & Roy C (1992). Melanoma prevention: behavioral and nonbehavioral factors in sunburn among an Australian urban population. *Prev Med*, **21**(5):654–69.

35 Baranowski T, Cullen KW, Nicklas T, Thompson D, & Baranowski J (2003). Are current health behavioral change models helpful in guiding prevention of weight gain efforts? *Obes Res*, **11**(Suppl):23S–43S.

36 Maibach EW, Rothschild MR, & Novelli WD (2002). Social marketing. In Glanz K, Rimer BK, Lewis FM (eds) *Health Behavior and Health Education: Theory, Research, and Practice*. 3rd edn. pp. 437–61. Jossey-Bass, San Francisco, CA.

37 Hastings G (2007). *Social Marketing: Why Should the Devil have all the best tunes?* Elsevier/Butterworth-Heinemann, Oxford.

38 Wakefield MA, Durkin S, Spittal MJ, et al (2008). Impact of tobacco control policies and mass media campaigns on monthly adult smoking prevalence. *Am J Public Health*, **98**(8):1443–50. Epub.

39 Dixon H, Borland R, Segan C, Stafford H, & Sindall C (1998). Public reaction to Victoria's '2 Fruit 'n' 5 Veg Every Day' campaign and reported consumption of fruit and vegetables. *Prev Med*, **27**(4):572–82.

40 Pollard CM, Miller MR, Daly AM, et al (2008). Increasing fruit and vegetable consumption: success of the Western Australian Go for 2&5 campaign. *Public Health Nutr*, **11**(3):314–20.

41 Grunfeld E, Zitzelsberger L, Evans WK, et al (2004). Better knowledge translation for effective cancer control: a priority for action. *Cancer Causes Control*, **15**(5):503–10.

42 Hill D, Borland R, & Karazija B (1991). Centre for Behavioural Research in Cancer. *Br J Addict*, **86**:257–62.

Chapter 4

Early diagnosis and screening in cancer control

Anthony Miller[1]

The relationship of screening to other cancer control strategies

The theory underlying cancer control implies strategic planning to ensure a rational, cost-effective approach to prevention, early detection and screening, treatment, rehabilitation and palliative care of cancer, in the context of the magnitude of the cancer problem, the resources available, and the other priorities for disease control in the country. Those interventions with demonstrated effectiveness should be promoted; those without an evidence base should not [1].

The effectiveness of screening is entirely dependent on the effectiveness of treatment for the lesions identified by screening, and the availability of facilities for the administration of a screening test, diagnosis of the abnormalities identified and treatment for the cancer precursors or invasive cancers identified. Without these pre-requisites, screening will not result in its desired objective, reduction in mortality from the cancer for which screening is conducted, and, if cancer precursors are detected, reduction in incidence of the cancer.

Screening is one component of early detection for cancer. It may seem self-evident that the early detection of cancer by screening will result in reduction of mortality from the cancer. However, this is not necessarily so, and it is the purpose of this chapter to try and place screening into context, and justify the concept that it is impossible to justify screening just because a cancer is found early, in fact cancer detection per se is not sufficient evidence that the individual has been benefited.

Definitions

Screening is one part of early detection; the other is achieving early diagnosis through health promotion (education). The World Health Organization (WHO) [2] proposed the following definitions:

- *Early diagnosis* is the awareness (by the public or health professionals) of early signs and symptoms of cancer in order to facilitate diagnosis before the disease becomes advanced, thus enabling more effective and simpler therapy.

- *Screening* is the systematic application of a screening test in a presumably asymptomatic population in order to identify individuals with an abnormality suggestive of a specific cancer who require further investigation.

[1] Anthony B. Miller, MD, FRCP, Associate Director, Research, Dalla Lana School of Public Health, University of Toronto, Toronto, Ontario Canada.

Education as a part of early detection – the foundation of screening

Early detection programmes must be preceded by education, both of the public and health care professionals, in order to increase awareness and achieve high response rates of the target population.

Public education programmes have been one of the main approaches to the promotion of screening, with emphasis on the belief that cancer, when diagnosed early, is far more likely to respond to effective treatment. The early programmes, especially by the American and Canadian Cancer Societies, emphasized the possible significance of lumps, sores, persistent indigestion or cough, and bleeding from the body's orifices, and the importance of seeking prompt medical attention if any of these occur. More recently, the cancer non-government organizations have emphasized the importance of screening tests, especially mammography.

However, that is not sufficient. Professional education of primary health care practitioners may also be essential before a programme can be successful. This may be required at all levels of health care organization, at primary care, at the district general hospital, and even at the tertiary care (referral, oncology centre) level. But we are gradually beginning to understand that education as such cannot secure the success of screening. Even though screening has to be a voluntary activity, initiating mechanisms to ensure that those in the target group are screened, and if the test is found to be abnormal, diagnosis and if necessary treatment follows, is essential to ensure the success of screening within a comprehensive cancer control programme.

Determination of the rationale for screening

There are two important concepts that need to be considered before initiating a screening programme [3]

- *The value of a screening test needs to be determined before it is introduced into practice.* There is a need to determine quantitatively, how much disability and how many premature deaths can be prevented by screening. The benefits can then be set against the financial costs and the human costs to the screenee of anxiety, discomfort, adverse effects, follow-up investigations, and treatments so that a rational decision can be made.

- *Early detection of disease is not an end in itself.* Screening should be concerned only with the detection of diseases or disorders that are known to cause significant suffering, disability or death if detected at a later stage. Identification of either trivial or untreatable conditions can cause anxiety and waste resources with no practical outcome.

It is essential to define a strategy for the introduction of screening in order to ensure maximal use of sometimes scarce resources. Both in the United Kingdom and Canada, for example, major efforts went into planning the introduction of breast and colorectal screening, and in the United Kingdom, the re-organization of screening for cancer of the cervix precursors, but far less effort went into the re-organization of cervical screening in Canada, in spite of repeated recommendations that this should be done [4–6]. Such re-organization was desirable, not because the programme was failing (indeed there is good evidence that it has been at least as effective as in the United States and Finland), but because success has been achieved by far too frequent screening, and over-treatment of most women diagnosed with cervical cancer precursors, in spite of evidence that the majority of these lesions regress [7, 8]. Thus too much money has been expended for a relatively unimportant cause of morbidity for the women who attend such screening. Indeed, the self-selection for participation in cervix screening is largely of low risk women.

Strategic planning

The World Health Organization (WHO) [9] has proposed a series of planning steps, and within them, various activities. Although proposed for middle and low-income countries, they are worth considering when a developed country decides to review, and strengthen, its National Cancer Control Plan. With some modification, these steps include:

Planning step 1: where are we now?

- Assess the cancer problem
- Assess the evidence-base for screening
- Consider alternative strategies to reach the same objectives (primary prevention or improved treatment)
- Assess the existing early detection plan and ongoing activities

Planning step 2: where do we want to be?

- Define the target population for early detection of frequent cancers
- Identify gaps in early detection services
- Set objectives for early diagnosis and screening
- Assess feasibility of screening interventions
- Set priorities for screening

Planning step 3: how do we get there?

- Plan procurement of key resources
- Determine activities for early diagnosis and screening
- Work with multi-disciplinary and multi-sectoral teams
- Move from policy to implementation

Working through these steps in relation to each priority cancer site provides the basis for the re-organization of screening and enables strategic decisions to be made to start or stop screening for a specific site.

Resources

The resources needed for screening are human as well as technical and financial. Although some screening tests can be self-administered, e.g. the faecal occult blood test for colorectal cancer screening, there have to be trained people who will instruct the screenee in the details of its use (e.g. a nurse or a family physician), and for all others, personnel have to be specially trained in the administration of the test. The skills required are varied, ranging to the ability to conduct a speculum examination of the vagina, recognize the transformation zone, and take an adequate smear for cervical cytology, to appropriate positioning and administration of compression for mammography. But the need for training does not stop there, laboratory technologists need to be trained for cervical cytology and interpreting faecal occult blood tests, radiologists for interpreting mammograms, nurse or physician endoscopists for flexible sigmoidoscopy, etc. The approach needed for reading screening mammograms is very different from that required to read diagnostic mammograms, and these skills can only readily be acquired by attending special training courses, something a qualified clinical radiologist may sometimes resist. Wherever possible, there is a great deal to be said for training a group of health care workers to administer specific screening tests, rather than leaving the task to the generalist. Nurses can be trained to perform excellent screening breast examinations [10], preferably following a defined protocol [11]. Nurses can be trained to perform endoscopy, and were successfully used for this purpose in a large US screening trial, with video cameras used as training devices [12]. We learnt long ago that cytotechnologists, specially trained to read cervical smears, will perform as well if not better than cytopathologists, providing the laboratory is of adequate size with adequate staffing to examine at least 25,000 smears a year, incorporating appropriate quality controls [4]. It seems likely that we have not taken this process far enough. Radiographers could perform the initial screening of mammograms, for example, and even non-nurses, such as social workers, trained to do breast examinations. The important thing is not the previous background of the person who will report on the screening test, it is the fact that they receive special training to perform the required task, and that an adequate system of quality control is put in place to ensure that high standards are maintained. [13].

The facilities required for a screening programme are dependent upon the cancer site and the test used. These should be as accessible to the target population for screening as possible. Many tests can be administered from the primary health care centre, advantageously, because the centre is already likely to be familiar to the target population, and they should not need to travel far. Even if the screening programme requires special equipment, or specially trained personnel to administer the test, they can sometimes be brought to the primary health centre, rather than expecting the target population to travel to a special centre or hospital. Special sessions can then be advertised to the target population when they can come for the screening test at the primary health centre.

Screening becomes far more complex and difficult to administer if special equipment is needed, e.g. mammography screening for breast cancer, endoscopy screening for colorectal cancer. This is one of the reasons why simpler tests may be selected rather than more sophisticated, though in the case of screening for colorectal cancer it has to be accepted that currently, the evidence base is far stronger for the simpler test, i.e. for the guaiac faecal occult blood test, rather than flexible sigmoidoscopy or colonoscopy.

The other type of facilities required are for diagnosis of abnormalities identified by screening, recognising that a screening test is not diagnostic; rather the test is intended to identify an abnormality that may represent a cancer precursor or an early cancer, but that other tests will be required to make a determination of this. These facilities, depending on the cancer site, will preferably be sited in a special diagnostic centre, often at the district general hospital. These range from special imaging, e.g. diagnostic mammography or ultrasound for breast cancer, to facilities for open, core, or needle biopsies for breast cancer and cervix cancer precursors, to colonoscopy for colorectal cancer. Once again, it is important that specially trained staff operate these facilities.

It cannot be too strongly emphasized that in planning for cancer control, it is inappropriate to introduce screening without the provision of the required trained personnel and facilities for screening and diagnosis, and subsequent treatment of confirmed abnormalities.

The evidence-base for screening

It has become usual only to recommend interventions for cancer control that are 'evidence-based'. However, the extent to which the evidence is sufficient, limited, or inadequate (to use the terminology of the International Agency for Research on Cancer – IARC) is often a function of the expert group that reviewed the evidence. Therefore, some system is desirable to stratify studies by the strength of the evidence they provide.

The US Preventive Services Task Force (USPSTF) grades its recommendations according to one of five classifications (A, B, C, D, I) reflecting the strength of evidence and magnitude of net benefit (benefits minus harms) [14].

+ The USPSTF strongly recommends that clinicians provide (the service) to eligible patients. *The USPSTF found good evidence that [the service] improves important health outcomes and concludes that benefits substantially outweigh harms.*

+ The USPSTF recommends that clinicians provide (this service) to eligible patients. *The USPSTF found at least fair evidence that [the service] improves important health outcomes and concludes that benefits outweigh harms.*

+ The USPSTF makes no recommendation for or against routine provision of (the service). *The USPSTF found at least fair evidence that [the service] can improve health outcomes but concludes that the balance of benefits and harms is too close to justify a general recommendation.*

+ The USPSTF recommends against routinely providing (the service) to asymptomatic patients. *The USPSTF found at least fair evidence that [the service] is ineffective or that harms outweigh benefits.*

+ The USPSTF concludes that the evidence is insufficient to recommend for or against routinely providing (the service). *Evidence that the [service] is effective is lacking, of poor quality, or conflicting and the balance of benefits and harms cannot be determined.*

The USPSTF also grades the quality of the overall evidence for a service on a 3-point scale (good, fair, poor):

+ Good: Evidence includes consistent results from well-designed, well-conducted studies in representative populations that directly assess effects on health outcomes.

+ Fair: Evidence is sufficient to determine effects on health outcomes, but the strength of the evidence is limited by the number, quality, or consistency of the individual studies, generalizability to routine practice, or indirect nature of the evidence on health outcomes.

+ Poor: Evidence is insufficient to assess the effects on health outcomes because of limited number or power of studies, important flaws in their design or conduct, gaps in the chain of evidence, or lack of information on important health outcomes.

For screening, the first accepted screening approach, for cervical cancer, was based on very indirect evidence. Indeed, initially the evidence was less than 'Fair', but with time, better evidence at the population level accumulated. However, randomized trial evidence of the efficacy of cervical cytology has never been obtained. For breast and colorectal screening, however, 'Good' evidence is available, as it is against screening for lung cancer by chest X-ray, but for prostate cancer, screening was largely introduced, especially in the United States, on the basis of only 'Fair' evidence, and still consistent 'Good' evidence is not available even though randomized screening trials have been in progress for over 10 years (see discussion later in this chapter) [15,16]. In Australia, screening for malignant melanoma of the skin has become widely used without 'Good' evidence, and a planned randomized trial has not been supported. This has resulted in an increase in the incidence of superficial spreading melanoma (the lesion that tends to be readily detected by inspection of the skin) but it is still not certain that the programme has resulted in reduction in mortality from the disease.

In general, however, randomized screening trials are accepted as the only unbiased method to evaluate the efficacy of screening [17–19]. In spite of the fact that many commentators have decried the high cost of such trials, and the length of time it takes for them to achieve their endpoint, no methodology of equivalent validity has yet been developed. I have set out elsewhere the requirements for such trials, and will not repeat these here [20].

Special consideration, however, needs to be given to the evidence needed for the introduction of new screening tests. If a test is shown to be of equivalent or superior sensitivity to a test already established as effective, many would regard the evidence on sensitivity alone as being sufficient to use the new test in substitution to the old. However, there are a number of caveats. Because of the often reciprocal relationship between sensitivity and specificity, improved sensitivity could imply reduced specificity, and this, as pointed out many years ago by Cole and Morrison [21], will mean increased costs to the screening programme. Further, the improved sensitivity may be spurious, if all that was achieved was the increased detection of precursor lesions destined to regress. Hakama et al. [22] have discussed these issues, and explained why we prefer to use the incidence method for determination of sensitivity, and as far as possible avoid making decisions on evaluation of relative sensitivity of two tests in the same individual.

Natural history

The success of screening is dependent on an understanding of the natural history of the detectable pre-clinical phase (DPCP), either cancer precursors as for cervix and colorectal cancer screening or early stages of the cancer itself (as for breast cancer screening), and a recognition that this natural history does not result in an inevitable progression between the development of the DPCP and an invasive cancer. Rather, there may be different forms of precursors or early cancers that may not necessarily all be on the same trajectory to cancer, nor that they progress at the same rate, or to the same extent. It is even possible in some instances for some of the early stages to be bypassed, or at least not be detectable, in an individual destined to develop cancer. So the demonstration that a screening test will detect a precursor, and that it can be ablated, or find an early cancer, that can be cured, does not necessarily mean that the individual has been benefited.

There is a distribution of cancers by severity, ranging from those that progress very slowly, if at all, to those that progress rapidly and soon metastasize and result in death. It is the rapidly progressive cancers, or the precursors of such cancers, that we should most like to detect with screening and subsequently cure. It could be argued that if screening finds or prevents the emergence of the cancers that are most easy to treat, and which only result in death under circumstances of major clinical delays or failure to treat, then we shall have achieved little. Indeed, off-setting any benefit from the detection by screening of easy to treat cancers will be the necessity for a large number of people to be screened who in the event will not benefit at all.

Obtaining the necessary information on natural history is best done through randomized screening trials, though cohort studies of the precursors of cancer of the cervix [7,8] combined with case-control studies designed to determine the efficacy of screening in those screened enabled analyses that were instrumental in demonstrating the futility of annual screening [23]. Long-term follow-up of the Mayo lung screening trial confirmed that overdiagnosis had occurred, with no benefit, which many found difficult to accept for a cancer as malignant as lung cancer [24]. Long follow-up of the Canadian Breast Screening trial [25] suggested overdiagnosis had occurred from mammography screening, and also that the detection and excision of a number of in situ cancers had had no impact upon the subsequent incidence of breast cancer, suggesting that these lesions are not precursors in the classic sense, but just markers of risk [26]. Relatively early during the prostate screening trials it was also recognized that overdiagnosis was substantial as a result of PSA testing [27].

Organization of screening

Organized screening is distinguished from opportunistic screening primarily on the basis of how invitations to screening are extended. In organized screening, invitations are issued to those at risk in a defined target population, usually through population registers, and measures instituted to facilitate their attendance for screening. In this context, risk is usually defined by age and sex.

In opportunistic screening, invitations to screening are extended to individuals when they encounter health care providers for reasons unrelated to cancer. Opportunistic screening is often inefficient, because many who are screened are not at high risk of cancer, many in the population who should be screened are not, and those that do receive screening may be screened either too frequently or too infrequently. All screening programmes require some degree of organization to be successful, and as the extent of the organization of the various elements of screening increases, so too does the impact of the programme. Important elements of organization include:

◆ An identifiable target group or population, with accompanying population registers
◆ Implementation measures available to guarantee high coverage and participation
◆ Access to high-quality screening
◆ Effective referral system in place for diagnosis and treatment
◆ Measures in place to monitor and evaluate a programme [28]

What screening is currently justified for cancer
Breast screening

There is sufficient evidence from randomized screening trials (RSTs) that mammography screening is associated with a significant reduction in deaths from breast cancer in women age 50 to 69 [19]. However, the evidence in women age 40 to 49 was judged by IARC [19] to be limited, the point estimate of effect being less and the reduction in breast cancer mortality non-significant. Since then, no new evidence has accrued on screening women age 50 or more, but for younger women, the UK Age Trial, in which women age 39 to 41 received annual mammography for 7 years, found a non-significant reduction in breast cancer mortality of similar order to the IARC meta-analysis [29]. In most countries that have introduced organized mammography screening, invitations are made every 2 years to women age 50 to 69, though in the United Kingdom screening is offered every 3 years and in the United States, the recommendation from most organizations is for annual mammography from the age of 40. The different recommendations on re-screening frequency represent in part different interpretations of the evidence, and as far as the United States is concerned, a different approach to screening, where there are recommendations for screening, but no organized programmes. There has been one trial comparing annual versus 3-yearly screening, which used indirect indicators of effectiveness as endpoints [30]. Only marginal additional benefit was estimated from the more frequent screening.

The question as to whether mammography adds a significant benefit to screening by good clinical breast examinations was regarded as critically important by the expert group that reviewed the US Breast Cancer Detection Demonstrations Projects [31] but only one trial was designed to answer this question, the Canadian National Breast Screening Study (CNBSS) (2) [25]. Even though nearly half the breast cancers detected by screening were found by mammography alone, the majority as expected being small and node negative, there was no reduction in breast cancer mortality consequent on the use of mammography screening. This null result led to accusations of poor mammography quality, but in fact the sensitivity of mammography was at least as good as that in other trials [32]. A model-based analysis suggested that both arms (both with and without mammography) had achieved a 20 per cent or more reduction in breast cancer mortality [33]. Although these results have not influenced breast screening policy in developed countries, they have led to attempts to evaluate the role of screening by clinical breast examination in some developing countries [34].

Breast self-examination (BSE) has long been advocated, but evidence that it is effective has been difficult to obtain. Although two observational studies suggest it can contribute to breast cancer mortality reduction [35,36], this has not been confirmed in two randomized trials, one in China and the other in Russia [37,38]. However, it has been insufficiently appreciated that the Russian trial, which was initiated in both St Petersburg and Moscow [39], has only reported results on the St Petersburg component, and that component only assessed the addition of BSE teaching to annual breast examinations, rather than the effect of BSE alone. One of the observational studies was a case control study nested within both components of the CNBSS, where all participants were instructed in BSE as part of their clinical breast examinations. It was the women who practiced BSE well (as judged by the examiners) who seemed to derive the benefit [37]. The other observational study was based on the Mama programme in Finland, of which a major feature was that women were informed of a designated radiologist to whom they could self-refer it they were concerned over changes in their breasts [36]. This avoided the difficulties often encountered by women who practice BSE that the primary care practitioner they see may not recognize the signs of early breast cancer.

Mammography is a technology that has been available for decades, and although improvements in processing have occurred, resulting in better images to be interpreted by trained radiologists, these improvements seem to have resulted in improved sensitivity and specificity of the technique, but no apparent improvement in the mortality benefit as determined by the RSTs. This has led to interest in new technologies. Unfortunately a major trial comparing digital with standard mammography was only able to assess relative sensitivity, as both tests were performed in the same women [40]. Hence, although interpreted as showing better sensitivity in younger women, this may not be true, the trial being unable to assess the effectiveness of the screens in detecting progressive disease, for the reasons given earlier. A study of two concurrently observed cohorts of women age 50 or more in Florence, Italy, found higher recall rates in the digital mammography group, and higher rates of in situ cancer detection. However, there was only a small difference in invasive cancer detection rates [41]. The other new technique, MRI, does seem to offer advantages to younger women because of the absence of radiation, and therefore is being advocated particularly for screening women at increased genetic risk of breast cancers [42].

An important question for cancer control is whether the breast screening programmes are producing the expected benefits in the populations where they have been applied. This question has been addressed by a number of 'before and after' analyses in different populations [e.g. 43,44]. A difficulty with these analyses is that in nearly all countries, the introduction of breast screening coincided with or followed the improvements in treatment of breast cancer that has resulted from adjuvant chemotherapy and hormone therapy. Only a few analyses have adequately addressed this. In one, in the United Kingdom, Blanks et al. [45] estimated that the 21 per cent reduction in breast cancer resulted from 14 per cent reduction due to improved treatment and 7 per cent due to screening. Berry et al [46], in the United States, used a series of models to attempt to address the same question. Although the models varied in the extent they attributed the reduction in breast cancer mortality since 1990 to treatment or screening, on average the conclusion was that about half the fall was due to each. This conclusion, however, was dependent on the assumption that the increase in incidence of breast cancer that had been observed in the United States would have been followed by an increase in mortality in the absence of screening. That this is unlikely is suggested by the fact that much of the increase was due to the use of mammography, while the rest, it became apparent after incidence fell, was due to the use (and then cessation by many women) of hormone replacement therapy – known to selectively increase the incidence of good prognosis breast cancers [47]. Further, the reduction in breast cancer mortality in the United States was exactly paralleled by a fall in Canada, whereas many of the

Canadian breast screening programmes did not start until after 1990. Thus in Canada and probably in the United States also most of the reduction had to be due to improved treatment, not the screening programmes.

Colorectal screening

The only other cancer for which there is RST evidence of the effectiveness of screening is from the use of the faecal occult blood test (FOBT). The three reported trials had different levels of efficacy, ranging between 15 and 31 per cent reduction in colorectal cancer mortality, from 10 to 18 years after initiation of screening [48]. The differences were in part due to lesser effectiveness of biennial versus annual screening, directly seen in the US trial [49], but also due to rehydration of the FOBT in the US trial, but not in the European, though both of them screened every two years and had lower compliance than in the US trial. This evidence base has been judged to be sufficient to initiate organized colorectal screening in the United Kingdom and many parts of Canada and elsewhere, using a FOBT test every 2 years, though it is recognized that major efforts are needed to ensure that diagnostic colonoscopy is available for those with positive screens. It remains to be seen whether sufficient compliance with screening will be obtained to ensure success.

In the United States, a recent expert report has recommended screening using immunological or DNA-based stool tests [50]. Unfortunately, this recommendation is based on the apparent greater sensitivity of these tests than the guaiac-based FOBT, with no evidence that the increased sensitivity will be followed by greater mortality reduction. It is conceivable that overdiagnosis will be increased, with little improvement in efficacy.

The other screening tests under evaluation are either endoscopic- or imaging-based. Flexible sigmoidoscopy for screening is being evaluated in trials in Europe and the United States. In the United States, there has been an increasing tendency to use colonoscopy for screening, but no RST of colonoscopy efficacy has been reported. In addition, virtual colonoscopy using CT scanning has been shown to be almost as sensitive to detection of polyps (the main target of endoscopy screening) as standard colonoscopy [51]. However, this still requires extensive preparation of the bowel (a major disincentive for individuals to accept colonoscopy), and if abnormal, would still have to be followed by diagnostic endoscopy, so it is not certain that this will prove to be an important advance.

Although most expert groups reached the conclusion that screening was needed in addition to primary prevention, it is still not clear that on a long term basis screening will be as cost-effective as prevention for colorectal cancer control. This will have to be carefully evaluated over the next decade.

Screening for cancer of the cervix uteri

Cervix cancer screening was introduced before the evaluation needs for screening was appreciated. Thus correlation type analyses [52], time sequence analyses [53], and eventually case control studies [e.g. 54,55] were used to reach the determination that screening using the Papanicolaou smear resulted in a reduction in both cervix cancer incidence and mortality. Modelling the understanding gained by studies of the natural history of precursors of invasive cancer [7,8,23,56] gradually led to a recognition that three or even 5-yearly screening was effective. An IARC working group [57] concluded that there was sufficient evidence that screening by conventional cytology has reduced cervical cancer incidence and mortality rates and also concluded that screening need not commence until age 25 and that there is no evidence that screening annually results in much greater efficacy than 3 to 5 yearly screening. For women who have been screened and who have never had an abnormality detected, screening can be stopped from the age of 64.

Many programmes have now switched from the standard cytology (Pap) smear to liquid-based cytology. An advantage of this is that the numbers of unsatisfactory smears are reduced, and also the specimens can be used for HPV DNA testing, but there is no evidence that the efficacy of liquid-based cytology is greater than standard cytology smears in reducing cervical cancer incidence and mortality.

The recognition that a necessary cause of cervix cancer is infection with one of several types of oncogenic human papillomaviruses (see Chapter 6 in this book) led to the introduction of tests for viral DNA in cervical samples (obtained in a liquid medium), and the recognition that many women can test positive after initiating sexual activity, but for the majority, the infection is rapidly cleared with no long-term sequelae. However, women with persistent evidence of infection are at risk of developing precursors of invasive cancer, and cytological evidence of high-grade lesions, usually confirmed after a diagnostic colposcopy. Although the sensitivity of the HPV test for such lesions seems superior to cytology, it is not clear that this comprises superior sensitivity to those lesions that are likely if untreated to progress to invasive cancer. This is now being evaluated in randomized trials comparing the application of the two forms of testing. In the interim, the IARC working group concluded that there was sufficient evidence that testing for human papillomavirus infection as the primary screening modality can reduce cervical incidence and mortality rates [57].

With the introduction of HPV vaccination programmes there has been concern over the screening policy to apply to the cohorts of women who are vaccinated. As the current vaccines protect only against infection with HPV types 16 and 18, and there is uncertainty over the degree of cross-protection against other oncogenic types, it must be assumed that vaccinated women will have their risk of cancer of the cervix reduced, but not abolished. One approach might be to test such women from the age of 25 at 5-year intervals for evidence of HPV infection. Those negative can be reassured, those positive, evaluated by colposcopy. Continued surveillance probably at least to the age of 55 would be required. In a model-based cost-effectiveness analysis, the best strategy for girls vaccinated before age 12 years was triennial cytology with HPV test triage beginning at age 25 years and switching at age 35 years to screening every 5 years by HPV testing with cytology triage [58]. We have recently outlined the short-, medium- and long-term requirements of a strategy to evaluate the impact of HPV immunization and defined a framework to facilitate planning and evaluation [59].

Cancers with uncertain evidence of screening efficacy

Prostate cancer

There are two tests currently advocated for screening for prostate cancer, the digital rectal examination (DRE) and a blood test for prostate specific antigen (PSA); for neither, until recently, was there randomized trial evidence that prostate cancer mortality is reduced secondary to their use in screening. However, the absence of such evidence did not prevent a number of professional organizations, especially in the United States, including the American Cancer Society, from recommending annual screening from the age of 50. This has led to widespread use of the PSA test in many countries, and a dramatic increase in the incidence of prostate cancer, clearly secondary to the lead time and overdiagnosis induced by the screening. The gap between incidence and mortality from prostate cancer is now very large (in Canada the incidence/mortality ratio is 2.6), and although there has been a small reduction in prostate cancer mortality in the population, which followed a small increase that accompanied the incidence increase, this is just as likely to be due to prolongation of life by hormone therapy, with death from competing causes of death, as due to an effect of screening.

Two randomized trials evaluating the effect of PSA screening, the Prostate, Lung, Colon and Ovary (PLCO) trial in the United States, and the European Randomized Study of Prostate Cancer screening (ERSPC) in several countries of Europe, were initiated in 1993 [60,61]. Recruitment into the PLCO trial was completed in 2001 (with 76,705 men randomized), and screening in 2006; follow-up of each participant is planned for at least 13 years. Recruitment into the ERSPC now exceeds 200,000, and is still continuing in some countries. These trials were planned with differences in the approaches to screening: annual in the PLCO trial, every 2 or 4 years in the ERSPC, and with a cut-off of 4 ng/mL for a positive PSA in the United States, and 3 ng/mL in Europe. However, it is anticipated that comparative analyses will be possible [62].

The early mortality results from both trials show there was no reduction in prostate cancer mortality in the first seven years after randomization in the screened groups compared to the control [15,16]. After that to ten years there was a slight difference between the trials. At ten years in the PLCO trial, with 67 per cent of those enrolled followed, there was, if anything, higher mortality from prostate cancer in the screened group than the control group; but the reverse was seen in the ERSPC. No data beyond 10 years were reported for the PLCO trial. In the ERSPC, all available data to a cut-off date of December 31, 2006 were reported, showing a difference in deaths from prostate cancer in the screened group compared to the control (261 vs. 363) with a rate ratio for their core age group (55–69 years) of 0.80 (95 per cent confidence interval (CI) 0.67–0.95), and 0.85 (95 per cent CI 0.73–1.00) for subjects of all ages included. Nearly all the reduction in prostate cancer deaths in the screening group was in men age 55 to 59 and 65 to 69. In practice, the confidence intervals surrounding the point estimates of the mortality rate ratios in the two trials overlap, so that chance cannot be excluded as an explanation for the apparent differences between them. If the separation of the mortality curves in ERSPC is confirmed with more data, it will still be necessary to be certain that other factors, especially treatment differences between the groups, are not responsible for this. Indeed, Appendix 7 of the ERSPC report shows major treatment differences that could explain their results [16]. However, it is important to note that both trials support the recommendation of the US Preventive Services Task Force [63] against screening men older than 69.

Draisma et al. [27] estimated from the Rotterdam component of the ERSPC that following a single PSA screening test at age 55, the lead time was 12.3 years and overdiagnosis was 27 per cent. Further, after a single screening test at age 75, the lead time was 6.0 years but overdiagnosis occurred in 56 per cent of the detected cases. On average, for a screening programme at 4-year intervals from 55 to 67, lead time is 11.2 years and overdiagnosis occurs in 48 per cent of cases. Similar estimates have not yet been derived from the PLCO trial, but they will probably be somewhat lower, given the higher cut-off level used for determination of PSA positivity. Nevertheless, it is clear that PSA testing results in substantial overdiagnosis, and that many men who are convinced their lives have been saved by PSA screening, even though many of them suffer from incontinence and impotence secondary to the unnecessary prostatectomy they had, have been deceived. This has been termed by Raffle and Gray 'The Popularity Paradox': 'The greater the harm through overdiagnosis and overtreatment from screening, the more people there are who believe they owe their health, or even their life, to the programme' [64].

Lung cancer

A cancer for which there is good evidence of no benefit, is lung, at least using chest X-rays. Indeed long-term follow-up of the Mayo lung trial has not only confirmed no benefit, but documented overdiagnosis as well [24]. Nevertheless, the advent of the low dose helical computerized tomography (CT) scan has led to considerable interest in the possibility that screening will reduce lung cancer mortality. The claims for improved survival following such screening [65] are, however, not soundly based, as there is no comparable unscreened control group. Indeed an attempt to compare the observed mortality in several studies with that expected, suggests little benefit [66]. Further, in many situations, the specificity of CT is so poor that a vast excess of diagnostic tests follows screening. A large US trial is underway evaluating CT screening in comparison with chest X-ray screening, while chest X-ray screening is also being re-evaluated in the PLCO trial [60]. There is also a European trial of CT screening underway, with unscreened controls. Fortunately at present, no major professional organization advocates lung screening, all being prepared to await the RST evidence that will be forthcoming.

Ovarian cancer

There are two major randomized trials evaluating screening for ovarian cancer, the PLCO and the UK Collaborative Trial in the United Kingdom. In the PLCO trial, annual CA125 blood tests and transvaginal ultrasound are used as first line screening tests, women with either test abnormal being further investigated. The UK trial has three arms, no screening, annual CA125 tests with ultrasound as the second line investigation, and annual ultrasound examination as primary screening. The results so far show that generally these two tests detect different cancers; the stage distribution of cancers detected by CA125 is not encouraging, as many tumours are late stage; ultrasound may be better in detecting earlier cancers, but at the cost of many false positives, unnecessary investigations, and oophorectomies [67,68]. Neither trial has yet reported on mortality results. At present, there is no evidence to support screening for ovarian cancer.

Conclusions

Screening is an expensive component of cancer control, which requires great care and efficient organization to ensure that the anticipated benefits are achieved. Screening has to be maintained, it can have no permanent effect on cancer occurrence, in contrast to the lasting impact of primary prevention.

Currently, screening makes a limited contribution to cancer control. In spite of some good evidence supporting mammography screening for breast cancer in women age 50 to 69, it is still not clear how much screening is contributing to the reduction in breast cancer mortality being seen in many countries. Screening for cervix cancer has been effective, but currently considerable care is needed to ensure the gains achieved are consolidated, and retained in an era with great enthusiasm for prevention by vaccination. There is randomized trial evidence to support screening for colorectal cancer, but organized population-based programmes are in their infancy, and their impact cannot be assessed. For no other cancer at present can screening be supported for cancer control in technically advanced Western nations.

References

1 National Cancer Control Programmes (2002). Policies and Managerial Guidelines. 2nd edn. World Health Organization, Geneva.

2 WHO Guide for Effective Programmes (2007). Cancer Control. Knowledge into Action: Early Detection. World Health Organization, Geneva,

3 Wald NJ (1994). Guidance on terminology. *J Med Screen*, 1:1–2.

4 Task Force appointed by the Conference of Deputy Ministers of Health (1976). Cervical cancer screening programmes. *Can Med Assoc J*, 114:1003–33.

5 Walton RJ, Allen HH, Anderson GH, et al (1982). Cervical cancer screening programmes: Summary of the 1982 Canadian Task Force Report. *Can Med Assoc J*, 127:581–589.

6 Miller AB, Anderson G, Brisson J, et al (1991). Report of a National Workshop on Screening for Cancer of the Cervix. *Can Med Assoc J*, **145**:1301–25.

7 Boyes DA, Morrison B, Knox EG, Draper G, & Miller AB (1982). A cohort study of cervical cancer screening in British Columbia. *Clin Invest Med*, **5**:1–29.

8 Holowaty P, Miller AB, Rohan T, & To T (1999). The natural history of dysplasia of the uterine cervix. *J Natl Cancer Inst*, **91**:252–58.

9 WHO Guide for Effective Programmes (2006). Cancer Control. Knowledge into Action: Planning. World Health Organization, Geneva.

10 Miller AB, Baines CJ, & Turnbull C (1991). The role of the nurse-examiner in the National Breast Screening Study. *Can J Public Health*, **82**:162–67.

11 Bassett AA (1985). Physical examination of the breast and breast self-examination. In Miller AB (ed) *Screening for Cancer*, pp 271–91. Academic Press, Inc., Orlando.

12 Weissfeld JL, Fagerstrom RM, & O'Brien B (2000). Quality control of cancer screening examination procedures in the prostate, lung, colorectal, and ovarian (PLCO) cancer screening trial. *Controlled Clinical Trials*, **21**:390–99S.

13 Miller AB (2002). Review: Quality assurance in screening strategies. *Virus Research*, **89**:295–99.

14 U.S. Preventive Services Task Force Ratings: Strength of Recommendations and Quality of Evidence. *Guide to Clinical Preventive Services, Third Edition: Periodic Updates*, 2000–2003. Agency for Healthcare Research and Quality, Rockville, MD. http://www.ahrq.gov/clinic/3rduspstf/ratings.htm, accessed June 2, 2008.

15 Andriole GL, Grubb RL, Buys SS, et al (2009) for the PLCO Project Team. Mortality results from a randomized prostate-cancer screening trial. *New Eng. J. Med*, **360**:1310–19.

16 Schröder FH, Hugosson J, Roobol MJ, et al (2009) for the ERSPC investigators. Screening and prostate-cancer mortality in a randomized European study. *New Eng J Med*, **360**:1320–28.

17 Prorok PC, Chamberlain J, Day NE, Hakama M, & Miller AB (1984). UICC workshop on the evaluation of screening programmes for cancer. *Int J Cancer*, **34**:1–4.

18 Miller AB (1996). Fundamental issues in screening for cancer. In Schottenfeld D & Fraumeni JF, Jr. (eds) *Cancer Epidemiology and Prevention*, 2nd edn. pp. 1433–52. Oxford University Press, Oxford, New York.

19 IARC Handbooks on Cancer Prevention (2002), *Breast Cancer Screening*. Vol 7, IARC Press, Lyon.

20 Miller AB (2006). Design of cancer screening trials/randomized trials for evaluation of cancer screening. *World J Surg*, **30**:1152–62.

21 Cole P & Morrison AS (1980). Basic issues in population screening for cancer. *J Natl Cancer Inst*, **64**:1263–72.

22 Hakama M, Auvinen A, Day NE, & Miller AB (2007). Sensitivity in cancer screening. *J Med Screen*, **14**:74–77.

23 Hakama M, Miller AB, & Day NE (eds) (1986). *Screening for cancer of the uterine cervix*. IARC Scientific publications no. 76. International Agency for Research on Cancer, Lyon.

24 Marcus PM, Bergstralh EJ, Fagerstrom RM, et al (2000). Lung cancer mortality in the Mayo lung project: impact of extended follow-up. *J Natl Cancer Inst*, **92**:1308–16.

25 Miller AB, To T, Baines CJ, & Wall C (2000). Canadian National Breast Screening Study-2: 13-year results of a randomized trial in women age 50–59 years. *J Natl Cancer Inst*, **92**:1490–99.

26 Miller AB & Borges AM (2001). Intermediate histological effect markers for breast cancer. In: Miller AB, Bartsch H, Boffetta P, Dragsted L, Vainio H. (eds) *Biomarkers in Cancer Chemoprevention*. IARC Scientific Publications No. 154. International Agency for Research on Cancer, Lyon, pp. 171–175.

27 Draisma G, Boer R, Otto SJ, et al (2003). Lead times and overdetection due to prostate-specific antigen screening: estimates from the European Randomized Study of Screening for Prostate Cancer. *J Natl Cancer Inst*, **95**:868–78.

28 Hakama M, Chamberlain J, Day NE, Miller AB, & Prorok PC (1985). Evaluation of screening programmes for gynecological cancer. *Br J Cancer*, **52**:669–73.

29 Moss SM, Cuckle H, Evans A, Johns L, Waller M, & Bobrow L (2006). Effect of mammographic screening from age 40 years on breast cancer mortality at 10 years follow-up: a randomized controlled trial. *Lancet*, **368**:2053–60.

30 Breast Screening Frequency Trial Group (2002). The frequency of breast cancer screening. Results from the UKCCCR randomised trial. *Eur J Cancer*, **38**:1458–64.

31 Beahrs O, Shapiro S, & Smart C (1979). Report of the working group to review the National Cancer Institute American Cancer Society Breast Cancer Detection Demonstration Projects. *J Natl Cancer Inst*, **62**:640–709.

32 Fletcher SW, Black W, Harris R, Rimer BK, & Shapiro S (1993). Report of the International Workshop on Screening for Breast Cancer. *J Natl Cancer Inst*, **85**:1644–56.

33 Rijnsburger AI, van Oortmarssen GJ, Boer R, et al (2004). Mammography benefit in the Canadian National Breast Screening Study-2: a model evaluation. *Int J Cancer*, **110**:756–62.

34 Boulos S, Gadallah M, Neguib S, et al (2005). Breast screening in the emerging world: High prevalence of breast cancer in Cairo. *The Breast*, **14**:340–46.

35 Gastrin G, Miller AB, To T, et al (1994). Incidence and mortality from breast cancer in the Mama programme for breast screening in Finland, 1973–1986. *Cancer*, **73**:2168–74.

36 Harvey BJ, Miller AB, Baines CJ, & Corey PN (1997). Effect of breast self-examination techniques on the risk of death from breast cancer. *Can Med Assoc J*, **157**:1205–12.

37 Thomas DB, Gao Dl, Ray, RM, et al (2002). Randomized trial of breast self-examination in Shanghai: Final results. *J Natl Cancer Inst*, **94**:1445–57.

38 Semiglazov VF, Moiseyenko VM, Manikhas AG, et al (1999). Interim results of a prospective randomized evaluation of self-examination for early detection of breast cancer (Russia/St Petersburg/WHO). *Vopr Onkol*, **45**:265–71.

39 Semiglazov VF, Sagaidak VN, Moiseyenko VM, & Mikhailov EA (1993). Study of the role of breast self-examination in the reduction of mortality from breast cancer. *Eur J Cancer*, **29A**:2039–46.

40 Pisano ED, Hendrik RE, Yaffe MJ, et al (2008). Diagnostic accuracy of digital versus film mammography: exploratory analysis of selected population subgroups in DMIST. *Radiology*, **246**:376–83.

41 Del Turco MR, Mantellini P, Ciatto S, et al (2007). Full-field digital versus screen-film mammography: Comparative accuracy in concurrent screening cohorts. *AJR*, **189**:860–66.

42 Schrading S & Kuhl CK (2008). Mammographic, US, and MR imaging phenotypes of familial breast cancer. *Radiology*, **246**:58–70.

43 Coldman A, Phillips N, Warren L, & Kan L (2006). Breast cancer mortality after screening mammography in British Columbia women. *Int J Cancer*, **120**:1076–80.

44 Sarkeala T, Heinavaara S, & Antilla A (2008). Organised mammography screening reduces breast cancer mortality: a cohort study from Finland. *Int J Cancer*, **122**:614–19.

45 Blanks RG, Moss SM, McGahan CE, Quinn MJ, & Babb PJ (2000). Effect of NHS breast screening programme on mortality from breast cancer in England and Wales, 1990–98: comparison of observed with expected mortality. *BMJ*, **321**:665–69.

46 Berry DA, Cronin KA, Plevritis SK, et al (2005). Effect of screening and adjuvant therapy on mortality from breast cancer. *N Eng J Med*, **353**:1784–92.

47 Ravdin PM, Cronin KA, Howlader N, et al (2007). The decrease in breast-cancer incidence in 2003 in the United States. *N Eng J Med*, **356**:1670–74.

48 Hewitson P, Glasziou P, Irwig L, Towler B, & Watson E (2007-1). Screening for colorectal cancer using the faecal occult blood test, Hemoccult. *Cochrane Database Syst Rev*, CD001216.

49 Mandel JS, Church TR, Ederer F, & Bond JH (1999). Colorectal cancer mortality: effectiveness of biennial screening for fecal occult blood. *J Natl Cancer Inst*, **91**:434–37.

50 Levin B, Lieberman DA, McFarland B, et al (2008). Screening and surveillance for the early detection of colorectal cancer and adenomatous polyps, 2008: A joint guideline from the American Cancer Society, the US Multi-Society Task Force on Colorectal Cancer, and the American College of Radiology. *CA Cancer J Clin*, http://caonline.amcancersoc.org/misc/guidelines.shtml, (accessed June 7, 2008).

51 Summerton S, Little E, & Cappell MS (2008). CT colonography: current status and future promise. *Gastroenterol Clin N Am*, **37**:161–89.

52 Miller AB, Lindsay J, & Hill GB (1976). Mortality from cancer of the uterus in Canada and its relationship to screening for cancer of the cervix. *Int J Cancer*, **17**:602–12.

53 Hakama M (1982). Trends in the incidence of cervical cancer in the Nordic countries. In Magnus K (ed) *Trends in Cancer Incidence, Causes and Practical Implications*, pp. 279–92. Hemisphere Publishing Corp., New York.

54 Clarke EA & Anderson TW (1979). Does screening by 'Pap' smears help prevent cervical cancer? *Lancet*, **ii**:1–4.

55 MacGregor JE, Moss SM, Parkin DM, & Day NE (1985). A case-control study of cervical screening in NE Scotland. *BMJ*, **290**:1543–48.

56 Yu SZ, Miller AB, & Sherman GJ (1982). Optimizing the age, number of tests, and test interval for cervical screening in Canada. *J Epidemiol Commununity Health*, **36**:1–10.

57 IARC Handbooks on Cancer Prevention (2005). *Cervix cancer screening*. Vol **10**, IARC Press, Lyon.

58 Goldhaber-Fiebert JD, Stout NK, Salomon JA, Kuntz KM, & Goldie SJ (2008). Cost-effectiveness of cervical cancer screening with human papillomavirus DNA testing and HPV-16,18 vaccination. *J Natl Cancer Inst*, **100**:308–20.

59 Howlett RI, Miller AB, Pasut G, & Mai V (2009). Defining a strategy to evaluate cervical cancer prevention and early detection in the era of HPV vaccination. *Prev Med*, **48**:432–37.

60 Prorok PC, Andriole GL, Bresalier R, et al (2000). Design of the prostate, lung, colorectal and ovarian (PLCO) cancer screening trial. *Controlled Clinical Trials*, **21**(6S):273S–309S.

61 Roobol MJ & Schroder FH (guest editors) (2003). European randomized study of screening for prostate cancer: Rationale, structure and preliminary results 1994–2003. *BJU Int*, **92**(Suppl 2):1–124.

62 The International Prostate Screening Trial Evaluation Group (1999). Rationale for randomised trials of prostate cancer screening. *Eur J Cancer*, **35**:262–71.

63 US Preventive Task Force (2008). Screening for prostate cancer: U.S. Preventive Services Task Force recommendation statement. *Annals of Int Med*, **149**:185–91.

64 Raffle AE & Gray JAM (2007). *Screening: Evidence and Practice*. Oxford University Press, Oxford, p. 68.

65 International Early Lung Cancer Program Investigators, Henschke CI, Yankelevitz D, Libby DM, Pasmentier DW, Smith JP, & Miettinen OS (2006). Survival of patients with stage 1 lung cancer detected on CT screening. *N Eng J Med*, **355**:1763–71.

66 Bach PB, Jett JR, Pastorino U, Tockman MS, Swensen SJ, & Begg CB (2007). Computed tomography screening and lung cancer outcomes. *JAMA*, **297**:953–61.

67 Partridge E, Kreimer AR, Greenlee RT, et al (2009). Results from four rounds of ovarian cancer screening in a randomized trial. *Obstet Gynecol*, **113**(4):775–782.

68 Menon U, Gentry-Maharaj A, Hallett R, et al (2009). Sensitivity and specificity of multimodal and ultrasound screening for ovarian cancer, and stage distribution of detected cancers: results of the prevalence screen of the UK collaborative trial of ovarian cancer screening (UKCTOCS). *Lancet Oncol*, **10**(4):327–340.

Part 3

Applying new knowledge

Chapter 5

Integrating science with service in cancer control: closing the gap between discovery and delivery

Jon Kerner[1]

The title of this chapter, originally proposed as 'Moving new discoveries into practice', implied that explicit knowledge from research (e.g. clinical trials) should influence cancer control programmes, practice, and policy. Underlying this 'should' is the assumption that evidence-based approaches, i.e. an intervention or policy that has resulted in improved outcomes in the context of scientific study, when implemented in a real world setting will increase the likelihood of improved outcomes. However, it has become increasingly clear that many in the public health, clinical practice, and public policy communities do not hold with this assumption, and that there are equal and often opposing forces to the dissemination and implementation of new knowledge gained from research. These include the mass of tacit knowledge gained from practitioner and policy-maker experience [1,2], as well as the complex service delivery and political policymaking contextual factors that constrain the acceptance, adaptation, and implementation of innovations based on research [3]. Thus, it has been posited that to close the gap between scientific discovery and service delivery, if we want more evidence-based practice, we need more practice-based evidence [4].

If we accept the premise that integrating the lessons learned from science with the lessons learned from service (public health, clinical, and public policy) may be key to closing the gap between discovery and delivery, then scientists, practitioners, policy makers, patients and their families, and the public at large will need to expand their understanding of the meaning of evidence from research and reality. Moreover, the innovations that emerge from our investments in cancer control science will need to be further evaluated through expanded investments in dissemination and implementation science as well as programme evaluation related to cancer control. These investments must focus more attention on the differences between the research context in which most cancer control science is produced (e.g. in the academy, biomedical industries) and communicated (e.g. peer-reviewed publication), and the public health practice, clinical practice, and policymaking contexts in which innovations that emerge from cancer control science are first observed and evaluated by potential practice and policy users, before adaptation and implementation are even, if ever, considered.

Similarly, carefully examining what evidence public health and clinical practitioners, as well as policymakers, want to help improve the effectiveness and efficiency of the cancer control services being provided and policies in place, or being considered in the future, is also critically important.

[1] Jon F. Kerner, Ph.D. Chair, Primary Prevention Action Group, Senior Scientific Advisor for Cancer Control and Knowledge Translation, Canadian Partnership Against Cancer, One University Avenue, Suite 300, Toronto, Ontario M5J 2P1.

Failures in understanding what evidence potential users of research want may help to explain the well documented delay in implementing into practice what is known from research [5]. Finally, bridging the scientific discovery, service delivery, and policy making communities may hold the key to addressing the confusion in terminology and misunderstandings across disciplines about the utility of research in different service and policy contexts. Each of these three broad issues will be addressed within this chapter.

Disseminating science in cancer control and the science of dissemination

Cancer control and its science

As reflected throughout this volume, cancer control covers a broad continuum of interventions ranging from primary prevention of the development of cancer (e.g. tobacco control), early detection of cancer or its precursor lesions (e.g. adenomas before they progress to invasive color-ectal cancer), prompt diagnosis of the signs and/or symptoms of cancer, optimal treatment, and supportive and palliative care. Further, cancer control emphasizes the application of new knowledge gained through research to achieve current best practice (see Chapter 1). The diversity of genomic and proteomic factors influencing the development and spread of the disease, the number of organ sites and physiological systems where primary tumours may first manifest themselves, and the diversity of research and practitioner disciplines whose work may contribute to improved outcomes (i.e. reduced cancer incidence and mortality and improved quality of life), while not unique to cancer, may make the ubiquitous application of best practices based on research across the cancer control continuum particularly challenging within the more general framework of chronic disease control.

These improved outcomes relate to a growing number of measures incorporated into the goals and objectives of national (and local) cancer control plans for which both the World Health Organization and the International Union Against Cancer are providing guidance to government and non-government organizations to develop and implement [6,7]. Relevant goals and objectives [8] include:

- ◆ Reduced cancer incidence through:
  - risk reduction behaviour change,
  - increased practitioner delivery of cancer prevention practices, and
  - policy and environmental changes that support both individual behaviour and practitioner behaviour change (e.g. increased tobacco product excise taxes and investment of these resources to support reimbursement for clinical preventive services).

- ◆ Earlier stage of disease at diagnosis of some cancers through:
  - increased awareness of, more positive attitudes towards, and use of screening services.
  - increased access to cancer screening services,
  - increased practitioner adoption of cancer screening practices, and
  - increased practitioner and patient follow-up of abnormal screening findings, as well as signs and symptoms of cancer.

- ◆ Reduced cancer-related morbidity and mortality through:
  - increased access to and provision of state-of-the-science cancer diagnostic and treatment services, including participation in clinical trials particularly where conventional care continues to prove ineffective (e.g. pancreatic cancer), and

+ Improvements in quality of life of cancer survivors:
  - increased access to and practitioner adoption of evidence-based cancer survivorship and palliation interventions leading to improved quality of life of cancer survivors and those terminally ill with cancer.

As previously noted, many different research disciplines contribute to the scientific cancer control evidence base, made up of research data and other forms of scientific information, which may be translated into actionable knowledge by an equally diverse set of practice and policy users. Much of this research is conducted in, or funded by, organizations based in high income countries where cancer has received considerable public attention and funding support because it is one of the major causes of mortality, morbidity and disease burden [9].

The multi-disciplinary scientific continuum begins with fundamental or basic research, usually based in laboratories conducting carefully controlled in vitro or in vivo (with laboratory animals) experiments, to explore the basic biological mechanisms for the development and spread of cancer. Basic research is complemented by observational research in human populations including epidemiology, surveillance, and survey research tracking the natural variation of biological, behavioural, and environmental risk factors and disease morbidity, mortality, and the differential burden of cancer within defined human populations. Intervention research focused on the general population, as well as cancer patients and their families, attempts to perturb the basic biological mechanisms and/or other observed risk factor (e.g. behavioural, environmental) and disease variation within defined populations to reduce the incidence and mortality of the disease, and to reduce the impact of the disease on patient quality of life. Finally, cancer health services and health policy research evaluates the utility and cost efficiency of different intervention approaches and policies as they are applied in real world health care and community settings.

In high income countries, the balance of cancer research investment tends to be skewed towards basic research, followed by intervention or applied research (usually clinically focused), with population science and health services research receiving proportionally the least amount of financial support [10]. Figure 5.1 summarizes this relatively large commitment to basic science and clinical research within Canada. Similarly, Figure 5.2 reflects the US government National Institute of Health's commitment to basic science in biomedical research. This research investment gradient leads to a premium being placed on discovering and testing new and improved technologies to control cancer (as well as other chronic diseases), relative to making it a priority to ensure that the technologies already available and shown to be effective in controlling cancer are delivered equitably and with high quality [11].

Another consequence of high income countries leading the way in supporting cancer research is that many of the cancer control technologies that emerge from this basic science discovery to intervention development process, supported by a government-industry-voluntary sector complex, are high-end technologies (e.g. Nuclear Magnetic Resonance Imaging), requiring major capital investments and mobilization of large human, physical, and administrative resources [12]. As cancer research continues to expand into new trans-disciplinary discovery and biotechnology development fields, the implications for the dissemination and implementation of these high-end technological approaches to cancer control, particularly for populations experiencing large disparities in cancer incidence and mortality (e.g. low socio-economic populations within high, middle, and low income countries) will need to be carefully evaluated from both a practice and policy perspective. The continued failure to ensure equitable access to new technologies for cancer control in and of itself contributes to growing cancer health disparities between the 'haves and have-nots' [2].

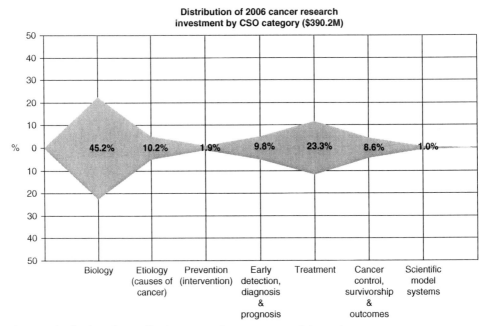

Fig. 5.1 Distribution of Canadian investment in cancer research by topic. From *Canadian Cancer Research Alliance 2006*, with permission [10].

Diffusing and disseminating cancer control science

Within the context of scientific discovery, the bulk of the communication and diffusion of cancer research information is carried out through discipline-specific peer-reviewed journal publications and conference presentations. The mass of scientific information communicated through peer-reviewed journal publication alone is enormous. For example, using the topic of cancer in a PubMed [13] search produced a total of 2,171,530 listings, of which 245,839 were review articles. Switching the search term to cancer control reduced the total number of listings to 137,617, of which 24,527 were review articles. Given the diversity of scientific findings reported across the cancer control continuum, the challenge of finding specific research information that can be easily translated into actionable knowledge for practitioners or policy makers in such a large mass of original reports or even review articles is daunting.

Communication and diffusion of scientific information have historically been relatively slow and deliberative processes that depended on the spoken or written word. In the scientific discovery context, this process permitted the replication and re-evaluation of research results, and the refinement of both methodological approaches to research as well as consideration and testing of alternative theoretical explanations for study findings. In the public health and clinical practice contexts, as well as in the public policy context, this slower pace of diffusion of information may have provided more opportunity to deliberate about new research information, place it in applied contexts and, as such, perhaps provided more time for new research information to be transformed into actionable knowledge. Nevertheless, the slow and deliberative pace of scientific inquiry, trickling into practice and policy considerations, no doubt contributed to the many historical examples of delayed incorporation of evidence-based interventions into practice [14].

Since the advent and wide dissemination of modern communication technologies (e.g. the Internet), more and more information from research is being transmitted to broader and more

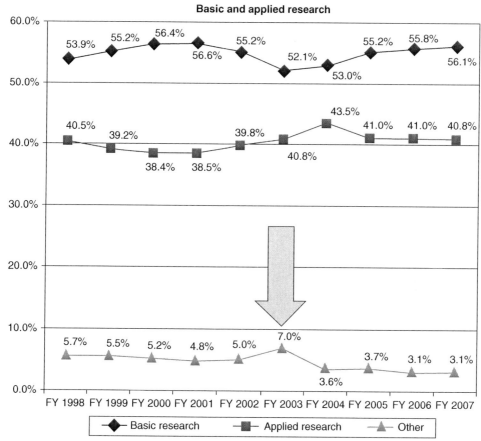

Fig. 5.2 NIH at the Crossroads: Myths, Realities, and Strategies for the Future. Presentation by Dr. Elias Zerhouni, Director of the National Institutes of Health (USA).
From http://www.drugabuse.gov/about/organization/nacda/powerpoint/NIHCrossroads506. ppt#369,5,Slide 5 (accessed 24 March 2009), with permission.

diverse audiences. On the one hand, this can be viewed as a positive development towards getting the lessons learned from science into practice. On the other hand, with less and less time to digest the information contained therein, one unintended consequence of the explosion of research information available through modern communication technologies is that there is a signal to noise ratio problem, with too much information being communicated and too little time to process the information into practice or policy contexts as knowledge that can be applied.

Given the pressure to speed new discoveries into new intervention technologies, given the concern about the equitable distribution of cancer control knowledge to benefit all populations that bear the burden of cancer, and given the rapidity with which discoveries are being reported and new technologies developed from them are either prematurely adopted [15] or are seen as superior to existing technologies that have been previously shown to be effective but are underutilized [16], there has been a growing interest in how best to manage new knowledge as it emerges from the translation of research information into practice or policy contexts and applications.

One approach to managing the plethora of new information from research has been the systematic evidence review process. While there has been a considerable growth in systematic reviews of research evidence in the past two decades, the conduct of such reviews is technically challenging, variable in quality, and in need of regular updating to keep the findings current with the constant publication of new original research reports [17]. Moreover, it is usually original research reports rather than systematic evidence reviews that capture the attention of the public and public officials, at least with respect to what is newsworthy from the media's perspective. As reported to the author by a Dallas (Texas) Morning News Health Reporter several years ago, 'the root of the word news is new and there is nothing new in a systematic evidence review' (personal communication)

The World Health Organization (WHO) has identified one issue for global public health as the 'know-do' gap, and has promoted a global knowledge management strategy targeted to national policymakers, WHO programmes, and health professionals. The strategy involves five strategic directions: (1) improving access to the world's health information, (2) translating knowledge into policy and action, (3) sharing and reapplying experiential knowledge, (4) leveraging e-Health in countries, and (5) fostering an enabling environment [18]. While the details of the five strategies are beyond the scope of this discussion, translating knowledge into policy and action, sharing and reapplying experiential knowledge, and fostering an enabling environment are all areas closely related to the three issues previously raised in the introduction to this chapter: (1) translating research information into actionable knowledge, (2) understanding what practice and policy communities know from their experience and want to learn from research, and (3) how variation in research, practice, and policy contexts can be bridged to increase the relevance of research information to practitioners and policy makers focused on cancer control.

The science of dissemination

To begin with, it should be recognized that within the dissemination and implementation scientific literature, there persists considerable confusion in terminology. Thus, in a recent study conducted with 33 applied research funding agencies in nine countries, 29 terms were used to refer to some aspect of translating knowledge into action [19]. Adding further to the confusion within the scientific literature is that the same terms can mean different things and different terms can refer to the same thing both within and across countries [20].

Second, the bulk of research on the dissemination and implementation of evidence-based interventions has not been specifically focused on cancer control. For example, in 2003, the National Cancer Institute (NCI), part of the US National Institutes of Health, contracted through the US Agency for Healthcare Research and Quality (AHRQ) evidence-practice centre programme at McMaster University in Hamilton, Ontario, to carry out a systematic review of dissemination and diffusion research that had been published, in relation to the number of systematic evidence reviews published on intervention efficacy in five cancer control domains [21]. The five cancer control domains were: (1) smoking cessation, (2) healthier diet, (3) mammography screening, (4) Pap smear screening, and (5) control of cancer pain.

With the exception of the control of cancer pain, the number of systematic evidence reviews of cancer control intervention efficacy was always larger than the number of published original scientific reports of the dissemination and diffusion of such interventions. As such, the authors were only able to draw limited conclusions from the available dissemination and diffusion research evidence base, within the context of cancer control that they examined. These conclusions included: (1) very few of the primary studies on dissemination and diffusion of cancer control interventions used randomized controlled designs to evaluate the dissemination strategy; (2) passive diffusion approaches, such as mailing of materials to targeted user populations, were generally ineffective; (3) more active dissemination approaches (e.g. train the trainer models, and educating opinion leaders) were more effective in promoting change in their knowledge, attitudes, and behaviours; and (4) the majority of the evidence for strategies to disseminate evidence-based interventions was directed to clinical providers as the primary audience for cancer control interventions.

A recent update and expansion of this evidence review, focused on dissemination and implementation research on community cancer prevention [22] concluded that while there has been a small increase in the number of dissemination and implementation publications focused on cancer prevention since 2005, there remain a number of challenges in the published literature. These challenges include: (1) a lack of uniform terminology, (2) studies targeting only a limited number of intervention delivery settings and target populations, (3) a limited number of valid and reliable measures of dissemination and implementation processes, (4) triangulation with and more practice-based evidence, (5) no standardized reporting criteria for dissemination and implementation research, and (6) the need for more active and multi-modal dissemination and implementation strategies.

Given the relative dearth of published dissemination and implementation research related specifically to cancer control, it behoves those concerned about getting the lessons learned from cancer control science into cancer control practice and policy, to look beyond the field of cancer control to a number of other research domains. These include the seminal social science work focused on fields other than health [23], and a growing body of health services research primarily focused on understanding how new clinical research evidence gets translated into clinical practice [24], as well as how innovations in health and other service delivery fields diffuse into organizations [25]. The scope of this research literature is very broad. For example, Greenhalgh et al. [25] identified 13 research traditions relevant to the diffusion of innovations in health service organizations.

They classified four of these traditions as coming from early diffusion research including rural sociology, medical sociology, communication studies, and marketing. Noting the important contributions that some of these research traditions had made (e.g. Roger's theories on the diffusion of innovations [23]), they also summarize several common limitations. These include the primary focus on the individual innovation and the individual adopter as the unit of analysis, and the implicit assumption that the findings of diffusion research are transferable to different contexts and settings. As will be discussed later, context counts a great deal, not only when considering how to disseminate and implement interventions based on research, but also in the design of the interventions and in the evaluation of their efficacy and effectiveness [26].

The next set of research traditions included development studies, in which the spread of innovations was viewed as pertaining to how appropriate a particular technology and/or idea is for particular situations at particular stages of development. Thus, for example, many high-end cancer control technologies developed in high income countries may have little or no meaning to, or applicability in, low income or even middle income countries. Moreover, the contextual fit between the innovation and the system that is asked to adopt it may be more important than the fixed properties of the innovation itself. Also included in this group of research traditions were health promotion and evidence-based medicine, with both research traditions evolving from one-way knowledge transfer models to more interactive partnerships between research producers and research users, as well as system and organizational change approaches to the adoption of innovations [23].

The final set of research traditions summarized by Greenhalgh et al. [25], come from the organizational and management literature and include: (1) studies of the structural determinants of innovation in organizations, (2) studies of the process, context, and culture of organizations, (3) inter-organizational studies, (4) knowledge-based approaches to organizational innovation, (5) narrative organizational studies, and (6) complexity studies derived from systems theory.

Given the scope and heterogeneity of the literature stemming from these different research traditions, there are three approaches to sorting through the breadth and depth of research on dissemination and implementation science. The one developed by Greenhalgh et al. [25] was entitled a meta-narrative review where the authors attempted to unfold the storyline of research from each scientific tradition and then compared and contrasted the storylines. While this did lead them to develop a conceptual model, they acknowledged that different researchers could generate a different set of literature and thus generate different storylines leading to a different conceptual framework.

Another method is to focus on a particular approach to knowledge translation and systematically review the empirical research from that tradition alone. Bero et al. [27] conducted a review of systematic evidence reviews of interventions to promote the implementation of research findings. Reviewing literature published from 1966 to 1995, they identified 18 systematic evidence reviews from which they categorized a number of broad strategies to promote the implementation of research findings. These included: (1) dissemination and implementation of clinical guidelines, (2) continuing medical education, and (3) particular strategies such as audit and feedback and computerized decision support systems. In general, more passive educational approaches were found to be generally ineffective and more specific strategies with greater intensity appeared more effective than more general approaches.

Looking at clinical practice guidelines as an example, guidelines have been developed as a strategy for translating clinical research findings in order to improve the quality of care. Cancer clinical practice guidelines have been developed and/or disseminated by many professional organizations (e.g. American Society of Clinical Oncology, European Society of Medical Oncology), government agencies (e.g. the National Cancer Institute, and the Agency for Healthcare Research and Quality in the United States), as well as independent organizations such as the National Quality Forum and the National Cancer Center Network in the United States, and the National Institute for Health and Clinical Excellence (NICE) in the United Kingdom. Clinical practice guidelines are being increasingly used to set practice standards [28], however the extent to which these standards are adopted is related both to the number and diversity of guidelines published, and the strategies used to disseminate and implement clinical practice guidelines.

With respect to the number and diversity of guidelines published, searching the US National Guidelines Clearinghouse [29], using the search term cancer, produced a listing of 847 related guidelines on a diverse set of cancer conditions, from a wide range of international sources. Narrowing the search to guidelines published between 2006 and 2008, focused on adult cancer treatment only, reduced the listing down to 204 related guidelines, but often representing more than one guideline for the same cancer condition from different international oncology organizations. This heterogeneity in cancer guidelines reflects different approaches to the development, structure, users, and end points of guidelines and suggests that without a systematic evaluation of their impact on health care practice their utility in broadly influencing cancer care remains largely unknown [30].

With respect to strategies used to disseminate and implement clinical practice guidelines, Grimshaw et al. [24] focused on a systematic literature review of research centred on the effectiveness and efficiency of clinical practice guideline dissemination and implementation strategies. A total of 235 studies, reporting 309 comparisons met the study inclusion criteria. In evaluating the quality of the studies, the authors judged them overall to be poor. Commonly evaluated single interventions included practitioner reminders, dissemination of educational materials, and audit and feedback. Seventy-three per cent of the comparisons involved multi-faceted interventions. For example, there were 23 comparisons of multi-faceted interventions that involved educational outreach. The majority of interventions observed modest to moderate improvements in care.

Thus, for example, there was a 14.1 per cent median absolute improvement for reminders, 8.1 per cent for dissemination of educational materials, 7 per cent improvement observed for audit and feedback, and 6 per cent for multi-faceted interventions involving educational outreach. No relationship was found between the number of intervention components and the effect of multi-faceted interventions.

From a practice perspective, there is limited research evidence available to support health system decisions about which guideline dissemination and implementation strategies are likely to be most effective within different service delivery contexts. Also, a relatively small percentage of studies and intervention comparisons (29.4 per cent) reported any economic data to help evaluate the cost-effectiveness of different guideline and dissemination/implementation approaches. From a research perspective, it was suggested that more studies are required to validate existing theories of health professional and organizational behaviour and behaviour change, to collect and analyze cost data, to develop and validate new and more coherent conceptual frameworks, and to estimate the effectiveness and efficiency of dissemination and implementation strategies in the varying contexts of barriers, facilitators, and modifiers of the effects of guideline adoption. Chapter 8 describes several examples from Canada and Europe of how guidelines are being expanded beyond the clinical practice context to influence health systems policies, and how users of guidelines are partnering with producers of guidelines to make them more 'locally' relevant.

As Graham et al. noted in their proposed framework for knowledge to action, there is no dearth of theories, models, and frameworks for taking the lessons learned from science and translating them into action [19]. In reviewing over 60 theories or frameworks, Graham et al. identified a number of commonalities among them. They included: (1) identifying a problem that needs addressing, (2) identifying, reviewing, and selecting the knowledge or research relevant to the problem, (3) adapting the knowledge or research to the local context, (4) assessing the barriers to using the knowledge, (5) selecting, tailoring, and implementing interventions to promote the use of the knowledge, (6) monitoring its use, (7) evaluating the outcomes of knowledge use, and (8) sustaining ongoing knowledge use. The knowledge to action process framework proposed by Graham et al. [19] incorporates three stages of knowledge creation (inquiry, synthesis, and tools production), in addition to the eight elements of the action cycle described earlier. This knowledge to action framework has been adopted by the Canadian Partnership Against Cancer (see Figure 5.3) as its framework for knowledge management related to cancer prevention and control [31].

The wide variety of conceptual frameworks that have been proposed for summarizing the many and varied processes of translating the lessons learned from science into practice, and vice-versa, combined with confusing diversity of terminology have contributed to the difficulties for the field to move forward and gain consensus on basic principles of knowledge translation (KT). Some frameworks focus on the individual decision maker, others look at the organizational context in which innovations may take place, while others view the process of integrating science with service from more of a complex systems perspective.

At the individual decision maker level, decision analysis has been proposed as a means of closing the gap between research and practice [32]. Thus, knowledge from research is based on scientific experiments, controlled clinical trials, and epidemiological studies, while knowledge used in practice is largely based on personal experience and from peers. It is posited that practitioners will respond quickly to new information from research when the research addresses issues close to the practice interests. However, since research is more often focused on uncovering 'truth' and researchers tend to put insufficient emphasis on the practical application of their work, research findings may be a priori rejected by practitioners as irrelevant to their service interests.

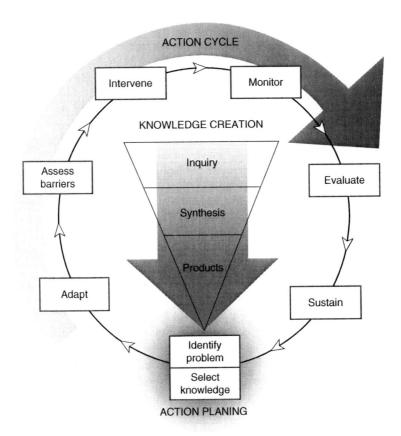

Fig. 5.3 Canadian partnership against cancer: knowledge to action framework.
Adapted from '*Lost in Knowledge Translation: Time for a Map?*' Graham et al. [19], with permission.

Thus, if new research/practice/policy partnerships can be developed, recognizing the legitimate differences between the tasks faced by practitioners and policy makers and those faced by researchers, then a shared decision-making model for integrating science with service may be possible.

From an organizational and systems perspective, some frameworks conceptualize the process as relatively linear, starting with research and ending up with adoption and institutionalization [33,34]. But even in the two linear frameworks referenced here, the end points of the process are viewed somewhat differently. In the Davis et al. framework [33], after stage 4 where an innovation becomes integrated into the routine and continuing practices and policies of the social system in which it was implemented, stage 5 is framed as diffusion of the innovation spreading to other social systems [23]. In contrast, Khoury et al. [34] discuss implementation, dissemination, and diffusion research as a third step in a continuum of translation research, with the final step (T4) focusing on outcomes research evaluating the impact of the adoption of the practice on health outcomes.

In the absence of a large body of dissemination, implementation, and knowledge translation research specific to cancer control, it may be important for cancer research funding agencies, concerned with getting more of their cancer control science to influence practice and policy, to increase funding of both observational studies of natural experiments in the diffusion and dissemination of prevention, early detection and treatment innovations, as well as dissemination, implementation and knowledge translation intervention studies to test specific elements of the many aforementioned theoretical frameworks that populate the broader health and organizational management literature. However, whether cancer research funding agencies can break with their 'addiction' to funding discovery research in order to fund more delivery research is an open question that current funding priorities suggest will be a great challenge.

What practitioners and policymakers want from science

To understand what practitioners and policymakers want from science, it is important to delineate the diverse audiences that make up these two classes of potential users of information generated by science. In the public health practice community, there are public health practitioners, whose focus is usually on promoting health and preventing chronic diseases like cancer within defined populations. Public health practice may be supported by government agencies and non-government organizations at local, state or provincial, or national levels. Within the context of government-funded public health services, what public health practitioners want from science may or may not align with what local, state or provincial, or national policymakers look for from science.

Within clinical practice, there are primary care practitioners who may also focus on disease prevention, but usually are concerned with dealing with both infectious illness and/or diagnosing and treating conditions (e.g. high blood pressure, rectal bleeding) presented by individual patients that increase the risk of developing or dying from chronic diseases like cancer. Moreover, primary care clinical practitioners are quite different from specialty care clinical practitioners, in that the former tend to deal with the whole person while the latter tend to focus on the specific illness or condition presented by the patient. Thus, in the primary care practice context, integrating the lessons learned from science with the lessons learned from practice may be more challenging because of the many and varied health conditions and illnesses confronted in everyday practice for which new research information is emerging on almost a daily basis.

For cancer care specialists, the scientific literature is more focused on specific cancers and/or modalities of diagnosis and treatments. On the one hand this can make the dissemination of scientific discoveries into practice simpler, because there is greater homogeneity of the clinical issues being addressed. On the other hand, given that much of the research on medical, radiological, and even surgical approaches to cancer care is conducted in relatively resource-rich academic environments, the dissemination potential of new cancer care technologies may be limited by the variation in resources within the diverse clinical care environments in which cancer patients are diagnosed and treated.

A key point made by Lomas [35] in his discussion of consensus recommendations as evidence for clinical practice, is that the messenger of the evidence may be as important as the message about the evidence. Thus, Lomas notes that in constituting panels to review evidence, medical specialty societies tend to constitute panels made up of clinical experts; research councils, universities, and research funding agencies favour scientific experts; and public foundations and government-sponsored panels are more likely to include non-experts in the content being reviewed. Thus, if the audiences to be reached with scientific evidence reviews include community practitioners and decision-makers, then ensuring visible representation of their viewpoints in consensus panels may be critical to the acceptability of the messages being disseminated. This specific observation for consensus panels has broader implications for ensuring that the messenger of the evidence is credible to the audiences to whom the evidence-based message is directed.

Moreover, engaging the practice and policy audiences of scientific evidence as to the best approaches to getting the research information to them in a form that is most likely to be assimilated increases the probability that new research evidence will be acted upon. Both detailing, as practiced by pharmaceutical representatives, and automated feedback to practitioners are methods that demonstrate that when feedback can be tailored to the individual practitioner and his/her practice context, the uptake and use of this new evidence is increased [36]. The challenge of tailoring messages to individual practice and policy decision-makers, and the contexts in which they work, is complex and resource intensive given the diversity which exists in the public health, clinical practice, and health policy contexts for health in general and cancer control in particular.

Turning to the public policy context, one of the most extensive studies of how academic research is used by which decision-makers in national and provincial government agencies was conducted by Rejean Landry and associates at the University of Laval in Quebec, Canada [37]. Landry et al. used survey study findings to answer three questions: (1) To what extent is academic research used in government agencies? (2) Are there differences across policy domains in regard to the extent of its use? (3) What determines use of academic research in government agencies? In the sample of 833 mail survey respondents (35 per cent response rate), 25 per cent of the sample represented agencies in the Canadian federal government while the remaining 75 per cent represented provincial government agencies with good geographic spread across Canada. With respect to types of agencies represented, 27 per cent of the respondents were in economic development, public finance, and taxation agencies; 18 per cent were in social services, health, and social security, 13 per cent worked in municipal and regional affairs, 11 per cent in environment, forestry, fishing and agriculture, 11 per cent in job creation and employment conditions, 9 per cent in education, communication, and technology, 9 per cent in language, culture, immigration, justice, and native affairs, and two per cent in other domains.

Looking across the six stages of knowledge utilization (1-reception, 2-cognition, 3-discussion, 4-reference, 5-adoption, 6-influence) [38], and across all types of agencies represented in the sample, approximately 12 per cent of respondents reported usually or always receiving academic research pertinent to their work and 9 per cent reported that the research received usually or always influenced decisions in their administrative units. Looking within the policy domains described earlier, the use of academic research reached its highest self-report levels in the domains of education and information technology, followed closely by social services, health, and social security.

In the social services, health, and social security domain the factors that increased the likelihood that academic research information would be utilized included: (1) acquisition efforts (e.g. personally making an effort to establish relationships with university researchers); (2) linkage mechanisms (e.g. meetings with colleagues in the respondent's field, congresses, conferences, scientific seminars involving university researchers); (3) user's context (e.g. university research results are considered pertinent by colleagues, university research work, studies, and reports reached the respondent at just the right time to be used). Across all policy domains, user's context was the best predictor of utilization of academic research information. User's acquisition efforts, linkage mechanisms, and adaptation of research products for users were also good predictors across all domains. However, of potential interest and relevance to cancer control and health policy domains, adaptation of research products to users was not a significant predictor of self-reported research information utilization in the social services, health, and social security domain.

Looking across all policy domains, Landry et al. come to several broad conclusions and make several broad recommendations to increase the utilization of academic research in public policy domains. First, the types of research (e.g. quantitative vs. qualitative) conducted to produce the research finding were not that important in predicting what research was utilized. Similarly, research focused on the advancement of scholarly knowledge was not a good predictor of the uptake of academic research. Thus, neither was considered a good lever for increasing the uptake of academic research in policy contexts. Second, the finding that user context positively influenced research information use means that the uses of research findings are contingent on the specific situation of the user. This creates a challenge for researchers and users alike to bridge the gap between a research discovery context and a policy decision-making application context. Finally, the importance of encouraging users to find and use research, expanding linkages between researchers and research users, and academics' efforts to tailor research products to users' needs and their context for action all lend themselves to interventions to increase the links between the lessons learned from science with the lessons learned from practice and policy.

Bridging communities of research, practice, and policy: context counts

As noted previously, one of the research frameworks to understand the role of context is from the organizational change literature as applied to the adoption of innovations [25]. For example, a study of the variation in adoption of respiratory diagnostic and treatment innovations in US hospitals, published over 30 years ago, continues to provide some important clues into the role of context in explaining the extent of hospital adoption of clinical innovations [39]. Looking at the adoption of 11 innovations for monitoring and treatment of patients with respiratory diseases in a sample of 295 hospitals surveyed, three sets of mechanisms that hospitals could use to expand the integration of new research-tested innovation information were examined: (1) extra-organizational mechanisms (e.g. hospital support for physician travel to external scientific meetings), (2) internal mechanisms (e.g. hospital support for outside speakers to present), and (3) joint mechanisms (e.g. hospital physician participation in research and publication).

A key contextual difference between the US hospitals in the study was whether or not they had a respiratory disease specialty care unit (i.e. department of inhalation therapy). Those hospitals with a specialty care unit on average adopted 5.84 of the 11 innovations assessed, while those hospitals without such a unit adopted a significantly smaller number of innovations (3.04). While this difference is not surprising, the factors that were correlated with the number of innovations adopted differed somewhat between the two groups of hospitals. While the number of paid outside speakers was positively correlated with adoption of innovation in both sets of hospitals, in hospitals with specialty care units the only other correlate of innovation uptake was hospital reimbursement for physicians participating in outside meetings. This factor was not a significant correlate of uptake in hospitals without a specialty care unit, but physician participation in laboratory research and physician publication were both significant correlates of the uptake of innovations in hospitals without a specialty care unit. The authors speculate that in hospitals with specialty care units the staff attending professional meetings act as conduits for and repositories of new technologies. In hospitals without specialty care units, physicians participating in research and publication may be more important because research is relatively less prevalent in these settings.

If these findings can be generalized beyond respiratory care, the implications for the adoption of innovations in cancer care are worth considering. For example, in the United States between 10 to 15 per cent of patients are estimated to receive their care in academic medical centres with specialty cancer care units [40]. An unknown percentage receives care in relatively high resource community hospital settings, again with specialty care units, and the remaining percentage receives care in resource-limited health care settings without specialty cancer care units. Thus, to increase the spread of cancer care innovations across these three different cancer care contexts, different approaches may be needed. Short of requiring that all cancer patients be seen in hospitals with specialty cancer care facilities, expanding research/practice partnerships in resource-limited health care settings may be a critical conduit for increasing the adoption of evidence-based practices in these contexts and thus reducing the disparities in outcomes experienced by the medically underserved.

To foster more research/practice partnerships, as well as research/policy partnerships, it is important to recognize the philosophical conflicts that exist between scientists versus practitioners and policy makers. The practitioner and policy maker are often under time pressure to act immediately, to solve complex problems with limited information, and to make judgments on whatever knowledge is available at the time. Conversely, scientists are trained to reserve judgment until all the data are in and analyzed, to test and refine hypotheses, to isolate variables and hold contextual conditions constant, and to continuously reinterpret observations and revise theories as new data become available [41]. There are often differences between the questions that interest practitioners and policy makers and the questions that interest researchers, and a variety of skills are required to communicate in common sense terms the findings from research and apply research to practical problems. To close the philosophical gap between research, practice, and policy, investments of time and energy need to be made by scientists, practitioners, and policy makers to help create a new 'culture' of trans-disciplinary collaboration.

Thus, research is more likely to have an impact on policy and practice when those involved in policy or practice have been involved in planning the research; and in these circumstances the results of the research are more likely to be reported directly to the relevant decision-makers. To foster a culture of trans-disciplinary collaboration new models of funding research/practice/policy partnership relationships rather than just specific research projects need to be developed. These can provide the longer term commitment to shared research priority setting which can enhance the chances that the findings will be influential. Finally, there is an advantage to developing context-specific local research initiatives in that these allow a much clearer linkage between research, practice, and policy [42].

To the extent that evidence-based medicine is focused on accelerating knowledge transfer from science into practice, it is also important to recognize that practitioners are not 'blank disks' waiting for the latest research findings to be downloaded into their 'RAMs'. Rather practitioners are subject to powerful contextual influences in their local practice environments. In broad terms Lomas [43] articulated these influences to include educational, administrative, personal, patient-based, community-based, and economic. Thus, even when research information has been synthesized and disseminated (e.g. as practice guidelines) by a credible body, its impact is likely to be limited to awareness, attitude, and perhaps new knowledge. However, for practice to change, implementation efforts must be made that are coordinated with the various contextual factors within which practitioners operate.

A very well delineated conceptual framework (see Figure 5.4) to coordinate the introduction of evidence-based approaches into cancer control practice contexts has been developed by the Cancer Prevention and Control Research Network jointly funded by the US Department of Health and Human Services (DHHS) Centers for Disease Control and Prevention (primarily focused on supporting evidence-based practice) and the DHHS National Institutes of Health National Cancer Institute (primarily focused on supporting cancer control research) [44]. The Cancer Prevention and Control Research Network (CPCRN) provides an infrastructure for applying relevant research to local cancer prevention and control needs. Its members conduct

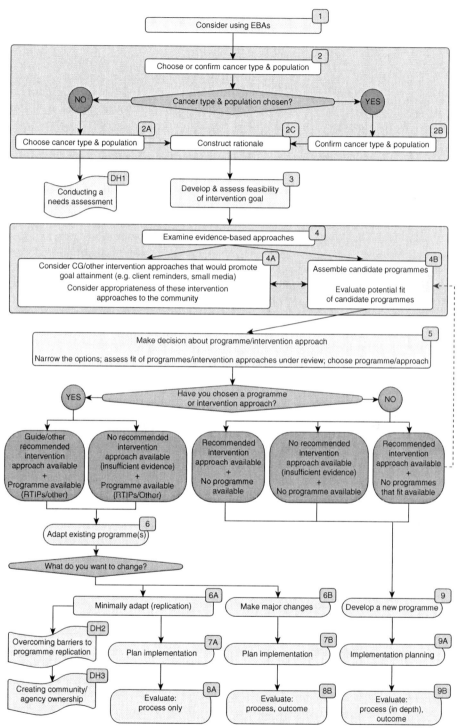

Fig. 5.4 Conceptual framework for adapting evidence-based approaches (EBA) to real-world contexts. From Fernandez ME et al. and the Cancer Prevention and Control Research Network, Evidence-based Approaches, workgroup [45], with permission.

community-based participatory cancer research across its eight network centres, crossing academic affiliations and geographic boundaries.

The conceptual framework is the basis of a new training programme for integrating evidence into practice entitled TACTIC (Tailored Assistance for Choosing Tested cancer control tools In Communities). As outlined in Figure 5.3 there are nine modules in the training programme: (1) deciding to use evidence-based approaches; (2) focusing on a cancer and a population (2a, 2b, 2c); (3) creating programme goals and objectives; (4) finding evidence-based programmes and approaches (4a & 4b); (5) choosing a programme or intervention approach; (6) programme adaptation; (7) implementation planning; (8) evaluation; and (9) programme development. As such, TACTIC can be seen as a set of decision support tools for community-based cancer control planners, decision-makers, and practitioners [45].

Whatever decision support tools may be made available for cancer control, there are many types of intervention programmes and intervention approaches from which to choose, with different levels of evidence applied to each. Exemplar questions that programme staff and policy makers often face when deciding how best to address a cancer control problem are: (1) Which programme or intervention approach has the strongest evidence of efficacy and effectiveness? (2) Which programme or approach has the best fit for the service delivery context in which we are operating? (3) Which programme or approach can most easily be adapted to improve the fit in our service delivery context or to meet the needs of our target populations? (4) How much flexibility do we have to adapt the programme or the approach without seriously undermining the impact on outcomes? (5) Which programme or intervention approach can we afford to implement within the resource base of our service delivery context? Researchers may be inclined to focus more on the first question while practitioners may be sensitive to the more practical questions 2 to 5 [2].

Recognizing that the answers to some of these questions may be in conflict with the answers to others, it should be recognized that for every context there is balance that must be reached between, for example, implementing an intervention with fidelity to ensure positive outcomes, and adaptation to help increase the contextual fit and implementation feasibility in real world settings. There is debate around the issue of implementation fidelity versus programme adaptation. Some argue that implementing the interventions with fidelity is the best way, perhaps the only way, to ensure comparable outcomes [46]. Adapting the intervention to help with contextual fit could be considered later, as long as core intervention elements were preserved intact. Others point out that unless programme implementers were able to adapt the intervention a priori to address contextual and population fit, and perhaps imbue a sense of programme ownership of the evidence-based intervention being implemented, there would be a much lower likelihood of initiating implementation in the first place.

Conceptual frameworks (like TACTIC) for engaging researchers, practitioners and policy-makers in working through a set of shared decisions about what research evidence is most relevant to the issues at hand that need to be addressed, may provide the greatest hope from moving away from passive diffusion and dissemination approaches, into knowledge exchange models that encourage an active dialogue and partnership between the producers of research evidence and the users of research evidence. However for such partnerships to be formed and sustained, all parties in the research, practice, policy cycle of knowledge to action and action back to knowledge must be provided the time to engage in these knowledge exchange partnerships and must be rewarded for their efforts in this regard. There are few if any incentives built into the academic, practice, or policymaking contexts that currently exist to support such a culture change. Absent such changes in priority setting and professional time management, the prospects for building and sustaining research/practice/policy partnerships are limited.

Conclusions

Cancer control practice and policies within and across countries can more quickly benefit from the substantial investment made in fundamental, intervention, and health services research if research and practice funding agencies, professional organizations, and policymakers commit to working together to close the gap between what we know and what we do. The balance between the enormous investments made in fundamental discovery research compared with the much more modest investments made in the more applied sciences, including dissemination and implementation research, must be re-evaluated if the lessons learned from science are to be better integrated with the lessons learned from practice and policy.

Expanded investments in dissemination and implementation research must be made if the process of integrating science with service is to be based on more than just who we know but also on what we know or need to know about these complex processes. In addition, intervention development and health services research on emerging cancer prevention and control technologies, based on discoveries from fundamental research, should reach out to the public health and clinical practice communities to engage them as partners in this applied research, rather than treating them as simply passive audiences waiting for the next novel technology to be handed to them. These participatory practice-based research approaches are particularly important in low and moderate income countries or regions, so that the dissemination and implementation potential of novel approaches to the prevention, diagnosis, and treatment of cancer can be considered early on in the intervention development and testing process. Without such participatory partnership approaches, the introduction of new technologies with limited dissemination potential will almost always exacerbate health disparities.

Finally, new models for research/practice/policy partnerships need to be developed, tested, and supported for those approaches that are shown to increase knowledge exchange and the adoption of evidence-based cancer prevention and control strategies. As communities of practice (COPs) are formed for international cancer control, supporting trans-disciplinary membership in these COPs, and supporting knowledge exchange forums among researchers, practitioners, and policymakers, can provide important exemplars for efforts within countries to increase the integration of science and service, and to accelerate the translation of knowledge into action.

References

1 Kerner J (2006). Knowledge translation versus knowledge integration: A funder's perspective. *J of Continuing Education in the Health Professions*, **26**:72–80.

2 Kerner J (2008). Integrating research, practice and policy: What we see depends on where we stand. *Journal of Public Health Management and Policy*, **14**(2):193–98.

3 Dopson S & Fitzgerald L (2005).The active role of context. In Dopson S, Fitzgerald L (eds) *Knowledge to Action? Evidence-based Health Care in Context*. pp. 79–103. Oxford University Press, Oxford.

4 Green LW (2007). The prevention research centers as models of practice-based evidence; two decades on. *Am J Prev Med*, **33**(1S):S6–S8.

5 Balas EA & Boren SA (2000). Managing clinical knowledge for health care improvement. *Yearbook of Medical Informatics*, pp. 65–70.

6 Burton R, Fitch M, Given LS, et al (2006). Planning. In Sepulveda C (ed) *Cancer Control – Knowledge into Action; WHO Guide for Effective Programmes; Module 1*. World Health Organization, Geneva.

7 Bekic AJ, Bhadrasian V, Black B, et al (2005). *National cancer control planning resources for non-governmental organizations*. International Union Against Cancer, Geneva.

8 Kerner JF, Myers B, Guirguis-Blake J, et al (2005). Translating research into improved outcomes in comprehensive cancer control. *Cancer Causes & Control*, **16**(Suppl. 1):27–40.

9 The Committee on cancer control in low- and middle-income countries board on global health (2007). *Cancer control opportunities in low- and middle-income countries.* Sloan FA, Gelband H (eds). National Academies Press, Washington, D.C.

10 Canadian Cancer Research Alliance (2006). *Cancer Research Investment in Canada: The Canadian Cancer Research Alliance's Survey of Government and Voluntary Sector Investment in Cancer Research in 2006.* CCRA, Toronto.

11 Kravitz RL (2005). Doing things better vs. doing better things. *Annals of Family Medicine,* 3(6):483–85.

12 Batista RN (1989). Innovation and diffusion of health-related technologies. *Int J. of Technology Assessment in Health Care,* 5:227–48.

13 National Library of Medicine, National Institutes of Health PubMed. *Cancer.* Available at: http://www. ncbi.nlm.nih.gov/sites/entrez (accessed 10 July 2008).

14 Berwick DM (2003). Disseminating innovations in health care. *JAMA,* 289(15):1969–75.

15 Woloshin S & Schwartz LM (2006). What's the rush? The dissemination and adoption of preliminary research results. *JNCI,* 98(6):372–3.

16 Woolf SH & Johnson RE (2005). The break-even point: when medical advances are less important than improving the fidelity with which they are delivered. *Annals of Family Medicine,* 3(6):545–52.

17 Grimshaw JM, Santesso N, Cumpston M, Mayhew A, & McGowan J (2006). Knowledge for knowledge translation: the role of the Cochrane collaboration. *J Cont Educ in the Health Professions.* 26:55–62.

18 World Health Organization (2005). *Knowledge Management Strategy.* WHO, Geneva.

19 Graham ID, Logan J, Harrison MB, et al (2006). Lost in knowledge translation: time for a map? *J of Cont Educ in the Health Professions.* 26:13–24.

20 Rabin BA, Brownson RC, Haire-Joshu D, Kreuter MW, & Weaver NL (2008). A glossary for dissemination and implementation research in health. *J Public Health Manage Pract,* 14(2):117–123.

21 Ellis P, Robineson P, Ciska D, et al (2003). *Diffusion and dissemination of evidence-based cancer control interventions.* Evidence Report/Technology Assessment Number 79. (Prepared by McMaster University Evidence Practice Center under Contract 290-97-0017). AHRQ Publication No. 03-E033. Agency for Healthcare Research and Quality, Rockville.

22 Rabin BA, Glasgow RE, Kerner JF, Klump PM, Kreuter MW, & Brownson RC (in Review). Dissemination and implementation research on community-based cancer prevention: a systematic review. *Am J Prev Med,*

23 Rogers EM (2003). *Diffusion of Innovations,* 5th edn. Free Press, New York.

24 Grimshaw JM, Thomas RE, Maclennan G, et al (2004). Effectiveness and efficiency of guideline dissemination and implementation strategies. *Health Technol Assess,* 8(6):1–72.

25 Greenhalgh T, Robert G, Macfarlane F, & Bate P, Kyriakidou O (2004). Diffusion of innovations in service organizations: systematic review and recommendations. *Milbank Q,* 82(4):581–629.

26 Glasgow RE, Lichtenstein E, & Marcus AC (2003). Why don't we see more translation of health promotion research to practice? Rethinking the efficacy-to-effectiveness transition. *AJPH,* 93(8):1261–67.

27 Bero LA, Grilli R, Grimshaw JM, et al (1998). Closing the gap between research and practice: an overview of systematic reviews of interventions to promote the implementation of research findings. *BMJ,* 317:465–68.

28 Wolff AC & Desch CE (2005). Clinical practice guidelines in oncology: translating evidence into practice (and back). Available at: http://jop.ascopubs.org *J Oncology Practice,* pp. 160–61 (accessed July 29, 2008).

29 National Guideline Clearinghouse. http://www.guideline.gov (accessed July 29, 2008).

30 Pentheroudakis G, Stahel R, Hansen H, Pavlidis N (2008). Heterogeneity in cancer guidelines: should we eradicate or tolerate? *Ann Oncol,* Jul 28 [Epub ahead of print].

31 Canadian Partnership Against Cancer (2008). *Annual Report 2007–2008.* CPACC, Toronto, Ontario.

32 Dowie J (1996). The research-practice gap and the role of decision analysis in closing it. *Health Care Analysis*, **4**:5–18.

33 Davis SM, Peterson JC, Helfrich CD, & Cunningham-Sabo L (2007). Introduction and conceptual model for utilization of prevention research. *Am J Prev Med*, **33**:S1–S5.

34 Khoury MJ, Gwinn M, Yoon PW, et al (2007). The continuum of translation research in genomic medicine: how can we accelerate the appropriate integration of human genome discoveries into health care and disease prevention. *Genetics in Medicine*, **9**(10):1–10.

35 Lomas J (1991). Words without action? The production, dissemination, and impact of consensus recommendations. *Ann Rev Public Health*, **12**:41–65.

36 Freemantle N & Watt I (1994). Dissemination: implementing the findings of research. *Health Libraries Review*, **11**:133–37.

37 Landry R, Lamari M, & Amara N (2003). The extent and determinants of the utilization of university research in government agencies. *Public Administration Review*, **63**(2):192–205.

38 Knott J & Wildavsky A (1980). If dissemination is the solution, what is the problem? *Knowledge: Creation, Diffusion, Utilization*, **1**(4):537–78.

39 Kimberly JR (1978). Hospital adoption of innovation: the role of integration into external informational environments. *J Health Social Behavior*, **19**:361–73.

40 Kerner JF & Coulter CH (1997). Partnerships for the delivery of cancer care. *HMO Practice*, **11**(2):56–8.

41 Chavis D, Stucky PE, & Wandersman A (1983). Returning basic research to the community, a relationship between scientist and citizen. *Am Psychol*, **38**(4):424–34.

42 Davis P & Howden-Chapman P (1996). Translating research finding into health policy. *Soc Sci Med*, **43**(5):865–72.

43 Lomas J (1993). Diffusion, dissemination, and implementation: Who should do what? *Annals of the New York Academy of Science*, **703**:226–37.

44 The Cancer Prevention and Control Research Network. Available at: http://www.cpcrn.org/ (accessed 31 January 2009).

45 Fernandez ME, Mullen PD, Kreuter M, Kegler M, & the CPCRN EBA Workgroup (Cancer Prevention and Control Research Network, Evidence-based Approaches). Development of a computer-based training and planning tool for increasing use of evidence-based approaches (EBAs) for cancer control. Poster presented to: American Society for Preventive Oncology, Bethesda. March 2008.

46 Elliott DS & Mihalic S (2004). Issues in disseminating and replicating effective prevention programmes. *Prevention Science*, **5**(1):47–53.

Chapter 6

The impact of immunization on cancer control: the example of HPV vaccination

Ann Burchell, Eduardo Franco[1]

Many types of cancer are aetiologically linked to infections with specific microbial agents. Taken together, such infections are responsible for about 18 per cent of all cancers worldwide and up to 25 per cent of cancers in developing nations [1]. Such a high attributable fraction is second only to that of tobacco smoking in cancer control. The realization that some cancers are caused by infectious agents means that vaccination can be considered as a primary prevention measure. Vaccination has substantial public health potential. No other preventive measure has such dramatic appeal, in terms of a successful track record in public health. Only vaccination has the ability to eliminate disease. Vaccination for cancer prevention has moved beyond theory and become a reality for two neoplastic diseases: liver cancer and cervical cancer. This chapter reviews briefly the role of infections as causal agents in cancer, describes anti-hepatitis B virus (HBV) immunization as the first cancer vaccine paradigm, and finally focuses on the latest paradigm of prophylactic vaccination against human papillomavirus (HPV) infection as the new front in cancer prevention.

Microbial aetiology of cancer and the example of HBV vaccination

Although many viruses, bacteria, and protozoan and metazoan parasites have been mentioned in the biomedical literature as potentially carcinogenic, conclusive epidemiologic and molecular evidence to date has been unequivocally demonstrated for only a few agents, relating to many forms of cancer. Simply finding pathologic or molecular evidence that an agent is present in the human host or that the latter was previously exposed to this agent is not sufficient to establish causation. The World Health Organization's International Agency for Research on Cancer (IARC) has developed valuable guidelines that can be used in deciding for policy purposes whether a biological, chemical, or physical agent (or an industrial process) can be deemed as causally related to cancer in humans. These guidelines are applied during expert review of the published evidence concerning a putative association. The conclusions of this process are published as part of IARC's monograph series on evaluation of carcinogenicity and can be accessed online in that agency's website (http://monographs.iarc.fr/ENG/Monographs/PDFs/index.php, accessed September 5, 2008).

Since its inception, the IARC monograph programme has evaluated several microbial agents. The list is summarized in Table 6.1. As shown, several infectious agents have been established as carcinogenic or probably carcinogenic to humans. For others, the evidence is less conclusive but

[1] Ann N. Burchell, PhD, Division of Cancer Epidemiology, McGill University; and Eduardo L. Franco, MD, DrPH, Professor of Epidemiology and Oncology, Director, Division of Cancer Epidemiology, McGill University, Montreal, Quebec, Canada.

Table 6.1 Microbial agents evaluated by the International Agency for Research on Cancer's monograph series with respect to the accumulated scientific evidence that they may cause cancer in humans

Monograph volume and year	Infectious agent	Evaluation	Group
59, 1994 [2]	Hepatitis B virus (HBV) (chronic infection)	Carcinogenic	1
	Hepatitis C virus (HCV) (chronic infection)	Carcinogenic	1
	Hepatitis D virus (HDV)	Not classifiable	3
61, 1994 [106]	Schistosoma haematobium	Carcinogenic	1
	Opistorchis viverrini	Carcinogenic	1
	Clonorchis sinensis	Probably carcinogenic	2A
	Schistosoma japonicum	Possibly carcinogenic	2B
	S. mansoni	Not classifiable	3
	O. felineus	Not classifiable	3
	Helicobacter pylori	Carcinogenic	1
64, 1995 [8]	Human papillomavirus (HPV) types 16 and 18	Carcinogenic	1
	HPVs types 31 and 33	Probably carcinogenic	2A
	HPVs, other types (except 6/11)	Possibly carcinogenic	2B
67, 1996 [107]	Human immunodeficiency virus (HIV) type 1	Carcinogenic	1
	Human T lymphotropic virus (HTLV) type I	Carcinogenic	1
	HTLV-II	Not classifiable	3
	HIV-2	Possibly carcinogenic	2B
70, 1997 [108]	Epstein-Barr virus (EBV)	Carcinogenic	1
	Human herpesvirus (HHV) type 8	Probably carcinogenic	2A
90, 2007 [16]	HPVs 16, 18, 31, 33, 35, 39, 45, 51, 52, 56, 58, 59, 66	Carcinogenic	1
	HPVs 6, 11	Possibly carcinogenic	2B
	HPV genus Beta	Possibly carcinogenic	2B

Groups 1, 2A, 2B, and 3 are the overall assessment, summarized as shown.

points to a possible carcinogenic role, whereas for some other agents the evidence is inconclusive. Among those for which the evidence is compelling are hepatitis B and C viruses (HBV and HCV; liver cancer), certain genotypes of human papillomavirus (HPV; cervical, anogenital, and oral cancers), Epstein-Barr virus (EBV; certain types of lymphomas and nasopharyngeal carcinoma), human T cell lymphotropic virus I (some forms of leukaemias), human immunodeficiency virus (HIV; AIDS-associated malignancies), human herpes virus 8 (HHV-8; Kaposi's sarcoma), *Helicobacter pylori* (stomach cancer and mucosa-associated lymphoid tissue lymphomas), *Schistosoma haematobium* (bladder cancer), and some forms of liver flukes (e.g. genus *Opistorchis*; liver cholangiocarcinoma). Altogether, it has been estimated that these agents cause 17.8 per cent of incident cancers worldwide (12.1 per cent, 5.6 per cent, and 0.1 per cent for viral, bacterial and parasitic infections, respectively) including as much as 5.2 per cent for HPV alone [1].

As shown in Table 6.1, the accumulated evidence for a causal role for chronic HBV infection in hepatocellular carcinoma was the first target among biological exposures assessed by the IARC monograph programme [2]. It is estimated that 54.4 per cent of global liver cancers are attributable to HBV, for a total of 340,000 cases in 2002 [1]. An HBV vaccine became commercially available in 1981 and was found to be highly efficacious in preventing chronic HBV carriage [3]. Further refinements to the vaccine preparation were made over the years, which also contributed to a reduction in production costs, thus making HBV vaccination affordable enough for inclusion in public health programmes. Long-term follow-up data from several countries has shown that symptomatic HBV infection is rare following vaccination, and that immunity persists for at least a decade [4].

British Columbia, Canada, was one of the first regions in North America to introduce universal HBV vaccination. In 1992, a school-based programme was initiated, offering HBV vaccine to all Grade 6 students (children aged 11 years). Following this introduction of adolescent vaccination, the annual incidence rate of acute hepatitis among those aged 12 to 20 years declined from 1.7 per 100,000 in 1992 to zero per 100,000 in 2001, suggesting elimination of HBV transmission within the targeted age group [5]. Similar impacts on rates of acute hepatitis B have been observed in other jurisdictions [4]. Furthermore, there is now evidence that HBV vaccination has the desired effect of preventing liver cancer. For example, a mass newborn vaccination programme was implemented in Taiwan in 1984, with later catch-up programmes for older children and adults [6]. Annual incidence rates of childhood (aged 6–14 years) hepatocellular carcinoma subsequently declined from 0.70 per 100,000 in 1981 to 1986 to 0.57 in 1986 to 1990, and further to 0.36 in 1990 to 1994. Mortality rates from childhood hepatocellular carcinoma also declined in the same period. The full impact of the Taiwanese programme will be verifiable once these vaccinated cohorts reach the peak age of onset of liver cancer.

The lessons learned from the implementation of HBV vaccination are extremely valuable as the first example of a successful prophylactic cancer vaccine. The rationale for adopting an HBV vaccine in clinical practice is simple; hepatitis B is an important disease in itself and is responsible for considerable morbidity and economic costs, even without factoring in the benefits in reduced risk of liver cancer later in life. However, affordability was an important issue; at $100 per course of immunization initially the vaccine was out of reach for most developing countries. Even in Western countries, cost considerations led to policies recommending immunization only of high-risk individuals and health workers, which unfortunately restricted the impact of vaccination to preventing only 5 per cent of the cases of liver cancer [7]. Subsequently, strong leadership by various agencies and the WHO permitted rapid technology transfer to multiple manufacturers, including those in developing countries. The end result was a remarkable reduction in vaccine production costs to about $1 per paediatric dose, which led to demonstration projects of mass immunization in several high-risk countries [7].

The experience with HBV vaccination has become particularly important also because we have now the opportunity to include a second cancer in the list of neoplastic diseases that can be prevented by immunization. Recently, two prophylactic vaccines against HPV infection have become available. HPV infection is recognized today as the necessary causal factor of all cervical cancer (squamous cell and adenocarcinomas) cases in the world, and the cause of a substantial proportion of many other anogenital neoplasms [8,9]. HPV has also been implicated in the genesis of head and neck cancer. The evidence for the oncogenic potential of HPV did not come easily, but resulted from a culmination of more than 25 years of vigorous multi-disciplinary research by molecular biologists, virologists, immunologists, clinicians, and epidemiologists. This realization paved the way for new exciting approaches for preventing cervical cancer, which is the second most common malignancy of women worldwide [10]. In the remaining of this chapter we summarize the scientific progress that led to the recognition of HPV as a cause of cervical and other cancers, the subsequent development of HPV vaccines, and how the implementation of these vaccines will result in a paradigm shift in the prevention and screening of HPV-related cancers.

The epidemiology of cervical cancer and HPV infection

Epidemiology of cervical cancer

Worldwide, cervical cancer is the second most common malignant neoplasm of women, accounting for nearly 10 per cent of all cancers (non-melanoma skin cancers excluded). It is estimated that 493,000 new cases of invasive cervical cancer were diagnosed in 2002, 83 per cent of which were in developing countries [10]. Cervical cancer can be characterized as a disease of poorer nations, with a disproportionate number of cases and the greatest proportion of deaths occurring in such regions. The highest risk areas for cervical cancer are in sub-Saharan Africa, Melanesia, the Caribbean, and Latin America, with average annual incidence rates above 30 per 100,000 women (rates standardized according to the world population of 1960) (Figure 6.1). Not surprisingly, in view of the substandard healthcare conditions, these areas also bear a disproportionately high mortality burden due to cervical cancer. Every year, an estimated 273,000 deaths from cervical cancer occur worldwide, with over three-fourths of them in developing countries [10].

One of the main reasons for the global heterogeneity in cervical cancer incidence and mortality is the implementation of Pap cytology screening in high-income countries over the past 50 years. In developed countries where universal organized or opportunistic screening was adopted, there was a 50 to 80 per cent reduction in cervical cancer rates [11]. Cervical cancer rates are now substantially lower in Western Europe and North America at less than 10 new cases annually per 100,000 women [12].

In developed countries, 66 per cent of women diagnosed with cervical cancer survive longer than five years whereas the 5-year survival rate in developing countries is less than 50 per cent [13]. The impact of this relatively low survival experience is increased by the fact that in high-fertility developing countries, cervical cancer generally affects women in the early post-menopausal years who often are the primary or sole caregiver for many school-age and teenage sons and daughters. The pre-mature loss of these mothers has a tremendous negative impact on the social structure of the local communities.

Epidemiology of HPV infection

The more than 100 HPV genotypes (types, for short) that have been catalogued so far are classified according to their DNA homology, which closely reflects tissue tropism (mucosal or cutaneous) and oncogenic potential [14]. About 40 types infect the epithelial lining of the anogenital tract and surfaces, as well as of other mucosal areas of the body, such as the upper aero-digestive tract. Among these mucosal HPVs, some 13 to 18 types have been identified as of probable or definite high-oncogenic risk (HR-HPV) on the basis of the frequency of association with cervical and other anogenital cancers and their pre-cancerous lesions. Over the years, the list of HR-HPVs has increased as a reflection of the continuous improvement in assay performance and the accumulated clinical literature on the distribution of HPV types in lesions from many parts of the world [15]. A recent conservative assessment by the IARC's Carcinogenicity Monograph Series referred to types 16, 18, 31, 33, 35, 39, 45, 51, 52, 55, 56, 58, 66 as HR-HPVs [16].

Infections with most mucosal HPV types that are not deemed as HR-HPVs are of no clinical consequence and cause no symptoms or visible lesions; such types are considered of

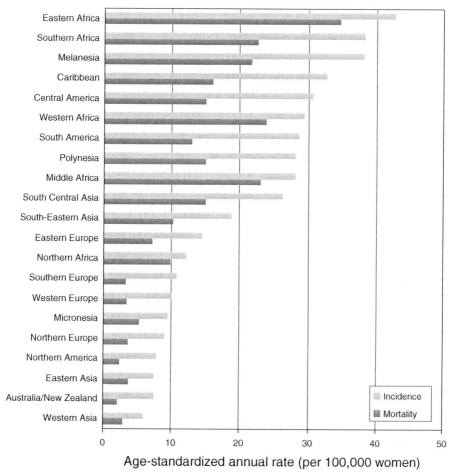

Fig. 6.1 Average annual incidence and mortality rates for cervical cancer by region, 2002. Standardization according to the age structure of world population of 1960.
Source: Globocan 2002 (Ferlay et al. [10]).

low-oncogenic risk (LR-HPV). Two LR-HPVs, however, HPVs 6 and 11, can cause benign lesions of the anogenital areas known as condylomata acuminata (genital warts), as well as a large proportion of low-grade squamous intraepithelial lesions (LSIL) of the cervix. Such LR-HPV infections are responsible for substantial morbidity and incur high costs associated with the treatment of the clinically relevant lesions. Perinatal transmission of HPV is also possible and can cause in rare instances recurrent respiratory papillomatosis in infants and young children [15].

Genital HPV infection is the most common sexually transmitted infection (STI) among women [17]. The prevalence of HPV infection varies greatly by age and by geography [18,19]. Among asymptomatic women in the general population or attending routine cervical cancer screening, prevalence rates are in the 2 per cent to 44 per cent range [15]. In a meta-analysis using data from 78 published studies, among women with normal cytology the age-adjusted global prevalence of any HPV type infection was 10.4 per cent, with considerable variation by age and region [19]. Prevalence was highest for young women and decreased in the middle age groups, followed by a second peak in prevalence in the older age groups. The two most common HPV types were HPV-16 (prevalence 2.5 percent) and HPV-18 (0.9 per cent).

HPV DNA has also been clearly identified in the male genitalia, anal mucosa, and oral cavity, but compared to women, fewer prevalence data exist. Depending on the population studied, sampling method and anatomic site, male genital HPV prevalence ranges from 0 to 73 per cent [20,21]. HR-HPV appears to occur in a higher proportion of male than in female infections [20]. Penile HPV prevalence increases with the number of sex partners and with the number of sex worker partners [21]. Men who have sex with men have been observed to have a particularly high prevalence of HPV [22].

Follow-up studies have documented high rates of HPV acquisition among young women; several studies have reported cumulative incidences of 40 per cent or greater after three years of follow-up [15]. High incidence among men has also been observed [21], although far fewer longitudinal studies have been conducted among males. Data supporting sexual intercourse as the primary route of genital HPV transmission include high incidence following sexual debut, documented transmission of genital warts between sex partners, concordance in sex partners for type-specific and HPV-16 variant-specific HPV DNA, the rarity of genital HPV infection in women who have not had vaginal intercourse, the strong and consistent associations between lifetime numbers of sex partners and HPV prevalence, and increased risk of HPV acquisition with new sex partners [23]. Many earlier studies did not observe a protective effect of condoms [24], but, in more recent studies specifically designed to address this question, consistent condom use does appear to reduce the risk of HPV infection [25,26].

Natural history of HPV infection and progression to cervical cancer

Following HPV acquisition, the natural history consists of either HPV clearance or development of a persistent HR-HPV infection and cervical neoplastic development. HPV infection triggers a slow process of disruption of the normal maturation of the transformation zone epithelium of the uterine cervix near its squamo-columnar junction [27]. This process of abnormal changes is initially limited to the cervical epithelium. These pre-invasive lesions, known in the old classifications as dysplasia or, more recently, as squamous intraepithelial lesions (SIL), can be discovered through cytological examination using the Papanicolaou technique ('Pap' screening test) and confirmed by colposcopic examination and biopsy as cervical intraepithelial neoplasia (CIN). They are invariably asymptomatic and if left untreated, they may eventually extend to the full thickness of the cervical epithelium (cervical carcinoma in situ (CIS)), and traverse the lining formed by the basement membrane to become invasive. This process may take a decade or longer but will eventually occur in a substantial proportion of CIS patients.

Although HPV infection is the central cause of cervical cancer, only a small percentage of women who are infected go on to develop cervical cancer or its precursors. Most HPV infections detected via molecular hybridization techniques are transient, and are no longer detectable within one to two years [15]. Even among women with persistent infection, HPV alone is not a sufficient cause and much work has been devoted to determining why certain HPV-positive women develop cervical cancer while others do not. The multi-factorial model of cervical cancer aetiology suggests an interplay of various cofactors. Smoking, high parity, long term use of oral contraceptives, co-infections and immunosuppression have been found to increase the risk of cervical cancer. Other factors such as genetic polymorphisms in the Human Leukocyte Antigen (HLA) system, polymorphisms in some oncogenes, nutrition, insulin-like growth factors (IGFs), and viral factors have also been identified as contributing to the overall cervical cancer risk [28].

Identification of the causal role of HPV in cervical carcinogenesis

Early on, cervical cancer was hypothesized to be related to sexual activity even before the advent of analytical epidemiologic studies. The simple premise was the widely held view that nuns did not develop this neoplasm whereas sex trade workers had an increased risk. Epidemiologic studies clearly identified specific sexual behaviours as key risk factors, such as age at first sexual inter-course and number of sexual partners [23]. During much of the 1960s and 70s, the consistency of epidemiologic findings pointing to a sexually-transmitted infection model propelled research efforts to identify the putative causal microbial agent or agents. Many sexually-transmitted agents were considered, and the herpes simplex virus (HSV-2), syphilis, gonorrhoea, and *Chlamydia trachomatis* were suspected. The evidence available at the time indicated that genital infection with HSV-2 was the most likely culprit. Although HSV was proven carcinogenic in vitro and in vivo, the evidentiary link to cervical cancer was mostly indirect [29].

In the 1980s the attention gradually turned to a new candidate, HPV, with the emergence of a consistent evidence base from molecular biology. Harald zur Hausen was the primary leader behind the long-standing hypothesis that proliferation of HPV in the cervical epithelium leads to disruption of cell maturation that develops as CIN, the pre-cancerous lesion; he was awarded the Nobel Prize in 2008 for this work. His initial insightful observations and experiments were made as early as in the late 1970s (reviewed in [30]). He and others subsequently conducted ground-breaking research that led to an understanding of how the early viral oncogenes E6 and E7 interfere with key regulators of the cell cycle, thus immortalizing cervical cells and preventing them from undergoing senescence and being lost by the normal exfoliation that regenerates the epithelium. The demonstration of this series of molecular events was essential for the scientific community to accept that HPV infection was the likely cause of cervical cancer, as shown in Figure 6.2.

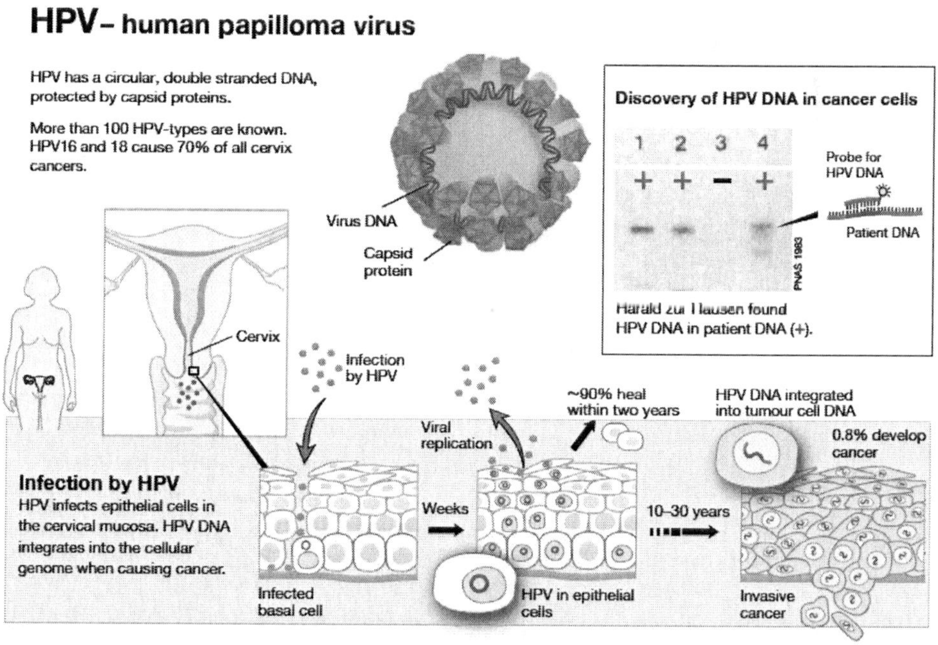

Fig. 6.2 Causation of cervical cancer by human papilloma virus.
Source: From The Nobel Foundation, 2008 in relation to the award of the Nobel Prize to H. zur Hausen (http://nobelprize.org/nobel_prizes/medicine/laureates/2008/press.html), with permission of the Nobel Foundation.

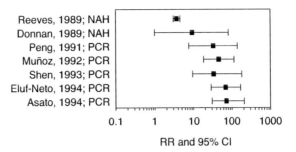

Fig. 6.3 Relative risks for associations between HPV and cervical cancer in case-control studies of first generation.

Abbreviations: NAH: non-amplified DNA hybridization; PCR: polymerase chain reaction; RR: relative risk; CI: confidence interval. Adoption of improved HPV DNA detection techniques such as PCR and better experience with laboratory procedures aiming at controlling contamination and other sources of measurement error led to a gradual increase in the RR estimates in successive studies.

Sources: Reeves et al. 1989 [109]; Donnan et al. 1989 [110]; Peng et al. [111]; Muñoz et al. 1992 [32]; Shen et al.1993 [112]; Eluf-Neto et al. 1994 [113]; & Asato et al. 1994 [114].

This acceptance did not come easily. There was much scepticism concerning the role of HPV infection. Reasons included observations that HPV infection was quite ubiquitous and, as such, it could not plausibly be a cause of disease. Contributing to the controversy were the weak to moderate associations that were observed in early molecular epidemiologic studies, unlike those one would expect from a key intermediate endpoint in cervical carcinogenesis (Figure 6.3). Later it was learned that measurement error in detecting cervical HPV DNA (thus leading to misclassification of the exposure) in these initial case-control studies had considerably underestimated the relative risk for the effect of HPV infection on cervical cancer (reviewed in [31]). As the experience with HPV DNA testing methodology led to the adoption of modern assays, such as polymerase chain reaction, the magnitude of the relative risks increased dramatically to near triple-digit point estimates (Figure 6.3).

It was a series of large and well-conducted case-control studies by the IARC using modern laboratory techniques that demonstrated that infection with certain HPV types is unequivocally one the one strongest cancer risk factor ever found (Figure 6.4) [32,33]. For example, the relative risk between tobacco and lung cancer is estimated between 7 and 15 [34], whereas the relative risk between HPV-16 and squamous-cell cervical cancer is 435 [32]. These studies also produced precise HPV type-specific estimates of relative risks, allowing for identification of specific types for prevention strategies [32,35].

In 1995, the IARC expert panel classified HPV 16 and 18 as 'Group 1, Human Carcinogens' in its Monograph series on carcinogenicity evaluation (Table 6.1) [8]. Following the 1995 IARC monograph was the recognition that HPV infection was not only the unequivocal central cause of cervical cancer but that it should also be viewed as a necessary cause [9]. No other cancer prevention paradigms (e.g. smoking-lung cancer, HBV-liver cancer) have this distinction [36]. Support for this assertion comes from the strong epidemiological evidence (Figures 6.3 and 6.4) and the detection of HPV DNA in up to 99.7 per cent of cervical cancers from all geographic areas [9,32,37,38]. As the evidence from new molecular epidemiologic studies came to light after 1995, the IARC decided to reconvene its HPV expert panel which resulted in an additional 11 HPV types to be classified as Group-1 carcinogens (Table 6.1) [16].

The empirical epidemiologic evidence concerning the carcinogenicity of different HPV types seen in the IARC studies [32] was consistent with what molecular virologists had predicted via phylogenetic relatedness analyses [39] and bioassays of oncogenic activity [40]. On the basis of the prevalence of the different HPV types in cervical cancers from different parts of the world it could be concluded that HPVs 16 and 18 were unequivocally the ones with the highest combined attributable proportion. HPV-16 is the most prevalent type causing approximately 54 per cent of cervical cancers worldwide, followed by HPV-18 which is associated with approximately 17 per cent of cervical cancers. As shown in Figure 6.5, in combination, HPV types 16 and 18 cause about 70 per cent of all cervical cancers [35]. Other HR types such as HPV-45, -31, and -33, albeit next in ranking, are responsible for less than 7 per cent of all cervical cancers, individually [41]. The ranking of the HR-HPV types shown in Figure 6.5 served as rationale for the development of the two initial prophylactic vaccines against HPV infection.

HPV vaccination

The human immune system is composed of an innate, non-specific component and an adaptive component. Adaptive immunity is conferred by a series of highly-specialized cells that process and prevent or eliminate specific pathogenic challenges. It may occur after either natural infection or vaccination, such that immunity is 'acquired'. Exposure to a particular pathogen or its antigen produces a primary immunological response involving B and T lymphocytes. This is

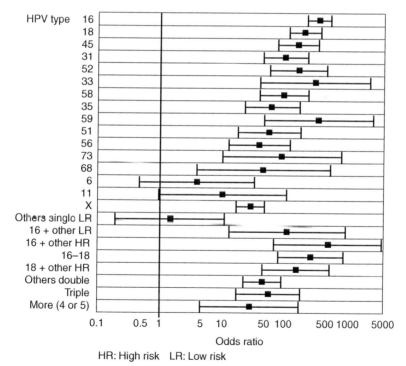

Fig. 6.4 Relative risks for the association between specific HPV types and invasive cervical cancer as estimated using the pooled data from the IARC case-control studies. These studies had improved HPV detection methods relative to the first generation of studies. In consequence, RR estimates are substantially higher than those in Figure 6.3.
Source of data: Muñoz et al. (2003).[33], reproduced with permission from HPV Today, issue no. 4, February 2004.

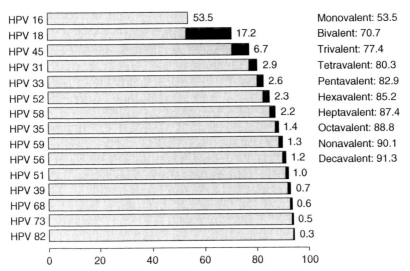

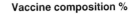

Fig. 6.5 Proportion of the global burden of invasive cervical cancers attributable to the incremental combination of different HPV types in a hypothetical prophylactic HPV vaccine of increasing valency. HPV 16 is the most common type, being detected in 53.5 per cent of all cervical cancers. The second most common type is HPV 18, at 17.2 per cent. Altogether, about 71 per cent of all cervical cancers are due to either HPV 16 or HPV 18, which forms the theoretical expectation for the preventive benefit from immunization with a bivalent HPV vaccine containing these two types. Source: Adapted with permission from Munoz et al. (2004). *Int J Cancer*. Aug 20. **111**(2):278–85.

followed by the development of immune memory cells, which can remember the pathogenic antigen and can launch a rapid protective response upon re-exposure.

A *vaccine* is a substance that contains antigen from a particular pathogen and is administered for the prevention or treatment of an infectious disease. Vaccine preparations may consist of live, attenuated, or killed micro-organisms or their antigenic proteins. Prophylactic vaccines aim to prevent infection by inducing neutralizing antibody response. Therapeutic vaccines aim to prevent proliferation of infected cells via cell-mediated immunity, thereby inducing regression. An ideal vaccine will provide at least the same degree and duration of protection as natural infection, without the accompanying clinical illness, with minimal side effects; and whose administration is simple, safe, acceptable, and cost-effective [4].

Development of HPV vaccine technology

As early as the 1980s, many laboratories worldwide were studying the immune response against HPV infection using linear epitopes, i.e. peptides derived from the nucleotide sequence of selected HPV genes that could be candidates for inducing a protective, neutralizing immune response. Today's successful prophylactic vaccines against HPV (see as follows) finally became a reality with the development of a technology that produces HPV virus-like particles (VLP) via expression of the major HPV capsid gene L1 in eukaryotic cell systems (yeast or insect cells). The expressed capsid protein self-assembles as pentamers and 72 of the latter spontaneously join to form a structure that resembles an intact HPV virion. The VLP does not contain the viral DNA and thus it is not infectious. However, the ordered arrangement of epitopes in the VLP makes this formulation highly immunogenic. The VLP technology has its roots in research by Robert Garcea in Colorado on polyomaviruses, which are closely related to HPVs [42,43]. Later, Zhou and colleagues in Brisbane, Australia, conducting work inspired and co-authored by Ian Frazer were the first to show in 1991 that the L1 (major) and L2 (minor) capsid genes of HPV 16, when expressed in a eukaryotic cell system, coded for the proteins that spontaneously self-assemble as VLPs [44]. Subsequently, the VLP technique was perfected and it was demonstrated that VLPs were highly immunogenic, inducing high titres of neutralizing antibodies. L1 alone can self-assemble into VLPs but L2 cannot; therefore, the first HPV vaccine candidates, including the current commercially available ones, consist of L1-based VLPs [45]. The historical account concerning the development of this research has been recently summarized by Frazer in a commentary [46].

The 1995 IARC monograph labelling HPV-16 and -18 as 'Group 1, Human Carcinogens' [8] gave pharmaceutical companies the needed body of evidence to allow them to take the financial risks in developing and field-testing candidate HPV vaccines. Variations of the L1-based VLP technology were subsequently adopted as formulations by Merck & Co., Inc. and GlaxoSmithKline Biologicals as candidate prophylactic vaccines against HPV in the mid-1990s. Following another decade of research and development, two highly efficacious vaccines that prevent HPV infection and cervical pre-cancers became available. These are Gardasil® (Merck & Co., Inc., NJ, USA) and Cervarix® (GlaxoSmithKline Biologicals, Rixensart, Belgium).

Table 6.2 describes the main characteristics of the two commercially available HPV vaccines. Cervarix® is a bivalent vaccine that targets the two HPV types (16 and 18) that are attributed to 70 per cent of cervical cancers worldwide. Gardasil® is a quadrivalent vaccine that targets types 16 and 18 as well as two additional types, 6 and 11, which are responsible for 90 per cent of genital warts. Both vaccines utilize recombinant technology to produce L1 VLPs but are based on different expression systems. The vaccines differ in their quantity of VLPs and their adjuvant systems. $AlSO_4$, the adjuvant used in Cervarix is supposed to yield an enhanced immunologic response with production of neutralizing antibodies [47]. The rationale behind the two vaccines also differs [48]. For the bivalent vaccine, the rationale was to focus on the oncogenic types 16 and 18 and produce a strong, sustained immune response. For the quadrivalent vaccine, the rationale was also to provide immunity to the two most important oncogenic types, and further to prevent infection with the two non-oncogenic types that cause most genital warts and recurrent respiratory papillomatosis.

Table 6.2 Characteristics of currently-available prophylactic human papillomavirus (HPV) vaccines

Characteristic	Cervarix®	Gardasil®
HPV types included	16, 18 (bivalent)	6, 11, 16, 18 (quadrivalent)
Dose of L1 protein	20/20 µg	20/40/40/20 µg
Expression system	Insect cells (baculovirus)	Yeast
Adjuvant	$AlSO_4$ (proprietary)	Aluminum hydroxy phosphate sulfate
Injection schedule	0, 1, 6 months (0.5 ml, intramuscular)	0, 2, 6 months (0.5 ml, intramuscular)
Follow-up data available	5.5 years (Phase II) 15 months (Phase III)	5 years (Phase II) 3 years (Phase III)

Clinical trial evidence for vaccine efficacy

Phase II and III randomized controlled trial results are available for both the bivalent and quadrivalent vaccines [49–54]. Because of the inherent differences in study designs and methods used by the two vaccine teams, it is a daunting task to summarize efficacy results for both virological and lesion endpoints. The following section and Table 6.3 provide a brief summary of interim results as of mid-2008. At this writing, all trials are still ongoing and final analyses have not yet been conducted. Recent in-depth reviews of the vaccine formulations, study methods, and trial findings have been published elsewhere [28,47,55–57]. In short, both vaccines have been proven to be highly efficacious.

The preventive impact of a vaccine is quantitatively expressed as 'vaccine efficacy', which is the percentage reduction in the number of cases among vaccinated individuals relative to placebo. An overview of vaccine efficacy results is provided in Table 6.3. The initial phase II trials were aimed at studying efficacy among healthy young women with no evidence of current or past infection with the HPV types included in the vaccine formulation. Exclusionary criteria for enrolment, randomization, and/or efficacy analysis included report of seven or more (bivalent) or five or more (quadrivalent) sex partners in lifetime, abnormal cytology (bivalent), presence of antibodies to the targeted HPV types, and presence of HPV-DNA of the targeted HPV types

Table 6.3 Overview of vaccine efficacy results in human papillomavirus (HPV) vaccine Phase II and III trials

Endpoint	Cervarix®			Gardasil®		
	Vaccine efficacy	Analysis	Reference	Vaccine efficacy	Analysis	Reference
Vaccine efficacy for various endpoints among susceptible women (i.e. with no evidence of current or past infection at study entry)						
4 month persistent cervicovaginal infection or disease associated with HPV 6/11/16/18	Not reported			90% (71–97) 89% (73–96)	ATP MITT	[51] [51]
6 month persistent cervical infection with HPV 16/18	96% (75–100) 94% (78–99) 80% (70–87)	ATP ITT MITT	[50] [50] [52]	Not reported		
CIN1+ caused by HPV16/18	89% (59–98)	MITT	[52]	100% (<0–100) 100% (32–100)	ATP MITT	[51] [55]* [51] [55]*
CIN2/3+ caused by HPV 16/18	90% (53–99)	MITT	[52]	98% (86–100) 95% (85–99)	ATP MITT	[54]
Vaccine efficacy regardless of infection status at study entry or during course of vaccination						
CIN2/3+ caused by HPV 16/18	Not reported			44% (26–58)	ITT	[54]

Vaccine efficacy shown as the percentage reduction in the number of cases among vaccinated individuals, with 95% confidence interval given in brackets.

CIN, cervical intraepithelial neoplasia. ATP, according-to-protocol analysis. ITT, intention-to-treat analysis. MITT, modified intention-to-treat analysis.

*95% confidential interval reported by Schiller et al. [55] using Phase II data [51].

(quadrivalent) or any HR-HPV types (bivalent) at or before study entry [57]. High (over 80 per cent) vaccine efficacies against incident HPV infection, persistent infection, abnormal cytology and disease were observed in both according-to-protocol (ATP) and (modified) intention-to-treat (ITT) analyses [49–51,57].

A Phase II efficacy trial of Gardasil® among young men was underway at the time of writing, but results are not yet available. This trial will assess vaccine efficacy, safety, and immunogenicity in young men using the endpoints of HPV infection, and genital warts [55]. Among participating men who have sex with men, a further endpoint of anal dysplasias will be evaluated [55].

Phase III trials among women have been considerably larger in size (>18,000) than the Phase II trials, and thus were better suited to investigate disease endpoints for vaccine efficacy [52,54]. Participants ranged from 15 to 26 years of age and reported four or fewer sex partners in their lifetime at enrolment. Unlike the phase II trials, women in phase III trials were not necessarily excluded if they had current HPV infection or evidence of past infection, indicated by detection of antibodies for the targeted HPV types. This inclusion allows for the assessment of vaccine efficacy as it might be expected in the general population, and according to a variety of characteristics related to infection status, serostatus and disease state [47].

Interim results from these phase III trials have been reported [52,54] and follow-up of participants for at least four years is going on. In the according-to-protocol (ATP) analyses, vaccine efficacy was greater than 90 per cent against persistent infection, abnormal cytology, and disease related to the targeted HPV types (Table 6.3). ATP analyses were generally limited to women who were DNA-negative and sero-negative to the vaccine-targeted types at study entry, who received all three vaccine doses, who had no protocol violations, and who remained DNA-negative during the full course of vaccination (bivalent) or until one month after the last injection (quadrivalent).

Modified ITT analyses of the phase III trials included women who received at least one dose but excluded women who were HPV DNA positive for a targeted type at enrolment. This modification to the ITT approach was done to investigate the effect of vaccine in a susceptible population. These analyses provided somewhat lower estimates of vaccine efficacy than the per-protocol analyses, likely due in part to the inclusion of women who did not receive all three injections. Nevertheless, most still indicated high efficacy (Table 6.3) [52,54]. Results from these modified ITT analyses reflect what might be achieved in a universal vaccination programme that opted to vaccinate girls prior to initiation of sexual activity, and thus prior to HPV exposure.

ITT analyses from the Phase III studies would be expected to have the lowest estimates of vaccine efficacy, since these included women regardless of their infection status at enrolment. These estimates give a sense of what might be expected upon administration of vaccine to the sexually-active general population irrespective of whether or not there has been exposure to HPV, which is not the intended policy for HPV vaccination guidelines. Results of such an analysis are available from the phase III trial for Gardasil® (Table 6.3) [54]. Twenty-seven per cent of study participants were HPV DNA-positive and/or sero-positive for the vaccine-related types at study entry. When these women were included in the analysis, vaccine efficacy was 44 per cent (95 per cent CI 26-58) against CIN2 or higher-grade lesions (CIN2+) caused by HPV 16/18 and 17 per cent (95 per cent CI 1-31) against CIN2+ caused by any HPV type [54]. These lower efficacy results are not surprising given that neither the bivalent nor quadrivalent vaccines showed evidence of efficacy against clearance or disease progression in women who were already infected with HPV 16 or 18 at enrolment [47]. That is, no therapeutic effect was observed. Nonetheless, even among women who were already infected with between one and three HPV types targeted in the quadrivalent vaccine, there was still protection against infection with the remaining type(s) [58].

The safety profiles of both vaccines have been shown to be similar to other non-infectious protein subunit vaccines such as tetanus or hepatitis B vaccine [47,55,56]. Immediate local adverse events were commonly pain, erythema, and swelling at the injection site. Systemic symptoms such as fever, myalgias, headaches, and gastrointestinal irritability were reported but did not significantly differ between study groups. The proportions of serious or pregnancy-related adverse events were also equivalent between study groups.

Both the bivalent and quadrivalent vaccines are highly immunogenic [47,55]. Seroconversion rates are 100 per cent one month after administration of all three doses, with peak geometric mean antibody titres (GMT) typically 100-fold higher than those resulting from natural infection. Over time, GMTs decline to a plateau at least 10-fold higher than that seen in natural infection, with no indication of a decline five years post-vaccination. Furthermore, there is evidence of a B cell memory response, which would be required for long-term immunity [47,55]. Immunogenicity as well as safety has also been documented among women outside the age range of the phase II and III clinical trials (i.e. girls aged 9–14 and women aged 27–55 years) [47]. The quadrivalent vaccine is similarly immunogenic and safe among boys aged 9 to 16 years [55].

The currently-available HPV vaccines were specifically designed to target a limited number of HPV types (bivalent: 16, 18; quadrivalent: 6, 11, 16, 18). Nevertheless, there is a biological basis for cross-protection against other types, and preliminary clinical evidence for cross-protection against types 31 and 45 is emerging [47,55,59]. Confirmatory evidence for the extent of cross-protective efficacy and its duration is eagerly awaited. The fact remains that an ideal HPV vaccine would be able to induce strong immunity against a broad spectrum of types.

Given the evidence for efficacy, safety, and immunogenicity that emerged from the phase II and III clinical trials and bridging studies, the two HPV vaccines have been licensed for use in over 80 countries in the world, including a US FDA license (Gardasil®) and European Medicines Agency (EMEA) licenses [48].

Implementation of HPV vaccination

The licensure of HPV vaccines prompted a broad discussion regarding the most appropriate public health policy for whether and how to implement these vaccines in many countries throughout the world [60,61]. The key issues are cost, target age for vaccination, and concerns regarding vaccination for a sexually-transmitted infection [48]. Currently, the cost of HPV vaccine far exceeds the financing abilities of developing countries and most middle-income countries, many of which have the highest rates of cervical cancer globally. Immediately following approval, the costs in the United States were around $300 to $500 for the three doses needed, but different purchasing agreements and competition from the second vaccine have led to costs of around $150 or perhaps lower; agreements in different countries are often confidential. International agencies (e.g. the Global Alliance of Vaccines and Immunization, the Pan American Health Organization Revolving Fund, UNICEF) will play an important role in easing the introduction and implementation of vaccines to developing countries [48,60,62]. Centralized procurement via these international mechanisms could result in far more affordable prices. Moreover, as seen with HBV, the cost of vaccination will gradually decline during the next decade, presumably to levels that will permit cost-effective deployment to developing countries.

The most appropriate age for vaccination must be balanced between what is expected to have the most health impact and what is most feasible given existing public health infrastructure. Currently, there is agreement that vaccination should occur prior to sexual initiation, or soon afterwards, i.e. pre-adolescent and adolescent girls [60]. This strategy is feasible in some developed countries that already have successful school-based vaccination programmes for this age group (e.g. HBV vaccine), but in other countries an adolescent programme would be a considerable challenge [60]. Conversely, infant vaccination programmes are universal and could have far greater impact for HPV and cervical cancer prevention, should immunity induced by these vaccines prove to be long-lasting [48].

Because HPV is a sexually transmitted virus, a unique set of concerns arise, particularly among conservative cultures in which sexuality among young people and/or the unmarried is taboo [48]. Some fear that HPV vaccines would increase sexual activity among youth, perhaps hastening sexual initiation, as it would send a message that society encourages or at least tolerates adolescent sex. These arguments against HPV vaccination are analogous to similar concerns that have been raised regarding sex education programmes or condom distribution among adolescents; however, there is strong evidence that such programmes result in safer sex behaviours or even delayed engagement in sexual activity [63]. This highlights the importance of incorporating broader sexual health counselling in adolescent-based HPV vaccination programmes, which could similarly address concerns that vaccination would adversely affect condom promotion and other safer sex messages [4]. Another argument against vaccination has been that a girl who would only have sex with one partner, her husband, would not be at risk of HPV infection and cervical cancer. Yet rates of acquisition are high in women's first sexual relationships [23]. Furthermore, in many parts of the world men report more partners than women, both before and after marriage, meaning that having sex with only one's husband does not eliminate the risk of HPV exposure [64]. A vaccine strategy targeted only towards women who have multiple partners (or other high-risk groups such as patients attending STD clinics) is likely to fail, given the lessons learned from attempts to implement hepatitis B vaccine in this fashion [4] and the fact that HPV vaccination is only maximally effective before HPV exposure. This past experience led to the conclusion that universal vaccination of young adolescent girls must be the goal of any HPV vaccine implementation strategy [48].

Long before efficacy data became available from clinical trials, public health researchers began to project the public health and economic impact of HPV vaccines under various implementation strategies [65]. As these vaccines became reality, research activity in this arena expanded exponentially [66–71]. Encouragingly, findings have been largely consistent across models. Models project that HPV vaccines would have a substantial impact on reducing HPV infections and cervical cancer, particularly in developing countries with no screening programmes. Vaccine implementation could be extremely cost-effective in scenarios in which the per-woman cost of vaccination is under $25, and/or when existing cervical screening strategies are modified (see next section). These mathematical models depend on a set of assumptions regarding the epidemiological parameters for HPV infection, progression to cervical pre-cancers and cancer, and long-term vaccine-induced immunity. Although many of these parameters have good estimates for various populations, uncertainties remain. One of the most influential parameters is the duration of protection that is provided by the vaccines, which is currently unknown. Observing the extent and duration of vaccine-acquired as well as naturally-acquired HPV immunity is a research priority.

Although vaccine efficacy among males is not yet known, the use of Gardasil among adolescent boys has been approved in the European Union, Australia, and elsewhere [55] for reasons of gender equity, although publicly funded vaccination is only available for girls. The benefit of vaccinating boys is a debated issue, which will only intensify should male vaccination prove to be efficacious. Prevention of HPV-related outcomes among males would be to their direct health benefit; nevertheless, HPV-related cancers are far rarer among men than they are in women. Male vaccination may also benefit women through herd immunity, in that it could break the chain of heterosexual HPV transmission in a population. Assuming 100 per cent protection in preventing HPV infection by the target types, models have only shown a cost-effective benefit of vaccinating boys when vaccine coverage among girls is low. Therefore, some argue that targeting resources to achieve high vaccine coverage in girls may prove to be more productive [55].

Cervical cancer screening and the projected impact of vaccination

Pap test screening as the mainstay of cervical cancer control

Following its introduction in or before the 1960s in many countries, the Papanicolaou cytology technique (Pap test) is undoubtedly the cancer screening test with the best record of accomplishments in contemporary medical practice [11]. Pap test screening targets the detection of pre-invasive cervical neoplastic lesions, thereby allowing close monitoring of equivocal or low-grade abnormalities on repeat tests or immediate referral for colposcopy, biopsy, and treatment of high grade or more severe lesions. This strategy permits preventing cervical cancer by arresting neoplastic development within the cervical epithelium before it becomes invasive.

Organized or opportunistic Pap screening has been the primary reason for the substantial reductions in cervical cancer morbidity and mortality in high-income countries. However, the economic burden imposed by cervical cancer screening is substantial. In most Western countries, for each new case of invasive cancer found by Pap cytology there are approximately 50 to 200 other cases of abnormal smears consistent with equivocal atypias or precursor lesions, which require triage and clinical management. Overall, these secondary screening activities impose a great financial burden on the health care system of countries that maintain cervical cancer screening programmes.

Most developing countries have yet to derive the same benefit from Pap test screening that developed countries have experienced, either because programmes have not been implemented at all or were instituted without the entire chain of components of quality assurance and follow-up procedures that are necessary for screening to be effective. As a result, incidence of cervical cancer has continued to increase in many Latin American, African, and Asian countries, possibly due also to the liberal changes in sexual mores that began in the 1960s that led to more widespread HPV transmission. Furthermore, the reductions in cervical cancer morbidity seen in many western countries have begun to stabilize which brings a sense of diminishing returns.

In spite of its success in developed countries, Pap cytology has important limitations related to the inherently subjective interpretation of morphologic alterations in cervical samples, sampling variation, and fatigue that results from the repetitive nature of reading smears. In consequence, the sensitivity of Pap cytology to detect high-grade CIN or invasive cervical cancer is relatively low at 51 per cent, whereas its specificity is considered high, at 98 per cent [72]. Therefore, the Pap test's high false negative rate is its most critical limitation. The advent of liquid-based cytology techniques has contributed to mitigate the problem of efficiency in processing cervical samples but the limitations of cytology remain the same [73]. This low sensitivity for an individual testing opportunity has to be compensated by the requirement to have women entering the eligible screening age-range with an initially negative smear to repeat their tests at least twice over the next 2 to 3 years before they can be safely followed as part of a routine screening schedule. This effectively brings a programme's sensitivity to acceptable levels but safeguards must be in place to ensure compliance, coverage, and quality; costly undertakings that have worked well only in western industrialized countries.

Cervical cancer screening post-vaccination

Despite the enthusiasm regarding the prospect from HPV vaccination, cervical cancer screening must continue after vaccination for a number of reasons. First, both vaccines are effective as pre-exposure prophylaxis for disease caused by HPV-16 and -18; however, women currently infected with these viruses may not derive any benefit [74]. Moreover, the target types included in the two vaccines are causally linked to about 70 per cent of all cervical cancers (Figure 6.5) [35]; therefore, even in a scenario of 100 per cent vaccine effectiveness and 100 per cent vaccine coverage, screening would still be necessary to detect lesions caused by other HR-HPV types. Although some degree of cross-protection against infection with phylogenetically-related HPVs (e.g. HPVs 45 and 31) has been observed [47], there is also a possibility of an increase in prevalence of other HPV types in vaccinated populations, as a result of the vacated ecologic niches following the progressive elimination of HPVs 16 and 18 (a yet unproven phenomenon known as type replacement). There is also the possibility that the type-specific immunity conferred by vaccination may wane over periods extending beyond five years.

Despite these caveats, a vaccinated woman may experience much lower risks of developing pre-cancerous lesions over a period that may extend for a decade or longer. Subsequent intensive screening via annual or biennial Pap cytology may waste resources while providing only marginal additional benefit beyond that conferred by immunization during a woman's main reproductive years. Implementation of HPV vaccination will impose a substantial burden on the health budgets of most countries. Proper planning of cervical cancer screening, an intervention that represents today a key healthcare expenditure, may help offset the costs that will stem from vaccination.

Expected impact of vaccination on screening practices

As the successive cohorts of vaccinated young women reach screening age there may be a gradual reduction in cervical lesion prevalence. Decreases in colposcopy referral rates to about 40 per cent to 60 per cent or less of the existing case loads in most Western countries are plausible, judging from attributable proportion estimates [75] and preliminary findings from vaccination trials [76]. Such reductions are likely to translate into initial savings to the health care system or to individuals. It is expected that the vaccine-induced decrease in cervical lesion prevalence may lead to a degradation of Pap cytology performance (because of a decreased expectation of abnormalities on a day's smear workload) and a decline in the positive predictive value of Pap cytology (due to reduced lesion prevalence) [77,78].

In the longer term, a statistically noticeable reduction of the burden of cervical cancer via HPV vaccination is unlikely to be observed for at least 10 to 15 years even if vaccine coverage is high because of the dual facts that vaccination below age 20 will not affect high grade CIN rates appreciably for 5 to 10 years and another 5 to 15 years will be necessary for this to be translated into reductions in cancer incidence. A paradoxical situation may arise if vaccine uptake is higher or happens exclusively among women who will eventually be adherent with screening recommendations. If adolescents and young women who are more likely to be vaccinated are also the ones destined to be screened regularly, the reduction in incidence of cervical abnormalities will happen nearly exclusively among such women. The fact they will benefit from screening makes them less likely to develop cervical cancer even if they had not been vaccinated, because any pre-cancerous lesions may eventually be found and treated. On the other hand, young women who were not vaccinated because of inability to pay may also be less likely to be screened and their undetected lesions will progress until invasion occurs, when the associated symptoms will then lead them to seek medical attention, which will then reveal cervical cancer [77]. This undesirable scenario of compounded social inequity is unlikely to occur in countries that already enjoy the benefits of an organized screening programme that reaches all women. Such high-income countries are also likely to adopt an organized and universal vaccination programme that benefits all segments of society.

New screening options following HPV vaccination: HPV DNA testing

HPV DNA testing in cervical cancer screening largely circumvents the limitations of Pap test screening, and has other advantages in a post-vaccination world [79]. HPV testing has much higher sensitivity than cytology but only slightly lower specificity in women 30 years or older [80–83]. Furthermore, HPV DNA testing is reproducible for large-scale implementation and eliminates the subjective interpretation of cytology. Adoption of this method could potentially lengthen the screening intervals and have fewer quality control requirements, which would result in more affordable and sustainable screening, particularly in developing countries. Randomized controlled trials of HPV testing in primary cervical cancer screening are currently ongoing and many have already provided results in support of this method's superior performance in detecting cervical cancer precursors with a greater margin of safety than Pap cytology (reviewed in [78]).

HPV DNA-based cervical cancer screening would also serve the purpose of a surveillance mechanism post-vaccine implementation, thus allowing an efficient and low-cost strategy to monitor long-term protection among vaccinated women while providing the benefit of continued screening. As HPV typing becomes incorporated in future HPV assays there will be an improved opportunity to manage HPV positive cases and to gain insights into the long-term effectiveness of vaccination [77].

Simply making cytology screening less frequent may not be a viable strategy to achieve a cost-effective combination of vaccination and screening. The anticipated reduction in the prevalence of pre-cancerous lesions requires rethinking the optimal screening approach. This decline in prevalence will necessarily result in a lower positive predictive value of both Pap and HPV screen tests. However, the accuracy of Pap tests is expected to be more adversely affected because it is prone to the vagaries of subjective interpretation, particularly in conditions of low lesion prevalence [78]. Conversely, HPV testing has the screening performance characteristics that would make it an ideal primary cervical cancer screening test in such conditions. Pap cytology should be reserved for triage settings, i.e. in assisting management of HPV positive cases. Among HPV-positive patients, the prevalence of pre-cancerous lesions will be high, leading to enhanced accuracy of the Pap test [78]. The advantages of the proposed approach have been described elsewhere [77,78] and are being evaluated in Finland [84], Northern Italy [85], and in British Columbia, Canada.

Expected impact on other HPV-associated cancers

HPV has been implicated in the development of malignancies of other anogenital sites besides the cervix including vagina, vulva, penis, and anus [20]. Unlike cervical cancer, in which 100 per cent of cancers are caused by HPV, cancers of other anogenital sites show lower risk attributions for HPV. It is estimated that 90 per cent of anal cancers, and 40 per cent of vaginal, vulvar, and penile cancers are attributable to HPV [1]. It is also thought that HPV may cause a substantial proportion of other anogenital malignancies and those of the upper aero-digestive tract [20].

Vaginal and vulvar cancers

Cancer of the vagina is extremely rare with an average incidence rate of approximately 1 new case per 100,000 women per year worldwide [86]. HPV seems to play a central role in the causal pathway. HPV-DNA is detected in 64 per cent to 91 per cent of vaginal cancers and 82 per cent to 100 per cent of their precursor lesions (vaginal intraepithelial lesions of grade 3) and HPV-16 appears to be the most prevalent type [87]. The model of vaginal cancer pathogenesis is very similar to that of cervical cancer and indicates the central role of HPV as the central sexually-transmitted agent [20]. Women with primary vaginal carcinoma are more likely to have been previously diagnosed with an anogenital tumour, particularly of the cervix [88].

Invasive squamous cell carcinoma of the vulva is relatively rare at slightly less than 5 per cent of all female genital tract malignancies but its incidence has increased over the past 30 years, especially in young women [89]. Approximately 60 per cent of vulvar cancers contain HPV DNA, particularly of HPV-16 [16,90]. However, there seem to be two distinct, age-dependent risk factor profiles for vulvar cancer [20]. Those affecting older women tend to be keratinizing squamous cell carcinomas and are rarely associated with HPV (less than 10 per cent). Vulvar cancers that have an early age of onset tend to be warty or basaloid carcinomas and constitute an HPV-related subgroup of tumours (60 per cent to 90 per cent are positive for HPV) [87]. These HPV-positive tumours seem to have become more frequent in recent decades and tend to have the same risk profile as other HPV-related anogenital cancers, i.e. association with high-risk sexual behaviours [20].

Findings on the efficacy of vaccination in preventing vaginal and vulvar pre-cancerous lesions with the quadrivalent vaccine [Gardasil®] are available [91]. Evidence suggests that the quadrivalent vaccine is highly effective against vulvar and vaginal intraepithelial neoplasia over a mean follow-up of 3 years. In the according-to-protocol analysis, vaccine efficacy was 100 per cent (95 per cent CI 72-100); this analysis was restricted to susceptible women who were HPV 16/18 DNA-negative and sero-negative to HPV 16/18 at study entry, who remained DNA-negative throughout the vaccination period, received all three doses, and did not violate the protocol [91]. The intention-to-treat (ITT) analyses estimated vaccine efficacy of 71 per cent (95 per cent CI 37-88) for lesions associated with HPV 16/18, and 49 per cent (95 percent CI 18-69) against lesions regardless of HPV type detected. These encouraging results suggest that the umbrella of protection conferred by HPV vaccination may be wide enough to potentially prevent all female lower genital tract cancers associated with the vaccine-targeted HPV types.

Penile cancer

Most penile cancers are squamous cell carcinomas and are a very rare disease in developed countries in Europe and North America, where incidence rates vary between 0.3 to 1 case per 100,000 men-years. Incidence is higher in parts of Africa (Uganda), Asia, and South America (Brazil and Colombia) at up to 4 cases per 100,000 men-years [92]. The exact etiologic mechanisms that lead to the development of penile cancer are largely unknown although the assumed attributable risk for HPV is 40 per cent [1]. Similarly to vulvar cancer, basaloid or warty penile carcinomas are most likely to contain HPV DNA (up to 100 per cent), whereas the more common keratinizing carcinomas have a lower HPV prevalence (30 per cent to 40 per cent) [93]. HPV-16 is also the most prevalent type in HPV-related penile cancer [94].

Clinical evidence for the efficacy of HPV vaccines in preventing penile cancer is not anticipated to become available from clinical trials among men due to the rarity of this cancer. Unlike pre-invasive lesions of the vulva and vagina, which serve as acceptable endpoints for judging vaccine efficacy, identification of penile intraepithelial neoplasia is yet to be widely used in practice, and thus no surrogate endpoints for vaccine efficacy are available for penile cancer. Any population-based impact will be documentable only during post-vaccination surveillance. Even in populations that opt to vaccinate only females, rates of penile cancer may decline as a secondary outcome of reduced HPV infection among women and less opportunity for transmission to male partners. It has been known that men are more likely to develop pre-cancerous lesions of the penis that are associated with HPV when their partners have cervical intraepithelial neoplasms [95].

Anal cancer

Anal cancer is relatively rare although the incidence among both men and women has increased by more than two-fold over the last 40 years [96]. Globally, nearly 100,000 new cases of anal cancer were reported in 2002 [10]. Rates of anal cancer are considerably higher among homosexual men [97]. Similarly HIV-positive men and women, transplant recipients, and women with cervical squamous intraepithelial lesions are at a higher risk than the general population [96,97].

HPV is detected in 83 per cent to 95 per cent of anal cancers, with an attributable risk estimate of 90 per cent [1]. As in cervical cancer, HPVs 16 and 18 are the most common types in anal carcinoma specimens. The model of anal cancer pathogenesis is very similar to that of cervical cancer. HPV infection is associated with the development of low- and high-grade anal precursor lesions, with eventual progression to invasive anal cancer.

Given the similarity between cervical and anal carcinogenesis, the efficacy of HPV vaccines in preventing anal pre-cancers and cancer is expected to be analogous to findings for cervical lesions, although clinical data are not yet available. Results from the ongoing Gardasil® vaccine trial in homosexual men will be particularly revealing regarding efficacy against anal pre-cancers [55].

Head and neck cancer

In 2002, head and neck cancer (cancers of the oral cavity, pharynx, and larynx) was ranked as the sixth leading cause of cancer deaths worldwide, with extensive variation by sex and geographic region [10]. However, the results of many studies suggest that head and neck cancer, particularly oral tongue cancer, is increasing in young adults internationally [98].

Evidence supports the idea that head and neck squamous-cell carcinoma is a multi-factorial disease with at least two distinct pathogenesis models, a dominating one involving smoking and alcohol consumption, and the other driven by HPV [99]. An average of 40 per cent of cancers of the oral cavity and pharynx are HPV-positive, and attributable risk per cents are 5 per cent and 16 per cent, respectively [1]. The association is strongest in the oropharynx, particularly in the tonsil [100,101]. Sexual activity has been associated with increased risk and husbands of women who had cervical cancer are more likely to be diagnosed with these cancers [102]. Among HPV-positive head and neck cancers, HPV-16 and HPV-18 are most prevalent [87].

Ongoing vaccination trials have not included a protocol for identifying the onset of oral pre-cancerous lesions among study participants. Moreover, classification schemes for such pre-cancerous lesions are not yet widely used, particularly among young women, the main group included in vaccine trials and demonstration projects. This population group has very low risk of developing such oral lesions. Therefore, it is only via cancer surveillance post-vaccination deployment that it will be possible to ascertain any possible impact on head-and-neck cancers. Any such impact is not expected to be verifiable before a decade or more has passed since HPV vaccination.

Future developments in HPV vaccines

Outstanding research questions for current HPV vaccines

A multitude of research questions regarding the current bivalent and quadrivalent HPV vaccines are being posed by researchers and public health officials. In the very near future, updated results from the phase III trials are expected to become available. These findings will be important for more precise estimates of vaccine efficacy with longer follow-up of trial participants. Results from the phase II efficacy trials of the quadrivalent vaccine among males are also eagerly anticipated.

One of the key research questions is the duration of vaccine-induced immunity, a most influ-ential variable in cost-effectiveness analyses. Only long-term follow-up of trial participants, large community-randomized trials, and phase IV surveillance post-introduction will determine whether induced immunity is long-lasting or if a booster will be required to maintain protective antibody titres. Such long-term data will also establish the minimum level of antibody titres required for immunity (a correlate of protection), which is unknown at this point. These studies will also provide data on long-term safety and cross-protection against HPV types not included in these vaccines.

Large community-randomized trials of HPV vaccination, such as those ongoing in Finland, will be ideal to investigate herd immunity [103], which is the phenomenon in which infectious disease spread may cease in a population, even though all are not immunized. As the proportion of immune individuals in a population rises, there are fewer opportunities for contacts between infected and susceptible persons. Therefore, less than 100 per cent vaccine coverage may still result in elimination of a pathogen. Many mathematical models have explored the extent of pro-tection that may be achieved with various levels of vaccine coverage among girls alone, or among girls and boys [103]. The large community-randomized trials will be instrumental to determine whether the modelled effects hold true with empirical data [103].

There has been theoretical concern that elimination of some, but not all, circulating HPV types could lead to type replacement, in which the ecological niche vacated by HPV types 16 and 18 would simply be filled by other HR-HPV types. Although there is little biological plausibility for type replacement, this must be verified empirically in long-term studies [103]. Thus far, epi-demiologic studies have not provided evidence that HPV types compete for specific ecological niches [104].

The most dramatic potential for an impact on cervical cancer rates will be in developing coun-tries, many of which have only partial, ineffective, or absent screening programmes. In addition to cost barriers, the current VLP vaccines require refrigeration at 4°C and this may challenge their implementation in some developing countries [45]. New vaccine technologies eliminating the need for cold chain storage will be helpful for global efforts.

Second generation vaccines

The two currently available vaccines, Gardasil® (Merck & Co., Inc., NJ, USA) and Cervarix® (GlaxoSmithKline Biologicals, Rixensart, Belgium), are based on L1 VLP technology and were designed to target specific HPV types 16 and 18 (and additionally 6 and 11 in Gardasil®). Although some evidence of cross-protection against HPV types 31 and 45 is emerging, it would be desirable to broaden protection to additional oncogenic types. Availability of an HPV vaccine that prevented the full spectrum of HPV types that can cause cancers would be the ultimate cancer control strategy by obviating the need for screening programmes in the future.

One option is using polyvalent L1-based VLP vaccines that would target additional HR-HPV types. Merck is exploring this possibility with an octovalent vaccine against types 6, 11, 16, 18, 31, 45, 52, and 58 but results are not available yet [45]. Another option is an L2-based VLP vaccine, which could generate broad-spectrum antibodies against all alpha-papillomavirus types, elimi-nating the need for an approach targeted to specific types; such an L2-based vaccine is currently in development [45].

A critical caveat of prophylactic HPV vaccination is that it is ineffective against infections that have already become established, either productive or latent. Therefore, development of thera-peutic HPV vaccines is a worthwhile pursuit. There is feverish research activity to this end, with many promising candidate vaccines, but, so far, few formulations have reached the stage of Phase II trials [45,105]. Ultimately, the availability of one or more efficacious therapeutic vaccines will contribute a key supplemental strategy towards the goal of cervical cancer eradication.

Conclusion

There is cautious optimism that universal implementation of HPV vaccination as pre-exposure prophylaxis of young adolescent women is likely to exert maximal impact on the future burden of cervical cancer in most countries. Optimism is without reservation when it comes to projections for developing countries, in which the beneficial impact is expected to be greater. There is also consensus that vaccination will not reduce risk of cancer for most women who are already genitally exposed to HPVs of the vaccine-targeted types.

Policymakers should not be misled by the promises of the new preventive technologies. A key objective for cervical cancer control is that the protection by HPV vaccination (based on today's technology which does not provide protection against all HR-HPVs) must be supplemented by the protection given by screening. Improper implementation of screening or relaxation of its safeguards may have a deleterious effect. As discussed in this chapter, worrisome scenarios may emerge as a result of misguided policies. For instance, uptake of vaccination mainly by the wrong age groups may occur if countries delay implementing universal vaccination of girls but aggressive marketing of vaccines leads to high uptake among older women who are already assiduous clients of screening. If the latter situation is eventually compounded by lower screening coverage, or relaxation of quality control activities required in screening programmes, cervical cancer rates may actually increase. Another concern is that countries may feel pressured to decrease expenditures needed to maintain cytology screening immediately following the investments committed to HPV vaccination. The cancer control dividends from HPV vaccination will take two or more decades to be realized via appreciable reductions in cervical cancer incidence. However, it is relatively easy to immediately lose the gains in reduction of disease burden that comes from screening. Policymakers in both high- and low-resource settings are urged to consider that primary (vaccination) and secondary (screening) prevention act by intervening at different points in the natural history of cervical cancer and imply actions in women of different ages. The constant changes in technology may pose a challenge to proper policy-making. As indicated in this chapter, the existing cytology screening paradigm will need to be re-considered post-vaccination in light of the strong evidence that is now available concerning the superiority of HPV DNA testing. To avoid missteps countries are urged to enforce only evidence-based decisions that are accepted by all stakeholders in the multi-disciplinary blend of disciplines that now characterizes cervical cancer prevention.

Acknowledgements

ANB is recipient of a pre-doctoral research studentship from the National Cancer Institute of Canada and the Canadian Cancer Society (NCIC/CCS). Funding for the HPV and cervical cancer research programme in the authors' unit has been provided by multiple grants from the Canadian Institutes of Health Research, US National Institutes of Health, and NCIC/CCS. Supplemental unconditional funding has also been provided by Merck-Frosst for projects unrelated to HPV vaccination.

References

1 Parkin DM (2006). The global health burden of infection-associated cancers in the year 2002. *Int J Cancer*, **118**(12):3030–44.

2 International Agency for Research on Cancer (IARC) (1994). *Hepatitis Viruses. IARC Monographs on the Evaluation of Carcinogenic Risks to Humans*. Vol. 59. IARC, Lyon, France.

3 Beasley RP, Hwang LY, Lee GC, et al (1983). Prevention of perinatally transmitted hepatitis B virus infections with hepatitis B virus infections with hepatitis B immune globulin and hepatitis B vaccine. *Lancet*, **2**:1099–1102.

4 Rekart ML & Brunham RC (2008). Chapter 99. STD Vaccines. In Holmes KK et al (eds) *Sexually Transmitted Diseases*, pp. 1913–16. 4th edn. McGraw Hill Medical, New York.

5 Patrick DM, Bigham M, Ng H, White R, Tweed A, & Skowronski DM (2003). Elimination of acute hepatitis B among adolescents after one decade of an immunization programme targeting Grade 6 students. *Pediatr Infect Dis J*, **22**(10):874–77.

6 Chang MH, Chen CJ, Lai MS, et al (1997). Universal hepatitis B vaccination in Taiwan and the incidence of hepatocellular carcinoma in children. *N Engl J Med*, **336**:1855–59.

7 Kane MA & Brooks A (2002). New immunization initiatives and progress toward the global control of hepatitis B. *Curr Opin Infect Dis*, **15**(5):465–69.

8 International Agency for Research on Cancer (IARC) (1995). *Human papillomaviruses. IARC Monographs on the Evaluation of Carcinogenic Risks to Humans*. Vol. 64. IARC, Lyon, France.

9 Walboomers JM, Jacobs MV, Manos MM, et al (1999). Human papillomavirus is a necessary cause of invasive cervical cancer worldwide. *J Pathol*, **189**:12–19.

10 Ferlay J, Bray F, Pisani P, & Parkin DM (2004). *GLOBOCAN 2002: Cancer Incidence, Mortality and Prevalence Worldwide*. IARC CancerBase No. 5, version 2.0. IARC Press, Lyon.

11 Franco EL, Duarte-Franco E, & Ferenczy A (2001). Cervical cancer: epidemiology, prevention, and role of human papillomavirus infection. *Can Med Assoc J*, **164**:1017–25.

12 Parkin D, Pisani P, & Ferlay J (1999). Estimates of the worldwide incidence of 24 major cancers in 1990. *Int J Cancer*, **80**:827–841.

13 Pisani P, Parkin DM, Bray F, & Ferlay J (1999). Estimates of the worldwide mortality from 25 cancers in 1990. *Int J Cancer*, **83**:18–29.

14 de Villiers EM, Fauquet C, Broker TR, Bernard HU, & zur Hausen H (2004). Classification of papillomaviruses. *Virology*, **324**(1):17–27.

15 Trottier H & Franco EL (2006). The epidemiology of genital human papillomavirus infection. *Vaccine*, **24**(S1):S1–S15.

16 International Agency for Research on Cancer (IARC) (2007). *Human Papillomaviruses. IARC Monographs on the Evaluation of Carcinogenic Risks to Humans*,Vol. 90. IARC, Lyon, France.

17 Aral SO & Holmes KK (2008). Chapter 5. The epidemiology of STIs and their social and behavioral determinants: Industrialized and developing countries. In Holmes KK et al (eds) *Sexually Transmitted Diseases*, 4th edn, pp. 53–92. McGraw Hill Medical, New York.

18 Clifford G, Herrero R, Muñoz N, et al (2005). Worldwide distribution of human papillomavirus types in cytologically normal women in the International Agency for Research on Cancer HPV prevalence surveys: a pooled analysis. *Lancet*, **366**:991–98.

19 de Sanjosé S, Diaz M, Castellsagué, et al (2007). Worldwide prevalence and genotype distribution of cervical human papillomavirus DNA in women with normal cytology: a meta-analysis. *Lancet Infectious Diseases*, **7**:453–59.

20 Giuliano AR, Tortolero-Luna G, Ferrer E, et al (2008). Epidemiology of human papillomavirus infection in men, cancers other than cervical and benign conditions. *Vaccine*, **26**(S10):K17–K28.

21 Partridge J & Koutsky L (2006). Genital human papillomavirus infection in men. *Lancet Infect Dis*, **6**:21–31.

22 Palefsky, JM Gillison ML, & Strickler HD (2006). Chapter 16. HPV vaccines in immunocompromised women and men. *Vaccine*, **24**(S3):S140–S146.

23 Burchell AN, Winer RL, de Sanjosé S, & Franco EL (2006). Epidemiology and transmission dynamics of genital human papillomavirus infection. *Vaccine*, **24**(S3):S52–S61.

24 Manhart LE & Koutsky LA (2002). Do condoms prevent genital HPV infection, external genital warts, or cervical neoplasia? A meta-analysis. *Sex Transm Dis*, **29**:725–35.

25 Winer RL, Hughes JP, Feng Q, et al (2006). Condom use and the risk of genital human papillomavirus infection in young women. *N Engl J Med*, **354**(25):2645–54.

26 Burchell AN, Hanley J, Tellier PP, Coutlée F, & Franco EL (2007). Evidence of HPV transmission among couples who recently initiated a sexual relationship: Results from the HITCH Cohort Study.

Oral presentation at the 24th International Papillomavirus Conference and Clinical Workshop, November 3–9, 2007, Beijing, China. Abstract 118.

27 Franco EL & Ferenczy A (2002). Part III, site-specific pre-cancerous conditions: Cervix. In Franco EL, Rohan TE (eds) *Cancer Precursors: Epidemiology, Detection, and Prevention*, pp. 249–86. Springer-Verlag, New York.

28 Franco EL, & Harper DM (2005). Vaccination against human papillomavirus infection: a new paradigm in cervical cancer control. *Vaccine*, 23:2388–94.

29 Franco EL (1991). Viral etiology of cervical cancer: a critique of the evidence. *Rev Infect Dis*, 13(6):1195–1206.

30 Zur Hausen H (2006). Perspectives of contemporary papillomavirus research. *Vaccine*, 24(S3):iii–iv.

31 Franco EL (1991). The sexually transmitted disease model for cervical cancer: incoherent epidemiologic findings and the role of misclassification of human papillomavirus infection. *Epidemiology*, 2:98–106.

32 Muñoz N, Bosch FX, de Sanjose S, et al (1992). The causal link between human papillomavirus and invasive cervical cancer: a population-based case-control study in Colombia and Spain. *Int J Cancer*, 52(5):743–49.

33 Muñoz N, Bosch FX, de Sanjose S, et al (2003). Epidemiologic classification of human papillomavirus types associated with cervical cancer. *N Engl J Med*, 6:348(6):518–27.

34 International Agency for Research on Cancer (IARC) (1986). *Tobacco smoking. IARC monographs on the evaluation of carcinogenic risk of chemical to human*. Vol. 38. IARC, Lyon, France.

35 Muñoz N, Bosch FX, Castellsague X, et al (2004). Against which human papillomavirus types shall we vaccinate and screen? The international perspective. *Int J Cancer*, 111(2):278–85.

36 Franco EL (1995). Cancer causes revisited: human papillomavirus and cervical neoplasia. *J Natl Cancer Inst*, 87(11):779–80.

37 Schiffman MH & Brinton LA (1995). The epidemiology of cervical carcinogenesis. *Cancer*, 76(S10):1888–1901.

38 Bosch FX, Manos MM, Munoz N (1995). Prevalence of human papillomavirus in cervical cancer: a worldwide perspective. International biological study on cervical cancer (IBSCC) Study Group. *J Natl Cancer Inst*, 87(11):796–802.

39 Schiffman M, Herrero R, Desalle R, et al (2005). The carcinogenicity of human papillomavirus types reflects viral evolution. *Virology*, 337:76–84.

40 Hiller T, Poppelreuther S, Stubenrauch F, & Iftner T (2006). Comparative analysis of 19 genital human papillomavirus types with regard to p53 degradation, immortalization, phylogeny, and epidemiologic risk classification. *Cancer Epidemiol Biomarkers Prev*, 15:1262–67.

41 Clifford GM, Smith JS, Plummer M, Muñoz N, & Franceschi S (2003). Human papillomavirus types in invasive cervical cancer worldwide: a meta-analysis. *Br J Cancer*, 88:63–73.

42 Salunke DM, Caspar DL, & Garcea RL (1986). Self-assembly of purified polyomavirus capsid protein VP1. *Cell*, 46(6):895–904.

43 Garcea RL, Salunke DM, & Caspar DL (1987). Site-directed mutation affecting polyomavirus capsid self-assembly in vitro. *Nature*, 329(6134):86–87.

44 Zhou J, Sun XY, Stenzel DJ, & Frazer IH (1991). Expression of vaccinia recombinant HPV 16 L1 and L2 ORF proteins in epithelial cells is sufficient for assembly of HPV virion-like particles. *Virology*, 85(1):251–57.

45 Huh WK & Roden RBS (2008). The future of vaccines for cervical cancer [review]. *Gynecol Oncol*, 109:S48–S56.

46 Frazer I (2006). God's gift to women: the human papillomavirus vaccine. *Immunity*, 25(2):179–84.

47 Harper DM (2008). Prophylactic human papillomavirus vaccines to prevent cervical cancer: review of the Phase II and III trials. *Therapy*, 5(3):313–324.

48 Bosch FX, de Sanjosé S, & Castellsagué X (2008). Evaluating the potential benefits of universal worldwide human papillomavirus vaccination. *Therapy*, 5(3):305–312.

49 Harper DM, Franco EL, Wheeler C, et al (2004). Efficacy of a bivalent L1 virus-like particle vaccine in prevention of infection with human papillomavirus types 16 and 18 in young women: a randomised controlled trial. *Lancet*, **364**:1757–65.

50 Harper DM, Franco EL, Wheeler C, et al (2006). Sustained efficacy up to 4.5 years of bivalent L1 virus-like particle vaccine against human papillomavirus types 16 and 18: follow-up from a randomised control trial. *Lancet*, **367**(9518):1247–55.

51 Villa LL, Costa RLR, Petta CA, et al (2005). Prophylactic quadrivalent human papillomavirus (types 6, 11, 16 and 18) L1 virus-like particle vaccine in young women: a randomized double-blind placebo-controlled multi-centre phase II efficacy trial. *Lancet Oncol*, **6**(5):271–78.

52 Paavonen J, Jenkins D, Bosch FX, et al (2007). Efficacy of a prophylactic adjuvanted bivalent L1 virus-like-particle vaccine against infection with human papillomavirus types 16 and 18 in young women: an interim analysis of a phase III double-blind, randomized controlled trial. *Lancet*, **369**:2161–70.

53 Garland SM, Hernandez-Avila M, Wheeler CM, et al (2007). Quadrivalent vaccine against human papillomavirus to prevent anogenital diseases. *New Engl J Med*, **356**:1928–43.

54 Villa LL, Perez G, Kjaer SK, et al (2007). Quadrivalent vaccine against human papillomaviruses to prevent high-grade cervical lesions. *New Engl J Med*, **356**:1915–27.

55 Schiller JT, Castellsagué X, Villa LL, & Hildesheim A (2008). An update of prophylactic human papillomavirus L1 virus-like particle vaccine clinical trial results. *Vaccine*, **26**(S10):K53–K61.

56 Rambout L, Hopkins L, Hutton B, & Fergusson D (2007). Prophylactic vaccination against human papillomavirus infection and disease in women: a systematic review of randomized controlled trials. *CMAJ*, **177**(5):469–479.

57 Koutsky LA & Harper DM (2006). Chapter 13. Current findings from prophylactic HPV vaccine trials. *Vaccine*, **24**(S3):S114–S121.

58 Villa LL, Perez G, Kjaer SK, et al (2007). Prophylactic efficacy of a quadrivalent human papillomavirus (HPV) vaccine in women with virological evidence of HPV infection. *J Infect Dis*, **196**:1438–46.

59 Nishida KJ, Pearson JM, & Twiggs LB (2008). Cross-protection from human papillomavirus 16/18 against types 45 and 31: fact or fancy? *Therapy*, **5**(3):265–68.

60 Wright TC, Bosch FX, Franco EL, et al (2006). Chapter 30. HPV vaccines and screening in the prevention of cervical cancer; conclusions from a 2006 workshop of international experts. *Vaccine*, **24**(S3):S251–S261.

61 Herzog TJ, Huh WK, Downs LS, et al (2008). Initial lessons learned in HPV vaccination. *Gynecologic Oncol*, **109**:S4–S11.

62 Andrus JK, Lewis MJ, Goldie SJ, et al (2008). Human papillomavirus vaccine policy and delivery in Latin America and the Carribean. *Vaccine*, **26**(S11):L80–L87.

63 Kirby DB, Laris BA, & Rolleri LA (2007). Sex and HIV education programmes: their impact on sexual behaviors of young people throughout the world. *J Adolesc Health*, **40**(3):206–17.

64 Bosch FX, Burchell AN, Schiffman M, et al (2008). Epidemiology and natural history of human papillomavirus infections and type-specific implications in cervical neoplasia. *Vaccine*, **26**(S10):K1–K16.

65 Garnett GP, Kim JJ, French K, & Goldie SJ (2006). Chapter 21. Modelling the impact of HPV vaccines on cervical cancer and screening programmes. *Vaccine*, **24**(S3):S178–S186.

66 Kulasingam S, et al (2007). A cost-effectiveness analysis of adding a human papillomavirus vaccine to the Australian National Cervical Cancer Screening Programme. *Sex Health*, **4**(3):165–75.

67 Brisson M, N Van de Velde, P De Wals (2007). The potential cost effectiveness of prophylactic human papillomavirus vaccines in Canada. *Vaccine*, **25**:5399–408.

68 Elbasha EH, Dasbach EJ, Insinga RP (2007). Model for assessing human papillomavirus vaccination strategies. *Emerg Infect Dis*, **13**:28–41.

69 Taira AV, Neukermans CP, Sanders GD (2004). Evaluating human papillomavirus vaccination programmes. *Emerg Infect Dis*, **10**:1915–23.

70 Goldie SJ, Kohli M, Grima D (2004). Projected clinical benefits and cost-effectiveness of a human papillomavirus 16/18 vaccine. *J Natl Cancer Inst*, **96**:604–15.

71 Sanders GD & Taira AV (2003). Cost-effectiveness of a potential vaccine for human papillomavirus. *Emerg Infect Dis*, **9**:37–48.

72 Nanda K, McCrory DC, Myers ER, et al (2000). Accuracy of the Papanicolaou test in screening for and follow-up of cervical cytologic abnormalities: a systematic review. *Ann Intern Med*, **132**:810–19.

73 Davey E, Barratt A, Irwig L, et al (2006). Effect of study design and quality on unsatisfactory rates, cytology classifications, and accuracy in liquid-based versus conventional cervical cytology: a systematic review. *Lancet*, **367**(9505):122–32.

74 Hildesheim A, Herrero R, Wacholder S, et al (2007). Effect of human papillomavirus 16/18 L1 viruslike particle vaccine among young women with pre-existing infection: a randomized trial. *JAMA*, **298**(7):743–53.

75 Clifford GM, Rana RK, Franceschi S, Smith JS, Gough G, & Pimenta JM (2005). Human papillomavirus genotype distribution in low-grade cervical lesions: comparison by geographic region and with cervical cancer. *Cancer Epidemiol Biomarkers Prev*, **14**:1157–64.

76 Ault KA & Future II Study Group (2007). Effect of prophylactic human papillomavirus L1 virus-like-particle vaccine on risk of cervical intraepithelial neoplasia grade 2, grade 3, and adenocarcinoma in situ: a combined analysis of four randomized clinical trials. *Lancet*, **369**(9576):1861–68.

77 Franco EL, Cuzick J, Hildesheim A, & de Sanjose S (2006). Chapter 20. Issues in planning cervical cancer screening in the era of HPV vaccination. *Vaccine*, **24**(S3):S171–S177.

78 Franco EL & Cuzick J (2008). Cervical cancer screening following prophylactic human papillomavirus vaccination. *Vaccine*, **26**(S1):A16–A23.

79 Franco E, Tsu V, Herrero R, et al (2008). Integration of human papillomavirus vaccination and cervical cancer screening in Latin America and the Carribean. *Vaccine*, **26**(S11):L88–L95.

80 Franco EL (2003). Primary screening of cervical cancer with human papillomavirus tests. *J Natl Cancer Inst Monogr*, **31**:89–96.

81 International Agency for Research on Cancer (IARC) Working Group (1995). *Cervix cancer screening. IARC Handbooks of Cancer Prevention*. IARC Press, Lyon, France.

82 Arbyn M, Sasieni P, Meijer CJ, Clavel C, Koliopoulos G, & Dillner J (2006). Chapter 9. Clinical applications of HPV testing: A summary of meta-analyses. *Vaccine*, **24**(S3):S78–S89.

83 Cuzick J, Mayrand MH, Ronco G, Snijders P, & Wardle J (2006). Chapter 10. New dimensions in cervical cancer screening. *Vaccine*, **24**(S3):S90–S97.

84 Kotaniemi-Talonen L, Nieminen P, Anttila A, & Hakama M (2005). Routine cervical screening with primary HPV testing and cytology triage protocol in a randomized setting. *Br J Cancer*, **93**(8):862–67.

85 Ronco G, Segnan N, Giorgi-Rossi P, et al (2006). New Technologies for Cervical Cancer Working Group. Human papillomavirus testing and liquid-based cytology: results at recruitment from the new technologies for cervical cancer randomized controlled trial. *J Natl Cancer Inst*, **98**(11):765–74.

86 Parkin DM, Whelan S, Ferlay J, Raymond LE, & Young J (1997). *Cancer incidence in five continents. Vol. VII. IARC Scientific Publications No. 143*. IARC, Lyon, France.

87 Muñoz N, Castellsagué X, Berrington A, & Gissmann L (2006). Chapter 1. HPV in the etiology of human cancer. *Vaccine*, **24**(S3):S1–S10.

88 Daling JR, Madeleine MM, Schwartz SM, et al (2002). A population-based study of squamous cell vaginal cancer: HPV and cofactors. *Gynecol Oncol*, **84**(2):263–70.

89 Judson PL, Habermann EB, Baxter NN, Durham SB, & Virnig BA (2006). Trends in the incidence of invasive and in situ vulvar carcinoma. *Obstet Gynecol*, **107**(5):1018–22.

90 Hampl M, Sarajuuri H, Wentzensen N, Bender HG, & Kueppers V (2006). Effect of human papillomavirus vaccines on vulvar, vaginal, and anal intraepithelial lesions and vulvar cancer. *Obstet Gynecol*, **108**(6):1361–68.

91 Joura EA, Leopolter S, Hernandez-Avila M, et al (2007). Efficacy of a quadrivalent prophylactic human papillomavirus (types 6, 11, 16, 18) L1 virus-like-particle vaccine against high-grade vulval and vaginal lesions: a combined analysis of three clinical trials. *Lancet*, **369**:1693–1702.

92 Parkin DM, Whelan SL, Ferlay J, et al (2002). *Cancer incidence in five continents. IARC Scientific Publications No. 155.* IARC, Lyon, France.

93 Rubin MA, Kleter B, Zhou M, et al (2001). Detection and typing of human papillomavirus DNA in penile carcinoma: evidence for multiple independent pathways of penile carcinogenesis. *Am J Pathol*, **159**(4):1211–18.

94 Heideman DA, Waterboer T, Pawlita M, et al (2007). Human papillomavirus-16 is the predominant type etiologically involved in penile squamous cell carcinoma. *J Clin Oncol*, **25**(29):4550–56.

95 Barrasso R, De Brux J, Croissant O, & Orth G (1987). High prevalence of papillomavirus-associated penile intraepithelial neoplasia in sexual partners of women with cervical intraepithelial neoplasia. *N Engl J Med*, **317**:916–23.

96 Spence A, Franco E, & Ferenczy A (2005). The role of human papillomaviruses in cancer: evidence to date. *Am J Cancer*, **4**:49–64.

97 Palefsky JM (2000). Human papillomavirus related tumors. *AIDS*, **14**(S3):S189–95.

98 Schantz SP & Yu GP (2002).Head and neck cancer incidence trends in young Americans, 1973–1997, with a special analysis for tongue cancer. *Arch Otolaryngol Head Neck Surg*, **128**(3):268–74.

99 Ragin CC, Modugno F, & Gollin SM (2007).The epidemiology and risk factors of head and neck cancer: a focus on human papillomavirus. *J Dent Res*, **86**(2):104–14.

100 D'Souza G, Kreimer AR, Viscidi R, et al (2007).Case-control study of human papillomavirus and oropharyngeal cancer. *N Engl J Med*, **356**(19):1944–56.

101 Pintos J, Black MJ, Sadeghi N, et al (2008). Human papillomavirus infection and oral cancer: a case-control study in Montreal, Canada. *Oral Oncol*, **44**:242–50.

102 Hemminki K, Dong C, & Frisch M (2000). Tonsillar and other upper aerodigestive tract cancer among cervical cancer patients and their husbands. *Eur J Cancer Prev*, **9**:433–37.

103 Lehtinen M, French KM, Dillner J, Paavonen J, & Garnett G (2008). Sound implementation of human papillomavirus vaccination as a community-randomized trial. *Therapy*, **5**(3):289–94.

104 Rousseau MC, Pereira JS, Prado JC, Villa LL, Rohan TE, & Franco EL (2001). Cervical coinfection with human papillomavirus (HPV) types as a predictor of acquisition and persistence of HPV infection. *J Infect Dis*, **184**:1508–17.

105 Kaufmann AM & Schneider A (2008). Therapeutic human papillomavirus vaccination. *Therapy*, **5**(3):339–48.

106 International Agency for Research on Cancer (IARC) (1994). *Schistosomes, Liver Flukes and Hellcobacter pylori. IARC monographs on the evaluation of carcinogenic risks to humans.* Vol. 61. IARC, Lyon, France.

107 International Agency for Research on Cancer (IARC) (1996). *Human Immunodeficiency Viruses and Human T-Cell Lymphotropic Viruses. IARC monographs on the evaluation of carcinogenic risks to humans.* Vol. 67. IARC, Lyon, France.

108 International Agency for Research on Cancer (IARC) (1997). *Epstein-Barr Virus and Kaposi's Sarcoma Herpesvirus/Human Herpesvirus 8. IARC monographs on the evaluation of carcinogenic risks to humans.* Vol. 70. IARC, Lyon, France.

109 Reeves WC, Brinton LA, García M, et al (1989). Human papillomavirus infection and cervical cancer in Latin America. *N Engl J Med*, **320**:1437–41.

110 Donnan SP, Wong FW, Ho SC, Lau EM, Takashi K, & Esteve J (1989). Reproductive and sexual risk factors and human papilloma virus infection in cervical cancer among Hong Kong Chinese. *Int J Epidemiol*, **18**:32–36.

111 Peng HQ, Liu SL, Mann V, Rohan T, & Rawls W (1991). Human papillomavirus types 16 and 33, herpes simplex virus type 2 and other risk factors for cervical cancer in Sichuan Province, China. *Int J Cancer*, **47**:711–16.

112 Shen CY, Ho MS, Chang SF, et al (1993). High rate of concurrent genital infections with human cytomegalovirus and human papillomaviruses in cervical cancer patients. *J Infect Dis*, **168**:449–52.

113 Eluf-Neto J, Booth M, Muñoz N, Bosch FX, Meijer CJ, & Walboomers JM (1994). Human papillomavirus and invasive cervical cancer in Brazil. *Br J Cancer*, **69**:114–19.

114 Asato T, Nakajima Y, Nagamine M, et al (1994). Correlation between the progression of cervical dysplasia and the prevalence of human papillomavirus. *J Infect Dis*, **169**:940–41.

Part 4

Optimizing patient care

Chapter 7

Improving cancer services: the approach taken in England

Mike Richards[1]

The overall goals of a national cancer control programme should be to reduce the burden of cancer in the population to a minimum and to provide optimal care to individual patients. To achieve these goals actions are required:

- ◆ To reduce the incidence of cancer (prevention)
- ◆ To improve survival rates through screening, early diagnosis and optimal delivery of treatments
- ◆ To reduce mortality through actions on incidence and survival
- ◆ To improve the quality of care, and thereby the quality of life, for those affected by cancer
- ◆ To optimize end of life care for those dying of cancer
- ◆ To build for the future through research

This chapter focuses on the approach taken to cancer control in one country. England was amongst the first jurisdictions to attempt to develop and implement a comprehensive national cancer programme. Many of the individual actions described here are similar to those being taken in other parts of the United Kingdom and in other countries including Denmark, France, and Canada. However, although the actions required are often similar, the delivery mechanisms may well need to be different, depending on the organization of health services within a particular jurisdiction. Indeed, even within one country the approach taken to implementation of a cancer strategy may need to change over time. This has been the case in England, where approaches to implementation have needed to respond to the evolution of the National Health Service (NHS). Although the focus of this chapter is on one country, many of the issues addressed are likely to be relevant elsewhere. These include:

- ◆ Why was a cancer control programme needed?
- ◆ What strategies have been adopted over the past 15 years and why?
- ◆ What has facilitated or impeded progress?
- ◆ What are the challenges for the future?

Background
The UK National Health Service

The NHS was established in the United Kingdom in 1948 with the aim of delivering a comprehensive service which was free at the point of delivery based on clinical need, not on ability to pay.

---

[1] Professor Mike Richards, CBE, MD, FRCP, National Cancer Director, England.

Since its inception it has been very largely tax funded, though limited charges have been payable for many years by some patients for prescriptions, dentistry, and some other services. Public expenditure accounts for almost 90 per cent of total expenditure on health in England.

Since the late 1990s responsibility for healthcare in Scotland, Wales, and Northern Ireland has progressively been devolved to relevant administrations, while that for England (population around 50 million) remains the responsibility of the UK government through the Department of Health in London.

Expenditure on healthcare in England lagged behind the European average in the 1980s and 1990s, though the gap has narrowed considerably in recent years. As a consequence, the infrastructure of the NHS in terms of workforce and facilities lagged behind that of other countries in the 1990s. This applied to the infrastructure for cancer services (e.g. CT scanners, MRI scanners, and linear accelerators) and to other aspects of healthcare. In the late 1990s Germany had twice as many doctors per head of population (3.6 per 1000) as the United Kingdom (1.8 per 1000).

The NHS has remained much loved by the population throughout its 60 years existence. Pride in the NHS was undoubtedly justified in its early years, but may have led to a degree of blindness to its deficiencies especially in the 1980s and early 1990s.

Cancer in England in the early 1990s

Like other western countries, the United Kingdom has a high death rate from cancer, with approximately one in three of the population developing cancer and one in four dying from cancer. Overall cancer mortality rates in England are broadly similar to those in comparator countries, though in the late 1980s and early 1990s mortality rates for lung cancer in men and breast cancer in women were amongst the worst in the world.

During the 1990s it became progressively more apparent that survival rates across a range of cancer types were inferior to those in most other Western European countries. The evidence for this came from the series of EUROCARE studies, which started with patients diagnosed in 1978 to 1985 and has most recently assessed outcomes for patients diagnosed in 2000 to 2002 [1–5]; see Figures 7.1 and 7.2. Initially the validity of these comparisons was questioned by clinicians in the United Kingdom and the results were greeted with disbelief by some. However, over time it has become generally accepted that the poor survival rates in the United Kingdom observed in the 1980s and 1990s were real and reflected a failure of the healthcare system to deliver optimal care.

What were these failures? In retrospect it is clear that the NHS was failing cancer patients in multiple ways: capacity was inadequate, new technology was only being adopted very slowly, few attempts had been made to streamline care delivery, few patients benefited from care being delivered by a coordinated team of professionals, many patients were being treated by generalists rather than specialists and there was poor communication between primary, secondary, and tertiary services. Taking breast cancer in the early 1990s as an example, it was possible for even a young woman not to undergo axillary node staging and for no attempt to be made to record the tumour size or pathological grade.

It is hard to understand why such a state of affairs had been allowed to exist. A fatalistic or nihilistic attitude towards cancer amongst both health professionals and the public, combined with a belief (pre EUROCARE) that outcomes in the United Kingdom would match those elsewhere may have been underlying factors. Importantly comparative data were unavailable and advocacy by patient groups and charities was, at that time, very weak.

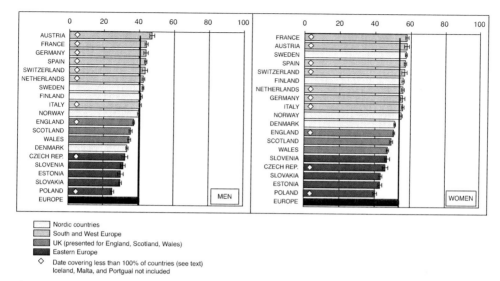

Fig. 7.1 5-year relative survival for all cancers combined, age standardized and incidence weighted, Europe, adults diagnosed in 1990 to 1994 and followed up to 1999.
Source: From *Eurocare 3* data. [3]

First steps to improve cancer services (1995–99)
The Calman-Hine report (1995)

The first wake up call on cancer services in England and Wales came in the mid-1990s. The Chief Medical Officers for England and Wales, Dr Kenneth Calman and Dr Deirdre Hine, commissioned a report by an expert advisory group on cancer which is now commonly called

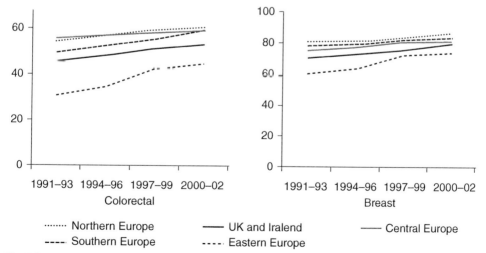

Fig. 7.2 5-year-period survival rates 1991 to 2002 for colorectal and breast cancer.
From *Eurocare 4* data [5].

the Calman-Hine report [6]. It is noteworthy that both chief medical officers had a pre-existing interest in cancer. The expert advisory group considered the evidence that was emerging at that time showing better outcomes for patients treated by specialists or in specialist centres for rare, uncommon, and common cancers. Alongside this a consensus was developing, at least amongst experts in breast cancer, that specialist breast units represented the optimal way forward [7].

The Calman-Hine report set out important principles regarding the provision of cancer care. Three levels of care working together as a network were recommended: primary care, cancer units in district general hospitals, and cancer centres which would normally service populations of at least one million. Multidisciplinary consultation and management was seen as essential.

The Calman-Hine report provided a much needed vision for the delivery of high quality care for all cancer patients. However, it did not cover prevention, screening or waiting times for hospital services. In addition it was not accompanied by any commitments on funding. It cannot therefore be considered as a comprehensive cancer control plan. Furthermore, implementation was not centrally directed.

Following publication of the Calman-Hine report progress was undoubtedly made, but the pace of change was variable. Different regions within England took different approaches. Some focused on the designation of cancer centres and cancer units, while others concentrated more on developing whole networks of care. Some pioneered approaches to accreditation of services.

Improving outcomes guidance

At a national level further work was commissioned to develop a series of guidance documents on services for different cancer sites (see Table 7.1). These 'Improving Outcomes Guidance Reports' were developed over a period of a decade (1996–2006). For each report proposals from a broad group of experts (including patients) were subjected to formal systematic reviews of the research

Table 7.1 Improving outcomes guidance reports

Breast cancers	1996 and 2002 (update)
Colorectal cancers	1997 and 2004 (update)
Lung cancers	1998
Gynaecological cancers	1999
Upper gastrointestinal cancers	2001
Urological cancers	2002
Haematological cancers	2003
Head and Neck cancers	2004
Supportive and palliative care	2004
Children's and Young Peoples' cancers	2005
Skin cancers	2006
Brain tumours	2006
Sarcomas	2006

These reports were published by the Department of Health until 2001 and by the National Institute of Health and Clinical Excellence (NICE) from 2002 onwards evidence and to wide consultation. The aim of each report is to set out the characteristics of a service which will deliver optimal outcomes. The reports are not designed as clinical guidelines which may inform decision making for individual patients. Instead they are aimed at the organizational level giving advice on the composition of multidisciplinary teams and on the relationship between volume or throughput of cases and outcomes. For several cancer types (e.g. gynaecologic, urological, upper gastrointestinal and head and neck cancers), the relevant Improving Outcomes Guidance report recommended that complex surgery should be consolidated in fewer hospitals than previously.

Steps taken by the new Labour Government (1997 onwards)

One of the first actions of the incoming Labour Government in 1997 was to raise the profile of waiting times for cancer, building on an election manifesto commitment. It is interesting to note that politicians had picked up on long-standing concerns amongst patients and the public about delays in diagnosis and treatment, even though this had not been addressed in the Calman-Hine report developed largely by healthcare professionals.

The initial commitment on waiting times was that 'everyone with suspected cancer will be able to see a specialist within two weeks of their GP deciding they need to be seen urgently and requesting an appointment. We will guarantee these arrangements for everyone with suspected breast cancer by April 1999 and for all other cases of suspected cancer by 2000' [8]. This commitment related solely to the interval between referral by a general practitioner (GP) and the first hospital visit. At this stage no commitments were made regarding the intervals to diagnosis or treatment.

In support of this commitment the Department of Health commissioned a retrospective baseline audit of waiting times for all patients diagnosed with cancer in England in the month of October 1997 [9]. This confirmed the size of the problem, with less than two thirds of patients who had been referred urgently being seen at a hospital within two weeks. To support implementation of the 'two week wait' target prospective monitoring arrangements were established and referral guidelines for suspected cancer were published by the Department of Health [10].

The late 1990s also saw the first injection of dedicated funds to improve the quality of cancer care. Implementation of each of the first three Improving Outcomes Guidance reports was undoubtedly assisted by the allocation of £10m of recurrent funding to support the development of teams and services for the relevant cancer. Progress towards the two week waiting time standard was also backed by the allocation of funds, which were used in some parts of the country to establish rapid access clinics (e.g. for patients with haematuria or postmenopausal bleeding).

Another important development at this time was the rise of advocacy related to cancer care. The National Cancer Alliance, which brought together patients and health professionals, undertook research based on focus groups of patients in different parts of the country, resulting in a report entitled 'Patient Centred Cancer Services: what patients say' published in 1996 [11]. This highlighted the importance of information and support, good communication between patients and professionals, and continuity of care amongst other issues. This type of market research had not previously been applied to cancer care in the UK.

At around the same time another cancer charity undertook a survey of health professionals working in different parts of the country to assess progress on implementation of the Calman-Hine report [12]. There is no doubt that advocacy by cancer charities has been an important catalyst for progress over the subsequent decade.

Despite all of these activities, a broad consensus emerged in early 1999 that the pace of change on cancer was not fast enough. Further evidence was emerging from the EUROCARE programme [2] on poor survival rates in the United Kingdom, along with strong evidence of differences in survival rates within England and Wales between NHS Regions and by socio-economic status [13]. In response to this the then Prime Minister, Tony Blair, convened a summit meeting on cancer at 10 Downing Street in May 1999. The fact that England and Wales generally lagged behind Europe on cancer survival rates was openly acknowledged by the government [14] and cancer was declared to be a top priority.

A number of actions followed the Downing Street summit. These included:

◆ A review of cancer research
◆ Establishment of a Cancer Action Team to promote implementation of cancer policy
◆ A review of cancer services by the Commission for Health Improvement [15]
◆ A large scale survey of the perceptions of cancer patients regarding their experience of care [16]
◆ Establishment of a Cancer Services Collaborative to support modernization of services at a local level
◆ Establishment of the post of National Cancer Director

The role of the National Cancer Director has been to lead the development of almost all aspects of cancer policy and to oversee implementation across the NHS. The only exception to this relates to the prevention of cancer, where there is clearly a great deal of overlap with other conditions such as cardiovascular disease. The National Cancer Director does, however, input to policy on prevention, particularly in relation to smoking and skin cancer.

On smoking the government set a target in 1998 to reduce smoking among adults from 28 per cent to 24 per cent by 2010 [17]. To achieve this, measures were introduced to increase taxation on tobacco, to end advertising and promotion of cigarettes, to reduce smuggling of tobacco and to assist smokers to quit. Much later (2007) legislation was introduced to make workplaces and public places smoke free. Adult smoking prevalence has now fallen to 21 per cent, with further reductions anticipated as a result of the smoke-free legislation.

A wider public health agenda was set out in 1999 in 'Saving Lives – our Healthier Nation' [18]. Included within this was a target to reduce the death rate from cancer in people under 75 years by at least a fifth by 2010, saving up to 100,000 lives in total. Mortality was already falling by the time the target was set. However, achievement of the target would require the existing trends to be continued over a period of 14 years.

The NHS Cancer Plan 2000

Development of the plan

One of the early tasks for the National Cancer Director was to secure agreement from the government for the development of a national cancer plan. This was agreed early in 2000 and it was made clear that the plan should be published as soon as reasonably possible.

The NHS Cancer Plan [19] was developed in parallel with the wider NHS Plan [20]. Both of these plans were developed in the context of a decision taken in March 2000 to make a sustained increase in NHS spending amounting to a real terms increase of a third over five years. Over time the aim was to bring health spending in England up to the EU average. Both plans carried the subtitle 'A plan for investment, a plan for reform'. Importantly both were launched by the then Prime Minister.

Given the timescale of less than 6 months from decision to develop a cancer plan to publication, it was not possible to establish a major formal consultative process. Instead, the National Cancer Director set up a small informal advisory group of experts and complemented this with extensive informal consultation at many different meetings and conferences. It might be argued that the product would have been better given more time and more formal consultation. However, in many ways, the actions required at that time were fairly clear cut, including the need to expand capacity in cancer services. It would certainly have been a mistake to delay and thereby risk any loss of political support.

Content and commitments

The NHS Cancer Plan [19] had ambitious aims, to raise the level of cancer services in England to be among the best in Europe and to save lives. It was the first comprehensive national cancer programme in England covering prevention, screening, community cancer services, cutting waiting times, improving treatment, and improving care including palliative care. The plan set out a number of key targets and commitments including new waiting time targets for diagnosis and treatment, extending cancer screening, and introducing nationwide peer assessment processes for cancer services to monitor implementation of the Improving Outcomes Guidance.

The Cancer Plan was backed with substantial extra funding and commitments to invest in staff, facilities, and research. The plan heralded the establishment of a National Cancer Research Institute (see next section). The plan made clear that cancer networks would be a major vehicle for local delivery of the commitments with oversight from the Regional Offices of the NHS. In addition a new Cancer Taskforce was established chaired by the National Cancer Director to oversee progress at a national level. Clear steps towards implementation were set out as part of the Cancer Plan with associated milestones for the early years.

Progress 2000 to 2005

Ideally progress would be measured in terms of clinical outcomes (survival, mortality, and patients' own reports of their experience of care and their health and wellbeing). However, some clinical outcomes are only measurable years after the event to which they relate (e.g. diagnosis and primary treatment). In addition if clinical outcomes improve it is not always clear what the change is attributable to (e.g. a change in service organization or the introduction of a new treatment).

It is therefore highly desirable to measure the structures and processes of care as well as the outcomes. For many of the potential measures of structure and process there is a strong evidential link with better outcomes. Examples of measures which have been used to monitor progress in implementation of the NHS Cancer Plan are shown in Tables 7.2 and 7.3.

Progress following publication of the NHS Cancer Plan has been monitored at a national level by the following bodies:

- A Cancer Programme Board at the Department of Health, chaired by the National Cancer Director. The Board meets monthly to review progress on all aspects of cancer policy.

- A Cancer Taskforce, with external representatives, met twice a year in the initial years after publication of the Cancer Plan. It has recently been replaced by an advisory board to monitor progress following the Cancer Reform Strategy.

- The National Audit Office, which scrutinizes public spending on behalf of parliament, undertook three detailed reviews into cancer in 2004 and 2005 [21–23].

- The Care Quality Commission (the successor body to the Commission for Health Improvement and the Healthcare Commission) monitors compliance against key targets by individual NHS organizations.

- Advisory groups established by the Department of Health and chaired or co-chaired by the National Cancer Director (e.g. for prostate, bowel, and lung cancer and for radiotherapy and chemotherapy) monitor progress on individual areas within the programme.

Table 7.2 Measuring structures and processes of cancer services

Smoking	Attenders at stop smoking services
	Numbers of quitters (e.g. at 4 weeks)
	Smoking prevalence in the population
Screening	Uptake/coverage rates
	Numbers and rates of cancers detected
	Size/stage of cancers detected
	Various quality assurance measures
Waiting times	Interval from urgent referral to first hospital visit
	Interval from urgent referral to first treatment
	Interval from diagnosis (decision to treat) to treatment
Multidisciplinary teams	Number of teams and throughput of cases
	Compliance with national peer review standards/measures
Treatment	Numbers of procedures (e.g. prostatectomies)
	Fractions/courses of radiotherapy
	Uptake of new drugs
Workforce	Numbers of consultants
	Numbers of nurse specialists
	Numbers of radiographers
	Participants in national training programmes
Facilities	Numbers of CT scanners
	Numbers of MRI scanners
	Numbers of PET/CT scanners
	Numbers of linear accelerators
Investment	Total investment in cancer services (nationally or locally)
	Additional investment in cancer services (year on year)
	Expenditure on specialist palliative care

Table 7.3 Outcome measures for cancer

Incidence	Incidence rates by tumour type
Survival	1-year survival rates by tumour type
	5-year survival rates by tumour type
Mortality	30 day mortality (e.g. following surgery)
	Overall mortality
	Mortality in socio-economically deprived areas
Patient Experience	Surveys of patients' reports of their experience of care

This level of scrutiny has been critical to maintaining momentum. The reports from the National Audit Office have shown that good progress has been made on virtually every aspect of the Cancer Plan, but that there is still more to be done to deliver optimal outcomes [21–23].

National drivers for change

The existence of a cancer plan sets a direction of travel, but does not in itself drive change. What are the drivers for change in a system as large and complex as the NHS? The National Cancer Director does not personally control local expenditure on cancer in England (currently estimated to be around £4.9 billion per annum), nor does he have direct authority over local commissioners or providers of services. He does, however, have influence vested in him by Ministers. This influence can be exercised directly through cancer networks and other organizations and through the performance management structure of the NHS. The latter includes the Department of Health, Strategic Health Authorities, and Primary Care Trusts.

The influence of the National Cancer Director is greatly enhanced by the existence of several relatively small but highly effective teams with different functions, but which work together as a National Cancer Programme, led by the National Cancer Director. These individual teams have evolved over time, but currently comprise:

- The Department of Health Cancer Policy Team (led by Ms Jane Allberry) – which provides advice to Ministers on all aspects of cancer and supports the National Cancer Director in developing and monitoring cancer policy

- The National Cancer Screening Team (led by Prof Julietta Patnick) – which oversees the introduction of new screening programmes, the extension of existing programmes, quality assurance of screening, and coordination of the national screening programmes

- The National Cancer Action Team (led by Ms Teresa Moss) – which has key roles in supporting the development of cancer networks, the development of standards/measures for cancer services, overseeing peer review appraisal of cancer services, and stronger commissioning amongst other functions

- NHS Improvement – Cancer (formerly the Cancer Services Collaborative) (led by Dr Janet Williamson) – which works with individual multidisciplinary teams and cancer services to streamline and modernize care for the benefit of patients and the NHS. NHS Improvement has had an important role in helping local cancer services to deliver reductions in waiting times. It is now focussing on transforming inpatient care and on the survivorship agenda

- The National Cancer Intelligence Network (led by Mr Chris Carrigan) – which was launched in 2008 and brings together the eight regional cancer registries in England, clinical reference groups for each tumour group, and a national cancer services analysis team

Support and encouragement from national teams are, however, not always sufficient on their own to deliver improvements in cancer services. The natural inertia in any large system should not be underestimated. Such inertia has certainly been observable in some NHS cancer services over the past decade. Hardworking clinicians often believe that improvements can only be brought about through substantial investment in additional staff, though the Cancer Services Collaborative has clearly demonstrated that major improvements can frequently be made with minimal investment by rationalising pathways of care. In addition, health service managers may not have sufficient insight into clinical processes or expertise in service improvement to help bring about change.

To overcome the barriers to change several complementary approaches were used following the publication of the NHS Cancer Plan. The key drivers were:

- Targets and rigorous performance management

- Guidance, standards, and peer review
- Support for service improvement
- Funding for national training initiatives

In addition financial incentives have been used to a very limited extent to enhance cancer services delivery in primary care through the Quality and Outcomes Framework (QOF). This is a voluntary annual reward and incentive programme for all GP practices. This has, for example, encouraged GPs to maintain registers of patients with cancer and to establish better care processes for people approaching the end of life.

Targets and rigorous performance management

Both the NHS Plan and the NHS Cancer Plan relied heavily on the combination of additional investment by local health services and targets as a driver for change. The targets made clear the areas in which investment and reform were most needed. In relation to cancer the key areas covered by targets were:

- Reductions in smoking rates in socio-economically deprived groups
- Extension of the breast screening programme
- Upgrading of the cervical screening programme
- Establishment of a colorectal cancer screening programme if and when pilot studies demonstrated that this was appropriate
- Reducing waiting times between referral and first treatment
- Reducing waiting times between diagnosis and first treatment
- Implementation of the Improving Outcomes Guidance recommendations
- Investment in hospices and specialist palliative care services
- Increased overall investment in cancer services

These areas were therefore regarded as 'must dos' for the NHS. This was reinforced through subsequent guidance documents from the Department of Health to the NHS regarding priorities for each year. The many other commitments in the Cancer Plan were seen as desirable but somewhat less essential.

Despite their 'must do' status achievement of the various targets required a considerable push from the centre. In the case of the extension of the breast screening programme, for example, most parts of the country achieved the target within the prescribed timescale. In the remaining areas strong pressure from the performance management team at the Department of Health was required.

In relation to the additional £50m promised for hospices and specialist palliative care services, it became clear that appropriate levels of additional funding were not being made by local Primary Care Trusts from their baseline allocations. As this was a high profile area involving a Cancer Plan target and the voluntary sector, a decision was made to establish a central fund of £50m for three years. This was then provided to localities on receipt of acceptable plans for service improvement. Spending on this area was rigorously monitored.

After the first full year of implementation of the Cancer Plan it also became apparent that progress towards the overall target to increase expenditure on cancer by £570m a year by 2003–2004 was unsatisfactory. However, it was not felt to be appropriate to establish a central fund for all new investment in cancer. Instead a rigorous investment tracking exercise was instituted. In the end investment was shown to be ahead of target (£639m) over the relevant time period [27].

More recently, programme budgeting has been introduced within the NHS, making tracking of investment much simpler. This provides a retrospective analysis of NHS resource utilization across 23 service areas, based on returns from Primary Care Trusts. Programme budgeting data has shown a further increase in expenditure of 27 per cent in the three year period 2003/04 to 2006/07.

The actions that were required to achieve the waiting time targets have been reported separately [28] and are summarized later in this chapter.

Guidance, standards, and peer review

Until the late 1990s no serious attempt had been made to assess the quality of local cancer services in England. Following the Calman-Hine report and the publication of the early Improving Outcomes Guidance reports, several NHS Regions (most notably Trent, Northern and Yorkshire) had started to develop their own approaches to appraisal or accreditation of services. By 2000 it was apparent that a national approach would be more desirable and that national standards (later referred to as measures) were needed, so that services could be assessed against common criteria.

A first national round of peer review was undertaken in 2001. This focused on four tumour groups (breast, colorectal, lung, and gynaecological) and involved nearly 700 multidisciplinary teams. Cross cutting services such as pathology, chemotherapy, radiotherapy, and specialist palliative care were also appraised [24]. Much of the learning from this initiative came from clinicians visiting services other than their own and gathering ideas on how their services might be improved.

The measures were revised and extended in 2004 [25] when a second round of peer review visits commenced. This involved a total of 1069 multidisciplinary teams (MDTs) across six tumour types (upper gastrointestinal and urological cancer services now being included), 1051 cross cutting services, and 8 cancer registries. The findings were all openly reported to individual NHS organizations and to local cancer networks and commissioners and published on a website (www.cquins.nhs.uk).

This second round of peer review confirmed that MDT working is now firmly embedded in this country and that considerable progress had been made since 2001 [26]. It showed that some teams were achieving very high levels of compliance with the measures of structure and processes of care. However, significant challenges were also highlighted. These included shortages of key staff groups such as clinical nurse specialists, histopathologists, and specialist palliative care staff in some teams. The publication of a national overview [26] has allowed individual cancer networks to benchmark the performance of their own services against those elsewhere in the country. Those with poorly performing services have been asked to confirm that remedial action has been taken.

There is a broad consensus that the peer review programme has been a valuable driver for service change. The programme will continue, but over time there will be a greater emphasis on measures of outcome and on self assessment, to reduce the burden of visits. There is no doubt that the combination of Improving Outcomes Guidance and peer review appraisal has pushed forward the consolidation of complex cancer surgical services.

Support for service improvement

The Cancer Services Collaborative was established in 1999, based on approaches developed by Don Berwick at the Institute for Healthcare Improvement in Boston, Massachusetts. More recently the collaborative has merged into NHS Improvement, which is undertaking similar initiatives in cardiac and stroke services.

In essence the approach involves gaining a detailed understanding of current care processes and then testing modifications. Often no single person will understand all the elements of a care process. For example, a consultant may have little knowledge of how referrals reach his office via a hospital post room or how bookings are made. Similarly, managers may have little understanding of the rationale for a sequence of diagnostic and staging investigations.

In relation to cancer services in England this approach has been demonstrated to reduce waiting times for radiological investigations and endoscopy and to facilitate achievement of both the two week waiting time target and the Cancer Plan targets for reducing waiting for diagnosis and treatment. More recently a similar approach has been shown to be effective in streamlining inpatient care pathways. The same principles are also being used to reduce the turnaround time between a woman having a cervical screening test and receiving the result.

The approach works well with enthusiasts and so-called 'early adopters'. Engaging other clinicians and managers remains a challenge. To a certain extent the combination of a service improvement approach showing what can be achieved and a performance management approach showing what must be achieved can be very powerful (see cancer waiting times in the following sections).

Funding for national training initiatives

The United Kingdom has a strong record of invention, but the NHS lags behind in the systemic uptake of innovations [29]. This is true for cancer and for other areas of healthcare. One of the clearest examples of this was the introduction of a new surgical procedure, total mesorectal excision (TME) for rectal cancer. This had been pioneered by a surgeon, Prof Heald, in Basingstoke, England in the 1980s. He had then trained surgeons in many other countries, but without significant uptake in the United Kingdom, despite evidence of lower recurrence rates and improved survival using the TME technique. Eventually, as a result of funding from the NHS Cancer Plan and a successful pilot programme funded by Macmillan Cancer Support, it became possible to institute a national training programme in England. This involved almost every colorectal cancer team in the country. Importantly the training was multidisciplinary involving radiologists, pathologists, oncologists, and nurse specialists as well as colorectal surgeons. In addition to the benefits for patients it is highly likely that the programme will be cost-saving over a small number of years, with fewer patients needing permanent colostomies and fewer needing treatment for recurrence.

Building on the success of the TME training programme comparable initiatives have now been undertaken or are underway relating to:

◆ Sentinel lymph node biopsy for breast cancer

◆ Colonoscopy – where major improvements in complete examinations have been observed

◆ Laparoscopic colorectal surgery

One of the key skills required by cancer clinicians is that they should be able to communicate effectively with their patients and with their colleagues. Prior to the publication of the NHS Cancer Plan a large survey of hospital consultants involved in cancer care had shown that less than half felt that they had had adequate training in communication. One of the commitments in the Cancer Plan was to provide such training. Based on models of training which have been proven to be effective in randomized controlled trials a training programme is now being rolled out across the NHS.

Local implementation through cancer networks

Cancer networks started to develop in the late 1990s in response to the Calman-Hine report. The NHS Cancer Plan subsequently made it clear that cancer networks would be the organizational model for implementation. Cancer networks bring together health service commissioners (Primary Care Trusts) and providers (primary and community care and hospitals, the voluntary sector and (ideally) local authorities). They are partnership organizations with no statutory authority but with a core team of dedicated staff. Their authority and influence comes from that vested in them by the relevant partner organizations (e.g. Primary Care Trusts in relation to commissioning). The funding for most aspects of cancer care is held by Primary Care Trusts serving populations typically of 300,000 to 500,000, though that for some complex services is held by specialized commissioning groups which cover the territories of a Strategic Health Authority (typically serving a population of around 5 million).

The key tasks of a cancer network are:

◆ To support PCTs in their role as commissioners of cancer services

◆ To assess the needs of the local population

◆ To develop and monitor local plans which are in line with national policy

◆ To support service reconfiguration in line with Improving Outcomes Guidance where necessary

◆ To support achievement of key targets and commitments

◆ To facilitate effective coordination of care across organizational boundaries

There are currently 28 cancer networks in England. Typically they serve populations of 1 to 2.5 million, though a few serve large populations (up to 3.2 million). In essence the boundaries of a network should reflect the natural flows of patients from the community to district

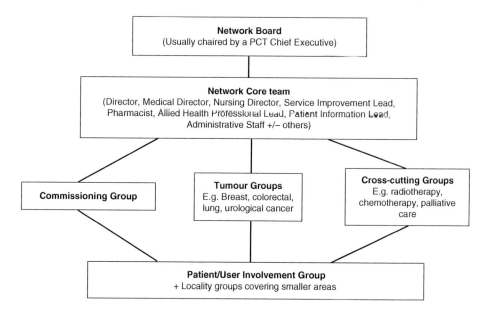

Fig. 7.3 Structure of a typical cancer network.

general hospitals and on to tertiary services. The structure of a typical cancer network is shown in Figure 7.3.

The study undertaken by the National Audit Office approximately four years after publication of the NHS Cancer Plan showed that cancer networks had helped to drive forward improvements in cancer services, but that there was more to do if they were all to become fully effective [23]. In part this was because of wider organizational changes in the NHS involving both Strategic Health Authorities and Primary Care Trusts. Further progress has undoubtedly been made over the subsequent four years, although some networks appear to be more effective than others. However, without networks it is extremely unlikely that some of the reconfiguration which has taken place would have been achieved.

The National Cancer Action Team (NCAT) has an important role in supporting cancer network development. NCAT organizes and sponsors three two-day meetings each year of around 10 representatives from each of the 30 networks. These Network Development Programme meetings provide a very useful opportunity for information and ideas to be shared between the centre and the networks and between networks themselves. The success of this initiative can partly be assessed by the keenness of participants to attend.

Problems and solutions

As has already been indicated, implementation of the Cancer Plan has not always been straightforward, even when a commitment was backed by a clear target. However, when problems have arisen, solutions have been found or progress towards a solution is underway.

Examples include:

- ◆ Achievement of the Cancer Plan waiting time targets
- ◆ Provision of world class radiotherapy services
- ◆ Provision of access to cost-effective new medicines

Achieving the waiting time targets

The waiting time targets set in the NHS Cancer Plan built on the two week wait target which had been set in the late 1990s. The two most important targets were:

1 A maximum of one month (31 days) wait from diagnosis to first treatment of all cancers. 'Diagnosis' was subsequently deemed to be the date of decision to treat.

2 A maximum two month (62 days) wait from urgent GP referral to first definitive treatment for all cancers.

Both of these targets had to be achieved by December 2005. By international standards these targets may be considered to be undemanding, though few countries can provide data on these time intervals. Nonetheless, the targets were considered demanding in England and proved to be so.

Although a great deal of work was done between 2000 and 2004 to expand the cancer workforce, to demonstrate through the Cancer Service Collaborative that reductions in waiting times could be achieved and to put monitoring systems in place, in practice progress remained very disappointing. At the end of 2004 less than 80 per cent of patients were being treated within the 62 day period, with virtually no improvement over the previous 12 months.

Recognising this and in response to media pressure and political concern, a National Cancer Waits Project (NCWP) was established at the end of 2004 bringing together the Cancer Policy Team and the Performance Management Team at the Department of Health, the Cancer Services Collaborative, and the National Cancer Action Team. An external reference group of clinicians

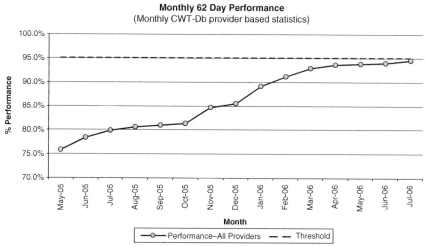

Monthly 62 Day Performance
(Monthly CWT-Db provider based statistics)

Fig. 7.4 Improvement in achievement of the 62 day cancer waiting time target.

and managers was also set up. The profile of cancer waiting times was raised throughout the NHS by making the targets a 'key deliverable'. The importance was stressed by Ministers, senior civil servants, the National Cancer Director, and by the Healthcare Commission who were responsible at that time for performance rating of NHS Trusts.

Weekly monitoring of performance from all hospitals was introduced ensuring that Trusts reported forward looking information on patients' progress through the care pathway, rather than simply reporting after the event that a patient had missed the target time. The Cancer Services Collaborative worked with demonstrator sites in each Strategic Health Authority and an intensive support team worked with Trusts with the poorest performance.

As a result of these initiatives the proportion of patients being treated with the target time rose rapidly, with a 95 per cent operational standard being achieved in the summer of 2006 (Figure 7.4).

Provision of world class radiotherapy services

During the 1980s and 1990s radiotherapy capacity in England had been allowed to fall substantially behind that in other developed countries, with inadequate numbers of staff (especially therapy radiographers) and linear accelerators. In recognition of this the NHS Cancer Plan made provision for a major increase in the number of therapy radiographers in training and provided central funding for an unprecedented number of new linear accelerators.

Despite successful implementation of these initiatives, it was clear by around 2005 that demand for radiotherapy was continuing to outstrip supply and that waiting times for radiotherapy were still unacceptably long. A National Radiotherapy Advisory Group (NRAG) was therefore established to assess future requirements and make recommendations on the way forward. The NRAG recommended that capacity should increase by around 80 per cent by 2016, with an immediate need to expand capacity by around one third. These recommendations were accepted by Ministers and form part of the Cancer Reform Strategy [27].

As a result of this each cancer network has been asked to draw up a plan consistent with the NRAG recommendations. Strategic Health Authorities (SHAs) have been asked to coordinate network plans. The National Cancer Action Team will then review all plans to ensure adequate capacity will be available across the country.

As a further driver for change the scope of the current waiting time standards is being extended to incorporate second and subsequent treatments for cancer, thereby capturing all radiotherapy treatments.

Provision of access to cost effective new medicines

In the late 1990s there was widespread concern that decision making by health authorities regarding funding for novel cancer drugs was very variable, creating a so-called 'postcode lottery' of care. This meant that funding decisions depended on where a patient lived rather than on clinical need. This applied to around 15 chemotherapy treatments licensed since 1993 (when paclitaxel first received a licence in England). As a result of this the Government asked the newly established National Institute for Clinical Excellence (NICE) to assess the cost effectiveness of these drugs.

Although the large majority of these drugs assessed in the first few years of NICE's existence received a positive appraisal, by 2003 it was apparent that despite NICE guidance there were unacceptable variations in the uptake of these drugs across the country [30]. This resulted in sustained media criticism partly fuelled by patient groups. A study undertaken by the National Cancer Director confirmed this [31]. However, the cause of the variation was not that some Primary Care Trusts (PCTs) were refusing to pay for NICE-approved drugs. Rather, there was poor local capacity planning and considerable variation in clinical practice [31].

Feedback of this benchmarking information to cancer networks almost certainly had a positive impact, as a follow up study in 2006 showed that uptake had increased markedly and variation between networks had decreased [32].

Despite these positive changes, concerns about access to new medicines reached a climax early in 2008. The main concerns were that:

- New cancer drugs which were available in other developed countries were not available in England.
- A small number of patients who were choosing to pay for drugs which were not funded by the NHS were being denied any NHS care.
- The interval between licensing and NICE providing guidance on drugs was unacceptably long.
- Primary Care Trusts were making varied judgements on funding of drugs which had not yet been appraised by NICE, creating a further 'postcode lottery'.

In response to these concerns, the Secretary of State for Health asked the National Cancer Director to undertake a review of these issues. His report made 14 recommendations which should improve access to new medicines and ensure that no patients are denied NHS care [33]. These recommendations have been accepted by the government, but it is still too early to judge how effective these measures will be.

The role of charities

The United Kingdom is fortunate to have three major cancer charities each with a distinctive profile, but each also having a commitment to work in partnership with the Department of Health and the NHS on cancer more widely. These are Cancer Research UK (research and information), Macmillan Cancer Support (information and support for patients and carers), and Marie Curie Cancer Care (End of Life Care). There are also multiple smaller charities which generally focus on single cancer types (e.g. Breakthrough Breast Cancer and the Prostate Cancer

Charity), on specific patient groups (e.g. Cancer Black Care and the Teenage Cancer Trust), or on end of life care (e.g. voluntary hospices).

The charities both individually and collectively have contributed very significantly to progress on cancer in England since 1995. These contributions include:

- Innovation and service development – for example, Macmillan Cancer Support has been very influential in establishing clinical nurse specialist posts; Marie Curie Cancer Care has pioneered new approaches to end of life care and the Teenage Cancer Trust has supported the development of specialist units for teenagers and young people with cancer.

- Ongoing service delivery – for example, voluntary hospices make a very substantial contribution to the delivery of specialist end of life care services for patients with cancer.

- Patient information – Many charities provide patient information, but of greatest significance is the partnership led by Macmillan Cancer Support (which now incorporates CancerBackup), Cancer Research UK, the National Cancer Action Team, and the NHS cancer networks. This partnership, which also involves other cancer charities, has the potential to provide information materials related to different phases of the cancer care pathway through a dedicated electronic platform to all health professionals and patients.

- Research – See next section.

- Advocacy – This has been an area of major development over the past decade. Charities have raised the general profile of cancer substantially through surveys that have shown it to be the most frequently reported concern amongst the public. Charities have also run effective targeted campaigns related to smoke-free legislation (Cancer Research UK) and the impact of cancer on individuals' financial position (Macmillan Cancer Support). Most recently charities have worked collectively to lobby for a second Cancer Plan (see following paragraphs).

Progress on research

Progress on cancer research in the UK over the past decade is an excellent example of partnership working between government and the voluntary sector. In response to concerns about the coordination of cancer research a Cancer Research Funders' Forum was established in 1999 bringing together the Department of Health, the Medical Research Council, and the major charities contributing to cancer research. An early success from that initiative was a review of opportunities for research into prostate cancer which resulted in increased investment and establishment of new research collaboratives.

Building on this a National Cancer Research Institute (NCRI) was launched in April 2001, as a partnership organization bringing together government, charities, and industry. This was never intended to be a large 'bricks and mortar' institute, but rather a largely virtual organization (with a small secretariat) to ensure greater coherence in research efforts.

Key outputs from the NCRI include:

- Establishment of a national cancer research network (largely funded by the Department of Health). The initial aim was to double the number of patients entered into clinical trials and other well designed studies from a baseline of 3.75 percent within three years. This was achieved ahead of target and accrual stood at 11.2 per cent in 2006-07. Provision of additional data managers and research nurses across the country has been one of the key factors in this achievement.

- Establishment of a cancer research database to which all partners contribute, using the same coding structure as that used by the National Cancer Institutes in the United States and

Canada. This led to the publication of a first strategic analysis in 2002 giving a comprehensive picture of research in the UK [34].

◆ Reviews into opportunities for research in under-funded areas including prevention [35], supportive and palliative care [36], lung cancer [37], and radiotherapy and radiobiology [38]. Each of these reviews had led to new research initiatives.

◆ Informatics and bio-banking initiatives.

◆ The establishment of a National Cancer Intelligence Network. This is a partnership organization involving regional cancer registries and clinical groups. The NCIN oversees collation and analysis of cancer data at a national level.

◆ A network of experimental cancer medicine centres.

◆ Enhanced consumer involvement in research.

◆ Improved international collaborations through the International Cancer Research Partnership.

◆ A successful annual NCRI conference.

◆ A strategic plan for 2008 to 2013 [39].

The cancer reform strategy

Development of a second cancer control plan

By late 2005 it was apparent that many of the targets and commitments from the NHS Cancer Plan had been achieved or were on track to being achieved. Concerns arose in the cancer community that momentum might be lost, despite there being much more to be done: a cancer community which had become stronger over the years of the plan. A Cancer Campaigning Group comprising around 30 cancer charities started lobbying for a second cancer plan [40]. In response to this, in December 2006 the government announced the development of a 'Cancer Reform Strategy' (CRS).

It is important to note that the NHS was facing a potential overspend at the time of this announcement. The government wanted to make it clear that this new national strategy would be different from the NHS Cancer Plan. Although it was recognized that expenditure on cancer would inevitably rise with increasing incidence and the introduction of new treatments, there should be no expectations that the strategy itself would contain commitments on additional expenditure.

Apart from the challenging financial position, the NHS had changed radically between 2000 and 2007. Any new cancer strategy would need to reflect this. In 2000 the NHS was a monopoly provider of clinical services as well as being the funder of services. By 2007 some elective surgery was being outsourced to independent sector treatment centres, as were some diagnostic services (e.g. some MRI scanning and PET CT scanning) with funding from the NHS. A system of standard tariffs for different procedures had been introduced and patients were expected to be given choice in relation to hospitals. The emphasis of government policy was starting to change from capacity building to improve access to a greater focus on fair, personalized, effective, and safe services [41]. There was also increased emphasis on supporting local change from the centre rather than instructing it and on making the best use of resources [41]. The Cancer Reform Strategy was also to be developed in parallel with a comprehensive End of Life Care Strategy, covering all conditions including cancer [42]. End of life care is therefore not a major theme of the CRS.

The approach to development of the CRS was much more inclusive and consultative than that taken in 2000 for the NHS Cancer Plan. Cancer charities, service users, cancer networks and health service managers played a major part alongside cancer experts. A formal advisory board was established along with working groups covering awareness and early detection, new service models, patient experience, clinical outcomes measurement, commissioning, and costs and benefits. Groups related to individual cancer sites were charged with developing visions for relevant services for the year 2012.

Contents and commitments

The CRS builds on progress achieved following the NHS Cancer Plan. It deliberately sets a direction for only five years (to 2012), as it was felt that it was realistic to predict what would be needed over that time scale. The strategy is unashamedly ambitious, aiming to deliver world class services and outcomes. It recognizes both the challenges related to the increasing incidence of cancer and the opportunities afforded by new scientific developments.

The NHS Cancer Plan had necessarily focused largely on the most pressing problems of its time, namely increasing capacity, reducing waiting times and the firm establishment of the infrastructure of MDTs and cancer networks. The CRS commits to going further in these areas, but gives new emphasis to what happens to patients before they are referred to hospital and after completion of primary treatment.

The CRS contains seven key areas for action:

1 Prevention: Consultation on the next steps for tobacco control following the introduction of smoke-free legislation in 2007 was announced, together with additional funding for the prevention of skin cancer. Other work on prevention (diet, obesity, and physical activity) is being dealt with separately.

2 Diagnosing cancer earlier: In addition to further improvements to the national screening programmes for breast, cervical, and bowel cancer, the CRS puts particular emphasis on earlier diagnosis of patients with symptoms. Over 90 per cent of all patients with cancer present symptomatically. There is a considerable body of evidence indicating that the poor survival rates observed in the United Kingdom [1–5] are to a large extent attributable to patients in the United Kingdom having more advanced disease at the time of diagnosis than their European counterparts. To take forward work in this area a National Awareness and Early Diagnosis Initiative has been launched.

3 Going further on cancer waits: The scope of the 31 day target set in 2000 has been extended to cover all treatments for cancer, not just the first treatment. The scope of the 62 day target has also been widened, so that more patients will benefit.

4 Better treatment: Commitments are made which will improve the quality of surgery, radiotherapy, and chemotherapy services.

5 Living with and beyond cancer: A new National Cancer Survivorship Initiative was announced.

6 Reducing cancer inequalities: A new National Cancer Equality Initiative was announced to tackle the inequalities in outcomes according to race, age, gender, disability, religion, sexual orientation, and socio-economic status.

7 Delivering care in the most appropriate setting: A major shift towards more ambulatory cancer care is envisaged. NHS Improvement is leading an initiative to transform inpatient care by reducing avoidable admissions to hospital and by reducing lengths of stay.

Two major drivers for implementation are set out in the CRS. These are:

1 Collection and publication of better information on clinical outcomes and on patient experience. The collection of defined datasets by MDTs will be mandated, with the relevant

information being sent to cancer registries and to the National Cancer Intelligence Network. A regular patient experience survey programme will also be instituted.

2 Stronger commissioning by PCTs working through cancer networks. It is recognized that commissioning of cancer services is highly complex.

National support for local commissioning is being strengthened. An electronic cancer commissioning toolkit has been made available to the NHS.

It is too early to assess the impact of the CRS. However, the strategy has been widely welcomed by stakeholders and progress in the first year has generally been judged to be satisfactory [43]. All the national initiatives announced in the strategy are now underway. The model of partnership working which characterized the development of the strategy is continuing into implementation, though this will not stop individual partners making their views known should progress not be satisfactory.

Personal reflections on change

Twenty years ago cancer services and outcomes in the United Kingdom lagged significantly behind those in other countries, but this was not recognized at the time. Since 1995 strenuous efforts have been made to catch up, with the direction being set first by the Calman-Hine report and subsequently by the NHS Cancer Plan and the Cancer Reform Strategy. There is no doubt that progress has been made, but it is not yet possible to say how much the gap with other developed countries has closed. Most knowledgeable observers in England believe that the gap will have been narrowed but not eliminated. In addition, though less frequent, I still hear too many individual reports of suboptimal care.

No single factor accounts for the progress that has been made. In my view the most important factors are:

◆ Direction: Having a clear national strategy and ensuring that it is both comprehensive and up to date.

◆ Political commitment: This has been consistent in this country for well over a decade and is reinforced by the high priority the public places on cancer care. The strong personal commitment of two Prime Ministers has been of enormous value.

◆ Leadership at national and local levels.

◆ Strong advocacy especially from the cancer charities.

◆ Relentless interest from the media.

◆ National support for local implementation through the National Cancer Action Team, The Cancer Screening Programme, NHS Improvement, and the National Cancer Intelligence Network.

◆ Targets and rigorous performance management of key deliverables.

◆ National guidance, standards and peer review.

◆ Funding to increase capacity where necessary and for national training initiatives.

◆ Monitoring: The data available now to monitor progress on cancer both nationally and locally is much better than it was a decade ago. However, further improvements are urgently needed so that meaningful comparisons of clinical outcomes can be made.

◆ Scrutiny, both internally within the Department of Health and externally by advocates, parliamentarians, the National Audit Office, and the Care Quality Commission.

Even with all these factors pushing in the same direction change has not always been straight-forward. It has required a great deal of very hard work by thousands of NHS staff to make the changes that are now benefiting patients. However, building on this progress and with the new initiatives now underway the goal of achieving world class outcomes is now realistic.

References

1 Berrino F, Sant M, Verdecchia A, Capocaccia R, Hakulinen T & Esteve J (1995). Survival of cancer patients in Europe – The EUROCARE study, IARC Scientific Publications No. 132 Lyon, France.

2 Berrino F, Capocaccia R, Esteve J, et al (1999). Survival of cancer patients in Europe – The EUROCARE-2 study, IARC Scientific Publications No. 151, Lyon, France.

3 Berrino F, Capocaccia R, Coleman MP, et al (2003). Survival of cancer patients in Europe – EUROCARE-3 study, *Ann Oncol*, **14**(suppl.5):1–155.

4 Berrino F, De Angelis R, Sant M, et al (2007). Survival for eight major cancers and all cancers combined for European adults diagnosed in 1995–99: results of the EUROCARE-4 study. *Lancet Oncol*, **8**:773–83.

5 Verdecchia A, Francisci S, Brenner H, et al (2007). Recent cancer survival in Europe: a 2000–02 period analysis of EUROCARE-4 data. *Lancet Oncol*, **8**:784–96.

6 A policy framework for commissioning cancer services (The Calman-Hine Report). Department of Health 1995.

7 Richards M A, Baum M, Dowsett, et al (1994). Provision of breast services in the UK: the advantages of specialist breast units, Report of a working party of the British Breast Group, The Breast (suppl.).

8 The New NHS: Modern, Dependable, Department of Health. December 1997.

9 Spurgeon P, Barwell F, & Kerr D (2000). Waiting times for cancer patients in England after general practitioners' referral: retrospective national survey. *BMJ*, **320**:838–39.

10 Referral guidelines for suspected cancer (1999). Department of Health.

11 Patient centred cancer services? What patients say (1996). National Cancer Alliance.

12 Taylor D & Mossman J (1997). Living with cancer: A discussion paper on the implementation of the Chief Medical Officer's Expert Advisory Group's recommendations on cancer services and the development of patient centred care (BACUP).

13 Coleman M P, Babb P, Damiecki P, et al (1999). Cancer survival trends in England and Wales, 1971–1995: deprivation and NHS Region. p. 695. The Stationery Office, London.

14 Challenging Cancer (1999). Department of Health.

15 NHS Cancer Care in England and Wales: National Service Framework Assessments No. 1 (2001). Commission for Health Improvement and the Audit Commission. The Stationery Office.

16 National surveys of NHS patients (2002) – cancer: National overview 1999–2000. Department of Health.

17 Smoking kills (1998). Department of Health.

18 Saving Lives: Our Healthier Nation (1999). Department of Health.

19 The NHS Cancer Plan: A plan for investment, a plan for reform (2000). Department of Health.

20 The NHS Plan: A plan for investment, a plan for reform (2000). Department of Health.

21 Tackling Cancer in England: Saving more lives (2004). National Audit Office.

22 Tackling Cancer: Improving the patient journey (2005). National Audit Office.

23 The NHS Cancer Plan: A progress report (2005). National Audit Office.

24 Peer Review of Cancer Services: A national overview (2002). Department of Health.

25 The Manual for Cancer Services, National Cancer Action Team (2004).

26 National Cancer Peer Review Programme 2004–2007. National Cancer Action Team 2008.

27 Cancer Reform Strategy, Department of Health. December 2007.

28 Waiting times for cancer: Progress, lessons learned, and next steps (2006). Department of Health.

29 High Quality Care for All: NHS Next Stage Review final report. Department of Health. June 2008.

30 The NHS Cancer Plan: Three year progress report (2003). Maintaining the momentum. Department of Health.

31 Variations in usage of cancer drugs approved by NICE (2004). Report of the review undertaken by the National Cancer Director. Department of Health.

32 [Variations report 2006]

33 Improving access to medicines for NHS patients: A report for the Secretary of State for Health by Professor Mike Richards (2008). Department of Health.

34 Strategic analysis: An overview of cancer research in the UK directly funded by the NCRI partner organisations (2002). National Cancer Research Institute.

35 Prevention and risk research in the UK: Report of the NCRI Strategic Planning Group on prevention and risk (2004). National Cancer Research Institute.

36 Supportive and palliative care research in the UK: Report of the NCRI Strategic Planning Group on supportive and palliative care (2004). National Cancer Research Institute.

37 Lung cancer research in the UK (2006). National Cancer Research Institute.

38 Rapid review of radiotherapy and associated radiobiology, National Cancer Research Institute 2008.

39 NCRI Strategic Plan 2008–2013. National Cancer Research Institute. 2008.

40 Preparing for a second plan: Maintaining the momentum in cancer policy. Cancer Campaigning Group. August 2006.

41 Our NHS, Our Future, NHS Next Stage Review interim report. October 2007.

42 End of Life Care Strategy: Promoting high quality care for all adults at the end of life. Department of Health. July 2008.

43 Cancer Reform Strategy: Maintaining momentum, building for the future – first annual report. Department of Health. December 2008.

Chapter 8

Population-based cancer control and the role of guidelines – towards a 'systems' approach

George P. Browman, Melissa Brouwers, Béatrice Fervers, Carol Sawka[1]

Clinical Practice Guidelines have been defined as 'systematically developed statements to assist practitioner and patient decisions about appropriate health care for specific clinical circumstances' [1]. This definition places guidelines within the context of healthcare decisions at the clinical level – that is, between a healthcare provider and an individual patient.

'Cancer control', on the other hand, the focus of this book, is defined as 'the development of integrated population-based approaches to reduce the incidence and mortality from cancer and to minimize its impact on affected individuals and on the community', signalling broader population-level concerns about disease control, and healthcare decisions at the organizational and policy levels.

In this chapter, we explore the role of guidelines beyond the clinician-patient context and profile several ongoing guideline initiatives to illustrate how cancer guidelines are being integrated into broader cancer control activities.

Practice guidelines in perspective: moving beyond the clinician-patient interface

The 'expectation' and the 'experience'

The expectation

The popularization of clinical guidelines was stimulated by documented unexplained geographic variations in clinical practice patterns that might jeopardize optimal outcomes [2], and by expectations that as the evidence-based movement advanced [3], there would be cost savings as unsubstantiated practices and premature dissemination of expensive technologies came under better control [4].

If such hopes were to be realized, then population-based cancer control would improve in two ways: first, through the aggregated improvements in individual outcomes to produce measurable

[1] George P. Browman MD, University of British Columbia and BC Cancer Agency, Vancouver Island Cancer Centre, Victoria, British Columbia, Canada; Melissa Brouwers, PhD, Associate Professor and Head of Health Services Research, Department of Oncology, McMaster University, and Provincial Director, Program in Evidence-based Care, Cancer Care Ontario, Hamilton, Ontario; Béatrice Fervers MD, PhD Centre Léon Bérard, EA 4129 "Santé, Individu, Société", Université de Lyon, Lyon, France; Carol Sawka MD, Professor of Medicine, University of Toronto, and VP Clinical Programs and Quality Initiatives, Cancer Care Ontario, Toronto, Canada.

improvements at the population level; and second, as freed-up resources were shifted from the inappropriate application of relatively ineffective interventions towards more effective population-based strategies.

The experience

The original promise of clinical guidelines has not been achieved to the extent expected, mainly because of the naïve hope that guidelines, once produced, would automatically have their intended influence.

In response, there is an emerging trend towards more proactive approaches to guidelines through implementation and monitoring their uptake. This has led to the design of instruments to measure their quality [5], emphasis on health and healthcare quality indicators and monitoring [6], and integrating the emerging field of 'knowledge translation'[2] into planning. Guideline programmes in the area of cancer are leading such initiatives. These programmes share a common feature – they treat guidelines as only one element of an 'integrated system' for improving cancer outcomes, and cancer control at the population level. They recognize that to be effective, guidelines cannot be passively relied on as stand-alone products, but must be considered within the context of a system-wide strategy for improved cancer outcomes at an affordable investment.

Here we provide a modified definition of guidelines for cancer control, and examples to illustrate the integration of guidelines with cancer control activities, including the contrasting roles that guidelines play when applied to population-based as opposed to clinical decision processes.

Contrasting the role of guidelines for individual practice versus population-level cancer control

Definition – guidelines for cancer control

For cancer guidelines to be applied effectively in population-based cancer control a broader definition is needed. We propose, 'Systematically developed statements, informed by research evidence, values and local/regional circumstances to assist fair decisions and judgments about cancer control at the clinical, management and policy levels'.

This definition acknowledges the more influential role of inputs other than research evidence into population level decisions, and highlights the importance of processes (fairness) for decision making at the broader level; however, the revised definition continues to support the notion of systemized processes that factor research evidence into recommendations for population-based cancer control.

Contrasting the utility of guidelines for informing decisions at the clinical (individual) and policy levels – the case of funding new and expensive cancer drugs

The funding of new and expensive cancer drugs is a topic dominating the agendas of patient advocacy groups, the media, oncologists, healthcare managers, and insurers, including government programmes, and serves to highlight the difference between individual level and population-based decisions based on the same evidence [7–9].

---

[2] The Canadian Institutes of Health Research define 'knowledge translation' as a dynamic and iterative process that includes synthesis, dissemination, exchange, and ethically sound application of knowledge to improve the health of Canadians, provide more effective health services and products and strengthen the health care system.

From the clinical perspective, guideline recommendations primarily intended to promote the most appropriate care for an individual would be based on evidence that maximizes the clinical benefit for the individual (survival, quality of life, recurrence-free interval) by a clinically 'meaningful' amount. Issues of cost are usually ignored.

However, if the intervention, such as an expensive drug, produced clinically meaningful but relatively small benefits for individuals, while using up resources that could be applied towards interventions with more impact then the population might be better off health-wise, if the dollars were shifted to these purposes. Such choices are particularly acute in publicly funded health care contexts.

Thus, the best clinical decision (for the individual patient eager to experience the potential benefit of the drug, even if small) would be to offer the treatment; but the most appropriate policy decision might be otherwise when the population's interests are considered. Which of these contrasting perspectives wins out depends on how various health systems and reimbursement mechanisms are arranged and on the fundamental values adopted by the society at large.

Up to now, policy makers have been appropriating guidelines originally developed to inform clinical decisions to make population decisions. This has led to some tension between the individual's interests and those of the population at large. In response, formal processes are needed to set priorities in a manner perceived by stakeholders as fair [10–18] and tools are required to better facilitate clinical level factors into population decisions [11,12,15,16]. Further, what both individuals and policy makers need to factor into such decisions is the 'value' attached to the benefit for both the individual and the population and the relative position of, or weight afforded to, each perspective in the decision-making process. 'Technology assessment', of which guidelines are an integral part, is one strategy to address this dilemma [19].

Guidelines and cancer control – integrating guidelines into cancer control – the 'cancer guidelines system'

We propose here that the effective use of guidelines for cancer control requires a shift of emphasis from the guideline per se 'as a stand-alone end product' towards its role as one element of a decision-informing 'system'.

Considering guidelines from a 'systems' perspective would call for better balancing investments in guidelines among their development, implementation, updating and monitoring phases, and achieving a better balance across clinical and programmatic/policy decisional needs (e.g. whether to implement a screening programme). Implementation would include strategies for knowledge translation, and monitoring the use of guidelines and their effects on population-level outcomes. Finally, the systems approach would pay heed to the ethical frameworks required for fair decision-making processes [e.g. 11,12,14–16,18].

Guidelines and cancer control – ongoing initiatives in industrialized countries

In this section, we describe four programmes in the guidelines movement that illustrate guidelines as a key component to advance cancer control 'system' activities:

1 The Canadian Partnership Against Cancer, Canadian Strategy for Cancer Control (http://www.partnershipagainstcancer.ca/)
2 The Cancer Care Ontario Program in Evidence-based Care [20] (www.cancercare.on.ca)
3 The French guidelines programme – SOR [21]
4 European cooperation – Co-CAN CPG (http://www.cocancpg.eu/)

These programmes illustrate, in practical terms, advancements in methods and procedures and the shift towards collaboration for integrating guidelines into systems approaches for cancer control.

The Canadian Partnership Against Cancer – a national cancer control strategy

The 'Canadian Strategy for Cancer Control' (the 'Strategy') was a grass-roots movement of stakeholders that recognized the need for the country as a whole to examine and prepare for the burgeoning cancer problem from a broader national perspective while respecting the political autonomy of the individual provinces that are ultimately responsible for health care delivery in their regions. The report produced by the 'Strategy' led to federal funding for the Canadian Partnership Against Cancer (the 'Partnership' – http://www.partnershipagainstcancer.ca/) to carry out the recommendations of the 'Strategy'. These recommendations called for action in several priority areas, one of which was 'guidelines'.

The 'Cancer Guidelines Action Group' (CGAG) is one of now eight Action Groups of the Partnership, and here we describe its approach to using guidelines as part of a cancer control strategy.

The CGAG vision and mission statements promote guidelines as vehicles for 'optimizing the use of evidence in cancer control'. In other words, the focus is not on guidelines as products per se, but rather as tools for a broader agenda around facilitating healthcare decisions in which research evidence plays an important role. In this context, the CGAG considered guidelines within the framework of knowledge translation approaches.

To promote the optimal use of evidence in decisions about cancer control from a broader pan-Canadian perspective, while respecting the authority of the regions, the CGAG decided to promote both cooperative and collaborative cross-jurisdictional activities using a 'bottom-up' rather than authoritarian approach. The approach involves the following elements:

Capacity enhancement: to achieve more equitable distribution of expertise and skills related to guideline activities across geographic regions – requires educational and knowledge transfer materials and venues

Technology platforms: to facilitate knowledge exchange and sharing, skills development, and real time collaboration – requires technological/communications infrastructures

Tools: in addition to technology platforms to facilitate affordable and uniform processes for locally relevant guideline activities,

'Social platforms': to promote sustainable interactions through functional social networks (communities of practice) [22]

Figure 8.1 presents a conceptual model of the relationship among the ongoing national projects of the CGAG, which are designed around the aforesaid elements.

A brief description of the projects follows. Foundational projects are the necessary platforms required for the success of other projects. The legacy project is intended to initiate a set of pan-Canadian relationships, both formal and informal, to promote sustainable collaboration based on equitable distribution of expertise across regions. Other projects are intended to produce more immediate benefits that can be measured over the first five years.

Social networking and measurement – foundational

This project will create and evaluate communities of practice as social platforms within and across regions to promote sustainable collaborations at the broader national level for the purpose of

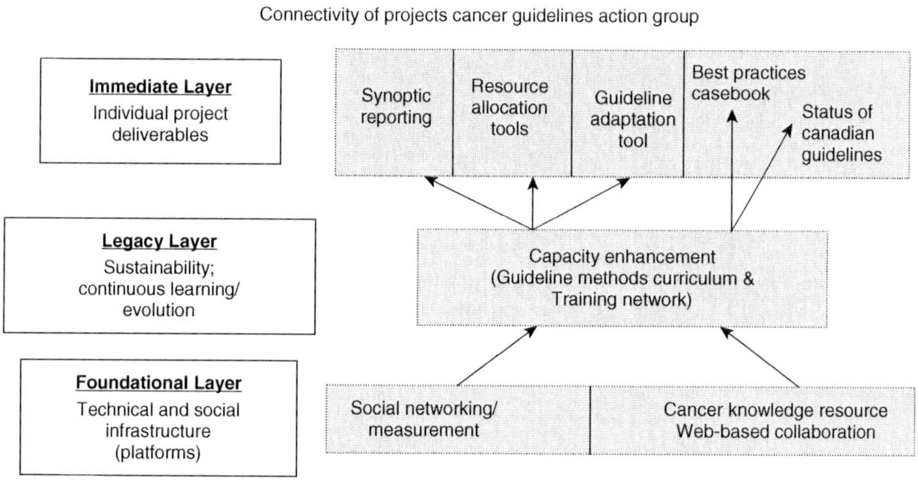

Connectivity of projects cancer guidelines action group

Fig. 8.1 Canadian Guidelines Action Group – diagram showing the relationships between program components, reproduced with permission.

shared cancer control strategies that transcend regional boundaries. The methods include social network analysis [23].

Cancer knowledge resource – foundational

The purpose of this project is to provide the technology/communications infrastructure (platform) for knowledge exchange and on-line collaboration using a suite of electronic tools. The *Resource* will not only link guideline development groups, but also link all other 'Partnership' action groups (surveillance, prevention, cancer journey, screening, standards, targets, and human resource planning).

Capacity enhancement – legacy

The purpose of this project is to take a lead in designing venues and strategies for transferring skills and knowledge from jurisdictions with a critical mass of expertise to those jurisdictions where such expertise is in shorter supply. It is hypothesized that a more equitable distribution of expertise related to guideline methods will accelerate national collaboration for a guidelines system required for cancer control. The capacity enhancement programme incorporates three sub-projects targeting curriculum and training objectives, formalized strategies for sharing best practices, and creating a status report of cancer guidelines to identify quality, gaps, and duplications of effort.

Synoptic reporting

This project builds on the considerable accumulating evidence that synoptic reporting in disciplines such as pathology, imaging, and operative reports in surgery improve information transfer for downstream clinical decision-making in contrast to traditional narrative reports [24–26]. The programme has started with five cross-jurisdictional projects in surgical oncology involving four cancer sites (colorectal, head and neck, breast, ovary); with guidelines and other evidence tools being integrated into point-of-care processes.

Resource allocation tools

Guidelines are being increasingly used and appropriated by policy makers to justify policy-level decisions, such as priorities about which new diagnostic tools or new and expensive cancer drugs to fund. The project aims to profile existing tools available to facilitate transparent and explicit (i.e. fair) decision-making and to enable participation of non-expert stakeholders in decision processes related to resource allocation decisions in cancer control.

Guideline adaptation

Currently, the most advanced project, guideline adaptation is part of an international collaborative (www.adapte.org) to allow guideline development groups to use already existing guidelines and adapt them for their own use. The purpose is to promote better awareness of the body of guidelines that exist, but more important, to avoid duplications of effort and expense involved in de novo guidelines development [27,28]. The project includes a manual and user guide that carries guideline development participants through critical evaluation and development steps that are intended to make development more efficient without compromising on the integrity of rigorous methodologies.

What the Canadian guidelines agenda is not, and why

Some would expect a national guidelines effort to be in the business of developing national guidelines, especially where there is a desire for uniform methods and quality of products, particularly around common issues of concern – such as cancer drug funding and access, and public health programming.

The CGAG has adopted a different strategy more targeted towards cancer control decisions for the following reasons. In the Canadian political context individual jurisdictions for the foreseeable future will reserve the right to make autonomous decisions, and because of the different political, social, and economic circumstances in which different jurisdictions operate, it is reasonable that recommendations from the same body of evidence could differ in important ways.

Second, the process of guideline development, properly done, is expected to produce secondary gains in terms of focusing local practitioners and other stakeholders on regional priorities in a disciplined way, leading to greater ownership of guidelines that are therefore more likely to be taken up. The process of critical evaluation of evidence and guideline development also serves as an invaluable educational tool that can further build local communities of practice and a learning culture [29].

Third, linking guideline development groups and other stakeholders, and providing them with tools to facilitate their work, likely will contribute to a more sustainable national culture of collaborative participation that also helps to disseminate expertise more widely.

Finally, in the critical area of policy decisions, such as those related to cancer drug funding, if uniform cross-jurisdictional processes are needed, then such processes should be developed around such priority areas, and in Canada they have been (see http://www.gov.sk.ca/news?newsId=78c1248b-7ed0-4f47-ba8d-c9d44f653728 and http://www.cancercare.on.ca/english/home/toolbox/drugs/ndfp/cancerdrugapprov/). The Partnership is contributing to such targeted national efforts through tools and social network development.

Program in Evidence-based Care, Cancer Care Ontario: experiences in transition from clinical guidelines to population-based cancer control guidance

(http://www.cancercare.on.ca/english/home/toolbox/qualityguidelines/pebc/).

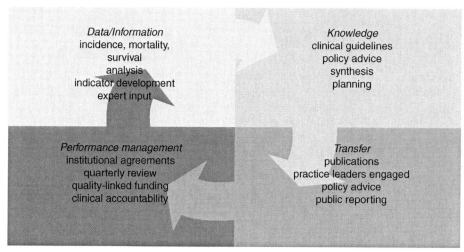

Fig. 8.2 Cancer Care Ontario (Canada): diagram of the quality improvement strategy, reproduced with permission of the authors.

Cancer Care Ontario, the advisory body to the Ontario government in matters related to cancer, has embraced a cancer control strategy of quality improvement at the patient and systems levels (see Figure 8.2). Four features characterize this strategy:

1 *Data*: routine and repeated monitoring of credible and meaningful population-based and system performance measures

2 *Knowledge*: identification of effective cancer control options and system strategies based on evidence

3 *Transfer*: design and implementation of tools and strategies to promote awareness and application of evidence-based knowledge

4 *Performance*: financial strategies and other incentives designed to better enable utilization of knowledge and increase awareness of accountability

Important to this model is the explicit integration of cancer guidelines to create a cancer care system informed by and accountable to evidence while recognizing the complexities inherent in changing a system and the behaviours of individuals within it. That guidelines alone do not necessarily result in change should not be unexpected; integrating them into an action – and results-oriented system increases the likelihood of success [29].

Program in Evidence-based Care – guidance then and guidance now

The Program in Evidence-based Care (PEBC), the guidelines programme of Cancer Care Ontario (CCO), has a long history of developing cancer guidelines primarily targeted at decisions made at the patient-provider interface (i.e. 'clinical' practice guidelines) [30,31]. Within the quality improvement strategy of CCO, the contributions of the PEBC are most evident in the knowledge and transfer quadrants in Figure 8.2.

More recently, the PEBC was challenged with creating advice documents designed to facilitate decisions by system leaders to influence organizational strategies and performance measurement. This led to new 'hybrid' guidance documents containing components to address either organizational issues only (e.g. the centralization of surgical services for complex surgical procedures with a steep volume: outcomes relationship); or both organizational and clinical issues relevant to a given topic (e.g. 'clinical' – is colorectal laparoscopic surgery as effective and safe as conventional surgery; e.g. 'organizational' – what organizational considerations are relevant for safe and effective delivery of laparoscopic surgery such as team complement, training of team members, space requirements, and managing surgical volumes?).

In creating hybrid documents targeted towards managers, the PEBC has retained its defining features – engagement of multidisciplinary panels, application of rigorous methodologies, and participation of stakeholders through formal review processes [32–34]. However, this venture into organizational and system guidance has had a significant impact on how PEBC determines priorities, who is involved in the guidance development process and the range of methodologies employed during guidance development – all lessons that highlight the transition from a clinical to a cancer control perspective.

Priorities

As reported elsewhere, multidisciplinary panels prioritize across candidate clinical practice guideline topics aided by explicit criteria [30,31] and by the experiences of the members. The once mainly clinical criteria for guideline priorities driven solely by the clinical community now include system criteria (e.g. ability to measure performance, availability of indicators, capacity to affect change), and incorporate priorities from administrators and policy makers.

Participation in the guideline enterprise

Since its inception the PEBC has engaged the 'users' of knowledge with its production, in order to create communities of stakeholders who understand evidence, can apply its methods, create recommendations and appreciate the importance of accountability between selected members of guideline development panels and the larger professional community. The philosophy was implemented by: creating teams of clinical and methodological experts working together; and using formal external review mechanisms that involved as much of the larger clinical community as possible [32–34].

The commitment to stakeholder engagement and its operationalization were generalized to the development of guidance documents geared towards organizational and system issues. However, for this transition the types of expertise required were more diverse, with the inclusion of administrators and managers as both guidance developers and external reviewers to place recommendations into the practical context.

Evolving methods for guidelines for population-based cancer control

The systematic review [35] has been the methodological foundation of all PEBC produced clinical guidelines. The formally structured reviews address explicitly framed questions formulated to be answered by analysis and interpretation of the synthesized evidence. This may also result in the adaptation of existing guidelines uncovered during the review, a strategy which has its own comprehensive and rigorous methodology (http://www.adapte.org/ – accessed August 14, 2008).

Despite the strength and continued relevance of systematic review for organizational and system guidance, the programme recognized the need to look beyond the published literature to consider additional methodologies for the cancer control toolbox, particularly in circumstances (which were often the case) where little evidence existed.

This led to exploration of the role of the *environmental scan* – an explicit and transparent search and review of the grey literature that features descriptions of, or data related to, solving an organizational or system problem that could be applied locally; and the development of more formalized consensus methods.

There are now several potential methodologies within the PEBC toolbox. Choice of method(s) is based on several factors including the quality and quantity of evidence, credibility of the evidence source, anticipated controversy and acceptability a guidance document might elicit, implementation plans, required change anticipated with the implementation of recommendations, and the urgency for implementation of recommendations.

Putting it all together: the case of thoracic surgery

The implications for this broader population-oriented approach to recommendations for cancer control are effectively illustrated in a commitment by CCO to improve quality of care for thoracic cancer surgery.

The Surgical Oncology Program (SOP) of CCO learned from clinical administrative databases that patient outcomes were worse for those receiving complex thoracic surgery in low volume institutions (data). This prompted the SOP to establish a formal partnership with the PEBC to create a guidance document with recommendations for surgical volumes (knowledge). A multi-professional panel worked together using systematic review, environmental scan, and engagement of the surgical community to create a final set of recommendations. The resulting document was disseminated on the CCO web site (http://www.cancercare.on.ca/english/home/toolbox/qualityguidelines/clin-program/surgery-ebs/ accessed August 14, 2008), published in a peer review journal [36], and distributed with tools to regional leaders (transfer). As a result, considerable negotiation has been undertaken to restructure and realign the delivery of complex thoracic surgery into fewer centres with introduction of formal pay-for-performance strategies (policy influence and performance).

Finally, use of the guidance document was adopted as one of the quality indicators monitored annually by the Quality Cancer System Index of Ontario (full circle of the quality improvement strategy to return back to data (http://www.cancercare.on.ca/english/csqi2008/ – accessed August 14, 2008). While more work is required, integrating higher level guidelines into a comprehensive integrated system of quality improvement has led to measurable improvements.

Conclusion

Cancer Care Ontario's experience illustrates the gradual evolution of a primarily clinically-oriented guidelines approach towards a guidance approach targeted at the system and organizational level. Throughout this evolution, the programme has remained true to its core principles of transparency and explicitness, methodological rigor, and engagement of key stakeholders.

France's SOR programme and coordination of cancer guideline programmes in Europe

The French 'Standards, Options: Recommendations' (SOR) programme

France's SOR guideline programme (www.sor-cancer.fr) was established in 1993 by the Federation of the Comprehensive Regional Cancer Centres (FNCLCC) (www.fnclcc.fr), as a primarily professional initiative within the quality improvement strategy of the 20 Comprehensive Regional Cancer Centres [37]. In 1995, universities, general hospitals, and professional societies began to collaborate within the programme and since 2003 guidelines have become integrated into the national cancer clinical governance strategies of the French National Cancer Plan. In this context, the SOR programme was transferred in 2008 to the French National Cancer Institute (INCa) (www.e-cancer.fr).

The SOR programme encompasses the development of national evidence-based oncology practice guidelines for the management of cancer and supportive care for adults and children as well as the provision of evidence-based patient information.

Evolving methods

The guideline development and updating methods of SOR [37] were developed almost simultaneously with, but independent of, the experiences described earlier for Cancer Care Ontario's Program in Evidence-based Care. The two programme leaders became aware of each other's efforts in 1994, and began sharing experiences at that time. The SOR and PEBC methods and principles are remarkably similar considering their independent programmatic development [38,39]. Both use rigorous evidence-based methods of systematic review, multidisciplinary guideline development panels, methodological experts as resources and educators, and formal community-level external review of guidelines to facilitate buy-in by practitioners. Incorporation of the patient perspective has been tried and continues to evolve in both programmes.

The lessons learned by both the SOR and Cancer Care Ontario Programs and their separate responses to barriers in guideline development and uptake were also similar. Like others, SOR found that developing and updating high quality guidelines is time consuming and expensive, requiring increasing resources over time as the inventory of guidelines (now numbering over 80) increased. To improve the efficiency of guideline production and updating, the SOR has increasingly customized existing guidelines instead of developing them *de novo* using guideline adaptation methods (www.adapte.org) [27], a strategy also promoted by the Canadian Partnership Against Cancer.

Guideline adoption and implementation

The SOR's evolving methods have, like Ontario's PEBC, shifted towards implementation and knowledge translation with the realization that cancer guidelines frequently lack applicability, which limits their effective use [40]. To improve acceptance of recommendations by practitioners the SOR programme has built a more formalized 'adoption' process into its guideline development activities.

Similar to the philosophy espoused by the Canadian Partnership, and for the same reasons, responsibility for implementation of SOR guidelines in France is regional with regional adaptation playing an important role. Guideline adaptation is intended not only to improve the efficiency of guideline development, but in France it is used by the regional cancer networks for tailoring national guidelines to the local care context. This participatory approach has been shown to be effective for changing practice, in particular for the regional cancer network of the Rhône-Alpes Region (ONCORA, http://oncoranet.lyon.fnclcc.fr/) [41,42], and it became mandatory for French cancer networks in 2007. Yet, not all regional networks currently possess the capacity and resources to successfully carry out this implementation process and some duplication of effort persists.

From a professional to systems perspective

Like other guideline development programmes, SOR has evolved over time to address issues of guideline implementation and utilization, both of which are important for promoting evidence-based clinical as well as broader cancer control interventions. The success of the 'bottom-up' approach has been acknowledged nationally by professional groups and by French national authorities. The transfer of the SOR programme from the FNCLCC (consortium of cancer centres) to the more broadly representative INCa, created in 2005, represents a shift in perspective with opportunities for a better focus on cancer control.

While cancer survival in France is among the highest in Europe, care varies significantly [44]. Hence, achieving uniform access to high-quality cancer care is a key purpose of the French national comprehensive cancer plan covering the full range of cancer control. Guidelines are central to several cancer control strategies of the plan – e.g. generation of regional networks, systematic multidisciplinary decision-making, elaboration of therapeutic protocols, and monitoring practice patterns. Nevertheless, in France guidelines remain predominantly clinically-oriented tools designed to promote the most appropriate care for the individual. Different from the evolution in Canada and some other countries, decisions about introducing new expensive cancer drugs in France are currently based primarily on evidence that focuses mainly on clinical benefit for the individual.

While the bottom-up approach of SOR has created the necessary collaborative culture and trust as well as widespread commitment to evidence-based principles, the transfer to INCa is expected to provide the structural component to reinforce the integration of SOR with national cancer control 'system' activities. Yet, it is too early to know how effective the shift from a disciplinary professional cancer system to a broader national approach will be.

International collaboration and research efforts

Taking advantage of the funding opportunities and the vision of the European Union, the SOR programme has made a second shift, towards international, European cooperative efforts [5,27,28,39,43], similar in many respects to the cross-jurisdictional efforts of the Canadian Partnership Against Cancer (described previously), and for similar reasons. The collaboration with Cancer Care Ontario since 1994 has provided good insights into the challenges encountered when different guideline programmes cooperate.

European cooperation – Co-Can CPG: coordination of cancer clinical practice in Europe (http://www.cocancpg.eu/)

Over the past decade most European countries have set up guideline programmes and infrastructures at the national or regional level. This has led to recognition of unnecessary duplications of effort and strategies for trans-national cooperation at the European level. Co-Can CPG (www.cocancpg.eu) is a European Union funded project (2006–2010) that aims to overcome existing duplications and fragmentation among cancer guideline developers in Europe [43]. Co-Can CPG is coordinated by France's INCa with 18 partners (Ministries of Health and key national or regional health institutes) from 11 countries (see Table 8.1).

Co-Can CPG strives to achieve its goals through the following activities designed for gradual improvements in the level of cooperation:

- Common framework for sharing knowledge, methods and skills
- Shared activities for guideline development and updating
- Assembling a critical mass for pertinent research into guideline methods
- Appropriate framework for long term cooperation

Similar to the situation as described in earlier sections for Canada, health systems and delivery of cancer services of the different European countries vary widely as well as outcomes achieved both within and between countries [44], and disparities grow as the Union expands. Within the European community there are different traditions of evidence-based guideline development and implementation, variability of where guidelines are located in the cancer control 'system' and different levels of accountability. Consequently, setting up cross-jurisdictional cooperation among guideline programmes involves carefully examining how trans-national activities can improve effectiveness of guideline development and utilization to maximize benefits for cancer control.

Table 8.1 Participants in the Co-Can CPG project (www.cocancpg.eu/)

Country	Organization
Belgium	Federaal kenniscentrum voor de gezondheidzorg – Centre Féderal d'Expertise des Soins de Santé (Belgian Health Care Knowledge Center)
Canada	Direction de Lutte Contre le Cancer du Québec
France	Institut National du Cancer (National Cancer Institute) – coordinator
	Fédération Nationale des Centres de Lutte contre le Cancer (French Federation of Comprehensive Cancer Centers)
	Haute Autorité de Santé (National Authority for Health)
Germany	Institute for Quality and Efficiency in Health Care
Hungary	Egeszegugyi Miniszterium (Ministry of Health)
	Orszagos Onkologia Intezet (National Institute of Oncology)
Israel	Ministry of Health
Italy	Agenzia Sanitaria Regionale – Regione Emilia Romagna
	Istituto Superiore de Sanità (National Institute for Health)
Lithuania	Institute of Oncology, Vilnius University
	Lietuvos Respublikos Sveikatos apsaugos ministerija (Ministry of Health)
Netherlands	Vereniging van Integrale Kankercentra (Association of Comprehensive Cancer Centres)
Spain	Agencia de Evaluación de Tecnologías Sanitarias de Andalucía (Andalusian Agency for Health Technology Assessment)
	Agéncia de Avaluacie de Tecnologia i Recerca Médiques (Catalan Agency for Health Technology Assessment and Research)
United Kingdom	NHS Quality Improvement Scotland
	National Institute for Health and Clinical Excellence

Joint activities for guideline development and updating

The Co-Can CPG collaborative has identified through surveys that evidence synthesis and monitoring for new evidence are considered the most costly and time consuming steps in guideline development, but also have the best potential for cooperation. For the reasons advanced by the Canadian Partnership Against Cancer (Cancer Guidelines Action Group), Co-Can CPG also decided not to engage in European guideline development, but to focus on regional enabling strategies for guideline uptake within socially, culturally, and economically diverse settings.

As a basis for implementing joint activities, Co-Can CPG has adopted international tools – e.g. the AGREE instrument (www.agreetrust.org) [5] and the ADAPTE process (www.adapte.org) [27, 28]. Formal comparison of methods has enabled Co-Can CPG members to develop common standardized processes to guarantee the quality of joint production as well as to define areas for joint research and development.

Similar to Canada's experience, capacity-building has been pursued through joint training activities and exchange of programme personnel in order to achieve more equitable distribution of expertise, and thus foster the trust in competence of others required for successful cooperation.

The future – identification of evidence gaps to inform future clinical research: 'closing the loop'

The experience of the Co-Can CPG members reinforces the importance of the linkage between guidelines and cancer treatment systems and the role played by research. One of the limitations of the evidence-based approach to guidelines is the lack of high-quality research evidence for so many interventions. To address this, Co-Can CPG, led by researchers at the UK National Institute of Health and Clinical Excellence, plans a systematic approach to explicitly identifying evidence gaps and uncertainties in a way that can usefully inform the development of future cancer clinical research.

Conclusion

Through the development of transnational cooperation Co-Can CPG is responding to current duplication of effort in guideline development. The elaboration of a common evidence-base at the European level will provide support for the coherent development of guidelines and policies at national and regional levels. The Co-Can CPG experience is intended to foster better under-standing of the regional and organizational circumstances and values that lead to legitimate inconsistencies between guideline recommendations based on the same evidence.

If the partners succeed in overcoming current barriers to effective cooperation – e.g. variability of settings and expertise, organizational 'system' commitment, and language barriers – Co-Can CPG has the potential to become a strong instrument to support cancer control activities through guidelines at the European level.

Summary

This chapter addresses the continuing transition of the cancer guidelines movement in North America and Europe to bring evidence to both clinical and higher level decisions for improved cancer control at the management and policy levels. The chapter highlights principles involved in shifting from the clinical to the population-based cancer control perspective when considering the utility of guidelines. Four examples are reviewed to illustrate programmatic initiatives designed around guidelines to advance 'cancer control'. These initiatives highlight future directions in the guidelines movement as part of a 'systems approach' to improving cancer control. We have pointed out the contrasting roles of guidelines intended to inform broader policy level as opposed to clinical level decisions and we have highlighted some of the issues to be faced in this transition.

The example of Cancer Care Ontario's Program in Evidence-based Care highlights a more advanced agenda committed towards the population perspective in which guidelines are being redefined, and deployed as part of broader quality monitoring and improvement strategies at the policy level. Canada's Partnership Against Cancer highlights attempts to incorporate guidelines as part of a national cancer strategy, while the experiences of France's SOR programme, still very much focused on guidelines as clinical tools, illustrates significant changes in administrative arrangements at the government level to coordinate guidelines as part of a national cancer plan. As described, there have been effective international collaborations among guideline programmes (Cancer Care Ontario and FNCLCC; Cancer Care Ontario and the American Society of Clinical Oncology), and there are emerging in Europe multinational cooperative efforts to make guide-lines more useful and more effective for cancer control.

Close examination by the reader of the stories told about how different guideline programmes are evolving should provide clear insights about the future of guidelines as an element of population-based cancer control strategies.

References

1 Field MJ & Lohr KM (eds) (1992). Institute of Medicine. *Guidelines for medical practice: From development to use*. National Academy Press, Washington, DC.

2 Wennberg JE (1999). Understanding geographic variations in health care delivery (editorial). *N Engl J Med*, **340**:52–53.

3 Sackett DL, Rosenberg WMC, Muir Gray JA, et al (1996). Evidence-based medicine: What it is and what it isn't. *BMJ*, **312**:71–72.

4 Fisher ES & Wennberg JE (2003). Health care quality, geographic variations, and the challenge of supply-sensitive care. *Perspect Biol Med*, **46**:69–79.

5 AGREE Collaboration (2003). Development and validation of an international appraisal instrument for assessing the quality of clinical practice guidelines: the AGREE project. *Qual Saf Health Care*, **12**:18–23.

6 Desch CE, McNiff KK, Schneider EC, et al (2008). American Society of Clinical Oncology/National Comprehensive Cancer Network Quality Measures. *J Clin Oncol*, **26**:3631–37.

7 Booth CM, Dranitsaris G, Gainford MC, et. al (2007). External influences and priority-setting for anti-cancer agents: a case study of media coverage in adjuvant Trastuzumab for breast cancer. *BMC Cancer*, **7**:110.

8 Foy R, So J, Rous E, & Scarffe JH (1999). Perspectives of commissioners and cancer specialists in prioritizing new cancer drugs: impact of the evidence threshold, *BMJ*, **318**:456–59.

9 Wilking N & Jonsson B (2005). *A pan-European comparison regarding patient access to cancer drugs*. Karolinska Institute in collaboration with Stockholm School of Economics, Stockholm, Sweden [as summarized in Stark CG, Special Report: Access to cancer therapy (2006). Market uptake of new oncology drugs. *EJHP*, 12:55–57].

10 Martin DK, Pater JL, & Singer P (2001). Priority-setting for new cancer drugs: a qualitative case study. *Lancet*, **358**:1676–81.

11 Pater JL, Browman G, Brouwers M, et al (2001). Funding new cancer dugs in Ontario: Closing the loop in the Practice Guidelines Development Cycle. *J Clin Oncol.*, **19**:3392–96.

12 Browman GP, Manns B, Hagen N, et al (2008). 6-STEPPPS: A modular tool to facilitate clinician participation in fair decisions for funding new cancer drugs. *J Oncol Practice*, **4**:2–7.

13 Sinclair S, Hagen NA, Chambers C, et al (2008). Accounting for reasonableness: Exploring the personal internal framework affecting decisions about cancer drug funding. *Health Policy*, **86**:381–90.

14 Daniels N (2000). Accountability for reasonableness: Establishing a fair process for priority setting is easier than agreeing on principles. *BMJ*, **321**:1300–01.

15 Giacomini M, Miller F, & Browman G (2003). Confronting the 'Grey Zones' of technology assessment: Evaluating genetic testing services for public insurance coverage in Canada. *Int J Technol Assess Health Care*, **19**:301–16.

16 Singer PA, Martin DK, Giacomini M, et al (2000). Priority setting for new technologies in medicine. A qualitative case study. *BMJ*, **321**:1316–19.

17 Wynia MK, Cummins D, Fleming D, et al (2004). Improving fairness in coverage decisions: Performance expectations for quality improvement. *Am J Bioethics*, **4**:87–100.

18 Giacomini M (2005). One of these things is not like the others: the idea of precedence in health technology assessment and coverage decisions. *Millbank Q*, **83**:192–223.

19 Banta HD, Battista RN, Gelband H, & Jonsson E (eds) (2004). Health Care Technology and its assessment in eight countries. DIANE Publishing, Available at http://www.dianepublishing.net/ProductDetails.asp?ProductCode=078812501X

20 Levine M, Browman G, Newman T, & Cowan DH (1996). The Ontario Cancer Treatment Practice Guidelines Initiative. *Oncology*, **10**(11 Suppl):19–22.

21 Durand-Zaleski I & Philip T (2001). SOR project: the French context. *Br J Cancer*, **84** (Suppl 2):4–5.

22 Wenger E, McDermott RA, & Snyder W (2002). *Cultivating Communities of Practice*. Harvard Business School Press, Boston.

23 Wasserman S & Faust K (1994). *Social Network Analysis: Methods and Applications.* Cambridge University Press, New York.

24 Edhemovic I, Temple WJ, de Gara CJ, & Stuart GCE (2004). The computer synoptic operative report – a leap forward in the science of surgery. *Ann Surg Oncol*, **11**:941–47.

25 Leslie KO & Rosai J (1994). Standardization of the surgical pathology report: formats, templates, and synoptic reports. *Sem Diagnostic Pathol*, **11**:253–57.

26 Qu Z, Ninan S, Almosa A, et al (2007). Synoptic reporting in tumor pathology: advantages of a web-based system. *Am J Clin Pathol*, **127**:898–903.

27 Fervers B, Burgers JS, Haugh MC, et al (2006). Adaptation of clinical guidelines: literature review and proposition for a framework and procedure. *Int J Qual Health Care*, **18**:167–76.

28 Graham ID, Harrison MB, Brouwers M, et al (2002). Facilitating the use of evidence in practice: evaluating and adopting clinical guidelines for local use by health care organizations. *J Obstet Gynecol Neonatal Nurs*, **31**:599–611.

29 Grimshaw JM, Thomas RE, MacLennan G, et al (2004). Effectiveness and efficiency of guideline dissemination and implementation strategies. *Health Technol Assess*, **8**:72.

30 Browman GP, Levine MN, Mohide EA, et al (1995). The practice guidelines development cycle: a conceptual tool for practice guidelines development and implementation. *J Clin Oncol*, **13**:502–512.

31 Brouwers MC & Browman GP (2003). The promise of clinical practice guidelines. In Sullivan T, Evans W, Angus H, & Hudson A (eds). *Strengthening the Quality of Cancer Services in Ontario*, pp. 183–203. CHA Press, Ottawa.

32 Browman GP, Newman TE, Mohide EA, et al (1998). Progress of clinical oncology guidelines development using the practice guidelines development cycle: The role of practitioner feedback. *J Clin Oncol*, **16**:1226–31.

33 Browman GP, Makarski J, Robinson P, et al (2005). Practitioners as experts: the influence of practicing oncologists 'in-the-field' on evidence-based guidelines development. *J Clin Oncol*, **23**:113–19.

34 Brouwers MC, Graham ID, Hanna SE, et al (2004). Clinicians' assessments of practice guidelines in oncology: the CAPGO survey. *Int J Technol Assess Health Care*, **20**:421–26.

35 Cook DJ, Mulrow CD & Haynes RB (1997). Systematic reviews: synthesis of best evidence for health care decisions. *Ann Int Med*, **126**:376–380.

36 Sundaresan S, Langer B, Oliver T, Schwarz F, Brouwers M, & Stern H (2007). Standards for thoracic surgical oncology in a single-payer health care system. *Ann Thorac Surg*, **84**:693–701.

37 Fervers B, Hardy J, & Philip T (2001). 'Standards, Options and Recommendations'. Clinical Practice Guidelines for cancer care from the French National Federation of Cancer Centres (FNCLCC). *Br J Cancer*, **84**:1–92.

38 Browman G (2001): 'Background to clinical guidelines in cancer': SOR, a programmatic approach to guideline development and aftercare. *Br J Cancer*, **84**(Suppl 2).1–3.

39 Fervers B, Philip T, Haugh MC, Cluzeau FA, & Browman G (2003). Clinical practice guidelines in Europe: time for European co-operation for cancer guidelines. *Lancet Oncol.*, **4**:139–40.

40 Castel P & Merle I (2002). Quand les normes de pratiques deviennent une ressource pour les médecins. *Sociologie du travail*, **44**:337–55.

41 Ray-Coquard I, Philip T, Lehmann M, et al (1997). Impact of a clinical guideline program for breast and colon cancer in a French cancer center. *JAMA*, **278**:1591–95.

42 Ray-Coquard I, Philip T, De Laroche G, et al (2002). A controlled 'before-after' study: impact of a clinical guidelines programme and regional cancer network organization on medical practice. *Br J Cancer*, **96**:313–21.

43 Fervers B, Remy-Stockinger M, Mazeau-Woynar V, et al (2008). CoCanCPG. Coordination of cancer clinical practice in Europe. *Tumori*, **94**:154–59.

44 Verdecchia A, Fransisci S, Brenner H, Gatta G, Micheli A, Mangone L, Kunkler I, & EUROCARE-4 Working Group (2007). Recent cancer survival in Europe: a 2000–02 period analysis of EUROCARE-4 data. *Lancet Oncol*, **8**:784–96.

Chapter 9

The optimal provision of cancer treatment services

Michael Barton, Geoff Delaney[1]

The optimal provision of cancer services to a population means that services such as screening, surgery, chemotherapy, or radiotherapy are delivered in the type and amount that meets local demand. Estimating demand requires knowledge of the types and numbers of cancers and the indications for services. For example, the demand for breast screening can be calculated by determining the number of women aged 50 to 70 years. It is more complicated to determine the demand for services such as radiotherapy or chemotherapy that have a large number of indications relevant to small proportions of the cancer population. Different populations will have different incidence rates of cancer, and the proportions of the common types of cancer may vary. In addition, factors relating to specific groups of patients such as performance status and co-morbidities may alter treatment recommendations. Studies have shown that control rates of cancer may be influenced when delays in treatment occur [1,2] and therefore the planning of sufficient services to meet the needs of the treatment population is vital to providing optimal care.

Approaches to estimating demand have included using expert opinion and examining well-serviced areas [3,4]. Expert opinion is subject to limitations of knowledge, bias, and lacks a strong evidence-based rationale. It is unknown how appropriate the levels of service provision and patient access are in well-provided areas. Without an evidence-based approach, it is not known whether apparently well-serviced areas are over-serviced, correctly serviced to meet demand, or under serviced.

This chapter describes an evidence-based approach to estimating the demand for cancer services and its application to different treatment modalities and different populations. The work was done mainly for Australia, but has been adapted and used in Europe and North America. Cancer services include all cancer control interventions such as screening, early detection, diagnosis, treatment, palliation, and rehabilitation. We will describe in detail the estimation of demand for radiotherapy and give examples of how this approach has been adapted to other modalities and other populations.

Background

The actual proportion of incident cases that receives radiotherapy varies almost two-fold within and between jurisdictions. In Ontario, Canada, in the period 1984 to 1991, the proportion

[1] Michael Barton, OAM, MBBS, MD, FRANZCR, Professor of Radiation Oncology, South West Sydney Clinical School, University of New South Wales, Sydney, New South Wales, Australia; and Geoff Delaney, MBBS, MD, PhD, FRANZCR, Professor and Director of Cancer Services, Sydney South West Area Health Service, Liverpool, New South Wales, Australia.

of cases that received radiotherapy varied between counties from under 19 per cent of cases to 32 per cent [5]. Greater variation was seen in New South Wales (NSW), Australia in 1998 when the proportion varied between health districts from 23 per cent on the mid north coast of NSW to 54 per cent in southern NSW [6].

Benchmarks for radiotherapy service provision have suggested that 50 to 55 per cent of new cases of cancer should receive radiotherapy at least once during the course of their illness. This has been based on expert opinion [3] and levels of service provision in well-resourced areas [6]. Based on this approach it has been estimated that in Australia over 10,000 cancer patients per year miss out on external beam radiotherapy [7].

A rational method of demand assessment

An alternative approach is to use the published evidence of indications for radiotherapy when it is the treatment of choice and integrate this with population-based data on the proportion of cancer patients with each treatment indication to develop a model of radiotherapy utilization. This concept was first described by Tyldsley et al. [8] for lung cancer. We have used a modification of this methodology and applied it to all cancer sites.

Indications for treatment

An indication for treatment is an oncological problem for which the treatment being examined is the treatment of choice because of superior outcomes in survival, local tumour control, quality of symptom relief, or side-effect profile when compared with alternative treatment approaches. For example, radiotherapy is the treatment of choice for nasopharyngeal cancer because it produces higher cure rates than the alternatives. For the purposes of calculating the proportion of patients who should receive a treatment at least once, the treatment could be used alone or in combination with other anti-cancer treatments. Treatment intent may be palliative or curative (including definitive and adjuvant intents).

In order for a treatment to be indicated, the patient must be suitable for treatment. They should be fit enough to undertake treatment. Patient choice is difficult to model because of the risk that patient choices in the real world will be influenced by their knowledge of local access. For example, 55 per cent of women with breast cancer in rural Australia have mastectomy compared to 45 per cent of women with breast cancer in metropolitan areas presumably because of the difficulties of accessing radiotherapy in rural Australia [9]. Hypothetical studies of patients or surrogates may yield results that are discordant with patients' actual behaviour [10].

Evidence for indications for treatment may be obtained from national and international evidence-based treatment guidelines. If these are not available, randomized and non-randomized studies can be examined. The quality of the evidence should be ranked using standard evidence rating scales [11] (Table 9.1).

The proportion of cancer cases with attributes for each treatment decision is determined from epidemiological databases and clinical reports. The quality of the epidemiological data is also ranked using the scale [12] shown in Table 9.2 and the highest level evidence should be used in constructing a model. Preference is given to population-based data because it is the most representative. National cancer incidence figures, such as those published by the Australian Institute of Health and Welfare [13] are used to determine the incidence of cancer types and tumour sites. However, data from other jurisdictions could easily be used to modify the estimates for other populations. Major attributes that describe large proportions of the population, such as cancer incidence and stage proportions, are usually able to be found from high-level population-based sources.

Table 9.1 Levels of evidence for indications for radiotherapy

Level	Description
I	Systematic review of all relevant randomized studies
II	At least one properly conducted randomized trial
III	Well-designed controlled trials without randomization. These include trials with 'pseudo-randomization' where a flawed randomization method occurred (e.g. alternate allocation of treatments) or comparative studies with either comparative or historical controls.
IV	Case series

Source: National Health and Medical Research Council of Australia [11].

Integration of indications and proportions

Indications can be mapped out in a 'tree' structure using standard decision evaluation software. The tree is broken into treatment decision points. Figure 9.1 shows a generic example. The example cancer is split into two stages; 80 per cent of cases are 'Localized' and 20 per cent are 'Metastatic'. Seventy per cent of 'Localized' cancers in the example have an indication for treatment and 30 per cent are not fit for treatment. Therefore in this example the proportion of all patients with localized cancers who are fit for treatment is $0.80 \times 0.70 = 0.56$ or 56 per cent. Similarly in this example the proportion of all cases with metastatic cancer with good performance status and symptoms is $0.2 \times 0.6 \times 0.5 = 0.06$. Overall the proportion of all cases with an indication for treatment at least once is $0.56 + 0.06 = 0.62$. For this example 62 per cent of cases have an indication for treatment.

A tree showing radiotherapy utilization for oesophageal cancer [14] is reproduced in Figure 9.2. Each branch of the tree ends with either radiotherapy being recommended (ends with outcome = 1) or radiotherapy not being recommended (outcome = 0). The numbers under each branch refer to the proportion of patients that the particular branch represents and the numbers on the far right refer to the overall proportion of that cancer that the entire branch represents. By summing the proportions for each branch with an indication for radiotherapy (those ending with '1') one may estimate the optimal radiotherapy rate. The model shows that radiotherapy is indicated for 80 per cent of oesophageal cancer patients, the largest proportion being patients

Table 9.2 Hierarchy of epidemiological data

Quality of source	Source type
α	National epidemiological data
β	State or Provincial Cancer Registry
γ	Epidemiological databases from other large international groups (e.g. SEER*)
δ	Results from reports of a random sample from a population
ε	Comprehensive multi-institutional database
ζ	Comprehensive single-institutional database
θ	Multi-institutional reports on selected groups (e.g. multi-institutional clinical trials)
λ	Single-institutional reports on selected groups of cases
μ	Expert opinion

Source: Tyldesley [8].

*Surveillance Epidemiology and End Results registry system, in the United States (www.seer.cancer.gov).

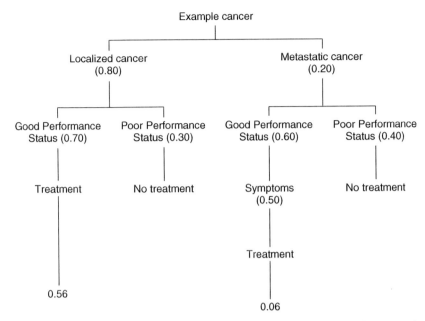

Fig. 9.1 Example of utilization tree. Figures in brackets below each attribute are the proportion of cases with that attribute.

without metastases and who do not undergo surgery (40 per cent of all patients) and those with metastases and symptomatic loco-regional disease (24 per cent).

Optimal radiotherapy utilization

We have examined the evidence for the efficacy of radiotherapy for all cancers and determined the proportion of cases of cancer with each attribute in the utilization tree from epidemiological data from which it is possible to calculate the proportion of cases that had each indication for radiotherapy. By summing the proportions of cases with indications for radiotherapy it is possible to calculate the overall radiotherapy utilization estimate for each cancer site and the overall utilization rate for all cancers. Table 9.3 summarizes the results for each of the cancers studied and represents the cohort eligible for radiotherapy, at least once during their illness, as a proportion of all cancer patients based on Australian data. Overall, 52.3 per cent of all cancer patients should ideally receive radiotherapy at least once during the course of their illness based on the best available evidence. The optimal radiotherapy utilization rates vary from a low rate of zero for liver cancer patients to a high of 92 per cent for central nervous system tumour patients [14–25].

The individual branches that represented the greatest proportion of cancer patients receiving radiation were early breast cancer treated by breast conserving surgery and post-operative radiotherapy (8 per cent of all cancer diagnoses), pre- or post-operative radiotherapy for T3-4 or N2-3 rectal cancer (1 per cent), early prostate cancer (2 per cent) and metastatic prostate cancer (2 per cent). In addition, there were many branches that ended in radiotherapy being recommended for symptom control for non-small cell lung cancer (3–6 per cent).

Robustness of demand modelling

The robustness of models should be tested to examine the assumptions on which the model is based and to test the sensitivity of the model to changes in uncertain variables. We have used both sensitivity analysis and peer review to examine the robustness of the model.

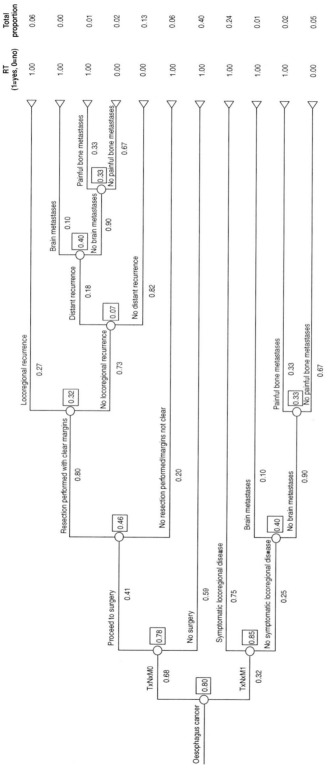

Fig. 9.2 Radiotherapy utilization tree for oesophageal cancer. Total proportion of patients needing radiotherapy is the total of the figures on the right relating to 'RT yes', coded 1.00; = 0.06 + 0.01 + 0.06 + 0.40 + 0.24 + 0.01 + 0.02 = 0.80.

Source: Delaney et al. [14], by permission.

Table 9.3 The overall optimal radiotherapy utilization rate by cancer type (Australian data)

Tumour type	Proportion of all cancers (%)	Proportion of *each* cancer with an indication for radiotherapy (%)	Sensitivity Analysis (%)	Proportion of *all* cancers with an indication for radiotherapy (%)
Breast	13	83	82.95–85.25	10.8
Lung	10	76	73–76	7.6
Melanoma	11	23	17–29	2.5
Prostate	12	60	55–67	7.2
Gynaecological	5	35	32–39	1.8
Colon	9	14	4–23	1.3
Rectum	5	65	NA*	3.3
Head and Neck	4	74	73–81	3.0
Gall Bladder	1	13	1–21	0.1
Liver	1	0	0	0.0
Oesophageal	1	80	73–81	0.8
Stomach	2	68	58–68	1.4
Pancreas	2	57	50–57	1.1
Lymphoma	4	65	65–66	2.6
Leukaemia	3	4	4–4.6	0.1
Myeloma	1	38	NA*	0.4
CNS	2	92	91.6–92.8	1.8
Renal	3	28	25–35	0.8
Bladder	3	58	44.5–58.3	1.7
Testis	1	49	49.3–49.5	0.5
Thyroid	1	10	NA*	0.1
Unknown Primary	4	61	53–70	2.4
Other	2	50	0–100	1.0
Total	100		51.6–53.1	52.3

*NA – Sensitivity Analysis was not conducted because there was no significant variation in the data.

Sensitivity analysis

Sensitivity analysis examines a range of realistic scenarios to estimate the effect of uncertainties on the results of utilization tree models. The uncertainties in a model may be due to variation in published estimates of the proportions of patients with particular attributes, different probabilities of benefit from treatment, which could be suggested by different data sources, or variations in the recommendations for the use of a treatment in different evidence-based guidelines because of a lack of evidence for one treatment approach or another.

One-way sensitivity analysis tests the effect of each uncertain variable on the final optimal treatment utilization rate. For the optimal radiotherapy utilization estimate of 52.3 per cent, analysis of the one-way sensitivity revealed that the estimate could vary between 51.6 per cent and 53.1 per cent, depending upon the data used in the calculation.

Monte Carlo simulations allow for assessments of uncertain data and their effect on the overall radiotherapy utilization rate in a multivariate fashion as opposed to the univariate method described earlier. Monte Carlo simulations are based upon the random sampling of variables from discrete and continuous distributions during individual trials. Observing the statistical properties of many trials using random sampled values allows additional insight into the performance of a model. A detailed description of the Monte Carlo analysis in this study is available [21]. The Monte Carlo analysis performed in this study involved 10,000 simulations. The number of simulations chosen was arbitrary but should be high to improve the power of the estimate. The result was an optimal radiotherapy utilization rate of 52.3 per cent (95 per cent confidence limits: 51.7 per cent, 53.1 per cent) [26]. The tightness of the confidence intervals demonstrates that the overall estimate is robust.

The final estimate is remarkably precise despite uncertainty in data when multiple sources of equal quality differed, uncertainty in some indications for radiotherapy, and uncertainty between treatment options of approximately equal efficacy such as radiotherapy, surgery, or watchful waiting for early prostate cancer. These tight confidence intervals may be explained by the fact that the overall estimate is most affected by attributes on the initial branches of the trees that affect many subsequent branches. Good quality data existed for the initial branches of the tree such as the type and stage of tumours which are collected by some population-based cancer registries. Most of the uncertainty existed in the distal branches of the tree and hence affected very small proportions of the cancer population and contributed very little to the overall estimate. In addition, the effect of these variations was such that some would increase the overall utilization rate while others would reduce it, so that to a large extent they would cancel each other.

External review

The results of this project had to be credible to all parties who may be affected by it, including, in Australia, State and Commonwealth governments, consumers, non-government organizations such as State cancer councils, and medical, surgical and radiation oncologists. To ensure that the project outcomes met expectations of rigour and that points of interpretation were resolved, an expert steering group was appointed. The steering group was convened by the Australian National Cancer Control Initiative (NCCI), with representation from major cancer organizations, consumers, epidemiologists, radiation and medical oncologists, surgeons, palliative care specialists, and experts in evidence and treatment guidelines, and was chaired by the Director of the NCCI. The steering group met with the investigators on a regular basis to review project scope, methodology, and results.

It was recognized that the indications for radiotherapy and the radiotherapy utilization trees for each cancer type and tumour site should be peer-reviewed. The draft results were scrutinized through a process of consultation prior to final adoption of the model. A Court of Reviewers was established comprised of experts drawn from the fields of surgical oncology, medical oncology, radiation oncology, palliative medicine, public health, and oncology nursing. Representatives of the guideline committees that were responsible for the existing Australian treatment guidelines were also invited to act as reviewers.

We collated 271 specific reviewer comments related to the review. This resulted in 139 changes to the text, trees, epidemiological data, or evidence cited. The review also resulted in major reconstructions of the radiotherapy utilization trees for two tumour sites.

Limitations of the model

Some limitations of this approach have been identified:

Quality of epidemiological data

The construction of these trees with so many branches required significant epidemiologic data to be available in order to accurately estimate the proportions of patients with particular attributes. Some data such as stage distributions were relatively easily obtained from central cancer registries but other attributes that have been poorly studied included performance status, and proportions of patients with specific symptoms that may warrant palliative radiotherapy and the proportion with relapse.

In some cases we have had to rely on less robust data or based our model on assumptions. We have dealt with this uncertainty by performing modelling and sensitivity analysis to assess the relative effect that any of these uncertainties might have on the overall utilization rate.

Indications for treatment outside the scope of the study

Most planning groups use the statutory cancer registry notifications as the basis for estimating workload. Notifiable cancers are cancers for which statutory requirements exist to notify a State cancer registry. Statutory notification in Australia excludes non-melanoma skin cancers and benign tumours but includes ductal carcinoma – in situ of the breast. However, there are indications for radiotherapy for some non-notifiable conditions such as benign tumours and other non-malignant conditions that are not included in these model-based estimates. These other conditions will need consideration when planning radiotherapy resources.

Radiotherapy has an established role for many non-melanoma skin cancers and this represents a moderate workload in most radiation oncology facilities, particularly in Australia where the incidence of non-melanoma skin cancers is relatively high compared with other countries [27]. In addition to the treatment of the primary disease, metastatic non-melanoma skin cancers are frequently treated with radiotherapy for nodal metastases. Radiotherapy also has an established role in the management of some benign tumours and non-cancerous conditions. These conditions include benign brain and parotid tumours, keloid, pituitary tumours, pterygia, heterotopic ossification, desmoid tumours, and exophthalmos from Grave's disease [28].

The overall demand for radiotherapy resources for these conditions is difficult to estimate as the incidence of these conditions is not reported and evidence-based treatment guidelines do not exist for most of non-malignant conditions. Alternative treatment options also exist.

It remains important to consider this additional workload in resource planning. Radiotherapy for benign disease and advanced non-melanoma skin cancers often require complex external beam radiotherapy and may add significantly to the radiotherapy resources required. In the absence of data, other methods can be used to estimate the workload. We found the best way was by assessing available data on current workloads in some Australian departments as a reflection of more widespread demand. Data from more than 40,000 patients treated over 10 years in two large Australian departments showed that 10 per cent of patients received radiotherapy for non-notifiable conditions [29].

Only external beam radiotherapy was considered

Inclusion of other forms of radiotherapy with radio-isotopes such as brachytherapy was beyond the scope of this original model as it was designed for external beam resource planning. However these other forms of radiotherapy should be considered when planning radiotherapy resources, and we describe results for brachytherapy below.

Controversies in the recommendations for radiotherapy

Despite using evidence-based treatment guidelines to determine indications for radiotherapy, there are areas where the role of radiotherapy remains poorly defined or where the indications for the use of radiotherapy remain vague. This is mainly due to poor evidence and the lack of good quality trials. The model is easily amended should new evidence for or against the use of radiotherapy for a specific clinical situation emerge.

The effect of patient choice considerations

We did not consider the effect of patient choice because of the risk that the studies reporting patient preference may have been confounded by the availability of radiotherapy to the study population. Very few patient choice studies provide information about whether resource constraints and displacement from home for patients were part of the discussion and decision-making process. It has been shown, for example, that Australian mastectomy rates increase in areas of radiotherapy remoteness [9].

Some of the studies do not discuss the context or framing of information presented to patients. In situations where descriptions of context were provided, the studies were usually hypothetical in that the subjects were not cancer patients or their treatment had been already determined (which may mean that they may have been influenced by discussion prior to the study). Patient choice studies do not address all of the patient choice issues for all radiotherapy situations. Due to these limitations, it was felt appropriate to not incorporate patient choice into the trees. This has the limitation that patients always have a choice in the treatment they receive and some will decline treatment even when it is strongly recommended. As this proportion cannot be obtained reliably it was felt best to omit it completely.

Rare indications for radiotherapy have not been included in the overall estimate

The methodology of this study involved studying indications for radiotherapy that would affect the overall radiotherapy utilization rate. However, data for some indications for radiotherapy were lacking or the proportion of cases is likely to be exceedingly small. Although only of small overall impact in their own right, the cumulative total of these indications might increase the overall radiotherapy utilization estimate by 1 to 2 per cent. Sufficient epidemiological data on the incidence of these metastatic manifestations do not exist to calculate a more accurate figure.

Application to radiotherapy service planning

The model of radiotherapy utilization may be used to plan new treatment services and to examine the adequacy of existing services.

Population-based radiotherapy service planning

This study estimated that the optimal radiotherapy utilization rate was 52 per cent using an evidence-based approach. The number of new cases of cancer may be obtained from a central cancer registry and hence the number of new cases with an indication for radiotherapy may be calculated from our benchmark. If the throughputs of megavoltage radiotherapy machines are known and workload capacities are also known then it is possible to calculate the number and distribution of staff and megavoltage radiotherapy equipment for benchmarking existing services or planning service expansion.

A number of Australian and international agencies have used the radiotherapy benchmark for planning radiotherapy resources. These include Victoria [29] and NSW [30] in Australia, and Scotland [31]. The International Atomic Energy Agency has also used the benchmark for estimating radiotherapy demand and service shortfall in low and middle income countries.

Some international planning and research groups have used the model described here to plan radiotherapy services. For example, Bentzen et al. [32] published an extensive review of the radiotherapy resource requirements in 25 countries in the European Union by using the model to calculate the current shortfall in radiotherapy resources. In only four European countries were radiotherapy resources sufficient to meet 80 per cent or more of demand. It was estimated that the required linear accelerators for each EU country ranged from 4 per million population (Cyprus) to 8 per million (Hungary) with an average of 5.9 linear accelerators per million to achieve the optimal radiotherapy utilization rate. The range was due to the wide variation in the crude incidence of various cancers because of differences in risk factors and the age structure of the population. For example, in 2002 the crude incidence of lung cancer in males varied from 41 cases per 100,000 in Moldova to 130 cases per 100,000 in Belgium [33].

Shortfalls between optimal and actual rates of radiotherapy utilization

The radiotherapy utilization trees that have been developed for each of the tumour sites are diagrammatic representations of optimal evidence-based cancer care from a radiotherapy perspective. They can be compared to actual radiotherapy utilization reported in patterns of care studies. Further details can be ascertained by analysing the distributions of tumour stage, histology, age, performance status, and other factors, in order to better define areas of discrepancy between the actual and ideal utilization rates.

Table 9.4 compares optimal radiotherapy utilization rates with available rates of actual radiotherapy utilization obtained from population-based data for each tumour site. The table highlights the paucity of the data on actual radiotherapy utilization, the high variability of the actual radiotherapy rates across different regions, and the general shortfall in radiotherapy use for most major tumour sites including the common tumour sites that have well-known evidence-based treatment guidelines such as breast cancer. These data are not subdivided by the various stages or other clinical attributes that would make a direct comparison between the optimal trees and the actual practice, although each of the tumour-site publications has detailed information by tumour stage [14–25].

Modelling changes in cancer incidence by type of cancer, tumour stage distribution, and treatment guidelines

One criticism of the model may be that the model will become out of date when new recommendations for treatment are made or when incidence or stage distributions change. However, one of the strengths of the model is that the trees are easily adapted when new information about cancer treatment comes to hand. Because new treatments will often only affect one branch in the overall utilization tree, the overall effect of any change is likely to be small and the estimate derived from this model is likely to remain valid for many years.

The software used to construct the radiotherapy trees can be readily used to change the overall model should there be changes in the incidence of certain cancers, a change in the stage distribution or a change in therapy recommendations based on clinical trials or revised clinical guidelines. For example, a change in stage distribution of cancer due to the development of superior staging investigations (such as the impact that positron emission tomography has had on non-small cell lung cancer staging or the impact that a new screening tool makes to stage distribution of

Table 9.4 Comparison of optimal and actual radiotherapy utilization rates for various geographical regions

| Cancer site | Optimal Radiotherapy utilization rate (%) | Actual radiotherapy utilization rates | | | | | | | |
| | | Sweden (%) 2001 | USA (%) | | UK (%) 1999 (NYCRIS)[7] | Australia (%) | | | |
			SEER[6] 1995–2000	ACS[1,5] 2001		National 1995	NSW[8] 2000	VIC[9]	SA[1,10] 1990–1994
Breast cancer	83	81	42.40	43.60	54	41	71	24	39.8
Lung cancer	76	71	39.35	35.52	NR4	NR4	49	44	37.6
Melanoma	23	23	1.87	1.13	NR4	NR4	13	NR4	1.8
Prostate	60	51	26.80	41.02	16	NR4	NR4	NR4	43.6
Kidney	27	63	7.82	3.64	NR4	NR4	NR4	NR4	11.0
Urinary Bladder	58	17	4.30	3.47	NR4	NR4	NR4	NR4	25.7
Testis	49	48	39.79	NR4	NR4	NR4	NR4	NR4	42.9
Oesophagus	80	73	54.33	NR4	31	NR4	NR4	NR4	47.1
Stomach	68	7	15.36	NR4	4	NR4	NR4	NR4	6.0
Pancreas	57	6	15.70	NR4	4	NR4	NR4	NR4	3.9
Liver	0	–	3.48	NR4	NR4	NR4	NR4	NR4	2.6
Gall Bladder	13	9	13.51	NR4	9	NR4	NR4	NR4	4.7
Colon	14	6	2.00	0.66	2	3	NR4	NR4	3.3
Rectum	61	56	37.59	41.20	33	38	NR4	NR4	16.5
Oral Cavity	74	94[3]	NR4	NR4	NR4	NR4	NR4	NR4	44.3[2]
Lip	20	22	7.63	NR4	NR4	NR4	NR4	NR4	2.0
Larynx	100	100	74.53	NR4	NR4	NR4	NR4	NR4	80.4
Oropharynx	100	100	70.41	NR4	NR4	NR4	NR4	NR4	NR4

(Continued)

Table 9.4 (Continued) Comparison of optimal and actual radiotherapy utilization rates for various geographical regions

Cancersite	OptimalRadiotherapy utilization rate (%)	Actual Radiotherapy Utilization Rates				Australia (%)			
		Sweden (%) 2001	USA (%) SEER 1995–2000	ACS[1] 2001	UK (%) 1999 (NYCRIS)[7]	National 1995	NSW[8] 2000	VIC[9]	SA[1,10] 1990–1994
Paranasal sinuses	100	100	NR[4]	NR[4]	NR[4]	NR[4]	NR[4]	NR[4]	NR[4]
Nasopharynx	100	100	84.02	NR[4]	NR[4]	NR[4]	NR[4]	NR[4]	NR[4]
Unk.prim (H+N)	90	NR[4]	NR[4]	NR[4]	NR[4]	NR[4]	NR[4]	NR[4]	NR[4]
Uterus	46	64	21.85	25.25	NR[4]	NR[4]	NR[4]	NR[4]	25.7
Cervix	58	83	43.84	32.88	NR[4]	NR[4]	NR[4]	NR[4]	40.9
CNS	92	37	59.03	NR[4]	NR[4]	NR[4]	NR[4]	NR[4]	51.9
Lymphoma	65	40	NR[4]	NR[4]	NR[4]	NR[4]	NR[4]	NR[4]	23.5
Leukaemia	4	8	NR[4]	NR[4]	NR[4]	NR[4]	NR[4]	NR[4]	5.6
Myeloma	38	82	NR[4]	NR[4]	NR[4]	NR[4]	NR[4]	NR[4]	33.8

[1]First treatment only
[2]includes salivary glands
[3]includes brachytherapy
[4]NR – Not reported
[5]ACS – American College of Surgeons
[6]SEER – Surveillance, Epidemiology and End Results database (National Cancer Institute)
[7]NYCRIS – Northern and Yorkshire Cancer Registry and Information Service
[8]NSW – the state of New South Wales
[9]VIC – the state of Victoria
[10]SA – the state of South Australia

a particular cancer), could easily be incorporated into the model provided that the new proportions of a particular attribute are known.

Other uses for the optimal treatment model

Optimum utilization for other treatments

The method described earlier is easily adaptable to other services, provided that evidence-based treatment recommendations are available. In Australia, the Collaboration for Cancer Outcomes Research and Evaluation (CCORE) has developed models for optimal referrals for genetic cancer risk assessment [34], chemotherapy delivery [35] and brachytherapy [36]. In addition, we have developed models of care for specific groups of patients such as screen-detected breast cancer patients [37] for surgery, radiation, chemotherapy, and hormone therapy for a defined sub-population.

Estimating optimal treatment for different populations

The data used represents an Australian population of cancer patients and the distribution of different types and stages of cancer are likely to be similar for other industrialized nations. Low or middle income countries have very different distributions of tumour types and stages due to differences in risk factors, access to screening, and lower median survival for the population. The model can be easily adapted to incorporate these differences in distribution of cancers as the recommendations for radiation remain the same. This is done by varying the proportions that appear in the tree. This has been done for low-middle income countries [38]. For example, the distribution of different types of cancers varies between the five broad regions of Africa [33]; cervix cancer is less common in North Africa and bladder cancer is more common than in other parts of Africa. These changes affect the optimum radiotherapy utilization rate so that the average rate for Africa (55 per cent) is higher than in Australia and has a wide range from 47 per cent in Middle Africa to 61 per cent in North Africa.

Estimating other end-points

The models described above, calculated proportions of a group that might receive treatment. The models can also be adapted to calculate other endpoints. These include using the models to calculate survival benefit or the average number of fractions of radiotherapy for each tumour type.

The number of daily radiotherapy treatments (fractions) varies with the tumour type and treatment intention from one fraction for palliation of bone pain to over 35 fractions for the curative treatment of prostate cancer. Thus the contribution of each indication to the demand for radiotherapy varies. In countries where the number of treatment fractions affects reimbursement there is evidence that higher numbers of fractions are used per course [39]. The average number of fractions per course of radiotherapy varies between radiotherapy departments. In NSW in 2004 the average number of fractions varied by 47 per cent from 15.7 to 23.1 [40]. By making the number of fractions the pay-off in the radiotherapy decision trees it is possible to determine the effect on demand for radiotherapy and to set a benchmark for appropriate fractionation. When there are several fractionation regimens for the same indication that have a similar effect on outcome it is possible to perform a sensitivity analysis to determine the effect of the variation.

By using survival benefit as the pay-off in the decision tree it is possible to calculate the overall survival benefit for an intervention. We have examined the survival benefit from radiotherapy for breast cancer [41]. Radiotherapy improved local control of breast cancer by 11 per cent and overall survival by 3 per cent.

Modelling optimal re-treatment rates

The models described in the earlier section only apply to the single use of a particular treatment. This is depicted in the trees as the terminal branch of the tree once a recommendation for treatment has been reached. One limitation is that there are many instances where patients undergo multiple courses of radiotherapy or chemotherapy due to recurrent or persistent disease. The proportion of patients that require greater than one treatment course needs to be incorporated into models of demand in order to plan treatment services.

It is estimated from actual practice that radiotherapy re-treatment represents up to 25 per cent of courses of radiotherapy [42]. Re-treatment assessment requires a different modelling process as the terminal branches need to be replaced by the possibility that the patient might re-enter the system. Once a patient has completed treatment they might then become disease free, relapse requiring further treatment, or die and these scenarios could occur after each episode of recurrence. The type of analysis that allows for this 're-entry' of the patient into a state that warrants further treatment is called Markov modelling or state transition.

Preliminary investigations of re-treatment by radiotherapy for lung cancer [43] showed 27 per cent of patients received two courses of radiotherapy, seven per cent received three courses and two per cent received a fourth course of radiotherapy. Because patients receiving two or more treatments were having palliative treatment for recurrence, re-treatment only accounted for 17 per cent of the number of fractions given for lung cancer.

Summary

It is possible to develop robust models of cancer service treatment from evidence-based guidelines and cancer incidence data. The proportion of cancer cases with an indication for a treatment can be calculated and proportions summed to give an overall estimate of service planning and bench-marking. Modelling deals with uncertainties by sensitivity analysis. Extensive peer review ensures that the indications are acceptable to oncology specialists and the study results are widely disseminated. Once a model is created it can be easily adapted if new information becomes available. Changes to one indication are unlikely to affect the overall estimate because each indication only affects a small proportion of cases. The model may also be used to examine complex endpoints such as survival, local control, and service use.

References

1 Huang J, Barbera L, Brouwers M, Browman G, & Mackillop WJ (2003). Does delay in starting treatment affect the outcomes of radiotherapy? A systematic review. *J Clin Oncol*, **21**:555–63.

2 Do V, Gebski V, & Barton MB (2000). The effect of waiting for radiotherapy for grade III/IV gliomas. *Radiother Oncol*, **57**:131–36.

3 Wigg DR & Morgan GW (2001). Radiation oncology in Australia: workforce, workloads and equipment 1986–1999. *Australas Radiol*, **45**:146–69.

4 Barbera L, Zhang-Salomons J, Huang J, Tyldesley S, & Mackillop W (2003). Defining the need for radiotherapy for lung cancer in the general population: a criterion-based, benchmarking approach. *Med Care*, **41**:1074–85.

5 Mackillop WJ, Groome PA, Zhang-Salomons J, et al (1997). Does a centralized radiotherapy system provide adequate access to care? *J Clin Oncol*, **15**:1261–71.

6 Barton M (2000). Radiotherapy utilization in New South Wales from 1996 to 1998. *Australas Radiol*, **44**:308–14.

7 Barton MB, Peters LJ, & Kenny L (2004). Radiotherapy in Australia one year after the Baume report: vision or mirage? *Med.J Aust*, **180**:55–56.

8 Tyldesley S, Boyd C, Schulze K, Math M, Walker H, & Mackillop WJ (2001). Estimating the need for radiotherapy for lung cancer: An evidence-based, epidemiologic approach. *Int J Radiat Oncol Biol Phys*, **49**(4): 973–85.

9 Hill DJ, Jamrozik K, White V, et al (1999) Surgical management of breast cancer in Australia in 1995. *NHMRC National Breast Cancer Centre*, Sydney.

10 Bremnes RM, Andersen K, & Wist EA (1995). Cancer patients, doctors and nurses vary in their willingness to undertake cancer chemotherapy. *Eur.J Cancer*, **31A**:1955–99.

11 National Health and Medical Research Council (1998). *Guide to the Development, Iimplementation and Evaluation of Clinical Practice Guidelines.* Commonwealth of Australia, Canberra.

12 Foroudi F, Tyldesley S, Walker H, & Mackillop WJ (2002). An evidence-based estimate of appropriate radiotherapy utilization rate for breast cancer. *Int J Radiat Oncol Biol Phys*, **53**: 1240–53.

13 Australian Institute of Health and Welfare and Australasian Association of Cancer Registries (2004). Cancer in Australia 2001 (Cancer Series no. 28). CAN 23. AIHW, Canberra.

14 Delaney G, Barton M, & Jacob S (2004). Estimation of an optimal radiotherapy utilization rate for gastrointestinal carcinoma. *Cancer*, **101**:657–70.

15 Delaney G, Jacob S, & Barton M (2004). Estimation of an optimal radiotherapy utilization rate for gynecologic carcinoma: part II–carcinoma of the endometrium. *Cancer*, **101**:682–92.

16 Delaney G, Jacob S, & Barton M (2004). Estimation of an optimal radiotherapy utilization rate for gynecologic carcinoma: part I–malignancies of the cervix, ovary, vagina and vulva. *Cancer*, **101**:671–81.

17 Delaney G, Barton M, & Jacob S (2004). Estimation of an optimal radiotherapy utilization rate for melanoma: a review of the evidence. *Cancer*, **100**:1293–1301.

18 Delaney G, Barton M, & Jacob S. Estimation of an optimal radiotherapy utilization rate for breast carcinoma: a review of the evidence. *Cancer*, **98**:1977–86.

19 Delaney G, Jacob S, & Barton M (2005). Estimation of an optimal external beam radiotherapy utilization rate for head and neck carcinoma. *Cancer*, **103**:2216–27.

20 Delaney G, Jacob S, & Barton M. Estimating the optimal external-beam radiotherapy utilization rate for genitourinary malignancies. *Cancer*, **103**:462–73.

21 Delaney G, Barton M, Jacob S, & Jalaludin B (2003). A model for decision making for the use of radiotherapy in lung cancer. *Lancet Oncol*, **4**:120–28.

22 Delaney G, Jacob S, & Barton M (2006). Estimating the optimal radiotherapy utilization for carcinoma of the central nervous system, thyroid carcinoma and carcinoma of unknown primary origin from evidence-based clinical guidelines. *Cancer*, **106**:453–65.

23 Featherstone C, Delaney G, Jacob S, & Barton M (2005). Estimating the optimal utilization rates of radiotherapy for hematologic malignancies from a review of the evidence: part I-lymphoma. *Cancer*, **103**:383–92.

24 Featherstone C, Delaney G, Jacob S, & Barton M (2005). Estimating the optimal utilization rates of radiotherapy for hematologic malignancies from a review of the evidence: part II-leukemia and myeloma. *Cancer*, **103**:393–401.

25 Delaney G, Jacob S, Featherstone C, & Barton M (2005). The role of radiotherapy in cancer treatment: estimating optimal utilization from a review of evidence-based clinical guidelines. *Cancer*, **104**:1129–37.

26 Delaney GP, Jacob S, Featherstone C & Barton MB (2003). Radiotherapy in cancer care: estimating optimal utilisation from a review of evidence-based clinical guidelines. CCORE/NCCI Canberra August 2003. http://www.canceraustralia.gov.au/media/3425/radiotherapyreport.pdf

27 Staples MP, Elwood M, Burton RC, Williams JL, Marks R, & Giles GG (2006). Non-melanoma skin cancer in Australia: the 2002 national survey and trends since 1985. *Med.J Aust*, **184**:6–10.

28 Donaldson, S. S (1990). *Radiotherapy of Benign Disease: A Clinical Guide.* Springer Verlag, Heidelberg.

29 Barton MB, Frommer M, Olver IN, Cox C, Crowe P, Wall B, Jenkin R, & Gabriel GS (2003). *A Cancer Services Framework for Victoria*, CCORE, Sydney.

30 Statewide Services Development Branch (2003). *Planning for Radiotherapy Services in NSW to 2006.* NSW Health, Sydney.

31 Radiotherapy activity planning group (2005). *Cancer in Scotalnd. Radiotherapy activity planning for Scotland 2011–2015*. NHS Scotland, Edinburgh.

32 Slotman BJ, Cottier B, Bentzen SM, Heeren G, Lievens Y, & van den BW (2005). Overview of national guidelines for infrastructure and staffing of radiotherapy. ESTRO-QUARTS: Work package 1. *Radiother Oncol*, **75**:349–56.

33 Ferlay J, Bray F, Pisani P, & Parkin DM (2004). GLOBOCAN 2002: Cancer Incidence, Mortality and Prevalence Worldwide. IARC CancerBase No. 5. (2.0). IARC Press, Lyon.

34 Featherstone C, Colley A, Tucker K, Kirk J, & Barton MB (2007). Estimating the referral rate for cancer genetic assessment from a systematic review of the evidence. *Br.J Cancer*, **96**:391–98.

35 Ng W, Jacob S, James M, Delaney G, & Barton MB (2008). *Chemotherapy in cancer care: estimating the optimal chemotherapy utilisation rate from a review of evidence-based clinical guidelines*. August. CCORE, Sydney.

36 Thompson S, Delaney G, Gabriel GS, Jacob S, Das P, & Barton M (2006). Estimation of the optimal brachytherapy utilization rate in the treatment of carcinoma of the uterine cervix: review of clinical practice guidelines and primary evidence. *Cancer*, **107**:2932–41.

37 Delaney G, Shafiq J, Chappell G, & Barton M (2008). Establishing treatment benchmarks for mammography-screened breast cancer population based on a review of evidence-based clinical guidelines. *Cancer*, **112**:1912–22.

38 Barton MB, Frommer M, & Shafiq J (2006). Role of radiotherapy in cancer control in low-income and middle-income countries. *Lancet Oncol*, **7**:584–95.

39. Lievens Y, Kesteloot K, Rijnders A, Kutcher G, & van den BW (2000). Differences in palliative radiotherapy for bone metastases within Western European countries. *Radiother Oncol*, **56**:297–303.

40. Statewide Services Development Branch (2006). *2004 Radiotherapy Management Information System Report*. NSW Health, Sydney.

41 Shafiq J, Delaney G, & Barton M (2007). An evidence-based estimation of local control and survival benefit of radiotherapy for breast cancer. *Radiother Oncol*, **84**:11–17.

42 Statewide Services Development Branch (2007). *2006 Radiotherapy Management Information System Report*. NSW Health, Sydney.

43 Estall V, Barton M, Vinod SK, & Liu Z (2007). Patterns of radiotherapy re-treatment in lung cancer patients: a retrospective, longitudinal study. *Journal of Thoracic Oncology*, **2**:531–6.

Chapter 10

Managing the costs of new therapies: the challenge of funding new drugs

Susan E. O'Reilly, Jaya Venkatesh[1]

The opportunities and the challenges

In developed nations, the growth in the number and variety of effective new cancer drugs, which improve cure rates, prolong life or improve quality of life for patients with cancer, has been one of the most exciting developments in modern medicine. Simultaneously, in many countries, the early twenty-first century is also the era of the aging 'baby boom' generation, born just after the Second World War. These population demographics will impose greater demands on the health care system over the next 25 years, as this group enters the highest risk age group for new cancer diagnoses. The collision of demographics and new technology (drugs) will force us to set priorities for investment in cancer care.

Until 10 to 20 years ago, progress in drug treatment of cancer had yielded slow but steady improvements, which typically emerged from the systematic approach, through clinical trials, to evaluate drugs and combinations of drugs in advanced disease. Where clinical benefit was evident, the promising treatments were then studied in newly diagnosed patients in the curative setting. Over time, chemotherapy drugs, which have broad cytotoxic or cytostatic effects on cancer cells, were shown to be dramatically effective in the curative treatment of childhood leukaemia, adult germ cell tumours of the testis and ovary, choriocarcinomas, Hodgkin's disease, and several subtypes of lymphoma. Substantial improvements were evident in failure-free and overall survival in women with breast cancer treated with anti-oestrogen hormones such as tamoxifen (the first of the 'targeted' therapies specific to hormonally sensitive cancers) and/or chemotherapy after surgery [1,2]. Other common cancers now benefit from adjuvant (curative) drug therapy at the time of initial surgery or radiation; e.g. oxaliplatin-based chemotherapy for Stage 3 colon cancer [3–6]. or hormones for high risk prostate cancer [7]. Incremental benefits in either disease control or survival have continued to be achieved in common advanced, incurable cancers, such as chemotherapy with bevacizumab (Avastin®) in colon cancer [8–11], pegylated liposomal doxorubicin (Caelyx®) in ovary [12–14], and erlotinib (Tarceva®) in lung cancer [15].

Although new chemotherapy drugs, alone or in combinations and with various schedules, remain an area of active research, the late 1990s and the first part of the twenty-first century have seen rapid growth in the understanding of the science of cancer development, growth and

[1] Susan E. O'Reilly, MB, FRCPC, Vice-President, Cancer Care, BC Cancer Agency, Vancouver, British Columbia, Canada, and Jaya Venkatesh, MHA, CMA, Director, Business Strategy and Operations, Provincial Systemic Therapy Programme, British Columbia Cancer Agency, Vancouver, BC, Canada.

metastatic behaviour. New laboratory techniques to determine molecular pathways in normal and cancer cells, the identification of inherited or acquired genetic mutations and their detection in cancer tissues, and the discovery of new biomarkers of disease prognosis or predictive behaviour in response to drugs, have all led to a multibillion dollar explosion of research and development in cancer drugs. Academic research organizations, especially universities, small biotechnology companies, and big multinational pharmaceutical companies are all in the race to discover and develop marketable therapies for cancer.

Nevertheless, to date only a handful of new drugs have proven to be breakthroughs in cancer care. Good examples of successful 'targeted' therapies are: imatinib (Gleevec®) for chronic myeloid leukaemia [16–18] and other Philadelphia chromosome positive leukaemias and c-kit positive tumours such as gastrointestinal sarcoma [19,20], trastuzumab (Herceptin®) [21–25] which targets the growth factor Her-2/neu in breast cancer and has demonstrated remarkable improvements in relapse-free survival in conjunction with chemotherapy after surgery, and a significant improvement in overall survival in the metastatic setting; erlotinib [15], (Tarceva®), an epidermal growth factor inhibitor in lung cancer, which prolongs survival in advanced disease; bevacizumab [8–11]; (Avastin®), an anti-angiogenesis drug, which reduces blood vessel growth and tumour nutrition and improves survival in metastatic colon cancer; and sunitinib [26] (Sutent®) and sorafenib [27]; (Nexavar®), tyrosine kinase inhibitors which prolong life in advanced renal cancer.

Despite the enormous scientific efforts underway, the course from discovery of a potentially effective cancer drug to its licensing for sale by national regulatory bodies such as the Food and Drug Authority (FDA) in the United States (http://www.fda.gov/) or, in Canada, the Health Canada Therapeutic Products Directorate (TPD) and Bureau of Biologicals (BB) (http://www. hc-sc.gc.ca/ahc-asc/branch-dirgen/hpfb-dgpsa/tpd-dpt/index-eng.php) is necessarily slow and very costly. Typically, once in vitro and animal efficacy and toxicity studies are completed, drugs progress through a progression of clinical trials in humans, involving Phase 1 trials of dosing and toxicity assessment, Phase 2 studies of efficacy in specific cancers, then Phase 3 randomized trials to compare patient outcomes with current best practices, in both the advanced disease setting, then subsequently in earlier, curative stages of cancer. Drug companies claim that they invest between 50 and 130 million US dollars to get one drug to market. The success rate for licensing a drug which enters clinical testing is estimated to be no more than 1 in 10, thus in the 'winner takes all' world of the 'Big Pharma' companies, potentially $500 million to $1.3 billion may have been invested overall, to see one successful product come to market. Pharmaceutical companies claim that they need to charge extraordinarily high prices for these new drugs during the years of patent protection, to defray their investment costs, reinvest in ongoing research and marketing, and reward their investors.

Health care providers, governments, and patients often exhibit healthy scepticism regarding drug pricing. The publicly funded health care systems and even insurance-company funded and managed care private systems in the United States creak under the strain of supporting the continuously escalating costs of overall health care, and, in particular, the skyrocketing costs of new drugs. It is highly probable that markets are approaching the limits of tolerance and affordability of the rate of growth in costs of new drugs. It is likely that there will be a more balanced approach to setting drug prices, particularly in the United States. Progress in pathology, which will limit the use of drugs to the subsets of patients most likely to derive benefit, will help limit the use of some drugs to patients with cancers exhibiting specific molecular and genetic profiles. This, in turn, will prove challenging for the drug development industry, as their risks are then proportionally higher, and returns lower. It remains to be seen whether this may adversely affect the tempo of drug discovery in the developed world.

The scale of the problem

Even in the world's wealthiest nation, the United States, concerns about the affordability and cost of drugs are finally being openly discussed by oncologists, health care providers, and the media. In the Sunday New York Times, July 6, 2008, the rising cost of cancer drugs and the conflicting evidence of efficacy from a variety of differing clinical trials was front page news; in particular, they quoted data from IMS Health, a health care information company, showing that cancer drugs constitute the second biggest category of drugs, behind cholesterol lowering drugs (for patients at risk of heart attacks and strokes), and accounted for $17.8 billion of the total prescription drug sales of $286.5 billion in the United States in 2007. Spending on drugs for cancer grew 14 per cent in the United States that year, but nevertheless, cancer was only fourth in the rate of growth in drug costs in relationship to other diseases.

Is cancer care consuming too much or too little of resources in the desire for better outcomes? Little comparative information is readily available on the costs of prevention, screening, diagnosis, and care across a spectrum of illnesses and disabilities, so it is challenging to attempt to benchmark against other diseases, such as cardiovascular, neurological, arthritic, or diabetic chronic diseases. Likewise, it is even more difficult, but relevant, to compare to the needs for governments to invest in other social services, education, and infrastructure, external to health.

The United States is a difficult model to analyse, as health care is funded by a smorgasbord of government funded Medicare, Medicaid, and Veterans programmes for the elderly, poor, or former military. Forty-five million people have no private health insurance, and the majority that do have a spectrum of coverage from limited and carefully managed coverage to more generous programmes. A health policy report by Dr. Peter Bach [28] describes the limits in Medicare's ability to control rising spending on cancer drugs. Complex legislation and regulations in the United States compromise the ability to restrict utilization to subsets of patients where the drugs are likely to be cost effective.

Oncology drug coverage in Canada

The Canadian health care system is predominantly publicly funded, and has many features relevant to other countries, and so we will discuss it in more detail. Each of the ten provinces and two territories funds and has governance over health care for its own population, but is expected to comply with the tenets of the Canada Health Act, which mandates that medically necessary care in a hospital setting is provided free of charge to the patients. Consequently, well organized provincial cancer agencies in most provinces fund all inpatient drug therapy, after suitable, but somewhat variable, reviews of benefits and costs. Oral drugs, or injectable hormones, such as LHRH (luteinizing hormone-releasing hormone) agonists for prostate cancer, may be funded either by provincial cancer agencies and dispensed through hospital pharmacies (as happens in British Columbia, Alberta, and Saskatchewan), or, in all other provinces, funded through provincial drug benefit plans which partially reimburse the cost of approved drugs dispensed through retail pharmacies. Consequently, formulary listing of individual drugs and financial coverage varies among provinces.

Both British Columbia and Ontario have well developed formal processes of technology review and economic evaluation for new drugs and for extended indications of existing drugs. In 2008 and 2009, all but one province (Quebec) have been collaborating in the development of a proposed Joint Oncology Drug Review, which may ultimately serve the needs of all provincial funding agencies. In the interim, the Ontario oncology drug preview processes, which are designed to advise their provincial government about both hospital and drug benefit plan listings, have been studied as a potential model for a national process. All participating provinces have observer status and receive copies of confidential drug company submissions and of preliminary and final Ontario recommendations. Nevertheless, all provinces then make their own internal decisions about funding priorities for cancer drugs.

British Columbia, Canada – An example of a comprehensive cancer drug system

It is helpful to gain an understanding of the growth in utilization and costs of cancer drugs by examining comprehensive data for a clearly defined population, such as British Columbia (BC). We can then extrapolate from this model to estimate the growth in costs and utilization throughout Canada and first world markets. Next, we can examine strategies in BC, Ontario, and elsewhere in the world for technology and economic review, before engaging in discussion of broader strategies to mitigate rising costs without major compromises in clinical efficacy.

In British Columbia, the westernmost province in Canada, the total population is 4.5 million, spread over an area equivalent to the size of France and Germany together, although most of the population is concentrated in the south, close to the border with the United States. The BC provincial Ministry of Health is responsible for the provision of free access to family doctors and to hospital care for all residents. It also operates a drug benefit plan (Pharmacare) which provides coverage for all outpatient drugs (subject to income-linked deductibles) except cancer drugs.

The British Columbia Cancer Agency (BCCA), a member organization of the BC Provincial Health Services Authority, has the mandate for cancer control in the province, and receives its funding from the provincial Ministry of Health. The BCCA manages and funds, from this public purse, all intravenous cancer drugs, administered in ambulatory clinics or inpatient services in cancer clinics and hospitals, and all oral, intramuscular, or subcutaneous cancer drugs required by patients in the province. Consequently, the BCCA is a monopoly provider for all publicly funded active cancer therapy, inclusive of chemotherapy, hormone therapy, immunotherapy, and targeted molecular drugs (in the same way, the BCCA is the only provider of radiotherapy services; but it has no monopoly on surgical services). All cancer patients in the province, regardless of whether they are seen at one of the five BCCA cancer centres or one of the 30 BCCA community cancer clinics, or have their medications prescribed by BCCA oncologists, community oncologists, surgeons or family doctors, are registered with the BCCA with demographic and diagnosis data, and are able to access free coverage of cancer drugs as long as these are given according to the more than 300 evidence-based guidelines and protocols published on the BCCA website www.bccancer.bc.ca. All demographics, drugs, doses, and dates are captured on an oncology drug data system, and data are available for analysis for utilization, monitoring for compliance with guidelines, and analysis of clinical outcomes.

Thus, the comprehensive BCCA cancer drug management system is a very powerful system in which we can examine oncology drug utilization and growth in a defined provincial population, where access to funded cancer drugs is managed by a single payer (the BC Cancer Agency) and provided free of charge to cancer patients. Drug utilization trends, financial management, communications, education, and compliance management strategies can be evaluated and extrapolated to larger national or international populations.

The BCCA oncology drug budget in fiscal 2008–09 was 130,000,000 Canadian dollars, which provides drug coverage for approximately 30,000 unique patients for their cancers (defining a 'unique patient' as a patient counted only once in a year, even if they have multiple treatments). Figure 10.1 shows that the annual drug budget for this province of 4.5 million increased by over 6 times in the last 11 years, an annual increase of about 20 per cent per year.

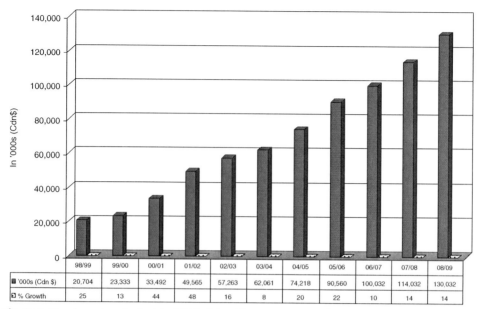

	98/99	99/00	00/01	01/02	02/03	03/04	04/05	05/06	06/07	07/08	08/09
'000s (Cdn $)	20,704	23,333	33,492	49,565	57,263	62,061	74,218	90,560	100,032	114,032	130,032
% Growth		25	13	44	48	16	8	20	22	10	14	14

Fig. 10.1 Oncology drug budget in British Columbia per annum, and growth compared to the previous fiscal year.

Figure 10.2 shows the growth in numbers of unique patients per year receiving cancer drugs in recent years, averaging 6.2 per cent per year since 1998–99. Future numbers are based on a conservative extrapolation at 4 per cent per year, predicting 46,500 unique patients by 2018–19, that is, a 50 per cent over the next 10 years. The growth in the numbers of patients on active therapy is a significant component of the increasing drug budget.

Notably, the growth in the incidence of cancer in the population is approximately 2.5 per cent per year (due mainly to population growth and ageing rather than to increases in incidence rates), but the prevalence of patients on active cancer therapy has grown at double or treble this rate. Why is growth greater in numbers of patients on active therapy than in incidence? There are several reasons:

1 Some of the curative 'adjuvant' regimens now last for many years (e.g. up to ten years for adjuvant breast cancer hormones).

2 Advanced, incurable cancer is now becoming a well managed chronic disease. Instead of patients having a brief episode of therapy for just a few months, and then succumbing to their disease, many are now living on active therapy for years; e.g. imatinib (Gleevec®) for chronic myeloid leukaemia, trastuzumab (Herceptin®) for advanced breast cancer, and LHRH agonists for prostate cancer.

3 Toxicity of therapy is now either better managed or less troublesome on new therapies, so compliance with recommended treatments is better.

4 Patients are well informed and often actively seek treatments, being informed from the plethora of information on the internet and other media.

The average cost per patient per year was $4,093 in 2008–09, a much more modest sum than the burgeoning costs of new drugs might suggest; it has increased from $1,142 in 1998–99 (Figure 10.3).

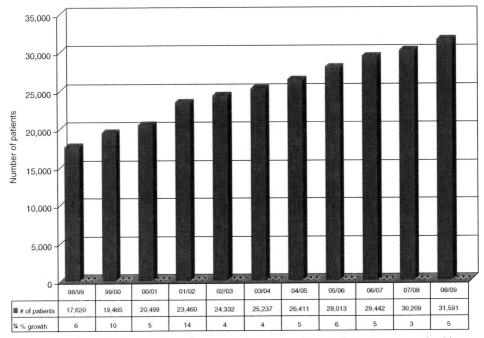

Fig. 10.2 Numbers of unique patients (i.e. counted once even if multiple treatments received in a year) accessing publicly-funded cancer drugs in British Columbia per fiscal year.

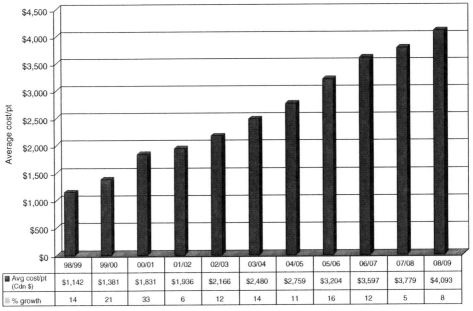

Fig. 10.3 Average cancer drug cost in Canadian dollars per patient per year in British Columbia, based on actual numbers of patients treated and drugs expenditure in a given year; and percentage growth per annum compared to previous year.

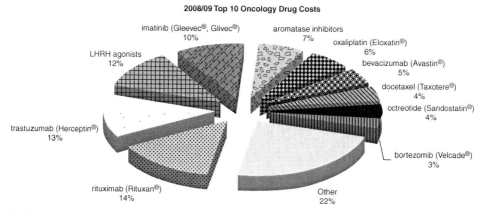

Fig. 10.4 Top 10 oncology drugs as proportions of the total 2008–09 oncology drug expenditure (Can $130 Million) for the British Columbia population.

In 2008–09, the top ten drugs were as shown in Figure 10.4; these typically comprise 75 per cent of the total budget.

Further data on the major types of cancer are regularly reviewed. Within each of 12 diagnostic categories of cancer, annual drug costs are shown in Figure 10.5, being highest for breast cancer, with lymphoma recently surpassing gastrointestinal and genito-urinary cancers. Annual numbers of unique patients receiving chemotherapy or hormonal drugs are shown in Figure 10.6, being highest for breast and genito-urinary cancers. Most interestingly, the average cost per patient per year for the major diagnostic groups is shown in Figure 10.7, being highest for sarcoma, central nervous system tumours, lymphoma, gastro-intestinal cancers, and leukaemias.

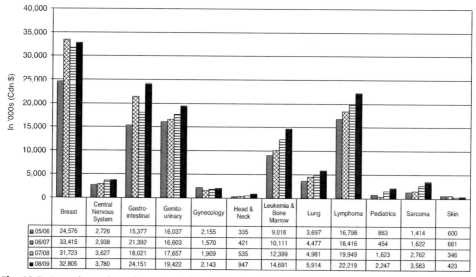

	Breast	Central Nervous System	Gastro-intestinal	Genito-urinary	Gynecology	Head & Neck	Leukemia & Bone Marrow	Lung	Lymphoma	Pediatrics	Sarcoma	Skin
05/06	24,576	2,726	15,377	16,037	2,155	335	9,016	3,697	16,798	883	1,414	600
06/07	33,415	2,938	21,392	16,603	1,570	421	10,111	4,477	18,416	454	1,622	661
07/08	31,723	3,627	18,021	17,657	1,909	535	12,399	4,981	19,949	1,623	2,762	346
08/09	32,805	3,780	24,151	19,422	2,143	947	14,691	5,914	22,219	2,247	3,583	423

Fig. 10.5 Annual oncology drug expenditure in British Columbia, thousands (Canadian dollars), according to diagnostic categories of cancer and year from 2005–06 to 2008–09.

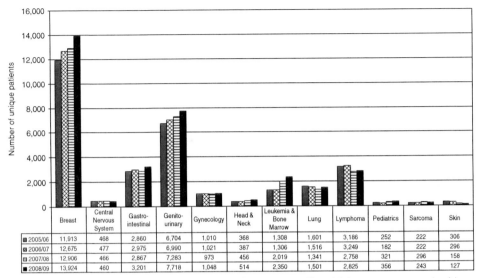

	Breast	Central Nervous System	Gastro-intestinal	Genito-urinary	Gynecology	Head & Neck	Leukemia & Bone Marrow	Lung	Lymphoma	Pediatrics	Sarcoma	Skin
2005/06	11,913	468	2,860	6,704	1,010	368	1,308	1,601	3,186	252	222	306
2006/07	12,675	477	2,975	6,990	1,021	387	1,306	1,516	3,249	182	222	296
2007/08	12,906	466	2,867	7,283	973	456	2,019	1,341	2,758	321	296	158
2008/09	13,924	460	3,201	7,718	1,048	514	2,350	1,501	2,825	356	243	127

Fig. 10.6 Numbers of unique patients (i.e. counted as one even if multiple treatments received in a year) by tumour group according to diagnostic categories of cancer accessing publicly-funded cancer drugs in British Columbia per fiscal year.

Oncology drug systematic review, utilization management, and cost control in British Columbia

As a vital component of its mandate to fund cancer drugs and other new programmes and technologies, the BCCA has conducted a 'Priorities and Evaluation' review on an annual basis for the last 13 years. The most frequent reviews are for new drugs, however, expanded indications

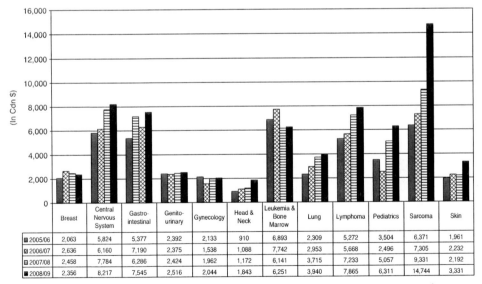

	Breast	Central Nervous System	Gastro-intestinal	Genito-urinary	Gynecology	Head & Neck	Leukemia & Bone Marrow	Lung	Lymphoma	Pediatrics	Sarcoma	Skin
2005/06	2,063	5,824	5,377	2,392	2,133	910	6,893	2,309	5,272	3,504	6,371	1,961
2006/07	2,636	6,160	7,190	2,375	1,538	1,088	7,742	2,953	5,668	2,496	7,305	2,232
2007/08	2,458	7,784	6,286	2,424	1,962	1,172	6,141	3,715	7,233	5,057	9,331	2,192
2008/09	2,356	8,217	7,545	2,516	2,044	1,843	6,251	3,940	7,865	6,311	14,744	3,331

Fig. 10.7 Average publicly-funded cancer drug cost per patient by tumour group per year in British Columbia (in Canadian Dollars).

for prevention, screening, radiation oncology, and other diagnostic or therapeutic programmes may also be reviewed. There are 12 provincial Tumour Groups spanning the range of major groups of cancers (e.g. breast, lung, gastrointestinal, genitourinary, lymphoma, leukaemia, brain, sarcoma, etc). These expert provincial tumour groups comprising oncologists from all subspecialties, pharmacists, and pathologists develop evidence-based clinical practice guidelines for each new drug or combination of drugs, or for a new indication for an existing drug. They then submit for each new drug or indication a formal application for drug funding to the Priorities and Evaluation Committee of the BCCA. This committee includes an administrative leader, oncologists from various professional disciplines, two pharmacists experienced in pharmacoeconomics and drug information, a health economist, and a statistician. All participants are experienced in technology review methodology.

The BCCA pharmacoeconomics team prepares a pharmacoeconomic model of the drug and delivery cost, based on a simple calculation of the cost per life year gained. This simple approach is a surrogate for preparation of more complex Quality Adjusted Life Year costs (where some assumptions may be difficult to quantify), but it does not take into account any additional costs to the health care system as a consequence of the treatment or prolongation of life. The inherent simplicity of this model, however, means that it is easy to apply in any health care system, does not rely on complex modelling, and can be applied reasonably quickly and in a consistent way to several potentially competing options. This is important as it is used as a practical management tool within the annual budget cycle, and often is based on very recent clinical advances. It is primarily influenced by the high acquisition costs of new drugs. It is essential to have information, either from published clinical trials data or from the pharmaceutical company, about the actual median (or mean) duration and dose of therapy; otherwise, the cost per patient will be overestimated as actual amount of drug used is often less than the prescribed intended amount. This simple model is feasible in circumstances where the cost of the drug greatly exceeds all other impacts on the health care system. It is reproducible over time, and thus contributes to consistency in decision-making. The BCCA annual cycle for oncology drug management is illustrated schematically in Figure 10.8.

The pharmacoeconomic team also estimates the cost of graduated uptake of a new drug in its first and subsequent years of use, based on BCCA provincial drug data or incidence data. Although this is not a requirement for the technology review step, it gives confidence in predicting the year by year budgetary impact and so builds confidence within the publicly funded Ministry of Health. Based on this review of clinical benefit and cost-effectiveness, the funding of a new drug can be implemented by the senior management of BCCA, within the overall total drug budget and annual increases agreed with the Ministry of Health. Where a new cancer drug replaces an existing one, the cost offsets are directly available to the BCCA drug budget; although if a new drug replaces surgery or radiotherapy the treatment of cost offsets is not straightforward.

The weaknesses in the BCCA drug review processes are that pharmaceutical companies cannot submit directly, as only those evidence-based treatment policies deemed worthy of a clinical practice guideline and submitted by the Tumour Group experts are reviewed. Industry may find this inherently unfair and typically prefers automatic review of all new drugs approved by Health Canada (http://www.hc-sc.gc.ca/index-eng.php). Likewise, it is challenging for industry to comprehend and interface with multiple different funding processes in the provinces of Canada. The BC review process does not utilize drug company prepared economic analyses, which typically use complex Quality Adjusted Life Year models and which endeavour to factor in the broad range of health cancer costs. The Ontario cancer drug review process, and some national organizations, such as the National Institute for Health and Clinical Excellence (NICE - http://www.nice.org.uk/) in the United Kingdom, have adopted an economic review process of clinical

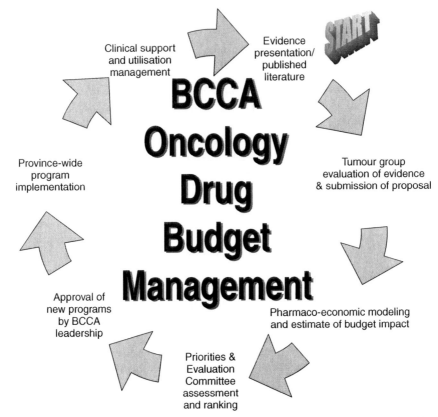

Fig. 10.8 Conceptual diagram of the annual oncology drug management cycle in British Columbia, Canada.

and economic evaluations submitted by industry. A further potential weakness is that the BCCA review process is internal, although arms-length from the Provincial Systemic Therapy Programme which funds and manages the drugs for the BCCA; there are no public volunteers or external experts participating in the review and ranking of new drugs. Finally, the reviews are conducted annually, usually well in advance of funding decisions for the next fiscal year, but problems arise occasionally when there is new evidence of substantial benefit from true 'breakthrough' drugs; in this uncommon situation, an out of cycle review is conducted and a request for funding made.

The BCCA process is based on a set of agreed principles, as follows:

1　New therapies depend, first, on evidence-based treatment guidelines, with clearly stated estimates of clinical benefits versus harms. Such guidelines should be based on 'level 1 evidence', ideally from well designed clinical trials enrolling large numbers of patients and showing important and statistically significant benefits, especially in overall survival, as well as quality of life outcomes, which have been assessed over an appropriate follow-up interval, usually several years.

2　There has to be a reasonable acceptance of lower levels of evidence in rare cancers or other clinical situations where large patient numbers are unachievable.

3 Health economic assessments, using pharmacoeconomics models, should have an equivalent level of scientific credibility to the clinical evidence. Good economic models facilitate ethically fair and consistent decision-making, over time.

4 The principle of distributive justice should apply; in that decisions should be fair across the spectrum of diseases (within cancer) and not driven by total budget impact in common diseases.

5 Decisions should be reasonably intuitive in regard to extrapolation of data in circumstances where no further data is likely to become available (e.g. trials within selected age groups, where broader use makes clinical sense).

6 Frank discussion around thresholds for funding, in light of clinical benefit and cost. This is a thorny problem, in light of the lack of valid data to determine optimal thresholds and lack societal consensus. Old 'thresholds' from decades ago, for example, renal dialysis costing $50,000 per life year gained, are unlikely to have a great deal of relevance in decision-making in 2010. Nevertheless, each publicly funded health care system needs to be able to set priorities within a window that is publicly affordable and tolerable to both patients and taxpayers.

Typically, 8 to 15 proposals for new or modified therapy programmes are reviewed annually, of which 70 per cent are funded. Only those programmes supported by BCCA evidence-based clinical guidelines are reviewed. The process is timely, as the guideline preparation and submission to the Priorities and Evaluation Committee typically begin prior to a new drug completing its review by Health Canada. The economic model is finalized when the drug has been approved by Health Canada and pricing information is available.

Communication and education

The BCCA implements funding for a new drug by posting on the professional section of its website www.bccancer.bc.ca the treatment protocol (with details of eligibility, toxicity, contraindications, dose, schedule, and dose reduction information), physician order sets for use throughout the province (developed by the oncologists, pharmacists, and nurses), and a patient information leaflet. A monthly 'Systemic Therapy Update' electronic newsletter is also posted on the website and e-mailed to all oncologist professionals in the province. The BCCA also provides educational forums for doctors, nurses, and pharmacists to support dissemination of new knowledge and safe practices.

The emphasis on prompt dissemination of information and the provision of useful tools such as protocols, cancer drug manuals, printable doctor's orders and patient information underpin the safe delivery of optimal therapy to all eligible patients. Optimal outcomes are a direct consequence of universal access to evidence-based therapy.

Optimising drug purchasing contracts

In Canada, when a new drug is approved for sale, the national Patent Medicine Price Review Board sets a price typically based on the median of prices in the United States and several European countries. The publicly funded provincial cancer agencies, or the health authorities or individual hospitals then endeavour to negotiate additional offsets, such as free product, discounts, or rebates. Several provinces now participate in common drug contracting and 'bundling' processes, in conjunction with drug contract management companies, to mitigate the impact of expensive single source products. There may be opportunities to develop this approach into national collaboration, over time. Once the period of patent protection for a new drug expires, opportunities for competitive bids from generic companies arise. Unfortunately, in Canada, even generic prices have remained high, despite their lack of investment in new drug development.

In the seven out of ten provinces in Canada where cancer hormones and oral drugs are reimbursed through provincial drug plans and dispensed through retail pharmacies, the opportunity for hospital-based drug contracting is lost, but the ability to limit reimbursement to the elderly or unemployed, and to apply income-linked deductibles to patients and families is gained. This strategy can control the financial risk to a publicly funded health care system, but at the cost of reducing compliance with optimal treatment. In circumstances where the clinical benefit is marginal and the cost is high, this is a reasonable approach. The difficulties arise when patients cannot afford highly effective, curative, or life-prolonging therapy. In Canada, the majority of families have some level of private health insurance (often provided by employers) in addition to publicly funded health care. Unfortunately, the majority of private plans have thresholds of maximum drug coverage, which frequently leave patients without the means to cover costs of 'catastrophic drugs'.

The BCCA purchases drugs through hospital contracts, which typically set lower prices than retail pharmacy prices, and uses the services of a multi-provincial, independent purchasing group for most of its drug contracting, to maximize cost savings. Other drugs are on individual contracts with the BCCA, and opportunities for discounts or other risk sharing strategies are optimized.

Monitoring use of drugs and compliance with protocols

The BCCA has close control of compliance with their evidence-based protocols; this is a key component of good fiscal and clinical management. All patients, whether treated at a BCCA facility or elsewhere in the province, are registered according to diagnosis; this first step opens a menu of treatments for that patient. Should more costly drugs be needed, then a second level of submission, including information such as staging or history of prior therapy, is required before a second tier of drugs is available. The most expensive drugs, or those most at risk of being prescribed in unapproved, unfunded clinical situations, require an online clinical submission, which goes through two levels of validation, at the expert tumour group level and by the Provincial Systemic Therapy Programme, before funding is approved.

Physicians submit clinical information online for approval for the most expensive drugs. BCCA pharmacists dispense only drugs approved for funding, and the community hospitals electronically submit their drugs dispensed for reimbursement. Drugs are only reimbursed to these hospitals if all criteria are met.

The BCCA oncology drug data warehouse 'Datamart' captures the demographic information, diagnosis, drug, date, and dose for all patients treated in the province. This system is used to facilitate periodic audits of compliance with molecular parameters (e.g. relating drug use to Her-2-neu over expression), dose, and duration of therapy. This data is also an invaluable resource for utilization management, financial monitoring and projections, and a research resource for clinicians and scientists. High level information routinely derived include the data shown in Figures 10.1 to 10.7: annual analysis of costs and utilization of specific drugs, especially the 'Top Ten' drugs, which typically comprise 75 per cent of the total budget; drug costs per patient; total expenditures, numbers of patients, and cost per patient according to diagnostic categories of cancer. This database is the essential framework for more detailed analyses, which may include assessing related costs such as diagnostic services and surgery, and predicting cost offsets, for example, where a drug reduces the risk of recurrence or may avoid procedures such as bone marrow transplants. Such analyses may use the economic methods described in Chapter 19 of this book. Although the BCCA drug utilization and compliance management system is electronically supported, countries where information systems may be unaffordable can also conduct similar close management through paper systems.

Validating the investment: population-based outcome analysis

In Canada, the ten provinces track and publish annual incidence and mortality statistics for broad categories of cancer, but this information is insufficiently detailed to evaluate the impact of costly drug programmes on specific diagnostic and staging sub-categories of cancer. Organized health care systems now have the advantage of clinical informatics to track overall survival in populations of patients receiving a specific therapy. In British Columbia, the availability of a variety of provincial databases including the tumour registry, the oncology drug Datamart, and pathology and stage information of cancer in patients referred to the BC Cancer Agency have facilitated tracking the population-based impact of cancer therapies. Published examples include the impact of rituximab when added to the previous standard chemotherapy combination CHOP in advanced staged aggressive histology lymphoma [29] (Figure 10.9), improvements in overall survival in four successive historical cohorts of patients with metastatic breast cancer who were eligible for new treatments [2]; current analysis has evaluated the impact of adding bevacizumab to chemotherapy in metastatic colorectal cancer [8–11]. The distinguishing feature of these analyses is that they assess the impact on clinical outcomes of all patients in the province, not only those

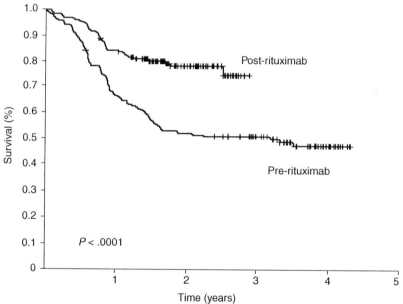

Fig. 10.9 Effect of a change in guidelines and drug funding on overall survival of all patients in British Columbia with advanced stage, diffuse large B-cell lymphoma (DLBCL).
On March 1 2001, the British Columbia (BC) Cancer Agency implemented a new policy recommending the combination of CHOP and rituximab for all newly diagnosed patients with advanced-stage DLBCL, regardless of age. The curves show the overall survival of all patients in the province diagnosed in the 18-month periods before the institution of this new policy (pre-rituximab, 140 patients), and after its introduction (post-rituximab, 152 patients).
From: Sehn et al., 2005, with permission.

who were treated in a particular centre. Analyses to date have validated that the impact of the population is consistent with the expected benefit from published clinical trials.

Canadian national developments in cancer drug review

Current regulatory process for all drugs

The developments in oncology drug review in Canada take place against the background of the regulatory process for drugs in general. In Canada (population 33 million) the Council of Federal, Provincial, and Territorial Ministers appointed a Board of Governors for the Canadian Association of Drug and Technology Assessment (CADTH), which is jointly funded (30 per cent federal, 70 per cent provincial) to conduct reviews of drugs and technology. The Board established a Common Drug Review (CDR) committee to review all new drugs indicated for ambulatory pharmacare programmes funded by the provincial and territorial governments. Industry submits to this process and the CDR, comprising clinicians, pharmacists, and economists with technology review expertise, evaluate the clinical benefit and cost-effectiveness. Significant resources are invested in health economic analysis and critiques, external experts are engaged to provide opinions, and industry is notified of the recommendations of the expert committee prior to the outcome being published on the website (http://cadth.ca/index.php/en/home).

CDR does not review intravenous drugs delivered in a hospital setting, nor does it have the benefit of established clinical guidelines from expert groups. In other respects, it provides high quality reviews in a timely fashion to participating provincial pharmacare plans. As such, it is not ideally positioned to take on the broad scope of review for oncology drugs in Canada.

Developments in oncology drug review

Canada, like many countries, has internal inconsistencies in drug funding, and is working towards a more consistent national approach. Nine out of the ten provinces have now embarked on collaborative planning for a joint interprovincial oncology drug review. The intent has been to achieve greater consistency in cancer drug review and funding, to develop one portal for industry, expert groups and publicly funded health care institutions to apply for reviews, to improve consistency of patient access to drugs, and to assist those provinces with limited human resources to access high quality reviews.

The provinces agreed in 2007 that there would be an interim Joint Oncology Drug Review (JODR) process, based on the Ontario model, which supports both Cancer Care Ontario for intravenous drug review, and the Ontario Drug Benefit plan for oral drugs reimbursed to retail pharmacies. In the Ontario model, submissions come principally from drug companies, after their drugs are approved by Health Canada (which does not deal with funding of the drugs). The Cancer Care Ontario Programme in Evidence-base Care then develops a clinical practice guideline, if deemed appropriate (http://www.cancercare.on.ca/toolbox/qualityguidelines/pebc/). Then a review of industry-supplied health economic data is done, by internal and external experts, leading to recommendations referred to the Ontario Ministry of Health through internal committees.

During the interim phase of the JODR, other provinces have observer status (http://www.health.gov.on.ca/english/providers/programme/drugs/drug_submissions/inter_oncology_drugs.html) and receive copies of industry submissions and reports from the committee. Individual funding decisions remain at the discretion of each province.

While the interim phase has been ongoing, the provinces have been collaborating in the design of an ideal Joint Oncology Drug Review, including defining principles, modelling governance and committee structures, including discussions regarding the development of national clinical practice guidelines, health economics, and ethics processes. An outcome is expected in 2009. If the model for cancer is implemented, it may be the forerunner of best practices in drug review in other diseases.

Those involved in planning the future Joint Oncology Drug Review for Canada have communicated the following principles:

The governance structure must ensure fair, objective, transparent processes and must be accountable to patients, payers, and public.

- Cancer drugs must be evaluated within a review process and decision-making framework which is consistent with those used for drugs in other diseases.

- The review process will be multidisciplinary, cross-jurisdictional, and collaborative in nature, with appropriate input from key stakeholders and linkage to other key national initiatives.

- The review process will reflect an ongoing commitment to excellence through best practices in a spirit of continuous quality improvement.

- The review process will have capacity for rigorous and consistent evidence-based clinical and pharmacoeconomic reviews to support evidence-based decision making.

- The review process will include an ethical framework.

- Review processes will be cost efficient, effective and streamlined to support timely decision making.

- The review process will have capacity for data capture and ongoing evaluation (decision monitoring/performance measurement) to support continuous improvements.

- There will be capacity for health outcomes and economic impact analysis to support decision making and planning.

Some other international models of oncology and general drug review and management

United Kingdom

In Britain, the National Health Service funds a variety of drugs in both the hospital and retail pharmacy settings for a population of approximately 60 million. In 1999, the National Institute for Clinical Excellence (NICE) was established to review drugs and technology, based on clinical benefit and cost-effectiveness, and to develop national guidelines. NICE will conduct a review of a drug on request from the Secretary of State for Health; typically, these comprise costly drugs. Both internal and external expert reviews from independent academic centres are submitted to the Technology Appraisal Committee, whose recommendations are reported to the NICE board for a final decision, which, in turn, is binding on the Primary Care Trusts in the United Kingdom. The NICE Board is appointed by an independent commission, on behalf of the Secretary of State for Health. The NICE Centre for Health Technology Assessment provides guidance on new or existing therapies; it works with academic centres and its Technology Appraisal Committee, which is advisory to NICE. Technology committee membership comes from cross sections of the National Health Service, patient or care organizations, industry, and universities.

In addition to clinical merit, a cost utility analysis, based on the British model of the cost of Quality Adjusted Life Years gained, is employed to determine fairly explicit thresholds for funding, in the region of 30,000 UK Pounds per QALY. Less cost-effective therapies are occasionally recommended, if there are compelling reasons to do so. All processes and outcomes are published on the NICE website (www.nice.org.uk/).

The NICE processes are well respected and based on accepted methods. A potential weakness in the UK system is that the NICE process is not directly linked to the funding processes within the Primary Care Trusts, thus health care providers may be challenged to balance budgets and provide broad-based health care services in an equitable manner when new drugs have a high overall budget impact. NICE has struggled to conduct reviews in a timely fashion and has recently implemented a fast track process for clinically important new drugs, when routine reviews were taking more than two years to initiate and complete. As with all local or national processes, the thresholds for clinical benefit and cost utility may not be readily transferable to other jurisdictions.

Australia

Australia has a national Pharmaceutical Benefits Scheme (PBS – http://www.pbs.gov.au/html/home) which operates a national formulary subsidizing drugs for coverage in the community setting for approximately 20 million people. An Advisory Committee (PBAC) reviews drugs for listing on the PBS. Submissions come from the pharmaceutical industry for all new drugs which will be dispensed in the community; hospital-delivered drugs are typically not reviewed through this process.

PBAC reviews both the clinical and the pharmacoeconomic evidence and submits a recommendation to the federal Minister for Health and Ageing for a decision to list the drug. Membership of PBAC includes community pharmacists, clinical pharmacologists, general practitioners, specialist physicians, health economists, and members of the public. The methods used are similar to NICE, but at present there is no fast track mechanism and reviews may take 17 months or more. Negative decisions appear difficult to reverse, even as clinical data matures, despite an appeals process. New intravenous cancer drugs are not typically part of the process, which introduces discordance between funding agencies and their review processes. Transparency for the public and for industry is considered very good. Final reports are published.

New Zealand

New Zealand (population 4.1 million) has a publicly funded Pharmaceutical Management Agency (PHARMAC – http://www.pharmac.govt.nz/) which manages a national drug formulary. Applications for funding are accepted from a variety of sources, such as industry, clinicians, or consumer groups. Industry typically initiates all new drug submissions; these are reviewed by the Pharmacy and Therapeutics Advisory Committee (PTAC), which considers clinical merit, cost-effectiveness and budget impact.

PTAC, with members from professional backgrounds in medicine, pharmacy, and economics, conducts internal economic reviews and is not reliant on industry QALY estimates. Submissions are prioritized for the timing of review depending on clinical benefit; there is no additional fast track process. There is a separate Consumer Advisory Committee to provide consumer input when requested by PHARMAC, but they do not participate in the drug review process. The PHARMAC Board is appointed by the Minister of Health and operates within a fixed annual budget, necessitating setting priorities for funding. The decision to list is made by the Board.

New Zealand is a small country, and a major role of PHARMAC is to set priorities for listing drugs to meet the needs of the population, within a constrained funding envelope. Although the emphasis has principally been on outpatient drugs, there is a gradual shift to reviewing intravenous drugs too. The focus is general and not specific to oncology.

Conclusions: Strategies to manage the costs of new therapies in a publicly funded system

The importance of evidence-based clinical guidelines

In Chapter 8 of this book, Dr. Browman and his colleagues discuss the processes of developing and using evidence-based guidelines. This is the fundamental building block of an effective population-based approach to better cancer outcomes. Locally, nationally, and internationally, considerable contributions of oncologists' professional time go into the intellectual effort of determining best practices. The consensus clinical guidelines produced are designed to represent the optimal use of available therapies to render the best outcomes at greatest efficacy and least toxicity. Nevertheless, most clinical guidelines do not overtly take into account the cost of therapies. Sometimes these standards and guidelines are regarded as too restrictive by hopeful patients with dire diseases, and by some of their physicians who are committed to being their advocates. In reality, the physician's role in advanced disease is to discuss all therapeutic choices in a balanced way with each patient, not to subject them to false hope or excess toxicity out of a reluctance to face the difficult transition from curative treatment to symptom control and palliative care. In a well managed system, patients should have access to all clinically important treatments that are affordable within the funding envelope of that jurisdiction. Evidence-based guidelines offer the best means of consistent, high quality practice and should be adhered to in the best interest of patient outcomes. Dissemination of guidelines and education about their use not only improves patient access and outcomes, but also indirectly contributes to good financial management and conserves scarce resources needed to implement other important innovations.

Technology reviews: Evaluation of clinical benefit, economic impact, and priority setting

Leaders of health care systems need to be able to choose which priorities to fund, based on reasonable expectations of benefit in relationship to ability to pay. Earlier in this chapter, we discussed several technology review processes which have had a profound impact on decision making in their national or regional milieus. In countries with limited financial resources, and limited human resources in time and expertise to conduct complex evaluations, any or all of these processes can be adapted to meet the health care and societal needs of that environment. Governments and Ministries need to address overall social welfare and health needs, starting with clean water, adequate food, basic housing, education, maternal and child health, prevention, immunizations and basic health care, and including beneficial medical interventions, depending on available resources; the threshold for funding cancer drugs can be adjusted to the reality of the environment and the reasonable expectations of its citizens.

Drug utilization management

Some issues in drug purchasing have been discussed in the Canadian context in the previous sections, and many countries are moving towards national or regional purchasing systems to lower costs. When a new drug is funded for a specific clinical indication (e.g. for advanced disease in one particular type of cancer), it is very tempting for doctors to prescribe it in other types of cancer, or sooner or later in the natural history of a cancer. Often, there may be ongoing clinical trials to see if the drug is effective in other cancers, so naturally, both patients and their doctors are keenly interested in broadening access in advance of confirmatory data from clinical trials. As a consequence, management utilization to comply with proven and funded indications is critical in protecting drug budgets from over-utilization and is a key aspect of fairness to all cancer patients to protect their access to treatments of proven efficacy. An effective drug utilization data system is essential for this, and a variety of paper-based and electronic systems have evolved to control utilization; the BC system is described earlier in this chapter. In the United States, managed care organizations such as Kaiser Permanente have been leaders in drug utilization management. The costs of such administrative systems are of course a major issue. It is relatively easy to develop drug utilization controls in a hospital system, but much harder to implement in the reimbursement of drugs to ambulatory patients, where full clinical information is typically lacking. Progress in linking clinical information and reimbursement is compromised both by lack of universal clinical informatics systems and the understandable barriers of privacy and confidentiality legislation.

In developing and middle-income countries with much more restricted resources, there needs to be a centralized, organized system to provide selected cancer drugs and supportive drugs, especially for pain relief; this is discussed further by Ian McGrath in Chapter 22 of this book. Careful selection of highly effective and cheap drug therapy in the majority of diagnostic groups is optimal. Countries such as Cuba have pursued this approach. Excellent examples of trade-offs might be restricting patients with hormone sensitive breast cancer to tamoxifen rather than the modestly more effective, but much more expensive, aromatase inhibitors; offering orchiectomy rather than expensive LHRH drugs for advanced prostate cancer; choosing the cheapest generic chemotherapy drug regimens for breast, ovary, colon, and other treatable cancers; and offering highly effective and quite affordable drugs for selected curable diseases such as Hodgkin's, some lymphomas and leukaemias, and testicular cancer.

Investment in molecular and genetic cancer pathology

The road to the future world of cancer drug management is considerably brightened by the gradual development of sensitive and specific markers of tumour susceptibility to treatment. Prognostic markers predict the risk of a poor or good outcome in an individual cancer patient, and, typically supplement the prognostic information given by clinical and pathology staging systems, which take into account the pathological diagnosis and grade of the tumour, as well as its size, location, lymph node involvement, and status of metastatic disease.

Predictive markers are specific to the likelihood of a tumour responding to a therapeutic intervention; some predictive markers are also prognostic markers, if they predict overall outcome. The best known examples are oestrogen and progesterone receptors in breast cancer, which have an impact on prognosis and specifically indicate that, where these receptors test positive, both curability in newly diagnosed breast cancer and disease control in metastatic cancer are very favourably influenced by drugs such as tamoxifen or aromatase inhibitors, which interfere with oestrogen metabolism. Likewise, the discovery of Her-2/neu testing in breast cancer and the development of Herceptin, which targets this growth factor, has had substantial clinical benefit for patients whose tumours strongly over-express Her-2/neu.

Very recent data in advanced colorectal cancers treated with epidermal growth factor target drugs (cetuximab (Erbitux®) or panitumumab (Vectibix®)) have demonstrated that 40 per cent of patients with the mutated K-ras gene do not benefit from therapy with these drugs, whereas those with wild-type K-ras have substantial benefit. Clearly, this predictive information is valuable both for patients who will benefit from the interventions, and also for those who will not, preventing unnecessary treatment and unwanted effects, as well as reducing costs.

There is much ongoing research to identify new biomarkers, and effective panels of oncology markers that can discriminate between prognostic groups of patients. The process of identification of potential markers, and their further evaluation in studies including clinical trials, to determine whether they have a reliable role in predicting benefit from various treatments is complex. It is strategically very important to incorporate acquisition of tumour tissue in the conduct of the majority of clinical trials, so that new biomarkers can be validated in such settings.

Although this field of predictive testing is only now coming to the forefront, organizations that fund health care would be penny wise and pound foolish if they did not invest appropriately in predictive testing of tumour tissue to mitigate the costs (and toxicity for patients) of using drugs in patients who would not benefit. These predictive molecular or genetic tests themselves may be costly, and the processes of critical evaluation of their usefulness must be applied in making decisions to fund them. Clearly, for a new drug with a proven predictive marker test, both drug and pathology test should be funded simultaneously; but in reality, nationally and internationally, 'stove pipes' of different governance or reimbursement systems for drugs versus laboratories can be an obstacle for this sensible approach. Rational application of good laboratory testing, ideally in a quality-controlled high-volume laboratory setting, offers the potential to revise clinical practice guidelines to conform to clinical benefit and holds the promise of sparing patient's toxicity from ineffective therapy, while reducing costs to the health care systems. The opportunity beckons to redirect costs saved and invest in effective new drugs or technology.

References

1 Early breast cancer trialists' collaborative group (2005). Effects of chemotherapy and hormonal therapy for early breast cancer on recurrence and 15-year survival: an overview of the randomized trial. Lancet, **365**:1687–1717.

2 Chia S, Speers D, Yachkova Y, et al (2007). The impact of new chemotherapeutic and hormone agents on survival in a population-base cohort of women with metastatic breast cancer. Cancer, **110**(5):973–79.

3 André T, Bonni C, Mounedji-Boudiaf, L, et al (2004). Oxaliplatin, fluorouracil, and leucovorin as adjuvant treatment for colon cancer. N Engl J Med, **350**:2343–51.

4 Kuebler JP, Wieand HS, O'Connell MJ, et al (2007). Oxaliplatin combined with weekly bolus fluorouracil and Leucovorin as surgical adjuvant chemotherapy for stage II and III colon cancer: results from NSABP C-07. JCO, **25**(16):2198–2204.

5 Goldberg RM, Sargent DJ, Morton RF, et al (2004). A randomized controlled trial of fluorouracil plus leucovorin, irinotecan, and oxaliplatin combinations in patients with previously untreated metastatic colorectal cancer. JCO, **22**(1):23–30.

6 Tournigand C, André T, Achille E, et al (2004). FOLFIRI followed by FOLFOX6 or the reverse sequence in advanced colorectal cancer: a randomized GERCOR study. JCO, **22**(2):229–37.

7 Bolla M, Collette L, Blank L, et al (2002). Long-term results with immediate androgen suppression and external irradiation in patients with locally advanced prostate cancer (an EORTC study): a phase III randomized trial. The Lancet, **360**:103–8.

8 Hurwitz H, Fehrenbacher L, Novotny W, et al (2004). Bevacizumab plus Irinotecan, Fluorouracil, and Leucovorin for Metastatic Colorectal Cancer. N Engl J Med, **350**(23):2335–42.

9 Giantonio BJ, Catalano PJ, Meropol J, et al (2007). Bevacizumab in combination with oxaliplatin, fluorouracil, and leucovorin (FOLFOX4) for previously treated metastatic colorectal cancer: results from the Eastern Cooperative Oncology Group Study E3200. JCO, **25**(12):1539–44.

10 Saltz LB, Clarke S, Diaz-Rubio E, et al (2008). Bevacizumab in combination with oxaliplatin-based chemotherapy as first-line therapy in metastatic colorectal cancer: a randomized phase III study. JCO, **26**(12): 2013–19.

11 Renouf D, Lim HJ, Speers C, et al (2009). Impact of bevacizumab (bev) on overall survival (OS) in patients (pts) with metastatic colorectal cancer (MCRC): A population based study. To be published.

12 Gordon AN, Fleagle JT, Guthrie D, et al (2001). Recurrent epithelial ovarian carcinoma: a randomized phase III study of pegylated liposomal doxorubicin versus topotecan. JCO, **19**(14):3312–22.

13 Ferrandina G, Ludovisi M, Lorusso D, et al (2008). Phase III trial of gemcitabine compared with pegylated liposomal doxorubicin in progressive or recurrent ovarian cancer. *JCO*, **26**(6):890–96.

14 Bookman MA, Brady MF, McGuire WP, et al. Evaluation of new platinum-based treatment regimens in advanced-stage ovarian cancer: a phase III trial of the gynecologic cancer intergroup. *JCO*, **27**(9):1419–25.

15 Shepherd FA, Rodrigues Pereira J, Ciuleanu T, et al. Erlotinib in previously treated non-small cell lung cancer. *N Engl J Med*, **353**:123–32.

16 Druker BJ, Guilhot F, O'Brien SG, et al (2006). Five-year follow-up of patients receiving imatinib for chronic myeloid leukemia. *N Engl J Med*, **355**(23):2408–17.

17 Baccarani M, Saglio G, Goldman J, et al (2006). Evolving concepts in the management of chronic myeloid leukemia: recommendations from an expert panel on behalf of the European LeukemiaNet. *Blood*, **108**(6):1809–20.

18 O'Brien SG, Guilhot F, Goldman JM, et al (2008). International randomized study of interferon versus STI571 7-year follow-up: sustained survival, low rate of transformation and increased rate of major molecular response in patients with newly diagnosed CML in chronic phase. *Blood*, **112**:76(a) abstract number 186.

19 Blanke C, Demetri GD, von Mehren M, et al (2008). Long-term results from a randomized phase II trial of standard- versus higher-dose imatinib mesylate for patients with unresectable or metastatic gastrointestinal stromal tumors expressing KIT. *JCO*, **26**(4):620–25.

20 Blanke C, Rankin C, Demetri GD, et al (2008). Phase III randomized, intergroup trial assessing imatinib mesylate at two dose levels in patients with unresectable or metastatic gastrointestinal stromal tumors expressing the kit receptor tyrosine kinase: S0033. *JCO*, **26**(4):626–32.

21 Romond EH, Perez EA, Bryant J, et al (2005). Trastuzumab plus adjuvant chemotherapy for operable her2-positive breast cancer. *N Engl J Med*, **353**:1673–84.

22 Joensuu H, Kellokumpu-Lehtinen PL, Bono P, et al (2006). Adjuvant docetaxel or vinorelbine with or without trastuzumab for breast cancer. *N Engl J Med*, **354**:809–20.

23 Smith I, Procter M, Gelber RD, et al (2007). 2-year follow-up of trastuzumab after adjuvant chemotherapy in her2-positive breast cancer: a randomized controlled trial. *Lancet*, **369**:29–36.

24 Viani GA, Afonso SL, Stefano EJ, et al (2007). Adjuvant trastuzumab in the treatment of her-2 positive early breast cancer: a meta-analysis of published randomized trials. *BMC Cancer*, **7**(153):1–11.

25 Piccart-Gebhart MJ, Procter M, Leyland-Jones B, et al (2005). Trastuzumab after adjuvant chemotherapy in her2-positive breast cancer. *N Engl J Med*, **353**:1659–72.

26 Motzer RJ, Hutson TE, Tomczak P, et al (2007). Sunitinib versus interferon alfa in metastatic renal-cell carcinoma. *N Engl J Med*, **356**(2):115–24.

27 Escudier B, Eisen T, Stadler WM, et al (2007). Sorafenib in advanced clear-cell renal-cell carcinoma. *N Engl J Med*, **356**(2):125–34.

28 Bach PB (2009). Limits on Medicare's ability to control rising spending on cancer drugs. *N Engl J Med*, **360**:626–633.

29 Sehn LH, Donaldson J, Chhanabhai M, et al (2005). Introduction of combined CHOP plus rituximab therapy dramatically improved outcome of diffuse large B-cell lymphoma in British Columbia. *JCO*, **23**(22):1–7.

Chapter 11

Community supports for people affected by cancer

Michael Jefford[1]

This chapter considers the supportive care needs of people affected by cancer – not just those who are told that they have a cancer diagnosis, but also their family members and friends, who are also often profoundly affected. The critical role of health care professionals in meeting the needs of all people affected by cancer is underscored. The many and varied sources of additional support provided outside the clinical setting are then described. The review focuses upon the needs of adults with cancer, though many of the issues and examples are also applicable to children, adolescents, and young adults with cancer. A critical issue is how to best integrate clinical programmes with the variety of supports outside the clinical setting.

Unmet needs and psychosocial distress in people affected by cancer

Cancer is a source of much stress; as noted by Mills and Sullivan, 'few words can evoke such an immediate, life threatening reaction as the word cancer' [1]. Patients and their families have to cope not only with the initial diagnosis of cancer and an uncertain outcome, but also with unfamiliar procedures and the presentation of treatment options. Patients may experience a range of physical, emotional, and psychological effects as a result of the disease and its treatment. Life can be changed in many practical ways for patients, their families, and friends. Patients and their carers may be unable to work, may have changed roles, and may experience significant financial impact.

Psychosocial distress, anxiety, and depression are common, not only in cancer patients, but in those close to them, particularly family members. In a large population study of people with various different types of cancer, Zabora reported a prevalence rate of psychological distress of 35 per cent [2]. In a study of 117 newly-referred outpatients, Ford and colleagues estimated that 26 per cent had significant anxiety and 7 per cent likely depression [3]. Several other studies report similar levels of anxiety and depression. Kissane and colleagues found that one third of cancer patients' spouses, and one quarter of their offspring, had clinical depression, compared with a prevalence of depression in the general population of just 6 per cent [4].

Patients report high levels of unmet needs – at diagnosis, through treatment, beyond treatment, when living with advanced disease, and towards the end of life [5,6]. Every person will have a

[1] Michael Jefford, MBBS, MPH, MHLthServMt, PhD, MRACMA, FRACP, Clinical Consultant, Cancer Council Victoria; Associate Professor of Medicine, University of Melbourne; Consultant Medical Oncologist, Division of Haematology and Medical Oncology, Peter MacCallum Cancer Centre, Melbourne, Victoria, Australia.

unique set of needs, which will vary throughout the cancer journey. Patients frequently report the need for additional information and for emotional support. The vast majority of cancer patients in Western countries prefer as much information as possible, regardless of whether it is good or bad. Providing information promotes understanding and increases psychological wellbeing [7]. However patients are often dissatisfied with the amount and quality of information they receive [8]. Patients who feel poorly informed are not only dissatisfied with their care, but also may have reduced wellbeing [9]. Lack of information can cause distress for both patients and their families.

Support provided in the clinical setting

Healthcare professionals are the most frequent, and preferred, source of cancer information [10,11]. Hospital medical specialists, general practitioners, nurses, pharmacists, and radiation therapists are all important sources of information. As well, social workers, pastoral care workers, psychologists, and psychiatrists are important sources of emotional and psychosocial support. The opportunity to discuss feelings with a member of the treatment team or with a counsellor can result in reduced levels of psychosocial distress [7].

Effectiveness of providing psychosocial care

There is good evidence that providing psychosocial support results in broad benefits for patients. A meta-analysis of 116 intervention studies found that educational and psychosocial interventions benefited patients in terms of all outcomes assessed: anxiety, depression, mood, nausea, vomiting, pain, and knowledge [7]. Meyer and Mark reported a meta-analysis of 45 randomized controlled trials showing that patients who received psychosocial interventions experienced significant and likely clinically important improvements in emotional adjustment, social functioning, treatment and disease-related symptoms, and overall quality of life [12].

Sheard and Maguire reported two meta-analyses considering the effect of psychological interventions on anxiety and depression [13]. They report that preventative psychological interventions have a moderate effect on anxiety, though a small to negligible effect upon depression. These interventions may be more successful if targeted to those at risk of, or suffering from, significant psychological distress. Whilst the majority of the above interventions were delivered within the clinical context, benefits may well be seen when non-clinicians, including well-trained peers and volunteers, deliver such interventions.

Clinical practice guidelines emphasize the need to check the amount of support available to the patient, to recommend additional support as required and provide information about where this is available [14]. A critical issue is the identification of people with unmet needs and those with, or at risk of, psychosocial distress. This is of course a major challenge.

Challenges in meeting all supportive care needs in the clinical setting

Supportive care is an umbrella term encompassing all services required to support people with cancer, as well as those close to them, throughout the cancer journey. Supportive care includes provision of information, self-help and support, psychological support, social support, symptom control, rehabilitation, spiritual support, palliative care, and bereavement care. For people affected by cancer, supportive care needs may include physical, psychological, social, information, and spiritual needs.

Different people will have a different set of supportive care needs, which will also likely change over time. Practical needs, such as the need for help with childcare assistance, or travel assistance, will apply only to some, for example. Similarly, the need for advice and self care strategies regarding symptoms will vary. There is considerable evidence to suggest that clinicians do not adequately identify and respond to the breadth of patients' needs.

Clinicians tend to underestimate the amount of information wanted by patients [15,16]. Similarly, much of the probable psychiatric morbidity experienced by patients with cancer appears to go unrecognized and is therefore untreated [17,18]. Numerous studies suggest that clinicians may ignore or fail to appropriately respond to and address emotional or other quality of life concerns [19]. Yet there is good evidence to suggest that providing information, emotional support, and counselling improves the well-being of people with cancer [7,12,13].

Of course, time is a major problem in almost all clinical encounters. Health care professionals, including medical staff, are often perceived to be too busy to provide all the information that patients, families, and friends may desire. Patients may not feel comfortable raising concerns with their doctor, they may not know how to express their concerns, may feel embarrassed, may feel that the doctor will discount their concerns, or believe that their doctor is unable to assist. Doctors and other health professionals may not ask about emotional issues or discuss 'difficult' issues because of concerns that such discussions might be too challenging or that they do not have the skills to assist.

There are major gaps between recommended psychosocial care [14] and current practice. With the growing number of people affected by cancer, the known high level of unmet needs, and the very limited oncology professional workforce, it is essential that all available resources and supports be rallied and coordinated to ensure best outcomes for people affected by cancer.

A process for the identification of supportive care needs is critical, though this must be coupled to a mechanism to respond to these needs. Efforts have begun to routinely screen patients for supportive care needs, recognising the full breadth of what constitutes supportive care [20]. Further work needs to be done to determine the most effective ways to regularly assess unmet needs. Routine collection of quality of life and unmet needs data, with feedback to physicians, may result in improved awareness of quality of life concerns and may impact upon symptom control [21,22]. Such a strategy may not, though, necessarily improve patients' emotional well-being [22]. Placing the sole emphasis upon doctors recognising and responding to all needs is unlikely to be a successful strategy.

Patients cannot gain benefit from the broad range of support services if they are unaware of them. Steginga and colleagues found that many people with cancer are unaware of available services [23], while a large number of people unaware of services believe that they would utilize and value these services if they were made aware of them. These authors note that patients less frequently receive advice about psychosocial support, compared with treatment-related information [23]. Again, we need a means to ensure that patients are aware of all the supports that are available for them.

Fitch points out that a fundamental challenge is to match a range of possible supportive care interventions to a patient's identified supportive care needs. A range of options should be available from which patients can choose [24].

Support in a broader context and the benefits of social support

Some people may feel that their health care team does not have the time or the capacity to deal with all of their needs. They may also prefer support away from the hospital or treatment centre. They may prefer the opportunity to obtain information and support where and when it suits them, rather than under the constraints of the clinical setting. This might include gaining support at home, over the telephone or using the Internet, or through face to face contact at home or in the community. Some patients may find the anonymity of telephone lines an easier way to discuss concerns or they may need support that can only be provided by a peer – someone who truly understands their own situation.

Patients gain significant support and also obtain information from family and friends [10,11]. Family and friends can provide an integral part in a patient's cancer care [25–29]. Patients also gain support from a broader social group, including neighbours, co-workers, clergy, and patient support groups. Raleigh reported that family, friends, and religious beliefs were the most commonly reported sources for supporting hopefulness [25].

Social support is considered to be a multidimensional construct that includes the provision of emotional, informational, appraisal, and practical, tangible support [30]. The adequacy of social support and social connectedness appear to impact upon patient quality of life, coping, and adjustment to illness [28]. This appears to be applicable across a broad range of cancer diagnoses [28]. People who perceive they have poor support are more likely to experience greater psychological distress [25,26,28,31]. Further, patients' adjustment to living with cancer can be shaped by the reactions of their family and intimate others. Descriptive data suggests that patient adjustment is enhanced by family and partner support [27,29].

A broad range of support programmes and services are available outside the clinical setting. Major challenges are ensuring that patients are aware of the services and determining how to integrate support provided in clinical and non-clinical, community settings.

Fitch points out the need to identify individuals' supportive care needs and provide a range of options to meet these [24]. Possible strategies will be determined as much by patient characteristics as by identified needs; a key to successful holistic care is coordination of a range of services, across different settings. While patients may receive diagnostic and treatment care in clinical settings (hospitals, cancer centres, clinics and doctors' rooms), they live in communities away from the clinic. Some may appreciate supportive care services being available in the clinic, but others may prefer to engage with services in their community. Likewise, some may appreciate professional support, whereas others might prefer information and support from friends, volunteers, or peers.

Fig. 11.1 considers three dimensions related to the provision of information and support: firstly, the complexity and specificity of information and support. While all people will appreciate some general information, many need information that is more tailored. A second dimension is the level of expertise of people providing information and support; this is relevant when considering planning and delivery of supportive care services. It does not suggest the value that people might gain from support providers at each level; someone may gain great value from a peer support volunteer, for example, yet in the same circumstance, gain little from a highly trained professional such as a psychiatrist. The third dimension is the setting of care.

Fitch has provided a useful model [24], depicted in Figure 11.2. It considers varying levels of need, relative numbers of patients, and emphasizes the need for a suite of services and resources that can be mobilized to address individual circumstances. Figure 11.2 suggests that supportive care needs may be met through a blend of providers and that many needs can be met through non-professional supports. As Fitch suggests, ideal care should seamlessly span different settings.

Support programmes and services in a community setting

The remainder of this chapter considers the various programmes and services that are commonly available to people affected by cancer, away from the clinical setting.

A   Tailoring of information and support to individual needs and circumstances

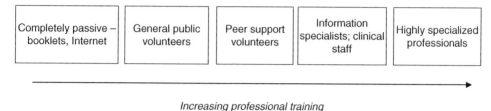

B   Level of expertise of people providing information and support

Fig. 11.1 Three dimensions in the process of providing information and support.

Educational programmes

Many patients report a need for further information to assist them in understanding their cancer experience as well as to adjust to living with the ongoing effects of treatment [5,6,8]. Family members often have similar needs. Structured education programmes play a major role in meeting these needs. Such programmes may be conducted in clinical or in non-clinical, community settings and may be facilitated by healthcare professionals, peers, or volunteers.

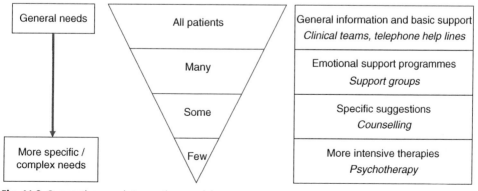

Fig. 11.2 Supportive care intervention model.
Source: From Fitch (2000) [24], with permission.

Educational programmes may be offered face to face, or provided via the Internet. Some patients may feel that an 'educational' programme is more appealing than a 'support' programme. Interestingly though, participants (cancer patients as well as family and friends) generally report improvements in knowledge and understanding, as well as emotional benefits.

As described previously, a meta-analysis of 116 intervention studies found that educational and psychosocial interventions benefit patients across a wide range of outcomes including anxiety, depression, mood, nausea, vomiting, pain control and knowledge [7]. A second meta-analysis reported by Meyer and Mark considered 45 randomized controlled trials and found that patients who received psychosocial interventions experienced a significant, and likely clinically important improvement in emotional adjustment, social functioning, treatment and disease-related symptoms, and overall quality of life [12].

Numerous reports describe results from various educational programmes. One example is the Australian Living with Cancer Education Program, which is described by Todd et al [32]. This programme has six broad aims: (1) to develop knowledge of cancer, (2) to encourage supportive discussions, (3) to meet with and learn from others who have had similar experiences, (4) to build on coping skills, (5) to foster self-acceptance, and (6) to encourage social action [32]. Typically, each programme involves between 10 and 15 participants with a range of cancer diagnoses and at various times since diagnosis, as well as family and friends. Sessions are run by two facilitators, who may have varied backgrounds. Facilitators have significant training and are supported by the resources of the Cancer Council's Cancer Information and Support Service. In general, the programmes consist of two hour sessions, held weekly, generally for four to eight weeks. Information is delivered using a range of media including written materials, video and through discussion. Emphasis is on interaction. The standard programme covers eight broad topics: (1) introduction, (2) what is cancer? (3) cancer treatments, (4) personal reactions, (5) communication, (6) self-esteem and intimacy, (7) self-care, and (8) where to from here? [32] Roberts and colleagues have reported an evaluation of the programme, involving 1460 participants [33]. There was high satisfaction with the programme and both patients and family and friends reported significant improvement in coping abilities, knowledge, and communication and relationships with significant others and with health professionals [33]. Further evaluation has shown positive changes in measures such as illness perceptions and emotional functioning. The programme may be particularly helpful for family and friends [34].

Telephone help lines

Many countries operate telephone information and support services for people affected by cancer. Accessing information and support via the telephone has a number of potential advantages. One is the broad availability of the service – essentially available to anyone with access to a telephone. Thus people living in geographically isolated areas may easily access support. Many services provide a free or toll-free number, removing cost as a barrier to obtaining information and support. Patients, family members, and friends can access the service at a time that suits them, and in their own environment. Time is less likely to be a significant constraint. For many people, the anonymity of a telephone service is a further advantage.

For many cancer control organizations, a telephone information line is a major element of a cancer information service (CIS). Morra and colleagues describe a network of CIS – the International Cancer Information Service Group (ICISG) [35]. The authors describe a CIS, as a programme that 'offers one-on-one personalized information to the public, patients, family members and friends, and health professionals; is staffed by qualified, trained information specialists; provides accurate, up-to-date cancer information; can provide information through multiple access points (mail, telephone, Internet, or face-to-face); and is usually part of an organization that already has some other programmes such as public education, patient information materials, or patient services' [35]. The ICISG has developed a web-based CIS Tool Box, designed to assist cancer organizations to set up or to improve a CIS [35]. The Tool Box can be accessed from the ICISG website – www.icisg.org.

Several reports have described the operation of cancer telephone information services [36–42]. Most services report that patients with a diagnosis of cancer tend to represent the minority of all callers [36,41,42]. Other callers include family and friends, health professionals, and members of the general public. Compared with non-callers, those who access CIS tend to be more seriously ill, are more stressed, and are more likely to be women, younger, and in treatment [36,40–42]. For patients with a cancer diagnosis, there is a relative over-representation of patients with breast cancer, and an under-representation of prevalent cancers such as lung and colorectal cancer. Callers tend to be better educated and reside in areas associated with medium to high socioeconomic status.

Patients with cancer, and family members, tend to call for information about the cancer diagnosis and about treatment options and to obtain emotional support [36,42]. Members of the general public are more likely to call about cancer prevention and early detection or for general information about cancer.

Accessing a cancer help line can help people to understand and feel better about their situation and can improve their confidence and interaction with their treating team. Manfredi et al. found that many callers share information supplied by the CIS with their doctors and consider the information to be helpful in making decisions about treatment [40]. The National Cancer Institute's (United States) CIS found that almost half of callers surveyed had discussed the information that CIS provided with a physician and that the information helped them make a treatment decision [43].

The vast majority of callers appear satisfied with the service, feel that their information needs are met, and feel that they gain emotional and psychological support from the interaction [36,40,41,44]. Interestingly, few callers appear to learn of cancer help lines through their health care team. This is of concern, as many people who might gain benefit from accessing the line cannot do so if they are unaware of the service (see Steginga et al [23]).

Peer support programmes

Peer support programmes are based on the premise that shared experience is a valuable resource that assists individuals to adjust to, and cope effectively with, stressful events [45]. Peer support can be provided in a variety of different formats: face to face (groups or one to one), over the telephone (group or one to one) or via the Internet (generally as a group). These programmes help by providing emotional and informational support from the perspective of shared personal experience. Several reviews suggest that peer support can improve personal relationships and social support, increase a sense of belonging, improve mood, and improve relationships with and satisfaction with health care professionals [46–48].

It has been suggested that peer support can impact positively on psychological adaptation to a cancer diagnosis and treatment, either directly (by decreasing feelings of isolation, encouraging health behaviours, and promoting positive psychological states), or by helping patients to reframe appraisals of their situations and improve coping responses [49].

Hoey and colleagues performed a systematic review to identify models of peer support for cancer patients and assess evidence of their effectiveness in improving psychosocial adjustment [46]. Only eight randomized controlled trials were identified in the review. These generally suggested that peer support programmes can lead to an increase in perceived social support and may reduce psychosocial distress. The authors of this and other recent reviews note significant methodological problems with studies including small sample sizes, lack of long-term follow-up, and limited outcome measures [46–48]. Also, relatively little research has been conducted with people with cancers other than breast cancer, and little work has considered the impact of peer support programmes for the volunteers providing support.

Group support programmes

An initial report by Spiegel suggested that cancer support groups might improve survival for people with advanced breast cancer [50]. This result has not been reproduced in subsequent studies [51,52]. However, there appears good evidence that support groups can improve psychological outcomes [52].

Several studies note that support group participants value being with others like them, sharing experiences, and gaining new knowledge, including information about cancer, treatments, coping, and self-care strategies [51,53–55]. Feeling alone and desiring information are common reasons for joining a cancer support group [54].

Ussher and colleagues have considered the unique features of support groups, compared with other supportive relationships [53]. Ninety three participants (75 women, 18 men) from nine representative Australian cancer support groups took part in participant observation and focus group interviews. Data was analysed using positioning theory. Participants indicated that support groups provide a sense of community, unconditional acceptance, and information about cancer and its treatment, in contrast to the isolation, rejection, and lack of knowledge about cancer experienced outside of the group [53]. As a consequence of group involvement, participants had increased confidence and sense of control in relation to self, living with cancer, and interactions with others, in particular the medical professionals. The support group was also positioned as facilitating positive relationships with family and friends. No difference was found between professionally-led and peer-led support groups.

An interesting observation, reported by Butow and colleagues is that support group participants desire that ideally the group be considered credible by the participant's treatment team [54]. Again, this emphasizes the need for professionals to be aware of, endorse, and refer their patients to support groups.

One to one support

Macvean and colleagues have conducted a systematic review of literature reporting on the use of volunteers in one to one support programmes for people with cancer [56]. Volunteers could be peers or not. Few (28) papers were suitable for review and the methodological quality of the studies was generally poor. However, regardless of whether volunteers were peers or not, one to one volunteer-based support programmes were generally well received and appeared to result in benefits, including improved well-being and/or reduced anxiety [56]. In accordance with other reviews, major benefits from this, and other modes of gaining peer support, were the opportunity to meet with someone who had survived the cancer, the opportunity to speak with someone who has a shared experience, and the sharing of information and coping and self-care strategies [47,48,56].

Many one to one face programmes exist. Reach to Recovery is one example. It is a peer programme in which women who have had treatment for breast cancer are trained as volunteers to provide information and support for women recently diagnosed with breast cancer. The volunteer is able to respond to the individual needs of the woman recently diagnosed.

The programme appears to be well received. Programme participants are generally satisfied and feel that the programme offers support and improves participants' quality of life [57].

Telephone-based peer support

Telephone-based peer support offers a number of advantages over face-to-face support. Firstly, the need for travel is avoided and people from rural or remote areas are able to participate. Secondly, participants can access support from the comfort of their own home and are able to access support even if they are feeling too unwell to leave their home. Some people do not feel comfortable meeting face to face [58]. Telephone-based peer support can be provided in a group or one to one. While a number of studies have described professionally-run telephone support (for examples, see Gotay and Botomley[58]) there is great opportunity for peers to provide telephone support for cancer patients and carers. There have been, to date, very few randomized controlled trials using this strategy [46].

Cancer Connect is an example of a one to one telephone-based peer support programme [45]. The Cancer Council in Australia runs this programme. It connects people who have cancer with volunteers who have had a similar experience and is free and confidential. This support is available at any stage throughout the cancer journey – at diagnosis, during, and after treatment. All volunteers undertake a training programme and are supported by a programme coordinator and the cancer nurses from the Cancer Council Helpline. Cancer Connect matches people according to type of cancer, but also can match according to gender, age, family circumstances, types and side effects of treatment, etc. Cancer Connect is able to match people with a cancer diagnosis, carers of someone with a cancer diagnosis, parents caring for a child with a cancer diagnosis, and people who carry a gene that increases their risk of developing cancer. Cancer Connect appears to be very well received. The majority of people responding to an evaluation of the programme were enthusiastic and felt that their experiences were positive [45].

Internet/online support

People with cancer very commonly access information about cancer and treatments from the Internet. Bass and colleagues considered Internet use in 498 people, newly diagnosed with cancer [59]. Patients were recruited from callers to a NCI CIS. Patients regarded the Internet as an important source of information. Internet use was significantly associated with several self-efficacy variables, including confidence participating in treatment decisions, asking physicians questions, and sharing feelings of concern [59].

Despite the widespread use of the Internet and suggestion that it has important potential benefits for patients, there is some reluctance from cancer clinicians regarding patient's use of the Internet to access information. In a survey of 333 health professionals belonging to the Victorian Cooperative Oncology Group, a group of mostly medical, oncology healthcare professionals, Newnham et al. found that many clinicians (68 per cent response rate) are concerned about the accuracy of information found on the Internet (64 per cent of respondents believed it accurate only sometimes, and 23 per cent rarely), and the vast majority (91 per cent) believed that information from the Internet had the potential to cause harm to patients [60]. Nevertheless, they generally supported patients' information-searching, believing it allowed them to be better informed (58 per cent), and did not affect their ability to cope with their illness (49 per cent), or their trust in, and relationship with, their doctor (69 per cent and 67 per cent, respectively) [60]. Clinicians' concerns about online information and support services may present an obstacle to patients accessing such resources: either because clinicians may not refer their patients to resources or because they may discourage access and participation.

Patients may also use the Internet to obtain support. There is growing use and availability of Internet-based support groups and online discussion boards and Internet mailing lists. While some online support services may be of high quality, limitations to accessing these include availability of Internet, cost, and time considerations.

In their recent systematic review of peer support programmes for people with cancer, Hoey and colleagues [46] identified two randomized controlled trials examining the impact of Internet support groups. In the study reported by Gustafson and colleagues, younger women with breast cancer were randomized to receive a booklet about breast cancer or to receive Comprehensive Health Enhancement Support System (CHESS), a home-based computer system providing information, decision-making, and emotional support [61]. Two hundred and forty six women were randomly allocated to each arm. At two- and five-month follow-up, the CHESS group had better perceived social support and greater confidence in their own involvement in their health care. No significant differences were seen in quality of life. The second study was reported by Winzelberg et al. [62]. In this study 72 women with breast carcinoma were assigned randomly to a 12-week, professionally-facilitated web-based support group (Bosom Buddies). Women could access discussion, post messages, and read answers and stories. The study found that this intervention could reduce depression, cancer-related trauma, and perceived stress. Effect sizes were moderate. This may be an effective strategy to reduce distress and provide support. Notably, this strategy was professionally facilitated. A challenge to the provision of this sort of approach may be the cost and availability of professional facilitators.

Online boards

Patients and caregivers access Internet mailing lists and participate in online discussion primarily to gain information – about types of cancer, treatments, effect of cancer and its treatment on others, and how to communicate with health care providers [63,64]. Participants also appear to gain some emotional support through these mechanisms.

Drop-in centres

Some hospitals and cancer centres operate drop-in centres or 'Cancer Information and Support Centres' (CISC) [65]. Other centres operate away from the treatment environment and may be operated by cancer charities or government agencies. Volunteers, health professionals, cancer survivors, carers, or a combination of these groups may staff a CISC. Such centres represent further opportunities for patients to gain information and support.

In a scoping study conducted prior to the development of a CISC in Belfast, 400 surveys were distributed to patients and carers [65]. A strongly expressed view was that the CISC should be 'a "medical" and "white coat" free zone' underscoring the need for patients to escape the clinical environment and emphasising the need for a broader consideration of needs [65]. Many felt that the CISC should offer counselling and emotional support, offer programmes to facilitate communication within families and with friends, and provide information and support programmes about sexuality and relationships. The majority of respondents wanted the CISC to establish support groups, provide access to spiritual and religious support, information and access to complementary therapies and offer financial advice also. There was a strong emphasis on provision of written and verbal information, presented in a manner that facilitates understanding.

Advantages of the CISC are that people can access information and support, away from the clinical setting, at a time that is convenient to the person. A CISC is available not just to patients, but also to family members, friends and the general public. The availability of counselling and complementary therapies may also be a benefit for many.

Other volunteer services and programmes

Volunteers have very varied backgrounds. In the cancer setting, they might include cancer survivors, past or current carers, current or retired health care professionals, or members of the general public. Volunteers with a personal cancer experience are a core part of peer support programmes and may facilitate educational or support groups or provide one to one support.

Macvean conducted a systematic review of literature reporting on one to one volunteer support programmes for people with cancer [56]. The review included both peer and non-peer support programmes. As described earlier, the review generally suggested that programmes are beneficial, though acknowledged the lack of rigour in both conducting and reporting studies [56].

An Italian report evaluated the activity and impact of volunteers, in the hospital and at home, as judged by patients with cancer, nurses, and the volunteers themselves [66]. Volunteers were particularly useful to improve a patient's mood (80 per cent) and to solve practical problems (47 per cent). The main form of intervention of all volunteers was to give psychosocial support to patients. Other activities of the volunteers were support for the family, assistance in social activities, and to give information [66].

Volunteers may thus represent a further means of providing support for patients, within and apart from the clinical setting. An innovative Australian volunteer-based intervention, the Pathfinder Programme, was designed to address unmet needs and potentially impact on anxiety and depression, in people with recently diagnosed colorectal cancer. Volunteers without a prior history of bowel cancer were trained to provide telephone-based information and support, tailored to the needs of patients, identified through self-report questionnaires [67]. Preliminary evaluation showed that the programme is acceptable to patients. Patients considered that telephone contact with the volunteers was beneficial and found that volunteers could understand their situation and could normalize concerns [67]. In a randomized controlled trial involving 482 patients, 227 patients received support from a Pathfinder volunteer and 255 received usual care alone [68]. Patients who had a Pathfinder volunteer reported fewer unmet needs and lower anxiety at 3 months follow up (though no significant change in depression), compared with patients in the usual care setting. Further follow up will be necessary, though this result suggests that such a volunteer programme may provide valuable support and improve psychosocial outcomes.

Issues beyond the initial cancer diagnosis and treatment

Earlier detection of cancer and improved treatments has resulted in a growing number of people cured of cancer. This, combined with the ageing population, has resulted in a greatly increased number of people living beyond cancer. Estimates suggest that there are more than 12 million cancer survivors in the United States alone. The majority of people who are cured of their cancer experience few major consequences of the disease and its treatments. But for a sizeable minority, the experience of cancer and treatment leaves significant physical, emotional, psychological, and practical impairments and changes [69,70].

Many survivors have ongoing unmet needs toward the end of treatment and during the phase of post-treatment survivorship. Traditionally, the major focus of clinical services, post treatment, has been upon the detection of disease recurrence. Services are not oriented toward the detection and management of late and long-term effects of cancer and treatment or to the identification and amelioration of psychosocial distress and need. Given the breadth of survivors' unmet needs a far broader approach needs to be developed. Provision of information about what survivors might expect following the completion of treatment is an essential minimum requirement [69].

Many survivors have ongoing needs for support and reassurance. Fear of recurrence is extremely common.

Cancer information and support services described in earlier sections need to ensure that they respond to the needs of survivors as much as the needs of people recently diagnosed and during treatment. Support groups are as relevant to survivors as to people newly diagnosed or having treatment. Likewise, cancer telephone help lines have a role in educating and supporting survivors beyond treatment completion. Again, patients will be optimally supported by integrating care in the clinical setting with the services and resources discussed previously.

Support for families, friends, and carers

Cancer affects more than just those who are told that they have a cancer diagnosis. Family and friends can be profoundly affected. Those close by may need to provide significant assistance with practical tasks as well as emotional support. Carers' lives can be changed significantly. Work situation and role functioning may be altered. There can be significant financial repercussions. Whilst providing emotional support, carers have to themselves deal with their own emotional reactions to the cancer diagnosis and threat to life.

In an Australian study, Kissane et al. found that one third of cancer patients' spouses were likely depressed, compared with a prevalence of depression in the general population of only 6 per cent [4]. Levels of stress experienced by partners of patients with cancer has been reported to be similar to, or higher than, that of patients themselves, yet carers receive less support [27,29,71–73]. There is growing recognition that carers' needs must be identified and addressed, ideally through consideration of the patient in a broader context and acknowledgement that the person with cancer is not the sole focus of attention [74,75]. Interventions need to start early in the course of illness and be family-focused. Caregivers need to be provided with appropriate instruction and guidance [75].

Carers are often ill prepared for the task of care giving [74,76]. In a study reported by Soothill and colleagues [76], 43 per cent of carers had significant unmet needs. People with unmet needs were more likely to be caring for someone with advanced disease and more likely to be in poor health themselves. Carers had unmet needs around aspects of managing daily life, emotions, and social identity [76]. Caregivers often require additional information and instruction in technical and care skills.

Issues for children who have a parent with cancer

Several studies with various types of cancers report that children of parents with cancer are susceptible to levels of stress and in need of support [77–79]. As previously described, Kissane and colleagues found that one quarter of cancer patients' children had clinical depression, compared with a prevalence of depression in the general population of just 6 per cent [4]. Several studies have suggested that children can experience problems as a consequence of their parent's cancer and its treatment. Usual school and social routines may be disrupted which can exacerbate children's worries. Difficulties with communication can further increase anxiety in children [79]. Parents may underestimate or may not recognize distress in their children at all [78].

A clinical approach to prevent distress and disruption in children is predicated on inclusion of children in the unit of treatment from the onset. Additional services can support parents and children. Telephone help lines can offer advice and assistance for parents to talk with their children about their cancer. Peer support programmes may also provide valuable advice. Furthermore, CISC may be able to offer parents support and counselling. Support services for young people with cancer are often also able to support young people who have a parent with cancer.

Conclusion

This chapter has focussed particularly on the supportive care needs of adults with cancer. Each person's needs are unique. How people cope with a cancer diagnosis will depend on a range of factors, including previous experiences dealing with illness and major life events, existing coping skills, and the availability of social support. Patients turn to their doctors and other healthcare professionals for information, support, and advice regarding treatments. People may still have a range of unmet needs. Many services exist for people affected by cancer, away from the clinical setting. These services offer the opportunity to help address the needs of patients, their families, and friends. Challenges are, firstly, to ensure that all people who might benefit from these services are aware of them and secondly, to determine how to coordinate supports in the clinical and non-clinical settings to meet the individual needs of all people affected by cancer.

References

1 Mills ME & Sullivan K (1999). The importance of information giving for patients newly diagnosed with cancer: a review of the literature. *J Clin Nurs*, **8**(6):631–42.

2 Zabora J, BrintzenhofeSzoc K, Curbow B, Hooker C, & Piantadosi S (2001). The prevalence of psychological distress by cancer site. *Psychooncology*, **10**(1):19–28.

3 Ford S, Lewis S, & Fallowfield L (1995). Psychological morbidity in newly referred patients with cancer. *J Psychosom Res*, **39**(2):193–202.

4 Kissane D, Bloch S, Burns WI, McKenzie DP, & Posterino M (1994). Psychological morbidity in the families of patients with cancer. *Psychooncology*, **3**:47–56.

5 Sanson-Fisher R, Girgis A, Boyes A, Bonevski B, Burton L, & Cook P (2000). The unmet supportive care needs of patients with cancer. Supportive Care Review Group. *Cancer*, **88**(1):226–37.

6 Whelan TJ, Mohide EA, Willan AR, et al (1997). The supportive care needs of newly diagnosed cancer patients attending a regional cancer center. *Cancer*, **80**(8):1518–24.

7 Devine EC & Westlake SK (1995). The effects of psychoeducational care provided to adults with cancer: meta-analysis of 116 studies. *Oncol Nurs Forum*, **22**(9):1369–81.

8 Jefford M & Tattersall MH (2002). Informing and involving cancer patients in their own care. *Lancet Oncol*, **3**(10):629–37.

9 Fallowfield LJ, Hall A, Maguire GP, & Baum M (1990). Psychological outcomes of different treatment policies in women with early breast cancer outside a clinical trial. *BMJ*, **301**(6752):575–80.

10 Rutten LJ, Arora NK, Bakos AD, Aziz N, & Rowland J (2005). Information needs and sources of information among cancer patients: a systematic review of research (1980–2003). *Patient Educ Couns*, **57**(3):250–61.

11 Mills ME & Davidson R (2002). Cancer patients' sources of information: use and quality issues. *Psychooncology*, **11**(5):371–78.

12 Meyer TJ & Mark MM (1995). Effects of psychosocial interventions with adult cancer patients: a meta-analysis of randomized experiments. *Health Psychol*, **14**(2):101–8.

13 Sheard T & Maguire P (1999). The effect of psychological interventions on anxiety and depression in cancer patients: results of two meta-analyses. *Br J Cancer*, **80**(11):1770–80.

14 National Breast Cancer Centre and National Cancer Control Initiative (2003). *Clinical practice guidelines for the psychosocial care of adults with cancer*. National Breast Cancer Centre, Camperdown, NSW.

15 Fallowfield L, Ford S, & Lewis S (1995). No news is not good news: information preferences of patients with cancer. *Psychooncology*, **4**(3):197–202.

16 Degner LF, Kristjanson LJ, Bowman D, et al (1997). Information needs and decisional preferences in women with breast cancer. *JAMA*, **277**(18):1485–92.

17 Fallowfield L, Ratcliffe D, Jenkins V, & Saul J (2001). Psychiatric morbidity and its recognition by doctors in patients with cancer. *Br J Cancer*, **84**(8):1011–15.

18 Cull A, Stewart M, & Altman DG (1995). Assessment of and intervention for psychosocial problems in routine oncology practice. *Br J Cancer*, **72**(1):229–35.

19 Detmar SB, Muller MJ, Wever LD, Schornagel JH, & Aaronson NK (2001). The patient-physician relationship. Patient-physician communication during outpatient palliative treatment visits: an observational study. *JAMA*, **285**(10):1351–57.

20 Pigott C, Pollard A, Thomson K, & Aranda S (2009). Unmet needs in cancer patients: development of a supportive needs screening tool (SNST). *Support Care Cancer*, **17**(1):33–45. Epub 2008 May 16.

21 Detmar SB, Muller MJ, Schornagel JH, Wever LD, & Aaronson NK. Health-related quality-of-life assessments and patient-physician communication: a randomized controlled trial. *JAMA*, **288**(23):3027–34.

22 Boyes A, Newell S, Girgis A, McElduff P, & Sanson-Fisher R (2006). Does routine assessment and real-time feedback improve cancer patients' psychosocial well-being? *Eur J Cancer Care (Engl)*, **15**(2):163–71.

23 Steginga SK, Campbell A, Ferguson M, et al (2008). Socio-demographic, psychosocial and attitudinal predictors of help seeking after cancer diagnosis. *Psychooncology*, **17**(10):997–1005.

24 Fitch M (2000). Supportive care for cancer patients. *Hosp Q*, **3**(4):39–46.

25 Raleigh ED (1992). Sources of hope in chronic illness. *Oncol Nurs Forum*, **19**(3):443–48.

26 Sollner W, Zschocke I, Zingg-Schir M, et al (1999). Interactive patterns of social support and individual coping strategies in melanoma patients and their correlations with adjustment to illness. *Psychosomatics*, **40**(3):239–50.

27 Morse SR & Fife B (1998). Coping with a partner's cancer: adjustment at four stages of the illness trajectory. *Oncol Nurs Forum*, **25**(4):751–60.

28 Ell KO, Mantell JE, Hamovitch MB, & Nishimoto RH (1989). Social support, sense of control, and coping among patients with breast, lung, or colorectal cancer. *J Psychosoc Oncol*, **7**(3):63–89.

29 Manne SL, Pape SJ, Taylor KL, & Dougherty J (1999). Spouse support, coping, and mood among individuals with cancer. *Ann Behav Med*, **21**(2):111–21.

30 Schaefer C, Coyne JC, & Lazarus RS (1981). The health-related functions of social support. *J Behav Med*, **4**(4):381–406.

31 Roberts CS, Cox CE, Shannon VJ, & Wells NL (1994). A closer look at social support as a moderator of stress in breast cancer. *Health Soc Work*, **19**(3):157–64.

32 Todd K, Roberts S, & Black C (2002). The Living with Cancer Education Programme. I. Development of an Australian education and support programme for cancer patients and their family and friends. *Eur J Cancer Care (Engl)*, **11**(4):271–79.

33 Roberts S, Black C, & Todd K (2002). The Living with Cancer Education Programme. II. Evaluation of an Australian education and support programme for cancer patients and their family and friends. *Eur J Cancer Care (Engl)*, **11**(4):280–89.

34 Sutherland G, Dpsych LH, White V, Jefford M, & Hegarty S (2008). How does a cancer education program impact on people with cancer and their family and friends? *J Cancer Educ*, **23**(2):126–32.

35 Morra ME, Thomsen C, Vezina A, et al (2007). The International Cancer Information Service: a worldwide resource. *J Cancer Educ*, **22**(1 Suppl):S61–69.

36 Jefford M, Black C, Grogan S, Yeoman G, White V, & Akkerman D (2005). Information and support needs of callers to the Cancer Helpline, the Cancer Council Victoria. *Eur J Cancer Care (Engl)*, **14**(2):113–23.

37 Meissner HI, Anderson DM, & Odenkirchen JC (1990). Meeting information needs of significant others: use of the Cancer Information Service. *Patient Educ Couns*, **15**(2):171–79.

38 Slevin ML, Terry Y, Hallett N, et al (1988). BACUP–the first two years: evaluation of a national cancer information service. *BMJ*, **297**(6649):669–72.

39 Ward JA, Baum S, Ter Maat J, Thomsen CA, & Maibach EW (1998). The value and impact of the Cancer Information Service telephone service. Part 4. *J Health Commun*, **3**(Suppl):50–70.

40 Manfredi C, Czaja R, Price J, Buis M, & Janiszewski R (1993). Cancer patients' search for information. *J Natl Cancer Inst Monogr*, (14):93–104.

41 Marcus AC, Woodworth MA, & Strickland CJ (1993). The Cancer Information Service as a laboratory for research: the first 15 years. *J Natl Cancer Inst Monogr*, (14):67–79.

42 Jefford M, Kirke B, Grogan S, Yeoman G, & Boyes A (2005). Australia's Cancer Helpline–an audit of utility and caller profile. *Aust Fam Physician*, **34**(5):393–94.

43 Davis SW, Fleisher L, Ter Maat J, Muha C, & Laepke K (1998). Treatment and clinical trials decision making: the impact of the Cancer Information Service. Part 5. *J Health Commun*, **3**(Suppl):71–85.

44 La Porta M, Hagood H, Kornfeld J, & Treiman K (2007). Evaluating the NCI's Cancer Information Service Contact Centers: meeting and exceeding the expectations of the public. *J Cancer Educ*, **22**(1 Suppl):S18–25.

45 Tilkeridis J, O'Connor L, Pignalosa G, Bramwell M, & Jefford M (2005). Peer support for cancer patients. *Aust Fam Physician*, **34**(4):288–89.

46 Hoey LM, Ieropoli SC, White VM, & Jefford M (2008). Systematic review of peer-support programs for people with cancer. *Patient Educ Couns*, **70**(3):315–37.

47 Campbell HS, Phaneuf MR, & Deane K (2004). Cancer peer support programs-do they work? *Patient Educ Couns*, **55**(1):3–15.

48 Dunn J, Steginga SK, Rosoman N, & Millichap D (2003). A review of peer support in the context of cancer. *J Psychosoc Oncol*, **21**:55–67.

49 Newell SA, Sanson-Fisher RW, & Savolainen NJ (2002). Systematic review of psychological therapies for cancer patients: overview and recommendations for future research. *J Natl Cancer Inst*, **94**(8):558–84.

50 Spiegel D, Bloom JR, Kraemer HC, & Gottheil E (1989). Effect of psychosocial treatment on survival of patients with metastatic breast cancer. *Lancet*, **2**(8668):888–91.

51 Gottlieb BH & Wachala ED (2007). Cancer support groups: a critical review of empirical studies. *Psychooncology*, **16**(5):379–400.

52 Goodwin PJ (2005). Support groups in advanced breast cancer. *Cancer*, **104**(11 Suppl):2596–601.

53 Ussher J, Kirsten L, Butow P, & Sandoval M (2006). What do cancer support groups provide which other supportive relationships do not? The experience of peer support groups for people with cancer. *Soc Sci Med*, **62**(10):2565–76.

54 Butow PN, Kirsten LT, Ussher JM, et al (2007). What is the ideal support group? Views of Australian people with cancer and their carers. *Psychooncology*, **16**(11):1039–45.

55 Docherty A (2004). Experience, functions and benefits of a cancer support group. *Patient Educ Couns*, **55**(1):87–93.

56 Macvean ML, White VM, & Sanson-Fisher R (2008). One-to-one volunteer support programs for people with cancer: a review of the literature. *Patient Educ Couns*, **70**(1):10–24.

57 Ashbury FD, Cameron C, Mercer SL, Fitch M, & Nielsen E (1998). One-on-one peer support and quality of life for breast cancer patients. *Patient Educ Couns*, **35**(2):89–100.

58 Gotay CC & Bottomley A (1998). Providing psycho-social support by telephone: what is its potential in cancer patients? *Eur J Cancer Care (Engl)*, **7**(4):225–31.

59 Bass SB, Ruzek SB, Gordon TF, Fleisher L, McKeown-Conn N, & Moore D (2006). Relationship of Internet health information use with patient behavior and self-efficacy: experiences of newly diagnosed cancer patients who contact the National Cancer Institute's Cancer Information Service. *J Health Commun*, **11**(2):219–36.

60 Newnham GM, Burns WI, Snyder RD, et al (2005). Attitudes of oncology health professionals to information from the Internet and other media. *Med J Aust*, **183**(4):197–200.

61 Gustafson DH, Hawkins R, Pingree S, et al (2001). Effect of computer support on younger women with breast cancer. *J Gen Intern Med*, **16**(7):435–45.

62 Winzelberg AJ, Classen C, Alpers GW, et al (2003). Evaluation of an internet support group for women with primary breast cancer. *Cancer*, **97**(5):1164–73.

63 Meier A, Lyons EJ, Frydman G, Forlenza M, & Rimer BK (2007). How cancer survivors provide support on cancer-related Internet mailing lists. *J Med Internet Res*, **9**(2):e12.

64 Fernsler JI &, Manchester LJ (1997). Evaluation of a computer-based cancer support network. *Cancer Pract*, **5**(1):46–51.

65 Manning DL & Dickens C (2007). Cancer Information and Support Centres: fixing parts cancer drugs cannot reach. *Eur J Cancer Care (Engl)*, **16**(1):33–8.

66 Fusco-Karmann C & Tamburini M (1994). Volunteers in hospital and home care: a precious resource. *Tumori*, **80**(4):269–72.

67 Macvean ML, White VM, Pratt S, Grogan S, & Sanson-Fisher R (2007). Reducing the unmet needs of patients with colorectal cancer: a feasibility study of The Pathfinder Volunteer Program. *Support Care Cancer*, **15**(3):293–99.

68 Sanson-Fisher R, White V, Grogan S, & Macvean M (2008). Reducing the needs, anxiety and depression of people with colorectal cancer in the Pathfinder Volunteer Program. In: Behavioural Research in Cancer Control Conference, Melbourne.

69 Institute of Medicine and National Research Council (2006). From cancer patient to cancer survivor: lost in transition. Committee on Cancer Survivorship: Improving Care and Quality of Life. National Academies Press; Washington, D.C.

70 Gotay CC & Muraoka MY (1998). Quality of life in long-term survivors of adult-onset cancers. *J Natl Cancer Inst*, **90**(9):656–67.

71 Northouse LL, Mood D, Templin T, Mellon S, & George T (2000). Couples' patterns of adjustment to colon cancer. *Soc Sci Med*, **50**(2):271–84.

72 Cliff AM & MacDonagh RP (2000). Psychosocial morbidity in prostate cancer: II. A comparison of patients and partners. *BJU Int*, **86**(7):834–39.

73 Couper J, Bloch S, Love A, Macvean M, Duchesne GM, & Kissane D (2006). Psychosocial adjustment of female partners of men with prostate cancer: a review of the literature. *Psychooncology*, **15**(11):937–53.

74 Thomas C, Morris SM, & Harman JC (2002). Companions through cancer: the care given by informal carers in cancer contexts. *Soc Sci Med*, **54**(4):529–44.

75 Given BA, Given CW, & Kozachik S (2001). Family support in advanced cancer. *CA Cancer J Clin*, **51**(4):213–31.

76 Soothill K, Morris SM, Harman JC, Francis B, Thomas C, & McIllmurray MB (2001). Informal carers of cancer patients: what are their unmet psychosocial needs? *Health Soc Care Community*, **9**(6):464–75.

77 Compas BE, Worsham NL, Epping-Jordan JE, et al (1994). When mom or dad has cancer: markers of psychological distress in cancer patients, spouses, and children. *Health Psychol*, **13**(6):507–15.

78 Welch AS, Wadsworth ME, & Compas BE (1996). Adjustment of children and adolescents to parental cancer. Parents' and children's perspectives. *Cancer*, **77**(7):1409–18.

79 Nelson E, Sloper P, Charlton A, & While D (1994). Children who have a parent with cancer: a pilot study. *J Cancer Educ*, **9**(1):30–36.

Chapter 12

Improving quality of life

Shirley Bush, Eduardo Bruera[1]

Oncological treatments aim for local and/or systemic control. They may be administered with a curative or palliative intent. If cancer in a patient cannot be cured, then the focus of treatment changes to achieving an improvement in survival time, reducing symptom burden, optimizing performance, and hence improving quality of life (QOL). Palliative care is the last of the four components of a cancer control programme, after prevention, early detection, and diagnosis and treatment [1].

Patients with advanced cancer may experience physical, psychosocial, and spiritual difficulties throughout their illness which impact on their overall QOL. The main objective of palliative care is to improve the QOL for both patients with life-threatening illness and their families [2]. Therefore, it is necessary to assess QOL to ascertain if this goal is being met.

Defining quality of life

> Therefore, one must practice the things which produce happiness, since if that is present we have everything and if it is absent we do everything in order to have it.

> Epicurus (341–271 B.C.) [3]

An initial challenge is how to define QOL. Depending on interpretation, it may be similar to the concepts of life satisfaction and happiness [4]. QOL is multi-dimensional and has been described in various ways in the literature [4, 5], although many authors do not give an explicit definition of QOL [6]. Ferrans used a definition of 'a person's sense of well-being that stems from satisfaction or dissatisfaction with the areas of life that are more important to him/her[7]. A consensus group used a definition based on the World Health Organization definition of health: 'QOL includes psychological and social functioning as well as physical functioning and incorporates positive aspects of well-being as well as negative aspects of disease and infirmity'[8]. In considering QOL as a broad concept, Kassa and Loge described it as 'how is your life, everything taken into consideration' [9].

The concept of QOL means different things to different people, and there may be cultural and geographical variations in its interpretation and expectation [10]. An online medical dictionary has defined QOL as: 'a patient's general well-being, including mental status, stress level, sexual function, and self-perceived health status'[11]. Well-being of the whole person encompasses not only health, but also the non-medical aspects of a patient's life. Many authors use the term of

[1] Shirley H Bush, MBBS, MRCGP, FAChPM, Assistant Professor, Division of Palliative Care, University of Ottawa and Palliative Care Physician, The Ottawa Hospital/Bruyère Continuing Care, Ottawa, Ontario, Canada; and Eduardo L. Franco, MD, DrPH, Professor of Epidemiology and Oncology, Director, Division of Cancer Epidemiology, McGill University, Montreal, Quebec, Canada.

'health-related QOL', but some have cautioned against the limitations in using this restrictive term as health concerns cannot be isolated from other contributors to QOL [12]. Patients with advanced cancer also consider more domains contributing to their life satisfaction compared with other patient populations and physically healthy people [13]. For the purpose of this chapter, the focus will be QOL in the global sense.

It is important to stress that an individual's perception of their own QOL is subjective in nature and changes with time. For this reason, the patient should be the primary source of information in its determination. If this is not possible, then it should be measured from the patient's perspective, without pre-conceived judgement (see later chapter section on measurement by proxy).

QOL is a complex multi-dimensional concept, which includes many domains or dimensions such as physical well-being, functional ability, emotional, and social well-being [5]. Sexuality is expressed in all these four domains. The importance of the existential domain and spiritual well-being has also been highlighted [14]. Other domains that have been proposed include cognitive function, control, financial, physical environment, and areas related to communication (provision and sharing of information, and decision-making) [4, 15]. Control refers to the ability of an individual to maintain command over the areas of their life that they can still influence. Effective communication impacts on emotional and physical well-being and enhances patient and healthcare professional satisfaction during a consultation [16]. Speech difficulties are common for patients who have been treated for head and neck cancer, especially after treatment with laryngectomy [17]. Patients with brain cancers or neuropsychiatric syndromes also commonly experience communication difficulties.

The term 'self-advocacy' encompasses some of the proposed domains. 'Self-advocacy' refers to an individual's ability to effectively communicate, convey, negotiate or assert his or her own interests, desires, needs, and rights. It involves making informed decisions and taking responsibility for those decisions (see Figure 12.1) [18].

The Gap theory of Calman described the concept of QOL as being the difference between present experiences and the hopes and expectations of how a person wants to be[19]. In order to estimate the 'gap', an assessment of the patient's concerns and priorities should be made. Realistic goals to improve QOL should be set with the involvement of both patient and family. The outcomes should be evaluated and the goals should be reviewed periodically and revised as needed, especially as disease progresses. Positive contributors to QOL may counteract, at least in part, the negative contributors. Narrowing the discrepancy between the patient's and family's expectations and the patient's current status or likely future reality may enhance QOL [19, 20]. (see Figure 12.2).

QOL is dynamic in its nature and will change with the impact of illness, treatment, support systems, and variations in other positive and negative contributors. Patients frequently have to adapt to their disease and the effects of treatments. A change in behaviour, such as dietary modification, may be needed or they may acquire new skills through adaptation to disability, such as using walking aids, and caring for a stoma or catheter. Both the mind and human spirit also have a fortunate ability to adapt in the presence of major life-threatening illness. This may be influenced by resilience, previous coping style, and also outlook on life. Patients may need to re-conceive their perception of self as in the role of a person with cancer. This leads an individual to review and change their expectations as they re-evaluate priorities for their remaining life.

In 1999, Sprangers and Schwartz proposed a theoretical model of 'response-shift' which may affect health-related QOL [21]. This model is not a rigid framework and not all QOL changes are affected by a 'response-shift'. It has five major components incorporating a change in health status of the individual (the catalyst), personal characteristics such as personality and background, mechanisms (behavioural, cognitive, and affective) to enable adjustment to the catalyst,

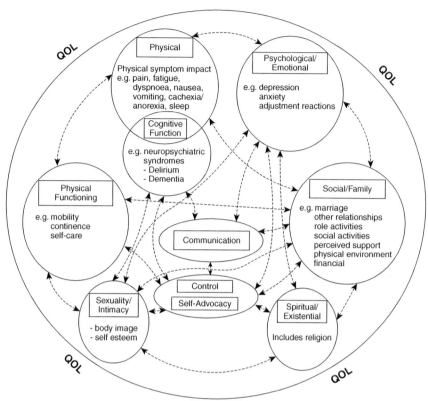

Fig. 12.1 A theoretical model for domains and factors that influence quality of life (QOL) – considering patients with advanced cancer.

the 'response-shift', and perceived QOL. The working definition for 'response-shift' was 'a change in the meaning of one's self-evaluation of QOL as a result of changes in internal standards, values, and the conceptualization of QOL'. There may also be a feedback loop if the perceived outcome QOL is felt to be suboptimal. This enables the mechanisms for adjustment to be reviewed in order to improve perceived QOL or for modification of the perception of QOL.

Challenges and advantages of measuring QOL

In clinical practice, health care professionals should routinely inquire about patients' QOL. As QOL is a dynamic process, it should be assessed on a regular basis to enable earlier detection of changes [12]. This systematic administration of a QOL instrument has been shown to open up communication between physician and patient, enabling discussion about personal and potentially difficult areas that are often neglected and avoided [22].

QOL measurement enables patients to make informed treatment choices to optimize their QOL. Assessments of QOL may aid prognostication for survival, with decreased survival predicted by higher burden of certain physical symptoms and lower performance status [23]. In addition to acting as a quality assurance measure to help improve an individual patient's care, QOL measured in more general terms can be used as an outcome measure, e.g. to demonstrate the impact of a particular intervention or treatment, or the effect of a palliative care service [24].

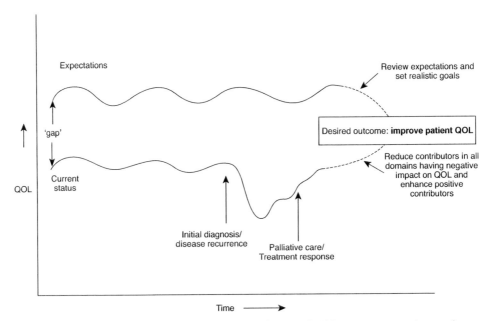

Fig. 12.2 Enhancing quality of life (QOL) by reducing the 'gap' [19] between expectations and current status.

Barriers have reduced the frequency of use of QOL instruments in the clinical setting, including the time needed for administration [25]. In addition, most QOL instruments have been developed for use in research and therefore may not be suitable for use in daily clinical practice. Computers with touch screens have been used with effect [26]. Clinical issues may also affect completion including the presence of pre-existing cognitive deficits, development of cognitive changes, and patients at the end of life who are too unwell. Instruments should not take too long to administer to avoid being burdensome, especially in frailer patients, for whom it is an advantage if the instrument can be administered by being read aloud (see later chapter section on measurement by proxy).

Global QOL instruments assess overall subjective QOL experience, e.g. with a single item question, 'How has your quality of life been'? QOL instruments may have subscales that inquire about specific domains or dimensions [9]. This is especially relevant when the disease is more advanced. Common specific dimensions that are assessed include fatigue, pain, anxiety, and depression. It is important to consider cultural variations. For example, patients may report depression in more semantic terms than emotional terms in some countries. Variations in population may be targeted depending on the instrument used. For example, a generic QOL instrument may be applicable to the whole population and other multi-dimensional instruments may be suitable for specific disease or diagnostic groups, such as cancer-specific or palliative care-specific instruments [9].

Traditionally it has been stated that since multiple dimensions impact on the construct of QOL, there is a need to use multi-dimensional assessments [5]. More recent authors have suggested that single-item global assessments can provide a reliable measure of QOL [27]. In practice, patient QOL assessments often include combinations of global and more detailed disease-specific and domain-specific instruments depending on the information required.

In addition to assessing QOL in patients, QOL of the family caregiver or family member should also be assessed by considering what is important for their own QOL as individuals. Acting on the information provided may help reduce burnout in the family caregiver. Family caregiver QOL is lower in most domains, as compared to the general population, especially in the psychological domain [28, 29]. The QOL for the family unit is also important but much more difficult to measure.

Overview of QOL assessment tools used in patients with advanced cancer

Multiple assessment tools are available, but currently there is no 'gold standard'. This section will briefly outline some of the available instruments that have been developed for patients with advanced cancer and their family caregivers.

Spitzer quality of life uniscale and Spitzer quality of life index (QL-Index)

These tools were designed for use by physicians to rate their patient's QOL but they can be self-administered and answered by patients [30]. The uniscale consists of a horizontal bar (with no gradations) that is marked with an X between anchors of lowest quality and highest quality to indicate rating of overall QOL during the previous week. (Further descriptors to these anchors are given in the tool).

The validated QL-Index has five categories: activities, daily living, health, support, and outlook. Each category has three items which score 0 (poor) to 2 (good QOL), providing a total QL-Index with a maximum score of 10. The QL-Index refers to a time frame of the previous week; the median completion time is one minute.

Edmonton symptom assessment system (ESAS)

In addition to the feeling of well-being, the multi-dimensional ESAS routinely records the patient's current subjective perception of multiple symptoms (pain, fatigue, nausea, depression, anxiety, drowsiness, appetite, and shortness of breath) [31]. The patient rates each of these symptoms on a scale of 0 to 10, where 0 indicates that the symptom is absent and 10 rates it at the worst possible severity. It should be noted, however, that a score of 0 out of 10 is the converse for appetite and feeling of well-being, as 0 out of 10 represents the best appetite or best feeling of well-being and 10 out of 10 represents the worst possible appetite or worst possible feeling of well-being. The ESAS was designed to be self-administered but, if needed, it can be completed with the assistance of the patient's caregiver (family or health care professional). The ESAS has been validated for internal consistency, criterion validity, and concurrent validity [32]. This is a practical tool to use in a busy clinical setting.

Rotterdam symptom checklist (RSCL)

This self-administered validated tool was developed to measure physical and psychological symptoms reported by cancer patients participating in clinical research [33]. The initial checklist consisted of 34 items with the addition of 8 items for activities of daily living. Completion time was 8 minutes. Subsequently, a revised version of the RSCL was produced with 31 items and a timeframe of 1 week compared with 3 days in the initial version. It consists of a four point, Likert-type rating scale (from not at all to very much) and there are no specific items for the social dimension. The 1996 RSCL manual [34] has a total of 30 items with 23 items covering physical symptom distress and 7 items covering psychological distress. The next section has 8 items on activity level (on a four point scale between unable and without help). The final item is an overall evaluation of life: 'All things considered how would you describe your quality of life during the past week'? This is a seven level Likert item (between excellent and extremely poor).

Functional assessment of cancer therapy - General (FACT-G)

This validated QOL measure was developed to evaluate patients receiving cancer treatment [35]. It is now a generic core questionnaire for the Functional Assessment of Chronic Illness Therapy (FACIT) measurement system [36]. These are copyrighted tools. The FACT-G (version 4) contains 27 items covering 4 primary QOL domains: physical well-being, social/family well-being, emotional well-being, and functional well-being. The measure has a 5-point scale from 0 to 4 for responses ranging from not at all to very much, and is to be answered in reference to the previous 7 days. The last statement on the FACT-G is 'I am content with the quality of my life right now'. The average time to complete the questionnaire is 5 to 10 minutes. It was originally developed for patient self-administration, but may be administered by an interviewer. The FACT-G needs an overall item response rate of over 80 per cent to be an acceptable indicator of a patient's QOL. There are now many FACIT subscales (cancer-specific and treatment-specific subscales, in addition to symptom-specific and non-cancer-specific subscales) to complement the FACT-G. As many of the questionnaires are now available in more than 45 different languages, cross-cultural comparisons can be made.

Two non-cancer-specific subscales for palliative care and spiritual wellbeing have recently been developed as part of the FACIT system. The FACIT-Pal (version 4) consists of the FACT-G as the core questionnaire followed by an additional nineteen items.

European Organization for Research and Treatment of Cancer – EORTC QLQ-C30 and EORTC QLQ-C15-PAL

The European Organization for Research and Treatment of Cancer (EORTC) developed the tool, EORTC QLQ-C30, to produce an integrated modular approach to evaluate the QOL of patients participating in international clinical trials [37]. The most recent version is QLQ-C30 Version 3.0 [38]. It is a copyrighted instrument that has been translated and validated into 81 languages. The current version contains 30 items and asks questions in reference to the past week, with a 4-point scale from 1 to 4 for responses ranging from not at all to very much. The last two items inquire about global health and global QOL (on a 1 to 7 scale ranging from very poor to excellent). As it is a modular tool, the QLQ-C30 core questionnaire can be supplemented with disease-specific modules and other specific questionnaire modules. The tool has been validated in patients with metastatic disease [39].

The EORTC QLQ-C15-PAL is a 15-item 'core questionnaire' for palliative care that was derived from the EORTC QLQ-C30 [40]. This questionnaire was developed to assess the QOL of palliative care cancer patients and is a copyrighted instrument [41]. Questions have been raised as to this questionnaire's sensitivity and lack of key questions covering existential and spiritual issues, and social support [42].

The McGill quality of life questionnaire (MQOL)

This differs from many other instruments in that it measures the existential domain and positive contributions to QOL [43]. This 17-item questionnaire measures overall QOL, and 5 distinct sub measures of physical well-being, physical symptoms, psychological symptoms, existential well-being and support [14]. The questions from the MQOL are in reference to the previous two days. It can be administered during disease progression as frequently as every two days. It takes 15 to 20 minutes for patients to complete (up to 35 minutes with verbal supervision). It has been validated [14], including in different languages [44]. The MQOL has been revised to Quality of Life in Life-Threatening Illness – Patient Version (QOLLTI-P) [15].

The schedule for the evaluation of individual quality of life (SEIQoL) and SEIQoL-direct weighting (SEIQoL-DW)

These two validated measures are interesting because they highlight the individual nature of QOL [45]. Both the SEIQoL and the shorter SEIQoL-DW consist of a three-stage semi-structured interview [46]. First, the patient identifies five areas that they consider to be important to their QOL. A shortlist of examples may be read to the patient if they have difficulty nominating the areas. In the next stage, the patient rates their current status or level of function for each nominated area. Finally, they give a weighting of importance to each area. The median time to complete the SEIQoL is 40 minutes so completion may not be possible in very fatigued patients. The full measure may be useful for in-depth exploration of individual QOL. The SEIQoL-DW takes approximately 15 minutes to complete.

Instruments to measure QOL in cancer survivors

The Quality of Life – Cancer Survivors (QOL-CS) instrument contains 41 items to be rated on a scale from 0 to 10. Four domains of QOL are covered: psychological, physical, social, and spiritual well-being [47]. The Quality of Life in Adult Cancer Survivors (QLACS) scale contains 47 items covering 12 domains with 7 generic and 5 cancer-specific domains [48]. A recent review concluded that there was a need for a psychometrically credible QOL instrument to evaluate cancer survivors one to five years post diagnosis [48].

Instruments to measure QOL in family caregiver

The Caregiver Quality of Life Index – Cancer (CQOLC) scale is a self-report consisting of 35 items using a 5-point Likert scale to assess QOL in the family caregiver of cancer patients [49]. It takes 10 minutes to complete. The Quality of Life in Life Threatening Illness – Family Carer Version (QOLLTI-F) was developed from family caregivers in a qualitative study. The final version contains 16 items and 7 different domains: state of caregiver, patient well-being, quality of care, outlook, environment, finances, and relationships. It also includes the caregiver's perception of the patient's condition [50].

Domain-specific instruments

These may be useful to focus on specific areas to provide a more detailed assessment. Examples include the Brief Pain Inventory (BPI) [51] and FACIT-Fatigue (FACIT-F) 13-item subscale from the FACIT measurement system [36].

Measurement by proxy

When patients are too unwell or fatigued, QOL assessments may be made using a proxy rater, such as family caregiver or healthcare professional. Many studies have compared the patient QOL assessment (which may not be reliable itself) directly with that of the proxy [52]. However, if proxy ratings are assessed independently, their reliability is similar or slightly better than patient ratings. Patient-proxy agreement tends to be moderate to high. It is positively influenced by the closeness of the relationship and with prospective assessments but may be less congruent with greater family caregiver burden [53]. There tends to be more agreement with physical function and symptoms that can be assessed objectively but less agreement in the psychological domain and with subjective symptoms, such as pain. There tend to be fewer discrepancies in patient-proxy agreement if the patient has extreme (very good or very poor) health status. Patient-healthcare professional proxy agreement may be less congruent. Cohen et al. in 1997 found that, more than 50 per cent of the time, palliative care staff did not identify those patients scoring severe distress on the MQOL [14].

Quality of life according to cancer trajectory

Diagnosis

When the initial diagnosis of cancer comes as a complete shock, the patient may experience acute psychological distress. Some patients may have already suspected the diagnosis from their presenting symptoms. Partners of patients with cancer also experience significant stress. The effect of a cancer diagnosis on QOL may be influenced by life circumstances at the time for the patient and their family.

After a cancer diagnosis, patients may experience depression, anxiety, and psychological distress, although a meta-analysis concluded that cancer patients as a group did not experience more psychological distress than the normal population, with the exception of an increased rate of depression [54]. Newly diagnosed breast cancer patients have been found to have the lowest QOL in both psychological and sexual domains [55]. Patients living alone had a significantly lower QOL than those cohabiting, especially in the younger age group 19 to 39 years.

Primary treatment

Treatment-related side effects negatively impact on both physical and psychosocial domains [56]. Post-surgical disfigurement may have enduring effects on body image and sexuality. QOL may initially decrease due to local and systemic side effects of therapies, such as chemotherapy induced nausea and vomiting. Fatigue is very common depending on the treatment regimen. However, overall QOL then often improves despite ongoing treatment. This may be related to the optimism and support provided by regular visits to health care professionals [57]. Education regarding the treatment regimen, anticipated side effects and psychosocial support are often provided.

Women with breast cancer aged 65 years and older have been shown to experience a decline in physical and mental health 15 months following breast cancer surgery [58].

Advanced cancer recurrence

Recurrence will often mar emotional, physical, and functional well-being of patients, as well as significantly affecting the emotional well-being of their family caregiver [59]. Social support and family hardiness have a positive effect on QOL. At this time, patients will often experience an increase in many physical symptoms, such as fatigue and pain, and a reduction in physical and social role functions, leading to a reduction in overall QOL [39].

Many patients will elect to undergo treatments with toxic side effects for the chance of increased survival at any cost over likely negative impact on QOL [60]. Their decision may be related to their own better expectations of prognosis or a need to be doing something rather than nothing and a sense of retaining control and hope. A mother with young children may continue treatment with adverse effects in the hope that this will buy more time with them for their well-being. QOL issues may not always be considered by physicians as a reason to modify or discontinue treatment in patients receiving palliative chemotherapy if there is no tumour progression or treatment toxicity [61].

Palliative care and end of life care

Towards the end of life, QOL for patients and their families is affected by poorly controlled symptoms, a further decline in physical function and social activity, and anticipatory grief. Patients may express concerns regarding the future for themselves and their family, increasing dependency, and 'being a burden' to others. At this stage, patients identify different diverse values as being important to them in the prelude to death. These include maintaining dignity, pain and symptom management, preparation for death, achieving a sense of completion (resolving conflicts, spending time with family and friends, saying goodbye to important people, as well as spiritual issues and meaningfulness at the end of life), participation in treatment decisions, open communication, being treated as a 'whole person', and avoiding inappropriate prolongation of dying [62, 63].

As a patient's condition deteriorates, overall QOL may remain the same, with those domains contributing most to QOL changing in both positive and negative directions. Some domains, such as social and family well-being, may not decline, but scores in the spirituality domain may improve [64] with existential issues becoming more important to patients towards the end of life. Hwang et al. in 2003 described a 'longitudinal terminal decline QOL model' with different QOL domains changing at different rates [65]. Their study in predominantly male Veteran Affairs patients showed three time points. Six months prior to death, slow declines in symptom distress, performance status, and QOL well-being (functional, emotional, and physical domains of FACT-G) started. Psychological symptom distress worsened three months prior to death. By two months prior to death, an accelerated decline in symptom distress, performance status, and most QOL parameters occurred.

Survivorship

With earlier diagnosis and improved treatment regimens, the population of cancer survivors is growing. Three stages have been described. Acute survival (from diagnosis to end of first year), extended survival (from end of first year to three years later) and permanent survival [66]. The majority of survivors fear recurrence with the probability of recurrence for most cancers being greatest during the extended survival phase.

Patients often describe positive benefits in surviving a life-threatening illness, including a re-prioritization of values and a determination to make the most of life. Living with a spouse or partner predicts a positive response to QOL [47]. However, there are also many negative after effects of the cancer diagnosis and treatment to be negotiated. These include: physical barriers to optimal function such as fatigue and cognitive changes; changes in body image and infertility and impact on sexuality; psychological sequelae including ongoing psychological distress, anxiety, and depression; socio-economic stresses and family distress [67]. Identifying and addressing these issues early with psychosocial interventions may help improve QOL.

Impact of supportive and palliative care

Supportive and palliative care strive to improve the QOL of patients and families facing life-threatening cancer, and other life-limiting illnesses, with holistic interdisciplinary care in a variety of settings (e.g. hospital, inpatient acute palliative care unit, inpatient hospice, and home) providing effective pain and symptom relief, spiritual and psychosocial support from diagnosis to the end of life. In addition, palliative care offers bereavement support to families.

The traditional model of supportive and palliative care involved late referral to the interdisciplinary team. Involvement of these teams usually occurred late in the illness trajectory after the failure of curative and palliative cancer treatments. The emerging model of supportive and palliative care programmes involves the integration of care from the moment of diagnosis to the moment of death/bereavement or survivorship. This emerging model allows for a contribution of supportive and palliative care to improve the QOL of cancer patients and their families throughout the whole trajectory of illness (see Figure 12.3).

By providing intensive symptom control, specialist palliative care has been shown to improve the QOL of patients, including existential well-being [68–70]. Although the majority of cases can be managed by the primary physician, patients and families with complex needs or refractory symptoms should be referred to the local specialist palliative care team for assistance. QOL of the family caregiver may be improved by the early provision of respite care and supportive counselling. Chapter 14 in this book discusses the contributions of supportive and palliative care teams in more depth.

Consideration of domains in improving QOL

For descriptive purposes, the common domains are reviewed separately in this section. However, in the clinical setting, domains should not be considered in isolation but with a multidimensional approach as they exert cross influences on each other. For example, treatment of psychological or existential distress will often lead to improved pain control.

Physical well-being domain

Patients with advanced cancer may experience a multitude of physical symptoms including pain, fatigue, delirium, dyspnoea, anorexia, nausea, vomiting, constipation, abdominal distension,

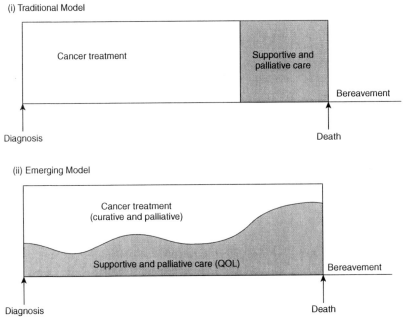

Fig. 12.3 Role of cancer treatment and supportive and palliative care in improving quality of life (QOL) in cancer patients.

and lymphoedema (see also Chapter 14). The number of physical symptoms has been shown to be associated with increased psychological distress and poorer overall QOL [71, 72]. Routinely assessing and effectively managing symptoms will help to improve QOL. As well as recording symptom intensity, it is important to measure the combined impact of symptoms, e.g. on sleep, function, and mobility. Treating uncontrolled physical symptoms will often improve other parameters such as psychological distress.

Fatigue is a very common symptom which is often overlooked. It occurs in over 80 per cent of patients undergoing treatment with chemotherapy and/or radiotherapy. Among all the physical cancer-related symptoms, fatigue impacts the most on a patient's QOL with 91 per cent reporting that it inhibited leading a 'normal' life [73]. During cancer treatment, an exercise programme has been shown to improve fatigue and QOL in breast cancer patients [74]. In advanced cancer patients, pain is usually due to the primary cancer itself or metastases, or as a side effect of oncological treatments. Pain severity is also associated with impaired QOL [75].

Delirium, an acute confusional state that results from diffuse organic brain dysfunction, frequently occurs in advanced cancer patients, with over 80 per cent of patients with advanced cancer developing delirium in their final days [76]. Delirium has a significant impact on patient's and family members' QOL because of loss of effective communication and potentially distressing symptoms [77].

Physical function domain

Physical functioning assessment currently plays a minor role in palliative care QOL instruments [78]. Patients often require assistance with physical activities of daily living, especially as disease progresses and frailty increases. Limitations due to fatigue are common. Referral to an occupational therapist and physiotherapist is invaluable, as is provision of suitable equipment to maximize function and reduce dependency on others. Wound dressing supplies and continence aids are frequently necessary. Community services may be accessed to provide assistance with personal hygiene, and domestic chores.

Psychological/emotional well-being domain

In addition to the emotional domain, the QOL of depressed patients is affected in other areas including social, cognitive, and physical domains [79]. It is important to detect and treat psychological distress as this will improve QOL. There is a higher likelihood of experiencing anxiety and depression with some cancer diagnoses, such as pancreatic cancer, and under the age of 30 years and over the age of 80 years [80]. Depression is also associated with a desire for hastened death in terminally ill cancer patients [81]. Patients with minimal social support may experience more anxiety and depression and a worse QOL than those with more support [82]. Psychosocial interventions and group psychotherapy may be beneficial. Expressive coping, allowing the active processing and expression of emotions, is related to improved QOL [83]. There is some evidence for massage and aromatherapy massage in reducing anxiety [84].

Social well-being and family domain

The social impact of advanced disease is wide ranging. Cancer and its treatment place an increased stress on personal relationships, and exacerbate pre-existing relationship difficulties. Family members are also likely to experience psychological distress. It is important to evaluate this, as they also need support and may require ongoing formal counselling to assist them in their care-giving role and during bereavement. The needs of children of parents with cancer can be overlooked at this demanding time. Parents may need assistance in communicating difficult issues with their children and preparing the child for life without them. In addition to family, peers, and counsellors, support to children and adolescents may be provided by schools, universities, and church and youth groups. Older patients and those who are married or living with others tend to have a higher QOL [82].

Financial issues are common and are often not captured by important QOL tools. (The EORTC QLQ-C30 has a single question specific to financial difficulties) [38]. Financial issues may be compounded if patients have no sickness entitlement or have exhausted their sickness allowance. Patients and their families may be self funding medical and pharmaceutical costs of treatment, including complementary and alternative therapies. Ongoing illness may have led to a permanent loss of employment and loss of regular income, especially if the patient was the sole income provider in the household, leading to financial stress and a risk of mortgage defaulting. An employed spouse or partner may also experience financial strain if they have taken unpaid leave in order to fulfil the carer's role at home. There may be outstanding business and legal issues, including preparation of a will and funeral arrangements. In addition, a single parent may wish to document their choice of responsible adult for the ongoing care and welfare of their children.

Referral to a social worker is fundamental in obtaining skilled assistance for patients and their families in accessing government and community supports, referral to other agencies, and providing supportive counselling to patients and their families. A social work component in a multidisciplinary team leads to improvement in QOL in the social domain [85].

Spiritual well-being and existential domain

There is a unique and significant association between spirituality and QOL [86]. Spirituality comprises the following dimensions: meaning of life, transcendence, higher power or source of energy, relationships, and religion [87]. Some patients experience death anxiety with fear of the unknown, fear of the state of non-existence, and the impending separation from loved ones. An existential crisis may occur with overwhelming spiritual suffering.

Religion may be an important component of an individual's spirituality, with specific beliefs and rituals, and ceremonies shared as a community. Use of religion in coping with the experience of life-threatening cancer improves overall QOL [88].

Chaplains and pastoral care workers are integral to a specialist palliative care team. Both patients and their families may benefit from their assistance with spiritual issues, especially if these are beyond the skills of the regular team. Other spiritual care interventions that have been used include psychotherapy, music, art, relaxation, therapeutic touch, and aromatherapy [89].

Sexuality and intimacy

> Yes, I haven't had enough sex[90].
>
> Sir John Betjeman CBE (1906–1984), British poet laureate, in an interview for the television
> documentary *Time with Betjeman* (February 1983), having been asked whether he had any regrets.

Sexuality and the ability to experience intimacy are also fundamental QOL issues [91]. Human sexuality is multi-dimensional and complex. In palliative care, sexuality is influenced by the impact of the cancer and its treatment, psychosocial distress, in addition to social and cultural norms, and will be affected by pre-existing problems in relationships. Sexuality should not be limited to the genital level of sexual function, sexual intercourse, fertility, and reproduction. Consideration of sexuality includes body image, self-esteem, mood, support, and sense of emotional connection and intimacy [17]. Sexuality means different things to different people, and may also vary according to life-stage [92]. Intimacy often refers to an emotional or physical closeness between partners, but can also be present in emotional and social interactions with other people.

Cancer survivors have a high incidence of altered sexuality, which is long lasting, or even permanent, and can impair QOL for both the cancer survivor and sexual partner [93]. Patients with localized prostate cancer report sexual and urinary symptoms negatively impacting on QOL [56]. Different modalities of treatments for a particular cancer may impact on QOL differently. Cervical cancer survivors treated with radiotherapy had worse sexual functioning and poorer QOL than those treated with radical hysterectomy [94]. Breast cancer survivors experience hormone changes and menopausal symptoms, especially vaginal dryness affecting sexual function, as well as body image changes. Information on spouses' behaviours and attitudes towards sexuality after treatment and formal sexual counselling may improve breast cancer survivors' QOL [95].

The commonly used QOL instruments cover the sexuality domain minimally. For example, on the FACT-G (version 4), there is one statement on satisfaction with sex life (with an option not to answer), and another on feeling close to partner or support person. The Rotterdam Symptom Checklist has only one question on sexuality (decreased sexual interest) and the EORTC QLQ-C30 has no questions addressing sexuality [34,36,38].

It is important for health care professionals to address issues of sexuality for all patients from diagnosis and through all stages of the cancer trajectory, regardless of their age [96] and independent of cancer site, as sexual problems are not limited to those patients with cancers directly affecting sexual organs. Physicians should inform all cancer patients about intimate and sexual changes after cancer and its treatment. Some patients will not wish to talk about this area of their personal lives, so health care professionals need to gain permission to discuss the topic first. Health care professionals should routinely assess, with sensitivity and without assumptions or prejudice, for intimacy and sexual needs of all patients whether they have a known partner or not, regardless of age, sexual orientation, sexual preferences, site of cancer, and type of cancer treatment [92]. Patients and their partners will vary in their desire for information and practical strategies for sexual intercourse and intimacy.

As cancer progresses, the focus of discussions may change to maintaining sexual and physical intimacy, especially when sexual intercourse is no longer possible. Towards the end of life, physical intimacy, and the need to touch and be touched remain important for QOL [91].

Barriers to discussing sexuality remain for many health care professionals. These include discomfort with the topic, lack of knowledge, and cultural issues, but the communication skills required for these discussions are the same as for any sensitive topic. The BETTER model was developed to assist nurses in discussing sexuality issues [97]. Resources written in familiar language are available for people affected by cancer, in the form of printed literature and websites (e.g. CancerHelp UK, the patient information website of Cancer Research UK (www.cancerhelp. org.uk), and National Cancer Institute, US National Institutes of Health, patient information, and comprehensive peer-reviewed information for health professionals (www.cancer.gov).

Conclusion

Systematic QOL evaluation is important in the management of advanced cancer patients and their families. A practical method in the clinical setting is to first measure QOL using a single global measure and then combine this with specific suitable multiple item instrument/s as appropriate to needs. Whichever assessment tool is used, the most important aspect in providing holistic care to our patients and their families is to identify and gain a deeper clarification and understanding of those factors that are important to their QOL at different points in time, without intrusion of the health care professional's own personal values and views on QOL. This will aid communication in the discussion of active treatment and symptom relief options and their prioritization, as well as end of life care wishes, with the overall aim of improving QOL for both patients and their families. Returning to Epicurus,

> It is not great sums of money or a mass of possessions(.....) which produce happiness and blessedness, but rather freedom from pain and gentleness in our feelings and a disposition of soul which measures out what is natural [3].

Acknowledgement

Eduardo Bruera is supported in part by National Institutes of Health grant numbers RO1NR 010162-01-A1, RO1CA122292-01, RO1CA124481-01.

References

1 WHO: *WHO Cancer Control Programme*. Available at: http://www.who.int/cancer/en/ (accessed 20 October 2009).

2 WHO 2002: *WHO definition of palliative care*. Available at: http://www.who.int/cancer/palliative/definition/en/ (accessed 20 October 2009).

3 Inwood B & Gerson LP (eds) (1994). *The Epicurus Reader. Selected Writings and Testimonia*. Hackett Publishing Company, Indianapolis.

4 Cohen SR (2001). Defining and measuring quality of life in palliative care. In Bruera E & Portenoy RK (eds). *Topics in Palliative Care*, vol.5, pp. 137–56. Oxford University Press, New York.

5 Cella DF (1994). Quality of life: concepts and definition. *J Pain Symptom Manage*, 9(3):186–92.

6 Gill TM & Feinstein AR (1994). A critical appraisal of the quality of quality-of-life measurements. *JAMA*, 272(8):619–26.

7 Ferrans CE (1990). Development of a quality of life index for patients with cancer. *Oncol Nurs Forum*, 17(3 Suppl):15–19; discussion 20-1.

8 Sloan JA, Cella D, Frost M, Guyatt GH, Sprangers M, & Symonds T (2002). Assessing clinical significance in measuring oncology patient quality of life: introduction to the symposium, content overview, and definition of terms. *Mayo Clin Proc*, 77(4):367–70.

9 Kaasa S & Loge JH (2003). Quality of life in palliative care: principles and practice. *Palliat Med*, 17(1):11–20.

10 Scott NW, Fayers PM, Aaronson NK, et al (2008). The relationship between overall quality of life and its subdimensions was influenced by culture: analysis of an international database. *J Clin Epidemiol*, 61(8):788–95.

11 *Stedman's Medical Dictionary*, 28th edition (2006) (accessed on line 26 June 2008)

12 Cohen SR (2006). Quality of life assessment in palliative care. In Bruera E, Higginson IJ, Ripamonti C, & von Gunten CF (eds). *Textbook of Palliative Medicine*, pp. 349–55. Hodder Arnold, London.

13 Kreitler S, Chaitchik S, Rapoport Y, Kreitler H, & Algor R (1993). Life satisfaction and health in cancer patients, orthopedic patients and healthy individuals. *Soc Sci Med*, 36(4):547–56.

14 Cohen S, Mount BM, Bruera E, Provost M, Rowe J, & Tong K (1997). Validity of the McGill Quality of Life Questionnaire in the palliative care setting: A multi-centre Canadian study demonstrating the importance of the existential domain. *Palliat Med*, 11(1):3–20.

15 Cohen SR & Leis A (2002). What determines the quality of life of terminally ill cancer patients from their own perspective? *J Palliat Care*, 18(1):48–58.

16 Fallowfield L & Jenkins V (1999). Effective communication skills are the key to good cancer care. *Eur J Cancer*, 35(11):1592–97.

17 National Breast Cancer Centre and National Cancer Control Initiative (2003). *Clinical practice guidelines for the psychosocial care of adults with cancer.* National Breast Cancer Centre, Camperdown, NSW. Available at: http://www.nhmrc.gov.au (accessed 18 July 2008)

18 VanReusen AK, Bos CS, Schumaker JB, & Deschler DD (1994). *Self-Advocacy Strategy for Education and Transition Planning.* Edge Enterprises, Lawrence, KS.

19 Calman KC (1984). Quality of life in cancer patients – an hypothesis. *J Med Ethics*, **10**(3):124-27.

20 Wan GJ, Counte MA, & Cella DF (1997). The influence of personal expectations on cancer patients' reports of health-related quality of life. *Psychooncology*, **6**(1):1–11.

21 Sprangers MA & Schwartz CE (1999). Integrating response shift into health-related quality of life research: a theoretical model. *Soc Sci Med*, **48**(11):1507–15.

22 Detmar SB, Muller MJ, Schornagel JH, Wever LD, & Aaronson NK (2002). Health-related quality-of-life assessments and patient-physician communication: a randomized controlled trial. *JAMA*, **288**(23):3027–34.

23 Vigano A, Dorgan M, Buckingham J, Bruera E, & Suarez-Almazor ME (2000). Survival prediction in terminal cancer patients: a systematic review of the medical literature. *Palliat Med*, **14**(5):363–74.

24 Paci E, Miccinesi G, Toscani F, et al (2001). Quality of life assessment and outcome of palliative care. *J Pain Symptom Manage*, **21**(3):179–88.

25 Davis K, Yount S, Wagner L, & Cella D (2004). Measurement and management of health-related quality of life in lung cancer. *Clin Adv Hematol Oncol*, **2**(8):533–40.

26 Velikova G, Booth L, Smith AB, et al (2004). Measuring quality of life in routine oncology practice improves communication and patient well-being: a randomized controlled trial. *J Clin Oncol*, **22**(4):714–24.

27 de Boer AG, van Lanschot JJ, Stalmeier PF, et al (2004). Is a single-item visual analogue scale as valid, reliable and responsive as multi-item scales in measuring quality of life? *Qual Life Res*, **13**(2):311–20

28 Persson C, Ostlund U, Wennman-Larsen A, Wengstrom Y, & Gustavsson P (2008). Health-related quality of life in significant others of patients dying from lung cancer. *Palliat Med*, **22**(3):239–47.

29 Bergelt C, Koch U, & Petersen C (2008). Quality of life in partners of patients with cancer. *Qual Life Res*, **17**(5):653–63.

30 Spitzer WO, Dobson AJ, Hall J, et al (1981). Measuring the quality of life of cancer patients: a concise QL-index for use by physicians. *J Chronic Dis*, **34**(12):585–97.

31 Bruera E, Kuehn N, Miller MJ, Selmser P, & Macmillan K (1991). The Edmonton Symptom Assessment System (ESAS): a simple method for the assessment of palliative care patients. *J Palliat Care*, **7**(2):6–9

32 Chang VT, Hwang SS, & Feuerman M (2000). Validation of the Edmonton Symptom Assessment Scale. *Cancer*, **88**(9):2164–71.

33 de Haes JC, van Knippenberg FC, & Neijt JP (1990). Measuring psychological and physical distress in cancer patients: structure and application of the Rotterdam Symptom Checklist. *Br J Cancer*, **62**(6):1034–38.

34 de Haes JCJM, Olschewski M, Fayers P, et al (1996). *Measuring the quality of life of cancer patients with the Rotterdam Symptom Checklist: A manual. (Appendix C).* Northern Centre for Healthcare Research (NCH), University of Groningen, The Netherlands.

35 Cella DF, Tulsky DS, Gray G, et al (1993). The functional assessment of cancer therapy scale: development and validation of the general measure. *J Clin Oncol*, **11**(3):570–79.

36 Functional assessment of chronic illness therapy (FACIT) Available at: http://www.facit.org/ (accessed 3 July 2008)

37 Aaronson NK, Ahmedzai S, Bergman B, et al (1993). The European Organization for Research and Treatment of Cancer QLQ-C30: a quality-of-life instrument for use in international clinical trials in oncology. *J Natl Cancer Inst*, **85**(5):365–76.

38 EORTC group for research into quality of life. *EORTC QLQ-C30.* Available at: http://groups.eortc.be/ qol/questionnaires_qlqc30.htm (accessed 26 June 2008)

39 Osoba D, Zee B, Pater J, Warr D, Kaizer L, & Latreille J (1994). Psychometric properties and responsiveness of the EORTC quality of Life Questionnaire (QLQ-C30) in patients with breast, ovarian and lung cancer. *Qual Life Res*, **3**(5):353–64.

40 Groenvold M, Petersen MA, Aaronson NK, et al (2006). The development of the EORTC QLQ-C15-PAL: a shortened questionnaire for cancer patients in palliative care. *Eur J Cancer*, **42**(1):55–64.

41 EORTC group for research into quality of life. *EORTC QLQ-C15-PAL*. Available at: http://groups.eortc.be/qol/questionnaires_qlqc15pal.htm (accessed 27 June 2008)

42 Echteld MA, Onwuteaka-Philipsen B, van der Wal G, Deliens L, & Klein M (2006). EORTC QLQ-C15-PAL: The new standard in the assessment of health-related quality of life in advanced cancer? *Palliat Med*, **20**(1):1–2.

43 Cohen SR, Mount BM, Strobel MG, & Bui F (1995). The McGill Quality of Life Questionnaire: a measure of quality of life appropriate for people with advanced disease. A preliminary study of validity and acceptability. *Palliat Med*, **9**(3):207–19.

44 Hyun Kim S, Kyung Gu S, Ho Yun Y, et al (2007). Validation study of the Korean version of the McGill Quality of Life Questionnaire. *Palliat Med*, **21**(5):441–47.

45 Joyce CR, Hickey A, McGee HM, & O'Boyle CA (2003). A theory-based method for the evaluation of individual quality of life: the SEIQoL. *Qual Life Res*, **12**(3):275–80.

46 Waldron D, O'Boyle CA, Kearney M, Moriarty M, & Carney D (1999). Quality-of-life measurement in advanced cancer: assessing the individual. *J Clin Oncol*, **17**(11):3603–11.

47 Ferrell BR, Dow KH, Leigh S, Ly J, & Gulasekaram P (1995). Quality of life in long-term cancer survivors. *Oncol Nurs Forum*, **22**(6):915–22.

48 Pearce NJM, Sanson-Fisher R, & Campbell HS (2007). Measuring quality of life in cancer survivors: a methodological review of existing scales. *Psycho-Oncology, published online in Wiley InterScience (www.interscience.wiley.com)*, DOI: 10.1002/pon.1281.

49 Weitzner MA, Jacobsen PB, Wagner H, Jr., Friedland J, & Cox C (1999). The caregiver quality of life index-cancer (CQOLC) scale: development and validation of an instrument to measure quality of life of the family caregiver of patients with cancer. *Qual Life Res*, **8**(1–2):55–63.

50 Cohen R, Leis AM, Kuhl D, Charbonneau C, Ritvo P, & Ashbury FD (2006). QOLLTI-F: measuring family carer quality of life. *Palliat Med*, **20**(8):755–67.

51 Daut RL, Cleeland CS, & Flanery RC (1983). Development of the Wisconsin Brief Pain Questionnaire to assess pain in cancer and other diseases. *Pain*, **17**(2):197–210.

52 Sneeuw KC, Sprangers MA, & Aaronson NK (2002). The role of health care providers and significant others in evaluating the quality of life of patients with chronic disease. *J Clin Epidemiol*, **55**(11):1130–43.

53 McPherson CJ & Addington-Hall JM (2003). Judging the quality of care at the end of life: can proxies provide reliable information? *Soc Sci Med*, **56**(1):95–109.

54 van't Spijker A, Trijsburg RW, & Duivenvoorden HJ (1997). Psychological sequelae of cancer diagnosis: a meta-analytical review of 58 studies after 1980. *Psychosom Med*, **59**(3):280–93.

55 Rustoen T, Moum T, Wiklund I, & Hanestad BR (1999). Quality of life in newly diagnosed cancer patients. *J Adv Nurs*, **29**(2):490–98.

56 Bacon CG, Giovannucci E, Testa M, Glass TA, & Kawachi I (2002). The association of treatment-related symptoms with quality-of-life outcomes for localized prostate carcinoma patients. *Cancer*, **94**(3):862–71.

57 Slevin ML (1992). Quality of life: philosophical question or clinical reality? *BMJ*, **305**(6851):466–69.

58 Ganz PA, Guadagnoli E, Landrum MB, Lash TL, Rakowski W, & Silliman RA (2003). Breast cancer in older women: quality of life and psychosocial adjustment in the 15 months after diagnosis. *J Clin Oncol*, **21**(21):4027–33.

59 Northouse LL, Mood D, Kershaw T, et al (2002). Quality of life of women with recurrent breast cancer and their family members. *J Clin Oncol*, **20**(19):4050–64.

60 Matsuyama R, Reddy S, & Smith TJ (2006). Why do patients choose chemotherapy near the end of life? A review of the perspective of those facing death from cancer. *J Clin Oncol*, **24**(21):3490–96.

61 Detmar SB, Muller MJ, Schornagel JH, Wever LD, & Aaronson NK (2002). Role of health-related quality of life in palliative chemotherapy treatment decisions. *J Clin Oncol*, **20**(4):1056–62.

62 Steinhauser KE, Christakis NA, Clipp EC, McNeilly M, McIntyre L, & Tulsky JA (2000). Factors considered important at the end of life by patients, family, physicians, and other care providers. *JAMA*, **284**(19):2476–82.

63 Singer PA, Martin DK, & Kelner M (1999). Quality end-of-life care: patients' perspectives. *JAMA*, **281**(2):163–68.

64 Sherman DW, Ye XY, McSherry C, Calabrese M, Parkas V, & Gatto M (2005). Spiritual well-being as a dimension of quality of life for patients with advanced cancer and AIDS and their family caregivers: Results of a longitudinal study. *Am J Hosp Palliat Med*, **22**(5):349–62.

65 Hwang SS, Chang VT, Fairclough DL, Cogswell J, & Kasimis B (2003). Longitudinal Quality of Life in Advanced Cancer Patients: Pilot Study Results from a VA Medical Cancer Center. *J Pain Symptom Manage*, **25**(3):225–34.

66 Bloom JR (2002). Surviving and thriving? *Psychooncology*, **11**(2):89–92.

67 Alfano CM & Rowland JH (2006). Recovery issues in cancer survivorship: a new challenge for supportive care. *Cancer J*, **12**(5):432–43.

68 Echteld MA, van Zuylen L, Bannink M, Witkamp E, & Van der Rijt CC (2007). Changes in and correlates of individual quality of life in advanced cancer patients admitted to an academic unit for palliative care. *Palliat Med*, **21**(3):199–205.

69 Cohen R, Boston P, Mount BM, & Porterfield P (2001). Changes in quality of life following admission to palliative care units. *Palliat Med*, **15**(5):363–71.

70 Rabow MW, Dibble SL, Pantilat SZ, & McPhee SJ (2004). The comprehensive care team: a controlled trial of outpatient palliative medicine consultation. *Arch Intern Med*, **164**(1):83–91.

71 Portenoy RK, Thaler HT, Kornblith AB, et al (1994). Symptom prevalence, characteristics and distress in a cancer population. *Qual Life Res*, **3**(3):183–89.

72 Chang VT, Hwang SS, Feuerman M, & Kasimis BS (2000). Symptom and quality of life survey of medical oncology patients at a veterans affairs medical center: a role for symptom assessment. *Cancer*, **88**(5):1175–83.

73 Curt GA, Breitbart W, Cella D, et al (2000). Impact of cancer-related fatigue on the lives of patients: new findings from the Fatigue Coalition. *Oncologist*, **5**(5):353–60.

74 Mock V, Pickett M, Ropka ME, et al (2001). Fatigue and quality of life outcomes of exercise during cancer treatment. *Cancer Pract*, **9**(3):119–27.

75 Smith EM, Gomm SA, & Dickens CM (2003). Assessing the independent contribution to quality of life from anxiety and depression in patients with advanced cancer. *Palliat Med*, **17**(6):509–13.

76 Centeno C, Sanz A, & Bruera E (2004). Delirium in advanced cancer patients. *Palliat Med*, **18**(3):184–94.

77 Gagnon P, Charbonneau C, Allard P, Soulard C, Dumont S, & Fillion L (2002). Delirium in advanced cancer: a psychoeducational intervention for family caregivers. *J Palliat Care*, **18**(4):253–61.

78 Jordhoy MS, Inger Ringdal G, Helbostad JL, Oldervoll L, Loge JH, & Kaasa S (2007). Assessing physical functioning: a systematic review of quality of life measures developed for use in palliative care. *Palliat Med*, **21**(8):673–82.

79 Grassi L, Indelli M, Marzola M, et al (1996). Depressive symptoms and quality of life in home-care-assisted cancer patients. *J Pain Symptom Manage*, **12**(5):300–07.

80 Zabora J, BrintzenhofeSzoc K, Curbow B, Hooker C, & Piantadosi S (2001). The prevalence of psychological distress by cancer site. *Psychooncology*, **10**(1):19–28.

81 Breitbart W, Rosenfeld B, Pessin H, et al (2000). Depression, hopelessness, and desire for hastened death in terminally ill patients with cancer. *JAMA*, **284**(22):2907–11.

82 Parker PA, Baile WF, de Moor C, & Cohen L (2003). Psychosocial and demographic predictors of quality of life in a large sample of cancer patients. *Psychooncology*, **12**(2):83–93.

83 Stanton AL, Danoff-Burg S, Cameron CL, et al (2000). Emotionally expressive coping predicts psychological and physical adjustment to breast cancer. *J Consult Clin Psychol*, **68**(5):875–82.

84 Fellowes D, Barnes K, & Wilkinson S (2004). Aromatherapy and massage for symptom relief in patients with cancer. *Cochrane Database of Systematic Reviews*, Issue 3. Art. No.: CD002287. DOI:10.1002/14651858.CD002287.pub2

85 Miller JJ, Frost MH, Rummans TA, et al (2007). Role of a medical social worker in improving quality of life for patients with advanced cancer with a structured multidisciplinary intervention. *J Psychosocl Oncol*, **25**(4):105–19.

86 Brady MJ, Peterman AH, Fitchett G, Mo M, & Cella D (1999). A case for including spirituality in quality of life measurement in oncology. *Psychooncology*, **8**(5):417–28.

87 Strang S & Strang P (2006). Spiritual care. In Bruera E, Higginson IJ, Ripamonti C, & von Gunten CF (eds). *Textbook of Palliative Medicine*, pp. 1019–28. Hodder Arnold, London.

88 Tarakeshwar N, Vanderwerker LC, Paulk E, Pearce MJ, Kasl SV, & Prigerson HG (2006). Religious coping is associated with the quality of life of patients with advanced cancer. *J Palliat Med*, **9**(3):646–57.

89 Chochinov HM & Cann BJ (2005). Interventions to enhance the spiritual aspects of dying. *J Palliat Med*, **8**(Suppl 1):S103–S115.

90 http://en.wikiquote.org/wiki/John_Betjeman (accessed 5 August 2008).

91 Cort E, Monroe B, & Oliviere D (2004). Couples in palliative care. *Sexual & Relationship Therapy*, **19**(3):337–54.

92 Hordern A & Street A (2007). Issues of intimacy and sexuality in the face of cancer: the patient perspective. *Cancer Nurs*, **30**(6):E11–E18.

93 Tierney DK (2008). Sexuality: a quality-of-life issue for cancer survivors. *Semin Oncol Nurs*, **24**(2):71–79.

94 Frumovitz M, Sun CC, Schover LR, et al (2005). Quality of life and sexual functioning in cervical cancer survivors. *J Clin Oncol*, **23**(30):7428–36.

95 Dorval M, Maunsell E, Deschenes L, Brisson J, & Masse B (1998). Long-term quality of life after breast cancer: comparison of 8-year survivors with population controls. *J Clin Oncol*, **16**(2):487–94.

96 Kleinplatz PJ (2008). Sexuality and older people. *BMJ*, **337**:a239.

97 Mick J, Hughes M, & Cohen MZ (2003). Sexuality and cancer: how oncology nurses can address it BETTER. *Oncol Nurs Forum*, **30**(abstr; suppl 2):152–53.

Chapter 13

Shifting the paradigm: from complementary and alternative medicine (CAM) to integrative oncology

Anne Leis, Stephen Sagar, Marja Verhoef, Lynda Balneaves, Dugald Seely, Doreen Oneschuk[1]

The profound desire by many patients to control cancer using a holistic, patient-centred perspective has been an important impetus for the rising popularity of complementary and alternative medicine (CAM) as an adjunct to biomedical conventional cancer treatments. More recently, the focus has shifted from single CAM modalities for cancer management to a more comprehensive approach called integrative oncology, which is 'an evolving, evidence-based specialty that uses CAM therapies in concert with biomedical cancer treatments to enhance its efficacy, improve symptom control, alleviate patient distress and reduce suffering' [1]. This chapter aims to explore the rationale for increased CAM utilization by cancer patients and survivors from a historical and ontological perspective, and to document the paradigm shift towards integrative oncology as a pivotal part of a cancer control framework. The scientific foundation of CAM has been difficult to establish, partly due to a lack of fit between the mainstream reductionist and positivist approach to health research, and because of the need to evaluate cancer control as a whole system of prevention, treatment, and care. However, evidence supporting the safety and efficacy of select CAM therapies is, slowly mounting through credible scientific enquiries, thus facilitating their incorporation into cancer control. Finally, we provide support for integrative oncology as a core component of cancer control, outline modalities to implement this vision, and discuss the implications for education, practice, research, and policy.

What is complementary and alternative medicine (CAM)?

The way CAM is defined and which professions, practices, and therapies are included under this label often depends on the point in time, the culture, and the socio-political forces at work within a country's health care system. Since the late 1980s, repeated attempts were made to develop discrete

[1] Anne Leis, PhD, Professor and Dr. Louis Schulman Cancer Research Chair, Dept of Community Health and Epidemiology, University of Saskatchewan, Saskatoon, Saskatchewan, Canada; Stephen Sagar, MBBS, MRCP, FRCR, FRCPC, DABR, Radiation Oncologist, Juravinski Cancer Centre and Associate Professor, Departments of Oncology and Medicine, McMaster University, Hamilton, Ontario, Canada; Marja Verhoef, PhD, Professor and Canada Research Chair in Complementary Medicine, Department of Community Health Sciences, University of Calgary, Alberta; Lynda Balneaves, RN, PhD, Associate Professor and CIHR New Investigator, University of British Columbia School of Nursing, Vancouver, British Columbia, Canada; Dugald Seely, ND, MSc, Research Director, Canadian College of Naturopathic Medicine, Toronto, Ontario, Canada; Doreen Oneschuk, MD, CCFP, Division of Palliative Care Medicine, Palliative Care Program, Grey Nuns Community Hospital, Edmonton, Alberta, Canada.

definitions and categories that would accurately describe this diverse field of health care [2–4]. The term 'complementary and alternative medicine' or CAM has been widely used during the past 10 years[5]. The popular use of this term is due in part to its uptake by the well-established National Institute of Health [NIH] National Centre for Complementary and Alternative Medicine [NCCAM], which is the US government's lead agency for scientific research on CAM. According to NCCAM, CAM refers to 'a group of diverse medical and health care systems, practices, and products that are not presently considered to be part of conventional medicine'. NCCAM defines *complementary medicine* as comprised of therapies and practices that are used alongside conventional medicine whereas *alternative medicine* is defined as being used in place of conventional medicine. CAM is further grouped by NCCAM into four domains to account for the wide diversity in therapies: (1) mind-body medicine, (2) biologically-based practices, (3) manipulative and body-based practices, and (4) energy therapies. Religious observance and prayer are usually excluded from the definition. Mind-body medicine includes those therapies that engage the ability of the mind to affect physiology and quality of life through sustained attention-focused techniques, or emotionally expressive and imaginative practices. Mind-body therapies include modalities such as hypnosis, imagery, meditation, yoga, music, and art therapy. Biologically-based therapies comprise a wide range of natural health products, vitamins and minerals, nutraceuticals, herbal products, and other biological substances. Therapies which involve the physical touching of an individual's body, such as massage or chiropractic techniques, are categorized as manipulative and body-based practices. Energy therapies are based on the conceptualization of the physiological body as being comprised of energy fields, which can be influenced through various techniques that may not include touching. Cutting across all four domains is the category called 'Whole Medical Systems'. These represent comprehensive systems of theory and practice that have developed prior to, or in parallel to, biomedicine. These systems usually have a history of effectiveness ascertained through many years of observation within a specific cultural context (e.g. traditional Chinese medicine, Ayurvedic medicine, and naturopathic medicine). At the 2004 European Forum for Complementary and Alternative Medicine – Promoting Integrated Healthcare, CAM was identified as the preferred label and defined as 'a diverse range of autonomous healthcare practices used for health maintenance, health promotion, disease prevention and for the treatment of ill-health' [6]. More recently, the newly formed National Institute of Complementary Medicine (NICM) in Australia adopted complementary medicine (CM) as 'an inclusive term that incorporates Complementary Medicines and Complementary Therapies (Modalities / Systems). The term complementary medicine is considered to be inclusive of historically used names such as alternative medicine, natural medicine, and traditional medicine. CM is concerned with both the maintenance of wellness and the treatment of illness' [7]. Over the years, the list of what is considered CAM has been a moving target as those therapies proven to be safe and effective tend to be integrated into conventional health care. Similarly, therapies considered to belong to conventional medicine may also vary depending on the paradigm and specialty area in which a health professional is trained, and how conventional medicine is itself defined.[8] For example, the increased emphasis on the potential impact of lifestyle behaviours, such as dietary changes, exercise, and sleep patterns, on cancer prevention and survivorship has broadened the scope of both CAM and conventional medicine [9], and further blurs the boundaries among different forms of medicine, thus impacting the scope of cancer control.

The relevance of CAM to cancer control

The interest in CAM in the Western world primarily focuses on CAM as an adjunct to mainstream oncology treatments rather than as an alternative to conventional medicine.

Notwithstanding the difficulties in defining CAM and accurately measuring CAM use, population-based prevalence studies suggest that at least one-third of patients in developed countries use CAM therapies during their cancer experience [10,11] and that CAM utilization is increasing within specific cancer populations [12,13]. To enhance cancer control strategies it is important to know the types of CAM cancer patients use, who is using CAM in terms of sociodemographic and personality characteristics, as well as reasons for use.

CAM modalities commonly used by cancer patients and survivors

According to a number of surveys conducted in many countries over the past years, the most popular modalities for cancer patients are natural health products, supplements, and vitamins followed by mind-body therapies and massage therapy [14]. These represent thousands of products and therapies with varying levels of regulations in the western world, and for the most part with no conclusive evidence for cancer [15,16]. A few reports of interactions with conventional oncology treatments have been published [17]. Mind-body approaches and body manipulation are often perceived as supportive therapies that may be helpful and innocuous. Rarely will oncology patients use a single modality; rather they mostly combine therapies to manage their cancer [18].

CAM users

CAM use is particularly common among younger [19], well-educated women [20,21] as well as within specific cancer populations (i.e. breast and prostate cancer) [22]. Moreover a trend is observed towards increased CAM use among younger cancer patients who wish to play an active role in the healing process and are less satisfied with treatment options [23,24]. CAM utilization is also influenced by belonging to an ethnic and cultural minority [25]. According to Sirois, psychological factors such as need perception, desire for control, motivation, and health beliefs also drive CAM use [26,27]. However no correlation between depression, anxiety, and the use of CAM was found [28]. Rather, CAM use has been described as a sign of active coping behaviour and can change as a function of the cancer journey [29].

Why are people using CAM?

'. . . you just don't know . . . I thought, 'I've gotta increase my odds. I have to do it all. I have to do complementary and conventional [treatment]'

Patient's quote

Studies exploring the reasons for cancer patients' use of CAM have repeatedly shown that patients are often 'pushed' towards CAM therapies and practitioners because of dissatisfaction with the quality of care provided within mainstream health care [30–32]. Limited time available during consultations, lack of respect for patient's beliefs and values, failure to involve patients in treatment decisions, as well as, for some individuals, poor treatment outcomes, have been cited as factors that are associated with cancer patients seeking alternative forms of health care [33]. Cancer patients are attracted towards integrating conventional and CAM treatments, as this allows cancer management to be more person-centred and more supportive of the body's ability to heal itself [34–38]. For many individuals, CAM therapies provide them with a sense of control over their illness as well as the opportunity to be a more active participant in their overall cancer care. Patients also prefer treatments that concur with their belief systems, such as the growing belief in the role of the mind in cancer [39]. Interest in CAM therapies shifts across the cancer trajectory, with individuals facing more advanced disease and limited treatment options being more likely to report the use of CAM [40]. Indeed, perceived risk of recurrence and advanced disease were shown to be strongly associated with CAM use [41]. Such treatment decisions may be motivated by the desire to maintain hope when faced with a poor prognosis as well as the need to achieve healing when cure is not possible. However, CAM use is not only a matter of balancing push and pull factors. Making such decisions is a complex process that is not linear and depends on the individual person's context [42].

Costs associated with CAM

Insurance coverage for CAM interventions varies between and within countries. Generally, patients must pay from their own financial resources regardless of the evidence-based status of the modality, and the out of pocket expenditures are most often underestimated. For CAM modalities, the reimbursed amount is generally modest and often does not include all costs related to CAM care [43]. Unfortunately when faced with a lack of universal healthcare in countries including the United States, some CAM therapies may become the first line of action because they represent the more affordable supportive care option.

Historical context and societal trends

The increasing use of CAM in Western society is part of important societal and cultural trends. With the publication of the Flexner Report [44] in 1910, a new era promoting scientific rigor, analytic reasoning, and sophisticated technology was born. This report was designed to address the lack of standards in medical education common in many schools in the United States, which were teaching various types of medicine including homeopathy, chiropractic, and osteopathic medicine [45]. Much needed reforms in the standards, organization, and curricula of North American medical schools took place with the effect of precipitating the closure of training programmes not focused on biological, disease-oriented models (e.g. homeopathy and naturopathy). At the same time, research became more rigorous and promoted a reductionist approach to elucidate causal relationships. Considered 'unscientific' many CAM modalities slowly disappeared as health care options. Despite some dissident voices such as Sir William Osler's, a technology-focused, reductionist, and disease-oriented medical system came to rule the day with anything resembling CAM being labelled 'quackery', a term with powerful negative connotations.

A shift towards the bio-psychosocial model

As a reaction to the era of modernism characterized by beliefs in the existence of objective truth, causality, and impartial observation, the shift towards post-modernism opened the door to a medicine less reliant on science and technology. Individuality, complexity, and the subjectivity of personal experience were rediscovered [46,47]. Postmodernism was one of the many emerging movements in the 1970s that contributed to scepticism about the ability of a reductionist form of biomedicine to resolve all contemporary health care problems, and this phenomenon led to widespread discussions about the practice and role of medicine in our society and culture. An important marker of this shift was the articulation of the 'bio-psychosocial' model of health and disease, which was viewed as more comprehensive than the biomedical model [48]. In addition, the shift towards globalization [49] meant faster access to information, increased sensitivity to cultural practices, and the rediscovery of healing paradigms and therapies typically excluded from health care offered within Western societies. After an absence of approximately 75 years, therapies now labelled under the umbrella term of CAM, slowly reappeared on the public health scene.

In this changing climate, the field of psycho-oncology emerged as a means to address the unmet social, emotional, and psychological needs of cancer patients [50]. Over the past 35 years psycho-oncology has matured and is now a key oncology sub-specialty area that aims to understand

and address the social, psychological, emotional, spiritual, and functional aspects of cancer from prevention through bereavement. Many large cancer centres throughout Western Europe, the United States, Canada, and Australia started to dedicate some funds to psycho-oncology clinical resources in the form of patient counselling, psycho-education, or stress management. Despite the mounting evidence base, psycho-oncology remains often underfunded because it tends not to be considered as a core cancer control discipline.

Another development, not specific to cancer was the increasing number of patients using CAM approaches. This resulted in public pressure on the United States Congress to pass legislation to establish the Office of Alternative Medicine (OAM) at the National Institutes of Health in 1992, with the mandate to launch a research programme to develop an evidence base for CAM. In 1999, the OAM became the National Centre for CAM (NCCAM) and has become a hallmark of the growing public and professional acceptance of CAM. Around the same time, but initially as a separate movement, integrative oncology slowly began to emerge as an approach and later as a discipline, which combines evidence-based conventional and CAM cancer treatments. The first CAM-oriented support centres opened in North America and Europe (examples include the Commonweal Cancer Help Programme in the United States [51] and the Bristol Cancer Help Centre in the United Kingdom, now called the Penny Brohn Cancer Care [52]). Originally perceived as offering controversial therapies of questionable efficacy to a limited number of cancer patients, these programmes first struggled to find support within mainstream cancer care and later gained momentum with the re-emergence of philosophical movements in health care towards holism, self-care, and patient-centred care [53]. Such institutions have led to a significant body of evidence in the past 20 years that supports the possible efficacy of select CAM interventions and the potential synergism of a more complex whole systems approach to cancer management. This movement has encouraged the rediscovery of a more humanistic and comprehensive approach to cancer control and the paradigm shift towards integrative oncology.

Cancer patients as partners in cancer control

These shifts also resulted in cancer patients wanting to be more active partners in all aspects of cancer treatment decision making. Today many cancer patients desire treatment options and outcomes that go beyond the biological and physical domains. Patients often search for a profound healing experience from their care that includes: 'the restoration of harmony, balance and optimal functioning at all levels of a person'(p. 3) [54]. Beyond physical treatments, the psychological, social, spiritual, and quality of life domains are important to people with cancer and require a whole-person approach to cancer control. As more cancer patients choose to incorporate CAM therapies into their cancer management, oncology health professionals and institutions are increasingly pressured to acknowledge and examine the potential effects of CAM, both positive and negative, on cancer control outcomes [55]. The literature further shows that the integration of CAM therapies is significantly improving quality of life as well as disease and patient-centred outcomes.[56,57] However, patients need support around CAM information and decision-support services to meet their healing goals. The demand for person-centred cancer control requires a change of culture within existing cancer institution and providers, as more explicit knowledge and discussion of CAM therapies are expected. As described in a 2005 Institute of Medicine Report [58], the holistic person-centred approach should be seen within an ecological model of cancer control, as 'it assumes that health and well being are affected by interaction among multiple determinants, including biology, behaviour, and the environment (p. 211)', thus extending the holistic integrative cancer control movement to the system level. For example, in some major cancer institutions, truly integrative oncology practice models are being implemented, and evaluation of these models will have to take into account and measure the complex interactions within the cancer control system.

Shifts in health policies, regulations, and scopes of practice

With the increasing use and popularity of CAM, some conventional health professionals are beginning to express an interest in incorporating CAM into their own practice, either by offering select CAM therapies or by providing patients with information, treatment recommendations, or referrals to CAM practitioners. Such practices can be described as occurring at the 'borderland of medicine, ethics, public policy, and law' [59] and require regulations and policies for conventional health care providers, for CAM practitioners as well as for product regulations. The policies and regulations across Western countries vary widely and even within countries, states, and provinces there are substantial differences in how CAM is regulated. In addition, health care professionals are often unaware of local professional guidelines or position statements, policies, and regulations regarding how CAM can be addressed within their discipline. In several countries, including Canada and the United States, policies and regulations are only beginning to be developed and vary widely, as compared to some European countries in which there is often a longer history of specific CAM professions.

As a result, the scope of practice, regulatory and disciplinary structure, as well as training of select CAM practitioners, may vary considerably on a regional basis. Other challenges, such as cost constraints in many Western health care systems and diffuse boundaries between CAM and conventional health professions and scopes of practices, have made further regulation of CAM practitioners difficult [60]. The dominance of evidence-based practice within health care may further slow the progression of statutory regulation of CAM disciplines as currently unregulated CAM professionals struggle to find sufficient evidence to support the efficacy and safety of the care they provide [61].

Most problematic has been the regulation of natural health products, which remain among the most frequently used types of CAM in cancer populations. Efforts have been made by the federal governments of Canada and the United States to ensure that over-the-counter natural health products are safe, appropriately labelled according to content, dose, and intended use, and have been produced using good manufacturing practices. For example, in Canada, the Natural Health Product Directorate (NHPD) of Health Canada (http://www.hc-sc.gc.ca/dhp-mps/prodnatur/index-eng.php) was established with the task of developing a regulatory framework that would oversee the licensing of all natural health products sold [60,62].

The evidence base for CAM

Both safety and efficacy of individual complementary therapies need to be demonstrated before determining their suitability for integration into mainstream care. For the past 15 years, the evidence supporting CAM interventions has been steadily increasing. Following the hierarchy of evidence based on study design and stringent methodological requirements, CAM evidence-based clinical practice guidelines have recently been proposed to support this safe integration. [63]. For example, within oncology populations, the benefit of mind-body medicine, the physiological basis for acupuncture, the role of touch, and the importance of appropriate exercise and nutrition have been shown [64]. However the evidence for efficacy and safety of botanical agents and other natural health products remains limited despite a number of promising laboratory investigations.

Space limitation within this chapter prevents us from presenting an exhaustive list of CAM clinical interventions that are beneficial to cancer patients, and generally safe. Only examples of recent trials and systematic reviews of commonly used CAM treatments are provided in Table 13.1 to illustrate this rapidly growing field. Details are covered in many current publications and textbooks [65–69].

Table 13.1 Evidence-based benefits of complementary and alternative medicine (CAM) interventions

CAM intervention	Evidence

Mind-Body

Mind-body medicine includes those therapies that engage the ability of the mind to affect physiology and quality of life through sustained attention-focused techniques or emotionally expressive and imaginative practices. Mind-body therapies include modalities such as hypnosis, imagery, meditation, yoga, music, and art therapy.

Meditation	Significant improvement in mood disturbance and symptoms of stress, as well as improvement in overall quality of life and sleep quality [63]
Hypnosis	• Reduces pain sensation in breast cancer patients receiving group support [70] • Improves fatigue [71] • Reduces anxiety and stress [72] • Effective for mucositis pain [72, 73] • Vomiting and nausea reduction [73] • Post-surgery pain and distress reduction, reduced anxiety, and distress [63] • Alleviate acute and chronic cancer pain conditions in children [74]. Alleviates nausea and vomiting associated with chemotherapy [74]
Relaxation and guided imagery	• Reduces pain and analgesic use, diminishes analgesic side effects [72] • Decreases nausea, vomiting, and severity of fatigue [73] • Decreases anxiety and distress significantly, reduces tension, depression, anger, and fatigue. Improves sleep induction [63] • Decreases levels of stress and increases immune functioning, decreases pain [75] • Decreases anxiety, improves mood, and less suppression of emotions [76] • Alters putative anti-cancer host defences during and after multimodality therapy [77] • Helpful for: pain control [75,78–81], recovery from cancer surgery [82], decreasing nausea and vomiting associated with chemotherapy [77, 82, 83] and the distress of radiation [84], facilitating emotional expression, and enhancing quality of life [80, 85] as well as increasing the production and functioning of immune cells, including T cells and natural killer cells [77, 86]
Mindfulness-based stress reduction (MBSR)	• Decreases mood disturbances and stress symptoms [87] • Reduces cancer-related fatigue and increases vitality [88] • Improves mood, sleep quality, and reduces stress [89] • Improves fatigue [71] • Decreases mood disturbances and stress as well as shifts immune profiles associated with decreased depressive symptoms [74] • 'Altered cortisol and immune patterns…consistent with less stress and mood disturbance' as well as enhanced quality of life and decreased symptoms of stress [90]
Expressive therapies: music, art, and dance [91]	• Music therapy: decreases incidence of nausea and vomiting [73] and reduces mood disturbance [70]; reduces pain-intensity levels and opioid requirements [92] • Effective in addressing physical, emotional, and spiritual needs of palliative care patients. Reduces anxiety and improves quality of life of terminally ill patients. Also reduces pain, tiredness, and drowsiness in palliative care patients [93]

(Continued)

Table 13.1 (Continued) Evidence-based benefits of complementary and alternative medicine (CAM) interventions

CAM intervention	Evidence
	• Mindfulness-based art therapy decreases stress-based arousal, reduces mood disturbance, is used as a coping strategy, and a way to improve quality of life [91]
Yoga	• Better social functioning, enhanced emotional well being, and mood [94] • Yoga may be a viable therapeutic intervention for improving cancer-related fatigue [88] • Tibetan yoga lowers sleep disturbance, but does not significantly impact fatigue [71] • Improves sleep quality, decreases sleep disturbances [63]
Tai Chi	• Women with breast cancer practising tai chi have experienced significant improvements in psychological and physiological symptoms compared to a control group [95, 96]

Manipulative and body-based
Therapies which involve the application of controlled force to a joint or movement of one or more parts of the body in order to restore or enhance health such as massage or chiropractic techniques.

Therapeutic massage [91] Manipulation of the soft tissues of the body using the hands for the purpose of producing positive effects on the vascular, muscular, and nervous systems of the body [97]	• Reduction of pain and anxiety [72, 98] • Immediate short term pain relief in men [70] • Enhances mood [72] • Decreases fatigue, symptoms of distress, nausea, and state anxiety [71] • Reduce anxiety, mood disturbances, and chronic pain as well as fatigue and distress [63, 99] • Aromatherapy massage helps short-term management of mild-to-moderate anxiety and depression in patients with cancer [100]

Biologically based
Biologically-based therapies comprise the wide range of natural health products, vitamins and minerals, nutraceuticals, herbal products, and other biological substances. The most commonly used herbs and vitamins among cancer patients include echinacea, ginko, garlic, green tea, shark cartilage, grape seed, milk thistle, melatonin, fish oil, ginger, saw palmetto, St. John's wort, black cohosh, cranberry, and valerian. [101].

Vitamin C, E, and coenzyme Q10	• Inconclusive results for the efficacy of antioxidant supplementation such as vitamins C and E, and coenzyme Q10 to prevent or treat cancer [102] • In cases where interactions are highly suspected, Seely et al. propose a strategy to avoid a negative interaction or even possibly instigate a synergistic effect. [103]
St. John's wort (*Hypericum perforatum*)	• It should be completely avoided during chemotherapeutic regimes as St. John's wort was found to be an active inducer of the CYP3A4 enzyme [104]

Energy therapies
Energy therapies are based on the conceptualization of the physiological body as being comprised of energy fields, which can be influenced through various techniques that may not include touching. These include therapies such as Reiki and Johrei, both of Japanese origin, Qi gong, a Chinese practice, and healing touch. Energy therapies are also an integral part of traditional Chinese medicine.

Table 13.1 (Continued) Evidence-based benefits of complementary and alternative medicine (CAM) interventions

CAM intervention	Evidence
Acupuncture Insertion and manipulation of needles into the skin at precise locations [traditionally meridians of energy; these are now known to have neurophysiological correlates] to treat various diseases or symptoms and improve health [30, 96]	• Effective for reducing the incidence of chemotherapy-induced nausea and vomiting [105], reduces chemotherapy-related neutropenia [106], cancer fatigue [71,107], and radiation-induced xerostomia [108,109] • Contributes to the control of pain (acute and chronic) and other side effects as well as helps to reduce the levels of pain medication required [63,110]; appears to be less and inconsistently effective for cancer pain [70,96] • Shown to influence the production of endogenous opioid neurotransmitters and may reduce pre-operative anxiety, but there is no report of effect on general anxiety [72] • Acupressure may have some benefit in reducing delayed chemotherapy-induced nausea and vomiting in women with breast cancer [111]

Selection based on randomized controlled trials (RCTs) and systematic reviews in recent years

In closing this section it is important to realize that CAM interventions do not always lend themselves well to assessment by means of a RCT. CAM interventions are often complex as they can include multiple components and are often administered in an individualized manner, taking into account the patient-provider relationship and the context of the treatment, including the patient's characteristics and preferences. Evaluating such interventions using methodology that requires standardization of the treatment, randomization, control of placebo effects, and often blinding may therefore lead to results that do not generally apply to patients using CAM interventions. This does not mean that CAM research should not be systematic and rigorous; however, it signals that more complex methods than RCTs may be needed for some CAM interventions [112].

The perspective that scientific evidence obtained by means of RCTs may be limited is not new; in fact Sackett, one of the leaders in promoting evidence-based medicine [EBM], has also pointed out that evidence is not solely established from research but also includes clinical expertise and patient values [113]. In combination, scientific evidence, clinical expertise, and respect for patient values are key components of optimal, evidence-based, whole-person cancer care. The question therefore is first 'how is "best evidence" determined' and 'is it really the "best" evidence'? Innovative methodologies, such as mixed methods [114] and pragmatic trials, include multimodal, non-linear quantitative and qualitative investigative approaches and are more suitable to address the true potential of integrative care and cancer control. These approaches consider the researcher, the participant, and the context as an integral part of both the intervention and the outcome measurements, which is needed to develop a rich evidence base more reflective of holistic medicine [112].

New paradigms for cancer control

Integrative oncology is an approach that crosses the conventional categories of cancer control from prevention [115,116], through treatment [32], supportive care [117], rehabilitation [118], survivorship [119,120], and end-of-life care [121]. From this perspective, it has much in common with current models of palliative care, that emphasize that whole-person care should be introduced early in the care plan, rather than during the terminal phase. Integrative oncology emphasizes a whole person and lifestyle approach to cancer care, evaluating complex systems, and collaborative pathways of care, in contrast to single interventions alone.

A new paradigm for cancer control research

Cancer control including care is much more than a constellation of separate treatments. Whole-person care includes the complex interactions of the intervention placed within the patient's personal context, which includes social relationships, expectations and beliefs, activities, and behaviours. These contextual elements develop in an ongoing process related to the patient's life situation, including social, cultural, economic, and political factors [122]. Whole-person cancer care, inherently individualized, suggests that randomized controlled trials (RCT) are ill-suited to capture the complexity of whole-person interventions. For example, such uniquely tailored patient-management challenges that would be expected of a standardized intervention, and the mere randomization may impose choices on patients and practitioners that they are not prepared to follow. Moreover, blinding and placebo control are usually impossible to achieve. In addition, RCTs typically exclude potentially important and informative qualitative and observational data about the use and benefits of an intervention in real-world settings. Ideally quantitative research is complemented by qualitative research to understand patients' experiences, motives, and behaviours.

Whole person cancer care is, in fact, a system of cancer control which is composed of interconnected parts that as a whole exhibit one or more emergent properties not obvious from the properties of the individual parts [112,123]. In addition, systems adapt to change. In order to study such systems, programmes of research are needed using various methodologies. Aickin emphasized the need to focus on the earlier stages (Early Phase Research) to advance understanding of the role of CAM and integrative medicine, rather than prematurely conducting RCTs [124].

Such a programme may roughly be divided into five phases: [124]

1 The identification of underlying assumptions of cancer control, for example whole person care.

2 Careful exploration and description of all treatment and care, as well as its process and context. This also includes identifying patterns of treatment/care between patients and settings.

3 Identification of the intended and unintended outcomes.

4 Developing testable explanations of observed processes, contexts, and outcomes (theoretical models).

5 Testing these explanations, using RCTs or modifications of such designs.

A new paradigm in oncology health care professionals' education

Many patients expect their conventional health care providers to discuss the safety and evidence for complementary therapies and to evaluate their options [125,126]. However, research suggests that most health care professionals (e.g. physicians, nurses, and pharmacists) do not have sufficient knowledge about CAM to confidently advise their patients [127–130]. At the same time, there is widespread interest on the part of educators and students to incorporate CAM content into conventional education programmes [131]. In an editorial published in Academic Medicine titled 'Is There Wheat among the Chaff?', Arthur Grollman empathically concluded that teaching about CAM is important in training competent physicians [132]. In a Canadian survey that assessed first-year medical students' attitudes, knowledge, and experiences of CAM, 52% stated that they had used CAM and 84% wanted further education [133]. Moreover, the undergraduate deans of Canadian medical schools suggested that medical school curricula should include evidence-based CAM [134]. It is especially important to begin teaching about CAM early in the undergraduate years, as it has been noted that, as conventional medical training proceeds, medical students increase their scepticism about CAM [135]. Medical students should be effectively taught CAM using the principles of evidence-based medicine [136,137].

CAM curriculum materials and teaching approaches have been developed in medical schools in several western countries like the United States [138], Canada [139], and the United Kingdom [140]. The Consortium of Academic Health Centers for Integrative Medicine includes over 40 highly esteemed academic medical centres in the United States and Canada [141]. Its mission is to help transform health care through rigorous scientific studies, new models of clinical care, and innovative educational programmes that integrate biomedicine, the complexity of human beings, the intrinsic nature of healing, and the rich diversity of therapeutic systems. Its education working group facilitates the incorporation of teaching on integrative medicine into all levels of medical education. The CAM in Undergraduate Medical Education (UME) project is a Canadian medical education initiative established in 2003 by a team of conventional and CAM educators [142]. Its main objective is to help medical school instructors impart to students the knowledge, skills, and attitudes to discuss CAM with patients in an informed and non-judgmental manner. Both initiatives developed early on a set of competencies for undergraduate medical education that can serve as a template for schools across North America and elsewhere as they move to develop a curriculum in this area [143].

Several initiatives are also underway to develop training programmes for nursing and pharmacy students regarding CAM. Health professionals such as nurses and psychosocial workers counsel patients on integrative treatment programmes. They serve as advocates for patients, providing unbiased guidance on CAM, self-care, mind-body techniques, end-of-life planning, and spiritual connectivity. With their help, patients become knowledgeable about available resources and are empowered to cope with their challenges. This role has been variously labelled 'Navigator', 'Pathfinder', or 'Cancer Guide'. Special training in integrative care counselling, covering a wide scope of practice, is provided by postgraduate courses, such as 'CancerGuides' [144].

At the postgraduate level, the Society for Integrative Oncology is a non-profit, multi-disciplinary organization founded in 2003 for health professionals committed to the study and application of complementary therapies and botanicals for cancer patients[1]. It provides a convenient forum for presentation, discussion, and peer review of evidence-based research and treatment modalities in the discipline of integrative medicine for the management of cancer patients, organizes an annual research and education conference, publishes a peer reviewed journal, and issues evidence-based practice guidelines [65].

Following the integration of CAM modalities into cancer control, it is equally important that the various complementary therapy practitioners are trained to provide evidence-based CAM information to cancer patients and maintain standards in cancer treatment programmes. For example, massage therapy is increasingly used in the supportive care programmes of many cancer centres. Indications, contraindications, communication, informed consent, and record keeping are mandatory standards that are being taught to massage therapists who participate in hospital programmes [145,146].

Redefining comprehensive cancer care within an integrative cancer control system

Over the past years the National Cancer Institute (NCI) in the United States has actively promoted the development of 'comprehensive cancer centres' characterized by scientific excellence and the capability to integrate a diversity of practices and research approaches to address the burden of cancer. As more evidence became available on the potential of CAM to improve symptom control, increase quality of life, provide more rapid and effective rehabilitation, enhance cancer control with less adverse effects, and consider consumers' cultural values, these Cancer Centres have established integrative oncology services and research programmes [67]. These centres are a major source for understanding the nature of cancer and for developing more effective approaches to cancer prevention, diagnosis, and care. They provide information about the latest research developments to patients and their families, educate health-care professionals and the public, and reach out to under-served populations.

A comprehensive cancer programme should integrate surgery, chemotherapy, radiotherapy, and molecular targeted therapies with a wide variety of meaningful, evidence-based interventions that can improve cancer control such as psycho-spiritual support, psychological therapies, physical therapies, acupuncture, and an investigative programme of promising botanical agents and other natural health products. A comprehensive cancer control system may result in economic advantages through lifestyle modification and prevention, more rapid rehabilitation, and the teaching of positive lifestyle skills to empower change. International collaboration between North American, European, and Asian universities, along with pharmaceutical companies, is encouraging the development of multi-targeted therapies from traditional herbs [147–150].

The practice of integrative oncology is already beginning to be established within the management systems of leading cancer control institutions [151]. Within cancer care settings in North America and the European Union, integrative cancer care services exist within prominent institutions, such as Memorial-Sloan Kettering Cancer Centre, the M.D. Anderson Cancer Centre in the United States, and the Royal Marsden in the United Kingdom. These centres offer inpatient and outpatient clinical care including CAM and are also involved in research and education [152]. In December 2004 in Brussels, doctors, practitioners, patients, and stakeholder organizations of the CAM community from across the European Union (EU) joined forces to promote the integration of evidence-based CAM in healthcare and agreed to become the 'European Forum for Complementary and Alternative Medicine' [EFCAM]. Their aim was to create a permanent forum for the exchange of views and information and to act as a single point of reference for the EU institutions on policy and regulatory issues of relevance for CAM. Finally, at the World Health Organization (WHO) level, the November 2008 Beijing Declaration was adopted to promote the safe and effective use of traditional medicine (TM), and ask WHO members and other stakeholders to integrate TM/CAM into national health systems [153]. Overall, the future of cancer control lies in the successful integrative approach of CAM and mainstream medicine in collaboration with all health care providers and based on a common understanding of the need for efficacy, safety, and cost effectiveness.

Conclusion

The development of integrative oncology has arisen from both a place of caution regarding the potentially harmful effects that may be associated with CAM as well as the desire on the part of CAM practitioners to be recognized as credible and legitimate health professionals with comprehensive standards and scopes of practice. However, this could only develop in a context in which patients' needs for more comprehensive cancer control were strongly expressed, identified, and recognized. Increased research on the efficacy and safety of CAM and its impact on quality of life have contributed to this movement as well. Whole person cancer care as encompassed by the term 'integrative oncology' is a system of cancer control. It is an evolutionary system composed of interconnected parts. As a whole, these parts exhibit emergent properties not obvious from the properties of the individual parts. New programmes for cancer control will be complex and comprehensive, resulting in synergistic improvements in health outcomes. More complex research methodologies, such as the mixed methods approach, will be required to measure these outcomes and to reflect the complexities of real-life situations. Although more research is required, the current indicators suggest that integrative oncology will enhance the quality of life and the rehabilitation of patients, and contribute to preventing further cancers in survivors and their families within a coherent public health programme of cancer control [9]. Ideally, future strategies will include introducing these interventions earlier, in order to enhance the primary prevention of cancer, and the incorporation of long-term economic analyses to better substantiate the potential societal benefits achievable from implementing integrative oncology.

Acknowledgment

The authors are members of the Cancer and CAM Research Team of the Sociobehavioural Cancer Research Network, Centre for Behavioural Research and Program Evaluation. The team has benefited from the financial support of the National Cancer Institute of Canada, with funds from the Canadian Cancer Society. We wish to extend our thanks to Ms Julia Bidonde, MSc, Research Officer, for her competent assistance to the project.

References

1 Sagar SM (2006). Integrative oncology in North America. *J Soc Integr Oncol*, **4**(1):27–39.

2 Ernst E, Resch KL, Mills S, et al (1995). Complementary medicine – a definition. *Br J Gen Pract*, **45**(398):506.

3 Gray RE (1998). Four perspectives on unconventional therapies. *Health (London)*, **2**(1):55–74.

4 Panel on Definition and Description (1997). Defining and describing complementary and alternative medicine. CAM Research Methodology Conference, April 1995. *Altern Ther Health Med*, **3**(2):49–57.

5 Lerner M (1994). *Choices in Healing: Integrating the Best of Conventional and Complementary Approaches to Cancer*. MIT Press, Cambridge.

6 European Forum for Complementary and Alternative Medicine (EFCAM) (2008). EFCAM Declaration. EFCAM (cited 2008 Dec. 20). Available from: URL:http://www.efcam.eu/content/view/14/28.

7 The National Institute of Complementary Medicine (NICM) (2009). Understanding Complementary Medicine (CM). NICM (cited 2009 May 20). Available from: URL:http://www.nicm.edu.au/content/view/31/35/.

8 Shumay DM, Maskarinec G, Gotay CC, Heiby EM, & Kakai H (2002). Determinants of the degree of complementary and alternative medicine use among patients with cancer. *J Altern Complement Med*, **8**(5):661–671.

9 Demark-Wahnefried W, Aziz NM, Rowland JH, & Pinto BM (2005). Riding the crest of the teachable moment: promoting long-term health after the diagnosis of cancer. *J Clin Oncol*, **23**(24):5814–30.

10 Molassiotis A, Fernadez-Ortega P, Pud D, et al (2005). Use of complementary and alternative medicine in cancer patients: a European survey. *Ann Oncol*, **16**(4):655–63.

11 Cassileth BR & Vickers AJ (2005). High prevalence of complementary and alternative medicine use among cancer patients: implications for research and clinical care. *J Clin Oncol*, **23**(12):2590–92.

12 Boon HS, Olatunde F, & Zick SM (2007). Trends in complementary/alternative medicine use by breast cancer survivors: comparing survey data from 1998 and 2005. *BMC Womens Health*, **7**(4).

13 Ponholzer A, Struhal G, & Madersbacher S (2003). Frequent use of complementary medicine by prostate cancer patients. *Eur Urol*, **43**(6):604–08.

14 Eng J, Ramsum D, Verhoef M, Guns E, Davison J, & Gallagher R (2003). A population-based survey of complementary and alternative medicine use in men recently diagnosed with prostate cancer. *Integr Cancer Ther*, **2**(3):212–16.

15 Ferner RE & Beard K (2005). Regulating herbal medicines in the UK. *BMJ*, **331**(7508):62–63.

16 Ernst E (2003). Herbal medicines put into context. *BMJ*, **327**(7420):881–82.

17 Sparreboom A, Cox MC, Acharya MR, & Figg WD. Herbal remedies in the United States: potential adverse interactions with anticancer agents. *J Clin Oncol*, **22**(12):2489–2503.

18 Fouladbakhsh JM, Stommel M, Given BA, & Given CW (2005). Predictors of use of complementary and alternative therapies among patients with cancer. *Oncol Nurs Forum*, **32**(6):1115–22.

19 Gerson-Cwilich R, Serrano-Olvera A, & Villalobos-Prieto A (2006). Complementary and alternative medicine (CAM) in Mexican patients with cancer. *Clin Transl Oncol*, **8**(3):200–07.

20 Buettner C, Kroenke CH, Phillips RS, Davis RB, Eisenberg DM, & Holmes MD (2006). Correlates of use of different types of complementary and alternative medicine by breast cancer survivors in the nurses' health study. *Breast Cancer Res Treat*, **100**(2):219–27.

21 Kimby CK, Launso L, Henningsen I, & Langgaard H (2003). Choice of unconventional treatment by patients with cancer. *J Altern Complement Med*, **9**(4):549–61.

22 Patterson RE, Neuhouser ML, Hedderson MM, et al (2002). Types of alternative medicine used by patients with breast, colon, or prostate cancer: predictors, motives, and costs. *J Altern Complement Med*, **8**(4):477–485.

23 Hann DM, Baker F, & Denniston MM (2003). Oncology professionals' communication with cancer patients about complementary therapy: a survey. *Complement Ther Med*, **11**(3):184–190.

24 Montazeri A, Sajadian A, Ebrahimi M, Haghighat S, & Harirchi I (2007). Factors predicting the use of complementary and alternative therapies among cancer patients in Iran. *Eur J Cancer Care (Engl)*, **16**(2):144–49.

25 Kakai H, Maskarinec G, Shumay DM, Tatsumura Y, & Tasaki K (2003). Ethnic differences in choices of health information by cancer patients using complementary and alternative medicine: an exploratory study with correspondence analysis. *Soc Sci Med*, **56**(4):851–862.

26 Sirois FM & Gick ML (2002). An investigation of the health beliefs and motivations of complementary medicine clients. *Soc Sci Med*, **55**(6):1025–37.

27 Sirois FM & Purc-Stephenson RJ (2008). Consumer decision factors for initial and long-term use of complementary and alternative medicine. *Complement Health Pract Rev*, **13**(1):3–19.

28 Sollner W, Maislinger S, Devries A, Steixner E, Rumpold G, & Lukas P (2000). Use of complementary and alternative medicine by cancer patients is not associated with perceived distress or poor compliance with standard treatment but with active coping behavior: a survey. *Cancer*, **89**(4):873–80.

29 Leis A & Millard J (2007). Complementary and alternative medicine (CAM) and supportive care in cancer: a synopsis of research perspectives and contributions by an interdisciplinary team. *Support Care Cancer*, **15**(8):909–12.

30 Vincent C & Furnham A (1996). Why do patients turn to complementary medicine? An empirical study. *Br J Clin Psychol*, **35**(Pt 1):37–48.

31 Boon H, Brown JB, Gavin A, & Westlake K (2003). Men with prostate cancer: making decisions about complementary/alternative medicine. *Med Decis Making*, **23**(6):471–79.

32 Hann D, Allen S, Ciambrone D, & Shah A (2006). Use of complementary therapies during chemotherapy: influence of patients' satisfaction with treatment decision making and the treating oncologist. *Integr Cancer Ther*, **5**(3):224–31.

33 Verhoef MJ, Balneaves LG, Boon HS, & Vroegindewey A (2005). Reasons for and characteristics associated with complementary and alternative medicine use among adult cancer patients: a systematic review. *Integr Cancer Ther*, **4**(4):274–86.

34 Bishop FL & Yardley L (2004). Constructing agency in treatment decisions: negotiating responsibility in cancer. *Health (London)*, **8**(4):465–482.

35 Boon H, Stewart M, Kennard MA, et al (2000). Use of complementary/alternative medicine by breast cancer survivors in Ontario: prevalence and perceptions. *J Clin Oncol*, **18**(13):2515-21.

36 Correa-Velez I, Clavarino A, & Eastwood H (2005). Surviving, relieving, repairing, and boosting up: reasons for using complementary/alternative medicine among patients with advanced cancer: a thematic analysis. *J Palliat Med*, **8**(5):953–61.

37 Evans MA, Shaw AR, Sharp DJ, et al (2007). Men with cancer: is their use of complementary and alternative medicine a response to needs unmet by conventional care? *Eur J Cancer Care (Engl)*, **16**(6):517–25.

38 Helyer LK, Chin S, Chui BK, et al (2006). The use of complementary and alternative medicines among patients with locally advanced breast cancer – a descriptive study. *BMC Cancer*, **6**:39.

39 Spiegel D (2001). Mind matters – group therapy and survival in breast cancer. *N Engl J Med*, **345**(24):1767–68.

40 Ernst E (2001). Complementary therapies in palliative cancer care. *Cancer*, **91**(11):2181–85.

41 Rakovitch E, Pignol JP, Chartier C, et al (2007). Complementary and alternative medicine use is associated with an increased perception of breast cancer risk and death. *Breast Cancer Res Treat*, **90**(2):139–48.

42 Balneaves LG, Truant TL, Kelly M, Verhoef MJ, & Davison BJ (2007). Bridging the gap: decision-making processes of women with breast cancer using complementary and alternative medicine (CAM). *Support Care Cancer*, **15**(8):973–83.

43 Lafferty WE, Tyree PT, Bellas AS, et al (2006). Insurance coverage and subsequent utilization of complementary and alternative medicine providers. *Am J Manag Care*, **12**(7):397–404.

44 Flexner A (1910). Medical education in the United States and Canada; a report to the Carnegie Foundation for the Advancement of Teaching. Carnegie Foundation for the Advancement of Teaching (cited 2009 June 2). Available from: URL:http://www.carnegiefoundation.org/publications/pub.asp?key=43&subkey=705&printable=true.

45 Beck AH (2004). The Flexner report and the standardization of American medical education. *JAMA*, **291**(17):2139–40.

46 Rosenau PM (1992). *Post-Modernism and the Social Sciences: Insights, Inroads, and Intrusions*. Princeton University Press, Princeton.

47 Chan JJ & Chan JE (2000). Medicine for the millennium: the challenge of postmodernism. *Med J Aust*, **172**(7):332–34.

48 Engel GL (1989). The need for a new medical model: a challenge for biomedicine. *J Interprof Care*, **4**(1):37–53.

49 Eastwood HL (2000). Complementary therapies: the appeal to general practitioners. *Med J Aust*, **173**(2):95–98.

50 Holland JC (2002). History of psycho-oncology: overcoming attitudinal and conceptual barriers. *Psychosom Med*, **64**(2):206–21.

51 Commonweal Cancer Help Program (2009). Commonweal (cited 2009 Jan. 27). Available from: URL:http://www.commonweal.org/programs/cancer-help.html.

52 Penny Brohn Cancer Care (2009) (cited 2009 Jan. 27). Available from: URL:http://www.pennybrohncancercare.org/default.asp.

53 Straus SE & Chesney MA (2004). NCCAM: a new plan, new priorities, and an open invitation. *Altern Ther Health Med*, **10**(6):16.

54 Cunningham AJ (2005). *Can the Mind Heal Cancer?:A Clinician-Scientist Examines the Evidence*. Hushion House, Toronto.

55 Brazier AS, Balneaves LG, Seely D, Stephen JE, Suryaprakash N, & Taylor-Brown JW (2008). Integrative practices of Canadian oncology health professionals. *Curr Oncol*, **15**(Suppl 2):S87–S91.

56 Jacobson JS, Grann VR, Gnatt MA, et al (2005). Cancer outcomes at the Hufeland (complementary/alternative medicine) klinik: a best-case series review. *Integr Cancer Ther*, **4**(2):156–67.

57 Mansky PJ & Wallerstedt DB (2006). Complementary medicine in palliative care and cancer symptom management. *Cancer J*, **12**(5):425–31.

58 Institute of Medicine of the National Academies, Committee on the Use of Complementary and Alternative Medicine by the American Public (2005). Integration of CAM and conventional medicine. In *Complementary and Alternative Medicine in the United States*, pp. 196–225. National Academies Press, Washington DC.

59 Cohen MH (2000). *Beyond Complementary Medicine: Legal and Ethical Perspectives on Health Care and Human Evolution*. University of Michigan Press, Ann Arbor.

60 Boon H (2002). Regulation of complementary/alternative medicine: a Canadian perspective. *Complement Ther Med*, **10**(1):14–19.

61 Ernst E, Cohen MH, & Stone J (2004). Ethical problems arising in evidence based complementary and alternative medicine. *J Med Ethics*, **30**(2):156–159.

62 Boon H, Brown JB, Gavin A, & Westlake K (2003). Men with prostate cancer: making decisions about complementary/alternative medicine. *Med Decis Making*, **23**(6):471–479.

63 Cassileth BR, Deng GE, Gomez JE, Johnstone PA, Kumar N, & Vickers AJ (2007). Complementary therapies and integrative oncology in lung cancer: ACCP evidence-based clinical practice guidelines. 2nd edn. *Chest*, **132**(3 Suppl):340S–54S.

64 Schmitz KH, Holtzman J, Courneya KS, Masse LC, Duval S, & Kane R (2005). Controlled physical activity trials in cancer survivors: a systematic review and meta-analysis. *Cancer Epidemiol Biomarkers Prev*, **14**(7):1588–95.

65 Gary Deng, Moshe Frenkel. Lorenzo Cohen, Barrie R. Cassileth, Donald I. Abrams, Jillian L. Capodice, Kerry S. Courneya, Trish Dryden, Suzanne Hanser, Nagi Kumar, Dan Labriola, Diane W. Wardell, and Stephen Sagar. Evidence-Based Clinical Practice Guidelines for Integrative Oncology: Complementary Therapies and Botanicals. Journal of the Society for Integrative Oncology, Vol 7, No 3 (Summer), 2009: pp 85–120.

66 Abrams D & Weil A (2008). *Integrative Oncology*. Oxford University Press, New York.

67 Cohen L & Markman M (2008). *Integrative Oncology: Incorporating Complementary Medicine into Conventional Cancer Care*. Humana Press Totowa.

68 Mumber MP (2006). *Integrative Oncology: Principles and Practice*. Taylor & Francis, New York.

69 Ernst E, Pittler MH, Wider B, & Boddy K (2008). *Oxford Handbook of Complementary Medicine*. Oxford University Press, New York.

70 Pan CX, Morrison RS, Ness J, Fugh-Berman A, & Leipzig RM (2000). Complementary and alternative medicine in the management of pain, dyspnea, and nausea and vomiting near the end of life. A systematic review. *J Pain Symptom Manage*, **20**(5):374–387.

71 Sood A, Barton DL, Bauer BA, & Loprinzi CL (2007). A critical review of complementary therapies for cancer-related fatigue. *Integr Cancer Ther*, **6**(1):8–13.

72 Deng G & Cassileth BR (2005). Integrative oncology: complementary therapies for pain, anxiety, and mood disturbance. *CA Cancer J Clin*, **55**(2):109–116.

73 Lotfi-Jam K, Carey M, Jefford M, Schofield P, Charleson C, & Aranda S (2008). Nonpharmacologic strategies for managing common chemotherapy adverse effects: a systematic review. *J Clin Oncol*, **26**(34):5618–29.

74 Monti DA, Sufian M, & Peterson C (2008). Potential role of mind-body therapies in cancer survivorship. *Cancer*. **112**(11 Suppl):2607–16.

75 Syrjala KL, Donaldson GW, Davis MW, Kippes ME, & Carr JE (1995). Relaxation and imagery and cognitive-behavioral training reduce pain during cancer treatment: a controlled clinical trial. *Pain*, **63**(2):189–198.

76 Wallace KG (1997). Analysis of recent literature concerning relaxation and imagery interventions for cancer pain. *Cancer Nurs*, **20**(2):79–88.

77 Walker M, Walker LG, Simpson E, et al (2000). Do relaxation and guided imagery improve survival in women with locally advanced breast cancer? *Psycho-oncology*, **9**(4):355.

78 Lewandowski W, Good M, & Draucker CB (2005). Changes in the meaning of pain with the use of guided imagery. *Pain Manag Nurs*, **6**(2):58–67.

79 Sloman R (2002). Relaxation and imagery for anxiety and depression control in community patients with advanced cancer. *Cancer Nurs*, **25**(6):432–35.

80 Astin JA (1998). Why patients use alternative medicine: results of a national study. *JAMA*, **279**(19):1548–53.

81 Huth MM, Broome ME, & Good M (2004). Imagery reduces children's post-operative pain. *Pain*, **110**(1–2):439–48.

82 Haase O, Schwenk W, Hermann C, & Muller JM (2005). Guided imagery and relaxation in conventional colorectal resections: a randomized, controlled, partially blinded trial. *Dis Colon Rectum*, **48**(10):1955–63.

83 Wyatt G, Sikorskii A, Siddiqi A, & Given CW (2007). Feasibility of a reflexology and guided imagery intervention during chemotherapy: results of a quasi-experimental study. *Oncol Nurs Forum*, **34**(3):635–42.

84 Nunes DFT, Rodriguez AL, da Silva Hoffmann F, et al (2007). Relaxation and guided imagery program in patients with breast cancer undergoing radiotherapy is not associated with neuroimmunomodulatory effects. *J Psychosom Res*, **63**(6):647–55.

85 Yoo HJ, Ahn SH, Kim SB, Kim WK, & Han OS (2005). Efficacy of progressive muscle relaxation training and guided imagery in reducing chemotherapy side effects in patients with breast cancer and in improving their quality of life. *Support Care Cancer*, **13**(10):826–33.

86 Leon-Pizarro C, Gich I, Barthe E, et al (2007). A randomized trial of the effect of training in relaxation and guided imagery techniques in improving psychological and quality-of-life indices for gynecologic and breast brachytherapy patients. *Psychooncology*, **16**(11):971–79.

87 Speca M, Carlson LE, Goodey E, & Angen M (2000). A randomized, wait-list controlled clinical trial: the effect of a mindfulness meditation-based stress reduction program on mood and symptoms of stress in cancer outpatients. *Psychosom Med*, **62**(5):613–22.

88 Mustian KM, Morrow GR, Carroll JK, Figueroa-Moseley CD, Jean-Pierre P, & Williams GC (2007). Integrative nonpharmacologic behavioral interventions for the management of cancer-related fatigue. *Oncologist*, **12**(Suppl 1):52–67.

89 Smith JE, Richardson J, Hoffman C, & Pilkington K (2005). Mindfulness-based stress reduction as supportive therapy in cancer care: systematic review. *J Adv Nurs*, **52**(3):315–27.

90 Carlson LE, Speca M, Faris P, & Patel KD (2007). One year pre-post intervention follow-up of psychological, immune, endocrine and blood pressure outcomes of mindfulness-based stress reduction (MBSR) in breast and prostate cancer outpatients. *Brain Behav Immun*, **21**(8):1038–49.

91 Monti DA & Peterson C (2003). Mindfulness-based art therapy (MBAT). *Integr Cancer Ther*, **2**(1):81–83.

92 Cepeda MS, Carr DB, Lau J, & Alvarez H (2006). Music for pain relief. *Cochrane Database Syst Rev*, (2):CD004843.

93 Horne-Thompson A & Grocke D (2008). The effect of music therapy on anxiety in patients who are terminally ill. *J Palliat Med*, **11**(4):582–90.

94 Moadel AB, Shah C, Wylie-Rosett J, et al (2007). Randomized controlled trial of yoga among a multiethnic sample of breast cancer patients: effects on quality of life. *J Clin Oncol*, **25**(28):4387–95.

95 Lee MS, Pittler MH, & Ernst E (2007). Is Tai Chi an effective adjunct in cancer care? A systematic review of controlled clinical trials. *Support Care Cancer*, **15**(6):597–601.

96 Lee H, Schmidt K, & Ernst E (2005). Acupuncture for the relief of cancer-related pain – a systematic review. *Eur J Pain*, **9**(4):437–44.

97 Liu Y & Fawcett TN (2008). The role of massage therapy in the relief of cancer pain. *Nurs Stand*, **22**(21):35–40.

98 Fellowes D, Barnes K, & Wilkinson S (2004). Aromatherapy and massage for symptom relief in patients with cancer. *Cochrane Database Syst Rev*, (2):CD002287.

99 Mehling WE, Jacobs B, Acree M, et al (2007). Symptom management with massage and acupuncture in postoperative cancer patients: a randomized controlled trial. *J Pain Symptom Manage*, **33**(3):258–66.

100 Wilkinson SM, Love SB, Westcombe AM, Gambles MA, Burgess CC, & Cargill A, et al (2007). Effectiveness of aromatherapy massage in the management of anxiety and depression in patients with cancer: a multicenter randomized controlled trial. *J Clin Oncol*, **25**(5):532–39.

101 Oneschuk D & Younus J (2008). Natural health products and cancer chemotherapy and radiation therapy. *Oncol Rev*, **1**(4):233–42.

102 Block KI, Koch AC, Mead MN, Tothy PK, Newman RA, & Gyllenhaal C (2007). Impact of antioxidant supplementation on chemotherapeutic efficacy: a systematic review of the evidence from randomized controlled trials. *Cancer Treat Rev*, **33**(5):407–418.

103 Seely D, Stempak D, & Baruchel S (2007). A strategy for controlling potential interactions between natural health products and chemotherapy: a review in pediatric oncology. *J Pediatr Hematol Oncol*, **29**(1):32–47.

104 Mannel M (2004). Drug interactions with St John's wort: mechanisms and clinical implications. *Drug Saf*, **27**(11):773–97.

105 Ezzo J, Vickers A, Richardson MA, et al (2005). Acupuncture-point stimulation for chemotherapy-induced nausea and vomiting. *J Clin Oncol*, **23**(28):7188–98.

106 Lu W, Hu D, Dean-Clower E, et al (2007). Acupuncture for chemotherapy-induced leukopenia: exploratory meta-analysis of randomized controlled trials. *J Soc Integr Oncol*, **5**(1):1–10.

107 Vickers AJ, Straus DJ, Fearon B, & Cassileth BR (2004). Acupuncture for postchemotherapy fatigue: a phase II study. *J Clin Oncol*, **22**(9):1731–35.

108 Johnstone PA, Niemtzow RC, & Riffenburgh RH (2002). Acupuncture for xerostomia: clinical update. *Cancer*, **94**(4):1151–56.

109 Wong RKW, Jones GW, Sagar SM, Babjak AF, & Whelan T (2003). A Phase I-II study in the use of acupuncture-like transcutaneous nerve stimulation in the treatment of radiation-induced xerostomia in head-and-neck cancer patients treated with radical radiotherapy. *Int J Radiat Oncol Biol Phys*, **57**(2):472–80.

110 Alimi D, Rubino C, Pichard-Leandri E, Fermand-Brule S, Dubreuil-Lemaire ML, & Hill C (2003). Analgesic effect of auricular acupuncture for cancer pain: a randomized, blinded, controlled trial. *J Clin Oncol*, **21**(22):4120–26.

111 Dibble SL, Luce J, Cooper BA, et al (2007). Acupressure for chemotherapy-induced nausea and vomiting: a randomized clinical trial. *Oncol Nurs Forum*, **34**(4):813–20.

112 Verhoef MJ & Leis A (2008). From studying patient treatment to studying patient care: arriving at methodologic crossroads. *Hematol Oncol Clin North Am*, **22**(4):671–82.

113 Sackett DL, Straus SE, Richardson WS, Rosenberg W, & Haynes RB (2000). *Evidence-Based Medicine: How to Practice andTeach EBM*. 2nd edn. Churchill Livingstone, New York.

114 Creswell JW (2008). *Research Design: Qualitative, Quantitative, and Mixed Methods Approaches*. 3rd ed. Sage Publications, Thousand Oaks.

115 Allan J, Barwick TA, Cashman S, et al (2004). Clinical prevention and population health: curriculum framework for health professions. *Am J Prev Med*, **27**(5):471–476.

116 Gaynor M (2004). Environmental oncology: an emerging science in cancer prevention and treatment. Interview by Jennifer Repo. *Altern Ther Health Med*, **10**(3):80–85.

117 Sagar SM & Cassileth BR (2005). Integrative oncology for comprehensive cancer centres: definitions, scope and policy. *Curr Oncol*, **12**:103–117.

118 Vargo MM (2008). The oncology-rehabilitation interface: better systems needed. *J Clin Oncol*, **26**(16):2610–11.

119 Wesa K, Gubili J, & Cassileth B (2008). Integrative oncology: complementary therapies for cancer survivors. *Hematol Oncol Clin North Am*, **22**(2):343–53.

120 Rowland JH, Aziz N, Tesauro G, & Feuer EJ (2001). The changing face of cancer survivorship. *Semin Oncol Nurs*, **17**(4):236–40.

121 Lewis CR, de Vedia A, Reuer B, Schwan R, & Tourin C (2003). Integrating complementary and alternative medicine (CAM) into standard hospice and palliative care. *Am J Hosp Palliat Care*, **20**(3):221–28.

122 Verhoef MJ, Mulkins A, Carlson LE, Hilsden RJ, & Kania A (2007). Assessing the role of evidence in patients' evaluation of complementary therapies: a quality study. *Integr Cancer Ther*, **6**(4):345–53.

123 Leis AM, Weeks LC, & Verhoef MJ (2008). Principles to guide integrative oncology and the development of an evidence base. *Curr Oncol*, **15**(Suppl 2):S83–S87.

124 Aickin M (2003). Participant-centered analysis in complementary and alternative medicine comparative trials. *J Altern Complement Med*, **9**(6):949–57.

125 O'Beirne M, Verhoef M, Paluck E, & Herbert C (2004). Complementary therapy use by cancer patients. Physicians' perceptions, attitudes, and ideas. *Can Fam Physician*, **50**:882–88.

126 Richardson MA, Masse LC, Nanny K, & Sanders C (2004). Discrepant views of oncologists and cancer patients on complementary/alternative medicine. *Support Care Cancer*, **12**(11):797–804.

127 Cohen L, Cohen MH, Kirkwood C, & Russell NC (2007). Discussing complementary therapies in an oncology setting. *J Soc Integr Oncol*, **5**(1):18–24.

128 Winslow LC & Shapiro H (2002). Physicians want education about complementary and alternative medicine to enhance communication with their patients. *Arch Intern Med*, **162**(10):1176–81.

129 Verhoef MJ & Sutherland LR (1995). Alternative medicine and general practitioners. Opinions and behaviour. *Can Fam Physician*, **41**:1005–11.

130 Baugniet J, Boon H, & Ostbye T (2000). Complementary/alternative medicine: comparing the view of medical students with students in other health care professions. *Fam Med*, **32**(3):178–84.

131 Verhoef M, Best A, & Boon H (2002). Role of complementary medicine in medical education: opinions of medical educators. *Ann R Coll Physicians Surg Can*, **35**(3):166–70.

132 Grollman AP (2001). Alternative medicine: the importance of evidence in medicine and in medical education. Is there wheat among the chaff? *Acad Med*, **76**(3):221–23.

133 Duggan K, Verhoef MJ, & Hilsden RJ (1999). First-year medical students and complementary and alternative medicine: attitudes, knowledge, and experiences. *Ann R Coll Physicians Surg Can*, **32**:157–60.

134 Verhoef M, Brundin-Mather R, Jones A, Boon H, & Epstein M (2004). Complementary and alternative medicine in undergraduate medical education. Associate deans' perspectives. *Can Fam Physician*, **50**:847–49.

135 Furnham A & McGill C (2003). Medical students' attitudes about complementary and alternative medicine. *J Altern Complement Med*, **9**(2):275–84.

136 Forjuoh SN, Rascoe TG, Symm B, & Edwards JC (2003). Teaching medical students complementary and alternative medicine using evidence-based principles. *J Altern Complement Med*, **9**(3):429–39.

137 Wetzel MS, Kaptchuk TJ, Haramati A, & Eisenberg DM (2003). Complementary and alternative medical therapies: implications for medical education. *Ann Intern Med*, **138**(3):191–96.

138 Maizes V, Schneider C, Bell I, & Weil A (2002). Integrative medical education: development and implementation of a comprehensive curriculum at the University of Arizona. *Acad Med*, **77**(9):851–60.

139 Sierpina VS, Kreitzer MJ, Burke A, Verhoef M, & Brundin-Mather R (2007). Innovations in integrative healthcare education: undergraduate holistic studies at San Francisco State University and the CAM in undergraduate medical education project in Canada. Explore:*J Sci Healing* (NY), **3**(2):174–76.

140 Owen DK, Lewith G, & Stephens CR (2001). Can doctors respond to patients' increasing interest in complementary and alternative medicine? *BMJ*, **322**(7279):154–58.

141 Brokaw JJ, Tunnicliff G, Raess BU, & Saxon DW (2002). The teaching of complementary and alternative medicine in U.S. medical schools: a survey of course directors. *Acad Med*, **77**(9):876–81.

142 Verhoef M, Epstein M, & Brundin-Mather R (2004). Developing a national vision for complementary and alternative medicine in undergraduate medical education: report on an invitational workshop held September 27–28, 2003. *Complementary and Alternative Medicine Issues in Undergraduate Medical Education* (cited 2009 June 2). Available from: URL:http://www.caminume.ca/documents/visionworkshop.pdf.

143 Kligler B, Maizes V, Schachter S, et al (2004). Core competencies in integrative medicine for medical school curricula: a proposal. *Acad Med*, **79**(6):521–31.

144 Staples JK, Wilson AT, Pierce B, & Gordon JS (2007). Effectiveness of CancerGuides a study of an integrative cancer care training program for health professionals. *Integr Cancer Ther*, **6**(1):14–24.

145 Sagar SM, Dryden T, & Wong RK (2007). Massage therapy for cancer patients: a reciprocal relationship between body and mind. *Curr Oncol*, **14**(2):45–56.

146 Russell NC, Sumler SS, Beinhorn CM, & Frenkel MA (2008). Role of massage therapy in cancer care. *J Altern Complement Med*, **14**(2):209–14.

147 Yance DR, Jr. & Sagar SM (2006). Targeting angiogenesis with integrative cancer therapies. *Integr Cancer Ther*, **5**(1):9–29.

148 Sagar SM & Wong RK (2008). Chinese medicine and biomodulation in cancer patients-Part one. *Curr Oncol*, **15**(1):42–48.

149 Sagar SM & Wong RK (2008). Chinese medicine and biomodulation in cancer patients-Part two. *Curr Oncol*, **15**(2):8–30.

150 Sagar SM (2007). Future directions for research on Silybum marianum for cancer patients. *Integr Cancer Ther*, **6**(2):166–73.

151 Editorial: What makes a practice a standard of excellence in integrated care (2008)? *Hematol Oncol News & Issues*.

152 Sagar SM (2008). Clinical audit of an integrative oncology program: how should we measure outcome? *Focus Altern Complement Ther*, **13**(3):168–72.

153 World Health Organization (2009). Beijing declaration (adopted by the WHO Congress on Traditional Medicine, Beijing, China, 8 November 2008). World Health Organization (cited 2009 May 21). Available from: URL:http://www.who.int/medicines/areas/traditional/congress/beijing_declaration/en/index.html.

Chapter 14

Patient-centred supportive and palliative care

Genevieve Thompson, Carla Ens, Harvey Chochinov[1]

Born out of the desire to alleviate the suffering of cancer patients [1], Dame Cicely Saunders and her colleagues developed the modern hospice movement in the United Kingdom in 1967. Since then, palliative care has been adopted throughout the world as a humanistic approach to patient care. Within the empirical literature, authors' definitions of palliative care provide insight into its core components. The widely applied definition by the World Health Organization (WHO) proposes that palliative care gives relief from pain and other distressing symptoms, affirms life, and views death as normal, neither hastens nor postpones death; integrates both spiritual and psychological aspects into care, offers support systems to patients, supports families during illness and bereavement, applies a multi-disciplinary team approach, enhances quality of life, and is applied over the entire course of the illness [2]. A generally accepted view of palliative care is that it is the active total care of patients whose disease is not responsive to curative treatment. It encompasses all treatment modalities that are aimed at enhancing quality of life rather than curing disease [3]. Within the cancer context, clinical oncology may incorporate two distinct aspects when defining palliative care: on the one hand, palliative care is about pain control and symptom management and, on the other hand, it involves non-curative tumour-directed treatments [4]. Whatever the wording, the definitions of palliative care have one constant emphasis: consideration for the patient's quality of life.

A similar emphasis is noted in the definition of cancer control as a public health programme 'designed to reduce the number of cancer cases and deaths and improve quality of life of cancer patients' [5]. The cancer control model purports to include the spectrum of care from primary prevention, early diagnosis, optimal treatment, and supportive and palliative care [6]; it can be viewed as a four member team, with each player making critical contributions to patient care. Theoretically, this population-based cancer control team appears seamless and equitable. After all, each player is concerned with a patient's overall quality of life during his or her experiences with cancer. However, it is unclear from the empirical literature if this team is actually cohesive or if the palliative care player is viewed as the 'poor cousin', left to fend for him or herself as resources become available. Was the notion of the cancer control team, consisting of players 'primary prevention', 'early diagnosis', 'curative treatment', and 'palliative care', formed out of

[1] Genevieve N. Thompson, RN, PhD, Manitoba Palliative Care Research Unit, CancerCare Manitoba, Research Associate, Faculty of Nursing, University of Manitoba, Winnipeg, Manitoba, Canada; Carla D.L. Ens, MSc, PhD, Department of Community Health Sciences, University of Manitoba, Canada; and Harvey M.Chochinov, MD, PhD, FRSC, Distinguished Professor and Canada Research Chair in Palliative Care, Department of Psychiatry, University of Manitoba, Director, Manitoba Palliative Care Research Unit, CancerCare Manitoba, Winnipeg, Manitoba, Canada.

convenience, proposed to satisfy practitioners with a more psychosocial bent, or one of necessity, aimed to meet the defined needs of patients, families, and caregivers?

Global cancer statistics indicate that cancer incidence and mortality are on the rise [7,8]; in 2002, over 7.5 million people worldwide died of cancer [9]. With about half of the world's new cancer cases occurring in developing countries, and approximately 80 per cent of these cancer patients presenting at an incurable stage of the disease, palliative care cannot be considered optional [10]. Factors such as cancer survival rates, an ageing population, and the importance of alleviating suffering during illness, contribute to the necessity for palliative care as an integral and critical component of the cancer control team [11]. The purpose of this chapter is to expand on the role of palliative care within the framework of cancer control. In addition, the public health approach outlined by the WHO, including appropriate policy, adequate drug availability, education, and palliative care delivery at all levels of health care, will be discussed. Finally, the challenges in adapting these principles into high and low resource settings will be described.

Role of palliative care in cancer control

Consideration must be given to the nature and description of palliative care within the cancer control model. The following section describes the role of palliative care within the spectrum of cancer care. Furthermore, it expands on and defines the different types of palliative care within health care today.

What is cancer control?

To address the growing burden of cancer worldwide, the WHO has pioneered initiatives and policies aimed at reducing the incidence and mortality of cancer through primary prevention, early detection, and application of anticancer treatment strategies [12]. Despite significant advances in anticancer treatment strategies, an estimated 60 per cent of cancer patients will experience significant pain and worldwide, two-thirds will not be cured [13], thus placing significant numbers of persons at risk of suffering from physical, psychological, social, spiritual and existential distress. The prevention of suffering has become recognized as an integral aspect of cancer control. The WHO, as seen in Figure 14.1, has advocated that palliative care is a critical component of national cancer control programmes [14]. This model has been adopted worldwide as a framework guiding the development of comprehensive cancer control strategies [6,15].

Thus cancer control can be defined as an overall strategy with four goals: (i) preventing disease; (ii) identifying early disease; (iii) treating to cure, rehabilitate, or prolong the lives of patients with invasive cancer; and (iv) prevention of suffering through the anticipation, early detection, and palliation of physical, psychosocial, existential/spiritual, and social concerns of patients [16]. One of the challenges facing the incorporation of palliative care into a national cancer control strategy is defining what is meant by palliative care.

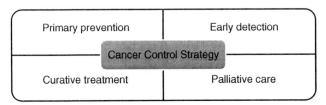

Fig. 14.1 The four integrated components of a comprehensive cancer control strategy
Source: From Stjernsward et al. (2007) [6].

What is palliative care?

Palliative care is 'an approach to care that improves the quality of life of patients and their families facing the problems associated with life-threatening illness, through the prevention and relief of suffering by means of early identification and impeccable assessment and treatment of pain, and other physical, psychosocial, and spiritual problems'[2]. The philosophy of palliative care espouses: (a) a patient and family focus; (b) active management of distressing symptoms; (c) total, individualized care of the patient; (d) an interdisciplinary team approach; (e) integration of the psychological and spiritual aspects of care; (f) supporting the family throughout the patient's illness and in their own bereavement; and (g) offering support to the patient so they may live as actively as possible until death [17,18]. Other tenets of palliative care include an open and positive attitude towards dying and death; viewing illness not as an isolated aberration in physiology, but rather in terms of the suffering it may cause [19].

Types of palliative care

As a pillar in any cancer control programme, palliative care is not limited to the final months of a patient's life [12]. Rather, it is vital to consider different modalities and intensities of care based on the unique needs of the individual and where along the illness trajectory they may be. In this regard, it is important to distinguish between a palliative approach, specialized palliative care, supportive care, hospice care, and end-of-life or terminal care [7,20].

A palliative approach

The principles of a palliative care approach are integral and intrinsic to all good clinical care, regardless of the nature or stage of the patient's illness [21]. In this manner, a patient undergoing active treatment for their disease may concurrently benefit from a palliative approach. The overall goal of a palliative approach is to improve the quality of life of the individual and reduce suffering, through improved comfort and level of function.

Specialist palliative care

Specialist palliative care services augment the palliative care approach, through targeted interventions delivered by multidisciplinary professionals with palliative care expertise. In this regard, the services provided by a specialist palliative care team serve as a resource to the primary care professionals [22]. When the care needs of the patient extend beyond the practitioner's level of expertise or when the patient is experiencing multiple or complex care needs, patients benefit from a referral to a palliative care specialist [21,23]. It is generally agreed that a small minority of patients will require specialized palliative care services during the course of their illness [20].

Supportive care

The phrase 'supportive care' emerged from chemotherapy clinical trial studies, describing the care provided to the comparison group; since then the term has become more frequent in the oncology literature to describe non-chemotherapeutic palliation [24,25]. Supportive care is not synonymous with palliative care but palliative care is an essential part of supportive care [26]. The objectives of supportive care are to manage the complications of cancer, cancer-related physical and psychological distress, and to alleviate the toxicities induced by anticancer treatments [27].

Hospice care

In many countries, hospice is the term used to define a place of care. In addition to being a place of care, hospice denotes a broader philosophy based on the principles of palliative care. Hospices are often funded by charities and act as specialized palliative care units, often focusing on end-of-life care [28] or delivering specialized services to patients in the community (e.g. home care, nursing homes). In countries with fewer resources, hospices are the primary source for palliative care services. These services include, but are not limited to: inpatient care, home care, hospital support teams, orphan support groups, and education [29].

End-of-life or terminal care

On the surface, the definition of end-of-life care is self-evident: the care that patients and their families receive when patients are dying or near death. End-of-life care is most frequently provided during the last days or weeks of life and focuses on preventing suffering by attending to the physical, emotional, and spiritual comfort of the patient and family. End-of-life care is the specific application of palliative care interventions in the last hours, days, or weeks of life [28].

Palliative care as a public health approach within cancer control programmes

Palliative care, like other aspects of cancer control, can be regarded as an exercise in prevention – prevention of suffering through timely diagnosis and expert management of physical symptoms and of psychosocial and spiritual concerns, at the earliest possible moment [19]. Ultimately, excellent palliative care is anticipatory in nature, rather than reactive. Evidence suggests that physical, emotional, or psychosocial symptoms not treated at the early stages of illness, become very difficult to manage later in the course of illness. In order to reduce patient and family suffering, implementing palliative care earlier in the course of disease as outlined by cancer control strategies is essential. The WHO's public health approach provides guidance in this endeavour by outlining four areas that are necessary for the integration of palliative care in cancer control: (i) appropriate policies; (ii) adequate drug availability; (iii) education of health care workers and the public; and (iv) implementation of palliative care services at all levels [30]. Each of these areas will be discussed in detail.

Policies to move palliative care ahead . . . barriers that stall progress

In the past four decades, there has been a steady growth in policy aimed at defining the core elements of palliative care programmes and their role within cancer care. Significant documents like the 'WHO Definition of Palliative Care' [2] along with their programme for Cancer Pain Relief – which introduced the three-step analgesic ladder with use of adjuvant treatment – have been significant markers in the global push to incorporate palliative care within cancer control models. An extensive review of international, national, and local policies is beyond the remit of this chapter. Several articles provide excellent reviews of policies in the United Kingdom [31], the United States [32], and the European Union [33]. The history of palliative care development in cancer is also available [29]. However, we will highlight key policy developments in palliative care and cancer control in order to further explore the integration of palliative care within a cancer control strategy.

Developing palliative care policy

Ensuring that appropriate policies are in place at the national and local level is a key requirement of the WHO public health approach to integrating palliative care within a cancer control strategy [12]. National policies are essential for facilitating the implementation of palliative care programmes within health care plans [6]. A significant step for many countries has been to declare palliative care as a right of its citizens. For example, in Canada, this was declared in June 2000 with the release of the Senate Subcommittee report 'Quality End-of-Life Care: The Right of Every Canadian' [34]. This foundational report detailed the importance of developing a Canadian strategy on palliative and end-of-life care, overseen by a national secretariat. This was established in 2001, within the federal department of Health Canada. As a result of these commitments, substantial progress in national end-of-life care policy has been made in Canada including: the development of Pan-Canadian Gold Standards for Palliative Home Care; National Norms of Practice and Accreditation Standards; and the Compassionate Care Benefit Program[2]. Similar declarations and policies have been made in the United Kingdom, Australia, and the European Union[3].

The role of non-governmental organizations

Worldwide, there has been a groundswell of activity by non-governmental organizations (NGOs) in the area of palliative end-of-life care. This is mainly due to the diligent work of national and local hospice palliative care organizations aimed at defining palliative care services, developing innovative models of care, standards of practice, accreditation standards, and guideline development. In the United States, for example, the National Consensus Project for Quality Palliative Care brought together multiple stakeholders to develop 'voluntary clinical practice guidelines to guide the growth and expansion of palliative care in the United States' [35, p.738]. Other countries have developed binding guidelines, recommending explicit service delivery models for palliative care [36]. On an international level, the WHO National Program against Cancer identified palliative care as a priority for national cancer programmes and suggested that governments revise their funding policies for the allocation of resources for palliative care [12].

Despite these constructive initiatives, several barriers exist that impede the development of palliative care policies within cancer care strategies. Firstly, the essential components of cancer care are not uniformly agreed upon or defined within legislation. While countries like the United States and Great Britain have a national cancer act outlining the essential elements of cancer care, others, such as Canada, are lacking an equivalent legislative mandate. In the United States, for example, the original National Cancer Act was declared in 1971; in 2007 and 2008, suggested amendments expanded the scope of care to include palliative and end-of-life care. An additional bill, the Comprehensive Cancer Care Improvement Act[4], was passed with hopes of expanding the traditional mandate of cancer care to include palliative and symptom management programmes. In the United Kingdom, the National Health Service (NHS) has developed a Cancer Plan, outlining actions that ensure patients receive the correct professional support, care, and treatment, along with aims to improve the palliative care and psychosocial support provided [37].

In the absence of a national cancer act or declaration, countries are left with little guidance or structure. In Canada, as an example, it is left to provincial jurisdictions to decide if palliative care is included within the mandates of provincial cancer centres or if it is defined as a core

....

2   This is an employment insurance benefit which pays up to a maximum of six weeks to a person who has to be absent from work to provide care or support to a gravely ill family member at risk of dying within 26 weeks [111].

3   In 1989 and 1992 the European parliament adopted resolutions on counselling and care of the terminally ill; the Council of Europe published a set of European guidelines on palliative care in 2003, describing this care as an essential and basic service for the whole population [29].

4   Introduced to the US Senate in March 2008, this bill seeks to provide coverage of comprehensive cancer care planning under the Medicare program and to improve the care delivered to individuals diagnosed with cancer by establishing a Medicare hospice demonstration program and grants for palliative care and symptom management programs, education, and related research [112].

health service. In one of the Canadian provinces for example, palliative care is a core health service within the provincial health department, but is not part of the programme objectives of Cancer Care Manitoba, the provincial cancer centre. Leaving provincial jurisdictions to decide if palliative care is part of cancer control results in the fractured delivery of palliative care services nationally and provincially, ultimately causing a disparity in the services provided for Canadians with cancer. In 2006, the federal government funded the Canadian Partnership against Cancer, which will oversee the implementation of the Canadian Strategy for Cancer Control [38]. Developing a coordinated national cancer control programme that incorporates palliative care throughout the cancer continuum along with public education, legislation, and action planning is a key to preventing undue suffering and providing dignified care to persons with cancer [39].

The other significant barrier to the development of policies concerning palliative care within a cancer control strategy is the lack of funding and reimbursement for the relief of suffering. Current physician billing structures are not geared towards remuneration strategies based on time spent with patients and families, beyond immediate treatment issues. As such, psychosocial and existential/spiritual dimensions of caring are particularly vulnerable and often sacrificed. One of the means to redress this may be to develop policies and billing codes, aimed at identifying the suffering experienced by cancer patients and the multifaceted approaches required within comprehensive, quality palliation. The current cancer staging system, for example, describes in detail the tumour type, location, and node involvement or metastasis (TNM system), yet does not capture the impact on quality of life, symptom load, or other burdens the patient may be experiencing. Only one cancer out of 49 staged by the TNM system includes symptoms as an important factor: lymphoma [40]. Adjusting this classification system to capture dimensions of suffering due to tumour burden, treatment effects, and symptom distress, would transform the field of oncology. This nosological approach would see palliative care principles applied to all patients, and reimbursement mechanisms based on tumour load and burden of suffering. Norway in 2003 developed a diagnosis-related group billing code for inpatient palliative care patients, to ensure more predictable and secure funding [41]. Appropriate billing structures for physicians will help ensure that more doctors will engage in preventative palliative care. This preventive approach addresses physical, psychological, existential, and spiritual distress of patients early in the trajectory of illness, which ultimately may ameliorate suffering at the end of life [42].

Finally, the current enrolment criteria of many hospice or palliative care programmes of six months of life expectancy or less, is a significant barrier to implementing palliative care within cancer control strategies. Physicians tend to be very poor at making accurate prognoses [43], and are often overly optimistic in their estimates of time left to live. Additionally, most hospice and palliative care programmes limit patients' options regarding life-extending treatment [44]. This places patients in the position of having to choose between curative intervention and palliation; a dichotomy that works against the principles of supportive health care. By moving away from prognosis-based criteria, to criteria based on holistic patient and family needs, a palliative model of care can emerge, responding to a broad spectrum of issues and concerns facing patients and families encountering life threatening or life limiting cancer [45].

Ensuring drug availability: a chain of command

Freedom from pain must be regarded as a human rights issue [46,47]. To redress inadequacies in pain control, in 1986, the WHO developed a three-step 'ladder' to guide clinicians in the management of cancer pain. Designed to be both effective and inexpensive, drug administration moves from non-opioids (aspirin and paracetamol) to mild opioids (codeine) and then to strong opioids (morphine) in response to patients' reported pain levels. The pain ladder also recommends adjuvant drugs be administered and that drugs should be given 'by the clock', opposed to on demand [48]. Over the past two decades, research has shown that WHO's pain control ladder has been applied in a multitude of settings with high rates of success [49–54]. It is highly regarded as a simple drug management plan that is easily transferable between different countries, and settings.

For the last three decades, the WHO has also published a 'Model List of Essential Medicines'. Essential medicines are those that satisfy the primary health care needs of the population [55] and are reviewed every two years. Medicines are selected 'with due regard to disease prevalence, evidence on efficacy and safety, and comparative cost-effectiveness' [55, p. 522]. At WHO's request, a working group was selected by the International Association of Hospice and Palliative Care (IAHPC) to formulate an essential medicines list for palliative care. This list, consisting of 33 medications – 14 of which were already included on the WHO Model List – is now publicly available and should increase access to appropriate medications for patients who have uncontrolled symptoms [55].

The assessment and treatment of symptoms is a cornerstone of palliative care. To be effective in this endeavour, palliative care programmes require national drug policies that allow for ready access to opioids, equitable distribution, fair pricing, and training in essential medications for health care providers [56]. Even with the excellent guidelines provided by organizations like the WHO and IAHPC, adequate symptom control through prescription of medications is difficult to ensure. The most commonly reported barriers are the availability of opioids, a lack of health care provider and public knowledge, and excessively strict national laws and regulations. These barriers are not limited to developing countries; examples of disparity in access exist in developed countries as well [57,58].

Opioid supply

Ensuring an adequate supply of opioids worldwide is a balancing act (see Figure 14.2). According to work by the Pain and Policy Studies Group (PPSG)[5], there should be an ongoing system of communication amongst various stakeholders within both the health care and the drug supply industry [59]; with inadequate information or poor communication, the balance to ensure adequate medication will be thrown off. For example, information that the International Narcotics Control Board receives ultimately determines poppy harvest and supply. The National Competent Authority's role is to estimate drug requirements and control the distribution chain whereas the importers, manufacturers, and distributors must produce and import sufficient quantities for retail distribution. Concurrently, the health care sector needs to be involved in ongoing training and the purchase of supplies to meet need while anticipating patients' drug needs. On the micro level, physicians and nurses work to assess patients' pain and prescribe according to need. Each element of the system must work together to ensure adequate supply and distribution of opioid analgesics.

A disparate consumption pattern has developed between resource-scarce and resource-wealthy countries: the lowest-income countries consume only a small proportion of opioids while a subset of developed countries consume the vast majority [59,60]. Quite simply, drugs are not consistently available in many countries [61]; a report by Help the Hospices indicated that over 20 per cent of palliative care service providers in Africa can never access strong opioids such as morphine [60]. The difference in consumption may be due, in part, to the excessively strict

---

[5] Based at the Paul P. Carbone Comprehensive Cancer Centre in the University of Wisconsin School of Medicine and Public Health and established in 1996. It is designated as a WHO Collaborating Centre [59].

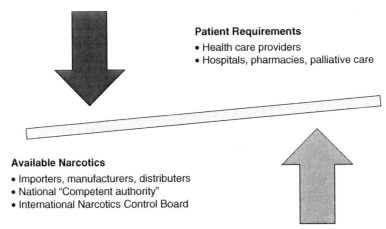

Patient Requirements
- Health care providers
- Hospitals, pharmacies, palliative care

Available Narcotics
- Importers, manufacturers, distributers
- National "Competent authority"
- International Narcotics Control Board

Fig. 14.2 Elements of opioid distribution system
Source: From Joranson and Ryan (2007) [59].

governmental regulations, cumbersome administrative procedures [62], or a lack of foreign currency to import the necessary drugs [63] that exist in many parts of the world.

Gap in knowledge

The extreme differences in opioid consumption patterns may also be due to the general (mis) understanding of opioids amongst health care providers. While there may be a 'gap between what is known about pain relief and what is actually done in terms of practice and care' [59, p. 531], it may simply be that best practices in palliative care – including pain and symptom control – are not part of many medical curricula. Without knowing the benefits and uses of opioids, it would be impossible for a doctor or nurse to include them in their management of patients [6,60,61,64]. Furthermore, this lack of knowledge by practitioners feeds into the imbalance of opioid availability; if health care staff do not document the patients' need for narcotics, then an increase in supply will not be realized [65].

For both health care practitioners and patients who have limited knowledge or understanding of morphine, the issue of morphine use is exacerbated by the myths related to morphine as the cause of death, fears of addiction, and fears of tolerance [60–62, 66, 67]. In South Africa, for example, morphine is not readily available in all health care centres [68]; the drug is typically only available in provincial hospitals and may only be available on certain days of the week [69]. Even in large centres where pain control medications are readily available, pain is still often under managed [70,71]. This reflects a general lack of knowledge in effective pain control techniques nationwide.

National laws and regulations

In many countries, national regulations are prohibitive regarding morphine use [61]. One report states that 'in some countries laws governing the handling of morphine and other controlled drugs are impractical or so stringent that they prevent health care workers using morphine when they feel it appropriate' [60, p. 20]. Although laws regulating morphine use were often created to prevent misuse and were adopted prior to advances in knowledge about pain and opioids [60], they still exist as barriers within the morphine chain of supply and demand. Other barriers expressed by health care workers were lengthy and prohibitive forms, stipulations on dosages, short lengths of supply, and a lack of qualified workers as deterrents to opioid prescription [60].

The issues surrounding drug availability are not without solutions. As the PPSG asserts, even with economic challenges, steps can be taken to enhance pain management. Several successes, such as the list of palliative care essential medicines and the continual support of palliative care by the WHO, are paving the way for improved pain management. While it is beyond the scope of this chapter to examine success stories in detail, a variety of articles are helpful when considering progress in various countries [59,64,72–74]. The way forward requires the collaboration of health care leaders willing to undertake public health reform. Through continued advocacy and education, adequate access to pain relief will become a required and expected component of cancer control.

Palliative care education: models of success

Palliative medicine plays a significant role in the improvement of care for people throughout the trajectory of illness, as well as when they are approaching death. This in and of itself is justification for ongoing palliative care education for all health care providers. However, a more persuasive argument for the inclusion of palliative medicine in training programmes may be that incorporating palliative care within the medical system could save resources; palliative approaches may reduce practices that are unnecessarily aggressive, costly, and unwarranted [75]. It has been estimated that the annual financial burden of pain in the United States is greater than $100 billion, including the cost of medical expenses, lost wages, and other associated costs [65]. Therefore, it is understandable that there has been a worldwide effort focused on increasing palliative care education.

Over a decade ago, the WHO challenged training institutions to make palliative care compulsory and give high recognition in institutions [75]. While progress is evident, reviews of education programmes in training institutions around the world have found palliative care programming to be patchy or non-existent [76–86]. This is true of the literature from developed [80–82, 85–87] and developing nations [76,83]. Case by case analyses of medical programmes around the world indicated that some university programmes have developed reasonable palliative medicine educational opportunities within both medicine and nursing faculties [88]. However, a variety of large-scale educational initiatives have been developed within resource-rich settings; several will be presented.

Canadian Pallium Project

This project, completed in September 2007, is described as an initiative to 'support, mobilize, and help individuals and organizations navigate the complexity of multiple systems and agents towards the constructive evolution of Canada's hospice palliative care capacity' [89, p. vi]. From its inception in late 2000, the Pallium Project has evolved from supporting primarily rural health care practitioners to collaborating with regional health authorities and community-based voluntary sector partners [89]. With federal funding, Pallium has focused on the use of innovative long distance technologies to support and enhance the education of health care professionals [90].

Educating future physicians in end-of-life care

With the advice and collaboration of many varied palliative care stakeholders across Canada, the goal of the EFPEC (Educating future physicians in end-of-life care) project was to design a common curriculum for medical students. The development of this national curriculum, based on common competencies for all undergraduate and clinical postgraduate trainees at all Canadian medical schools, facilitated the introduction of palliative and end-of-life care questions in licensing and certification exams. The project was completed in March, 2008.

End-of-life nursing education consortium

ELNEC (End-of-life nursing education consortium) programme, developed in 2000 and funded by the Robert Wood Johnson Foundation, is an education programme to improve end-of-life care in the United States [91]. The ELNEC curriculum has also been adapted for an international audience with positive results [92].

Comprehensive advanced palliative care education

CAPCE (Comprehensive advanced palliative care education) programme – a Canadian initiative – is a 120-hour programme designed for learners to extend their palliative care knowledge into the hospice workplace and act as resources for the palliative care team. Developed in 2002, a recent evaluation has shown that the CAPCE programme has effectively transferred palliative care knowledge to the workplace [93].

Support, education, assessment, and monitoring project

In 2003, the SEAM (Support, education, assessment, and monitoring project) service model was developed in Australia for use in rural palliative care delivery. The education component was delivered to health care professionals, clients, and family members. The primary goal of the model was to 'develop, implement, and evaluate an integrated service model of palliative care that would focus on improving rural people's access to services' [94, p. 2].

Palliative care education in developing countries

Palliative care education programmes, whether at the university or community level, in developing countries appear to be uncommon [95,96] but increasing in number [97]. The literature does contain descriptions of several education initiatives. For example, the University of Cape Town in South Africa has recently begun a post-graduate palliative care distance education programme. Prior to this programme, there were five South African doctors who had received training in palliative medicine, all from the University of Wales in Cardiff [83]. Since its inception in 2000, the programme, offering a diploma in palliative medicine or a master of philosophy degree in palliative medicine, has accepted up to 27 students per year [83]. Another example is seen in Uganda where palliative care education programmes have been in existence for over a decade; training was provided through Mildmay International and has been extended to the Hospice Association of Uganda as well as undergraduate medical education [97]. The African Palliative Care Association, an organization for all of Africa, facilitates training and education for member hospices and palliative care organizations. According to the APCA website, education and training objectives include developing standardized education and training programmes, providing educational resources for partners, and assisting with technical needs during training and education (www.apca.co.ug).

Implementation of palliative care

Historically, the organization of hospice and palliative care services has been predicated on two models. The first is a model of care where hospice denotes a place of care, in many instances separate from mainstream healthcare. Many of these facilities or home care programmes are run by charities or non-profit organizations, which rely on voluntary donations for a considerable part of their funding. This type of model is perhaps best illustrated in the establishment of St. Christopher's Hospice by Cicely Saunders and her colleagues in the United Kingdom. A second model arose from the development of inpatient units in acute care teaching hospitals such as those established in 1974 at St. Boniface General Hospital in Winnipeg and at the

Royal Victoria Hospital in Montreal. Although such units are closely linked with oncology, they remain separate from cancer centres and cancer control strategies. Indeed, cancer care in the United States and elsewhere has been structured as a delivery system for chemotherapy and radiotherapy, rather than as a comprehensive approach that addresses all patient concerns including psychosocial, spiritual, and social concerns [26].

To fully embrace a public health approach to implementing palliative care within cancer control strategies requires the extension of palliative care services beyond these two traditional health care delivery models. For public health strategies to be effective, they must be endorsed by governments and incorporated at all levels of the health care system; to be efficient, these strategies must be community-based and well coordinated [30,39]. MacDonald, in writing about this issue more than ten years ago, stated that coordination between institutions, family physicians, and palliative home care programmes is essential to providing a seamless flow of care and to preventing patient suffering [16]. There is general agreement that palliative care needs to be closely integrated with oncology services, and that it should be provided by an interdisciplinary team, commence early in the course of cancer treatment, and be tailored to the needs of the patient [98,99].

Using a health-promoting and population-based approach recognizes that not all people living with cancer need or want the same level and access to specialized palliative care services [100,101]. A model of care that is flexible, integrated through formal partnerships with different services and providers, incorporates generalist and specialist health professionals, has a single entry point and administrative structure, and is responsive to the level of patient need are factors expressed in the literature as integral to excellent palliative care provision [102–104]. Palliative care networks, modelled in several Canadian provinces [105–107] and in the United Kingdom [104], are comprised of local stakeholders who help develop and implement strategic priorities and service delivery models that will maximize resource utilization and integration to improve the delivery of palliative care [105]. Though these initiatives are commendable, they may not be fully integrated with treatment services such as cancer centres and other organizations that provide social services [108]. However, one such example is seen in Australia. To be fully responsive to the breadth of patient needs, Palliative Care Australia (see http://pallcare.org.au) developed a model that incorporated a population-based approach to planning for and providing palliative care services. This model, combined with the proposed best practices framework for organizing healthcare delivery systems by Hollander and Prince [109] has been adapted and is seen in Figure 14.3.

The acuity and complexity of patient and family needs defines the level of palliative care services delivered within this model. In this manner, patients may move between different levels of care throughout their illness trajectory. The vast majority of persons will fall into group A, whereby their needs are most easily and best met by primary health care providers including community nurses, family physicians, and medical specialists such as oncologists. Those patients who experience sporadic or occasional exacerbations of psychosocial, physical, or existential/spiritual distress will require expert consultation from specialist palliative care services, with ongoing care being provided by their primary care providers (Group B). A subset of these patients will have needs requiring more intensive care that is best achieved through ongoing collaboration and shared care arrangements between the primary care provider and palliative care specialist (Group C). A small sub-group of palliative care patients (Group D) will have complex care needs requiring direct ongoing involvement from specialist palliative care services either in the community or in designated inpatient/hospice beds.

This integrated model of collaborative care is built on a population-based approach with defined levels of care and clear role delineation. The model recognizes and respects the relationship between primary care providers, patients, and family members. Additionally, the expertise of

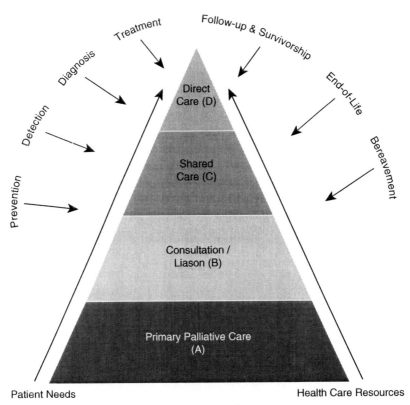

Fig. 14.3 Providing palliative care within a cancer control strategy.
Source: From Palliative Care Australia (p.13, [110])

specialist palliative care providers is used more effectively and provides opportunities for formalized education and collaboration with generalist providers. For successful implementation of the model, local needs and capacity must be taken into consideration when developing and delivering palliative care. Other pre-requisites that will enhance the uptake and implementation of this model include: (i) a positive philosophical and policy environment including sustainable funding, a commitment to the psychosocial model of care, and evidence-based decision making; (ii) administrative best practices including a single or highly coordinated administrative structure, single funding envelope, and integrated electronic information systems; (iii) clinical best practices such as standardized system-level assessment and care authorization, single system-level patient classification system, and case management; and (iv) linkages across systems of care including cross-appointments of staff [109].

Integration of palliative care and cancer control

There is little argument that palliative care has a rightful place within national cancer control strategies and that most cancer patients wish to receive dignified care focused on promoting comfort throughout the course of their illness. What is debatable, however, is how fully developed a nation's awareness of the principles of palliative care is and how well integrated these programmes are within models of cancer care. Although the WHO asserts that a national cancer control programme can be efficacious regardless of resources [5], a nation's resources have a tremendous impact on the level of integration and the extent of implementation in a national palliative care programme. Limiting factors such as a lack of public knowledge or support, shortage of health professionals educated in palliative care, limited access to opioids, and excess reliance on curative interventions, reduce the likelihood that cancer patients will have access to palliative care programmes throughout their cancer trajectory. Adopting the public health approach to implementing palliative care requires that developed and developing countries find creative ways to use their limited resources to overcome these barriers.

For rich countries, providing the full complement of services from primary care through to the direct care provided by palliative care practitioners is possible. Successful achievement requires national guidelines and accreditation standards, along with palliative care education that is standardized in all medical and nursing curricula. Well-resourced countries may also look at including palliative care measures such as quality of life or symptom distress in cancer surveillance systems as a means to monitor suffering within this population.

In countries with fewer resources, implementing national minimum standards for pain relief and palliative care is essential [12]. All cancer patients must be guaranteed access to primary care providers versed in the principles of palliative care. In this manner, medical and nursing education must encapsulate the core competencies of palliative care. Educational initiatives must meet local needs, and integrating palliative care within developing countries' cancer control strategies requires the use of local community resources and capacity. For example in Kerala, India, the Neighbourhood Network in Palliative Care provides training to community volunteers who work in conjunction with palliative care professionals and health facilities to plan and deliver services [72].

Regardless of the differences in resource intensity, leadership is required to demonstrate how palliative care and cancer care services must evolve within the context of national health care in order to ensure 'genuine cradle-to-grave care as a central tenet of a just and modern civil society' [89, p 6]. In order to achieve equitable, readily available, and accessible palliative care services for all cancer patients, palliative care must be viewed as an integral element of a comprehensive cancer control strategy.

References

1 Saunders C (2000). The evolution of palliative care. *Patient Educ Couns*, Aug;**41**(1):7–13.

2 World Health Organization (2008). WHO definition of palliative care. Available at: http://www.who.int.proxy2.lib.umanitoba.ca/cancer/palliatIve (accessed 26 Feb 2008).

3 Kim A, Fall P, & Wang D (2005). Palliative care: optimizing quality of life. *J Am Osteopath Assoc*, Nov;**105**(11 Suppl 5):S9–S14.

4 van Kleffens T, Van Baarsen B, Hoekman K, & Van Leeuwen E (2004). Clarifying the term 'palliative' in clinical oncology. *Eur J Cancer Care (Engl)*, Jul;**13**(3):263–71.

5 World Health Organization (2008). National cancer control programmes. Available at: http://www.who.int/cancer/nccp/en/ (Accessed 5 Oct 2009).

6 Stjernsward J, Foley KM, & Ferris FD (2007). Integrating palliative care into national policies. *J Pain Symptom Manage*, May;**33**(5):514–20.

7 Ahmedzai SH, Costa A, Blengini C, et al (2004). A new international framework for palliative care. *Eur J Cancer*, Oct;**40**(15):2192–2200.

8 MacDonald N (1993). Oncology and palliative care: the case for co-ordination. *Cancer Treat.Rev*, **19**(Suppl A):29–41.

9 Lingwood RJ, Boyle P, Milburn A, et al (2008). The challenge of cancer control in Africa. *Nat Rev Cancer*, May;**8**(5):398–403.

10 Torres Vigil I, Aday LA, De Lima L, & Cleeland CS (2007). What predicts the quality of advanced cancer care in Latin America? A look at five countries: Argentina, Brazil, Cuba, Mexico, and Peru. *J Pain Symptom Manage*, Sep;**34**(3):315–327.

11 Higginson IJ & Costantini M (2008). Dying with cancer, living well with advanced cancer. *Eur J Cancer*, Jul;**44**(10):1414–24.

12 World Health Organization (2002). National Cancer Control Programmes: Policies and Managerial Guidelines. 2nd ed. World Health Organization, Geneva.

13 Stjernsward J, Foley KM, & Ferris FD (2007). The public health strategy for palliative care. *J Pain Symptom Manage*, May;**33**(5):486–493.

14 Foley KM (2005). Improving palliative care for cancer: a national and international perspective. *Gynecol Oncol*, Dec;**99**(3 Suppl 1):S213–S214.

15 Kerner JF, Guirguis-Blake J, Hennessy KD, et al (2005). Translating research into improved outcomes in comprehensive cancer control. *Cancer Causes Control*, Oct;**16**(Suppl 1):27–40.

16 MacDonald N (1998). Palliative care – an essential component of cancer control. *CMAJ*, Jun 30;**158**(13):1709–16.

17 Meghani SH (2004). A concept analysis of palliative care in the United States. *J Adv Nurs*, Apr;**46**(2):152–61.

18 Ferris FD, Balfour HM, Bowen K, et al (2002). A model to guide patient and family care: based on nationally accepted principles and norms of practice. *J Pain Symptom Manage*, Aug;**24**(2):106–23.

19 MacDonald N (1991). Palliative care – the fourth phase of cancer prevention. *Cancer Detect Prev*, **15**(3):253–55.

20 Maltoni M & Amadori D (2001). Palliative medicine and medical oncology. *Ann Oncol*, Apr;**12**(4):443–50.

21 Doyle D, Hanks G, Cherny NI, & Calman K (2004). Introduction. In: Doyle D, Hanks G, Cherny NI, & Calman K (eds) *Oxford Textbook of Palliative Medicine*. 3rd ed, pp. 1–4. Oxford University Press, New York.

22 Jeffrey D (2003). What do we mean by psychosocial care in palliative care? In: Lloyd-Williams M (ed) *Psychosocial Issues in Palliative Care*, pp. 1–12. Oxford University Press, New York.

23 Ferris FD & Librach SL (2005). Models, standards, guidelines. *Clin Geriatr Med*, Feb;**21**(1):17–44.

24 Cullen M (2001). 'Best supportive care' has had its day. *Lancet Oncol*, Mar;**2**(3):173–175.

25 MacDonald N (1998). Best supportive care. *Cancer Prev Control*, Aug;**2**(4):191–192.

26 Ahmedzai SH & Walsh D (2000). Palliative medicine and modern cancer care. *Semin Oncol*, Feb;**27**(1):1–6.

27 Bosnjak S (2003). The importance of clinical practice guidelines (CPGs) for the quality and development of supportive care in Central and Eastern European (CEE) countries. *Support Care Cancer*, Dec;**11**(12):775–79.

28 Ahmedzai SH, Costa A, Blengini C, et al (2004). A new international framework for palliative care. *Eur J Cancer*, Oct;**40**(15):2192–2200.

29 Clark D (2007). From margins to centre: a review of the history of palliative care in cancer. *Lancet Oncol*, May;**8**(5):430–38.

30 Stjernsward J (2007). Palliative care: the public health strategy. *J Public Health Policy*, **28**(1):42–55.

31 Mathew A, Cowley S, Bliss J, & Thistlewood G)2003). The development of palliative care in national government policy in England, 1986–2000. *Palliat Med*, Apr;**17**(3):270–282.

32 Lorenz KA, Shugarman LR, & Lynn J (2006). Health care policy issues in end-of-life care. *J Palliat Med*, Jun;**9**(3):731–748.

33 Clark D & Centeno C (2006). Palliative care in Europe: an emerging approach to comparative analysis. *Clin Med*, Mar-Apr;**6**(2):197–201.

34 Carstairs S (2000). Quality end-of-life care: the right of every Canadian. Final report of the Senate Subcommittee to Update 'Of Life and Death' of the Standing Social Committee on Social Affairs, Science, and Technology. 37th Parliament, 1st session.

35 Ferrell B, Connor SR, Cordes A, et al (2007). The national agenda for quality palliative care: the National Consensus Project and the National Quality Forum. *J Pain Symptom Manage*, Jun;**33**(6):737–44.

36 Knight A (2006). Palliative care in the United Kingdom. In: Ferrell BR, Coyle N (eds) *Textbook of Palliative Nursing*. 2nd ed, pp. 1165–76. Oxford University Press, New York.

37 Richards MA (2003). Priorities for supportive and palliative care in England. *Palliat Med*, Jan;**17**(1):7–8.

38 Canadian Cancer Society (2008). Canadian Strategy for Cancer Control. 2007. http://www.cancer.ca (accessed 5 October 2009).

39 Martin WM (1998). Cancer in developing countries: Part II – Cancer control: strategies and priorities. *Clin Oncol (R Coll Radiol)*, **10**(5):283–287.

40 Joishy SK (2001). Palliative medical oncology. *Surg Oncol Clin N Am*, Jan;**10**(1):203–20.

41 Kaasa S, Jordhoy MS, & Haugen DF (2007). Palliative care in Norway: a national public health model. *J Pain Symptom Manage*, May;**33**(5):599–604.

42 MacDonald N (1992). Cancer centres–their role in palliative care. *J Palliat Care*, Spring;**8**(1):38–42.

43 Glare P, Virik K, Jones M, et al (2003). A systematic review of physicians' survival predictions in terminally ill cancer patients. *BMJ*, Jul 26;**327**(7408):195–198.

44 Werth JL & Blevins D (2002). Public policy and end-of-life care. *American Behavioral Scientist*, **46**(3):401–422.

45 Shugarman LR, Lorenz K, & Lynn J (2005). End-of-life care: an agenda for policy improvement. *Clin Geriatr Med*, Feb;**21**(1):255–72, xi.

46 Brennan F (2007). Palliative care as an international human right. *J Pain Symptom Manage*, May;**33**(5):494–99.

47 Brennan F, Carr DB, & Cousins M (2007). Pain management: a fundamental human right. *Anesth Analg*, Jul;**105**(1):205–21.

48 World Health Organization (1986). *Cancer Pain Relief*. World Health Organization, Geneva, Albany. WHO Publications Center USA distributor.

49 Otsuka K & Yasuhara H (2007). Toward freedom from cancer pain in Japan. *J Pain Palliat Care Pharmacother*, **21**(3):37–42.

50 Zyczkowska J, Szczerbinska K, Jantzi MR, & Hirdes JP (2007). Pain among the oldest old in community and institutional settings. *Pain*, May;**129**(1–2):167–176.

51 Barakzoy AS & Moss AH (2006). Efficacy of the world health organization analgesic ladder to treat pain in end-stage renal disease. *J Am Soc Nephrol*, Nov;**17**(11):3198–3203.

52 Azevedo Sao Leao Ferreira, K, Kimura M, & Jacobsen Teixeira M (2006). The WHO analgesic ladder for cancer pain control, twenty years of use. How much pain relief does one get from using it? *Support Care Cancer*, Nov;**14**(11).1086–93.

53 Klepstad P, Kaasa S, Cherny N, Hanks G, de Conno F, & Research Steering Committee of the EAPC (2005). Pain and pain treatments in European palliative care units. A cross sectional survey from the European Association for Palliative Care Research Network. *Palliat Med*, Sep;**19**(6):477–84.

54 Maltoni M, Scarpi E, Modonesi C, et al (2005). A validation study of the WHO analgesic ladder: a two-step vs three-step strategy. *Support Care Cancer*, Nov;**13**(11):888–94.

55 De Lima L, Krakauer EL, Lorenz K, Praill D, Macdonald N, & Doyle D (2007). Ensuring palliative medicine availability: the development of the IAHPC list of essential medicines for palliative care. *J Pain Symptom Manage*, May;**33**(5):521–526.

56 Sepulveda C, Marlin A, Yoshida T, & Ullrich A (2002). Palliative Care: the World Health Organization's global perspective. *J Pain Symptom Manage*, Aug;**24**(2):91–96.

57 Passik SD, Whitcomb LA, Kirsh KL, et al (2002). A pilot study of oncology staff perceptions of palliative care and psycho-oncology services in rural and community settings in Indiana. *J Rural Health*, Winter;**18**(1):31–34.

58 Schrader SL, Nelson ML, & Eidsness LM (2007). Palliative care teams on the prairie: composition, perceived challenges & opportunities. *S D Med*, Apr;**60**(4):147–49, 151–53.

59 Joranson DE & Ryan KM (2007). Ensuring opioid availability: methods and resources. *J Pain Symptom Manage*, May;**33**(5):527–32.

60 Adams V (2007). Access to pain relief: An essential human right. Journal of pain & palliative care pharmacotherapy 22(2):101–29, 2008.

61 Schrijvers D (2007). Should palliative care replace palliative treatment for cancer in resource-poor countries? *Lancet Oncol*, Feb;**8**(2):86–87.

62 De Lima L & Barnard D (2001). Advances in Palliative Care in Latin America and the Caribbean: Ongoing Projects of the Pan American Health Organization (PAHO). *J Palliat Med*, Summer;**4**(2):227–31.

63 World Health Organization. (2007). *A Community Health Approach to Palliative Care for HIV/AIDS and Cancer Patients*. Available: http://www.who.int/hiv/pub/prev_care/palliativecare/en/index.html (Accessed 5 October 2009).

64 Brown S, Black F, Vaidya P, Shrestha S, Ennals D, & LeBaron VT (2007). Palliative care development: the Nepal model. *J Pain Symptom Manage*, May;**33**(5):573–77.

65 Dahl JL (2002). Working with regulators to improve the standard of care in pain management: the U.S. experience. *J Pain Symptom Manage*, Aug;**24**(2):136–46.

66 Lickiss JN (2001). Approaching cancer pain relief. *Eur J Pain*, **5** (Suppl A):5–14.

67 Otsuka K, & Yasuhara H (2007). Toward freedom from cancer pain in Japan. *J Pain Palliat Care Pharmacother*,**21**(3):37–42.

68 Demmer C (2007). AIDS and palliative care in South Africa. *Am J Hosp Palliat Care*, Feb-Mar; **24**(1):7–12.

69 Gwyther E (2002). South Africa: the status of palliative care. *J Pain Symptom Manage*, Aug;**24**(2):236–38.

70 van Niekerk JP (2003). Palliative care–from dream to mainstream. *S Afr Med J*, Sep;**93**(9):625.

71 Uys LR (2003). Aspects of the care of people with HIV/AIDS in South Africa. *Public Health Nurs*, 2003 Jul–Aug;**20**(4):271–80.

72 Bollini P, Venkateswaran C, & Sureshkumar K (2004). Palliative care in Kerala, India: a model for resource-poor settings. *Onkologie*, Apr;**27**(2):138–42.

73 Gilson AM, Joranson DE, Maurer MA, Ryan KM, & Garthwaite JP (2005). Progress to achieve balanced state policy relevant to pain management and palliative care: 2000–2003. *J Pain Palliat Care Pharmacother*, **19**(1):13–26.

74 Gilson AM, Maurer MA, & Joranson DE (2005). State policy affecting pain management: recent improvements and the positive impact of regulatory health policies. *Health Policy*, Oct;**74**(2):192–204.

75 Scott JF, MacDonald N, & Mount BM (1998). Palliative medicine education. In: Doyle D, Hanks WC, MacDonald N (eds) 2nd ed, pp. 1169–1200. Oxford Medical Publications, Oxford.

76 Krasuska ME, Stanislawek A, & Mazurkiewicz M (2002). Palliative care professional education in the new millennium: global perspectives – universal needs. *Ann Univ Mariae Curie Sklodowska [Med]*, **57**(1):439–43.

77 Yuen K, Barrington D, Headford N, McNulty M, & Smith M (1998). Educating doctors in palliative medicine: development of a competency-based training program. *J Palliat Care*, Autumn;**14**(3):79–82.

78 Schulman-Green D, McCorkle R, Cherlin E, Johnson-Hurzeler R, & Bradley EH (2005). Nurses' communication of prognosis and implications for hospice referral: a study of nurses caring for terminally ill hospitalized patients. *Am J Crit Care*, Jan;**14**(1):64–70.

79 Oliver D (1998). Training and knowledge of palliative care of junior doctors. *Palliat Med*, Jul;**12**(4):297–99.

80 Lloyd-Williams M & Carter YH (2003). General practice vocational training in the UK: what teaching is given in palliative care? *Palliat Med*, Oct;**17**(7):616–20.

81 Kelley ML, Habjan S, & Aegard J (2004). Building capacity to provide palliative care in rural and remote communities: does education make a difference? *J Palliat Care*, Winter;**20**(4):308–15.

82 Cairns W & Yates PM (2003). Education and training in palliative care. *Med J Aust*, Sep 15;**179**(6 Suppl):S26–S28.

83 Bateman C (2002). GP'S vision kick-starts palliative training. *S Afr Med J*, **92**(12):936–37.

84 MacDonald N (1995). A proposed matrix for organisational changes to improve quality of life in oncology. *Eur J Cancer*, **31A**(Suppl 6):S18–S21.

85 Centeno C, Noguera A, Lynch T, & Clark D (2007). Official certification of doctors working in palliative medicine in Europe: data from an EAPC study in 52 European countries. *Palliat Med*, Dec;**21**(8):683–87.

86 Oneschuk D, Hanson J, & Bruera E (2000). An international survey of undergraduate medical education in palliative medicine. *J Pain Symptom Manage*, Sep;**20**(3):174–79.

87 Lloyd-Williams M & MacLeod R (2004). A systematic review of teaching and learning in palliative care within the medical undergraduate curriculum. *Med Teach*, **26**(8):683–90.

88 Kelly D, Gould D, White I, & Berridge EJ (2006). Modernising cancer and palliative care education in the UK: insights from one Cancer Network. *Eur J Oncol Nurs*, Jul;**10**(3):187–97.

89 Aherne M & Pereira J (2005). A generative response to palliative service capacity in Canada. *Int J Health Care Qual Assur Inc Leadersh Health Serv*, **18**(1):iii–xxi.

90 Fainsinger RL (2002). Canada: palliative care and cancer pain. *J Pain Symptom Manage*, Aug;**24**(2):173–76.

91 Coyne P, Paice JA, Ferrell BR, Malloy P, Virani R, & Fennimore LA (2007). Oncology end-of-life nursing education consortium training program: improving palliative care in cancer. *Oncol Nurs Forum*, Jul;**34**(4):801–07.

92 Paice JA, Ferrell BR, Coyle N, Coyne P, & Callaway M (2008). Global efforts to improve palliative care: the international end-of-life nursing education consortium training programme. *J Adv Nurs*, Jan;**61**(2):173–80.

93 Harris D, Hillier LM, & Keat N (2007). Sustainable practice improvements: impact of the comprehensive advanced palliative care education (CAPCE) program. *J Palliat Care*, Winter;**23**(4):262–72.

94 Buikstra E, Pearce S, Hegney D, & Fallon T (2006). SEAM – improving the quality of palliative care in regional Toowoomba, Australia: lessons learned. *Rural Remote Health*, Jan–Mar;**6**(1):415.

95 Omar S, Alieldin NH, & Khatib OM (2007). Cancer magnitude, challenges and control in the Eastern Mediterranean region. *East Mediterr Health J*, Nov-Dec;**13**(6):1486–96.

96 Abu-Saad Huijer H, & Dimassi H (2007). Palliative care in Lebanon: knowledge, attitudes and practices of physicians and nurses. *J Med Liban*, Jul–Sep;**55**(3):121–28.

97 Downing J (2006). Palliative care and education in Uganda. *Int J Palliat Nurs*, Aug;**12**(8):358–61.

98 Llamas KJ, Pickhaver AM, & Piller NB (2001). Mainstreaming palliative care for cancer patients in the acute hospital setting. *Palliat Med*, May;**15**(3):207–12.

99 Mitchell WM & von Gunten CF (2008). The role of palliative medicine in cancer patient care. *Cancer Treat Res*, **140**:159–71.

100 Phillips JL, Davidson PM, Jackson D, Kristjanson L, Bennett ML, & Daly J (2006). Enhancing palliative care delivery in a regional community in Australia. *Aust Health Rev*,. Aug;**30**(3):370–79.

101 Street AF (2007). Leading the way: innovative health promoting palliative care. *Contemp.Nurse*, Dec;**27**(1):104–06.

102 Lagman R & Walsh D (2005). Integration of palliative medicine into comprehensive cancer care. *Semin Oncol*, Apr;**32**(2):134–38.

103 McKinlay E & McBain L (2007). Evaluation of the palliative care partnership: a New Zealand solution to the provision of integrated palliative care. *N Z Med J*, Oct 12;**120**(1263):2745–57.

104 Travis S & Hunt P (2001). Supportive and palliative care networks: a new model for integrated care. *Int J Palliat Nurs*, Oct;**7**(10):501–04.

105 Dudgeon D, Vaitonis V, Seow H, King S, Angus H, & Sawka C (2007). Ontario, Canada: using networks to integrate palliative care province-wide. *J Pain Symptom Manage*, May;**33**(5):640–44.

106 Fainsinger RL, Brenneis C, & Fassbender K (2007). Edmonton, Canada: a regional model of palliative care development. *J Pain Symptom Manage*, May;**33**(5):634–39.

107 Morin D, Saint-Laurent L, Bresse MP, Dallaire C, & Fillion L (2007). The benefits of a palliative care network: a case study in Quebec, Canada. *Int J Palliat Nurs*, Apr;**13**(4):190–96.

108 Brazil K, Bainbridge D, Sussman J, Whelan T, O'Brien MA, & Pyette N (2008). Providing supportive care to cancer patients: a study on inter-organizational relationships. *Int J Integr Care*, Feb 11;**8**:e01.

109 Hollander MJ & Prince MJ (2008). Organizing healthcare delivery systems for persons with ongoing care needs and their families: a best practices framework. *Healthc Q*, **11**(1):44–54.

110 Palliative Care Australia (2005). A guide to palliative care service development: A population based approach. Canberra: PC Australia.

111 Service Canada. Employment insurance (EI) compassionate care benefits. Available at: http://www.hrsdc.gc.ca/en/ei/types/compassionate_care.shtml#tphp (Accessed 5 October 2009).

112 The Library of Congress (2008). Thomas – Legislative information from the Library of Congress. Available at: http://thomas.loc.gov/ (Accessed 5 October 2009).

Part 5

Integrated cancer control

Chapter 15

From cancer care to cancer control: organization of population-based cancer control systems

Simon Sutcliffe[1]

The cancer challenge

It is a common misperception that cancer is an unforeseen, unexpected, and unwelcome event abruptly interfering in an otherwise healthy life – the concept that a cancer diagnosis has no antecedent process. However, epidemiological and molecular studies identify that cancer is a process – a process that starts in health and progresses through events that cause normal cells to acquire the properties of malignancy (uncontrolled proliferation; abrogation of programmed cell death; failure to repair genetic damage; immortalization of cancer cells; and invasion of tissue and metastasis) [1]. The consequences of this process constitute a 'burden' expressed at a personal, family and community, societal, and economic level. Accordingly, to address the 'burden' requires that the process be addressed; that there be a strategy directed to the elements of the cancer process, from primary prevention to end-of-life care, and that the strategy be directed to the entire population.

A comprehensive, population-based strategy is based upon certain foundational premises:

◆ Cancer is an increasing burden for all nations, constituting approximately 30 per cent of deaths in developed nations largely as a result of population increase and aging, and an increasingly important component of population mortality in developing countries as improving longevity and the shift from communicable to non-communicable disease mortality takes place [2].

◆ Cancer affects all members of the population – there are no exceptions, only an enhanced or diminished probability of developing cancer based upon susceptibilities arising from genetic (hereditary), educational, socio-economic, behavioural, or circumstantial risks or exposures. Such factors may give rise to disparities of outcome as they predicate against equal opportunity to derive benefit from preventive or therapeutic interventions [3,4].

◆ The outcomes of cancer (such as mortality, 5-year survival, and functionality) are most affected by influencing adverse causal risk factors for cancer, by modifying exposures, often by communication, education, awareness, and personal or societal choice. In effect, the greatest impact upon mortality from cancer is exercised through control of incidence, or developing cancer.

[1] Simon B. Sutcliffe, MD, FRCP, FRCPC, FRCR, Board Chair, Canadian Partnership Against Cancer, Canada, and Past President, BC Cancer Agency, Vancouver, British Columbia, Canada.

- Cancer outcomes can be favourably influenced through therapeutic interventions, most successfully when applied earlier in the trajectory of the process.
- The outcomes of successful interventions depend greatly on accessibility, timeliness, quality and safety, as experienced by all members of the population.
- Notwithstanding the application of all that is known to be beneficial, the current proportion of patients who will die of their cancer is approximately 45 to 50 per cent in developed countries and 60 to70 per cent in the developing world, thereby reinforcing the necessity to know more about effective cancer control through research as a means of applying knowledge to improve cancer outcomes.

Population-based cancer control aims to reduce the incidence and mortality of cancer, and to enhance the quality of life of those affected by cancer, through an integrated and coordinated approach directed to primary prevention, early detection, treatment, rehabilitation, and palliation [4–6].

Cancer treatment, cancer care, and cancer control

The terms 'cancer treatment', 'cancer care', and 'cancer control' are frequently used synonymously, as if they have a common meaning. However, as explored by Caron et al. [7] (and described further in Chapter 17 of this book), the terms are quite distinct and present several contrasts in ways to reduce the impact of cancer:

- reducing incidence through prevention is included only in cancer control.
- reducing mortality is included in all, but the 'clock starts' with the diagnosis of cancer in the treatment and care paradigms, and with risk/susceptibility for cancer in times of health in the control paradigm.
- the other essential contrast is between the episode of care (treatment) and the continuum of care (care).
- the institutional response to care (treatment) is distinguished from 'shared care' across primary, community, and tertiary settings characterizing the continuum of care (care).
- contrasts between the health system response as a facility-driven approach (treatment), a community-driven approach through networks of care providers and support systems (care), and an integrated approach across systems applied to health and illness management, including education, transportation, environment, social services, health and illness services, etc. (control).

The distinction of treatment, care and control has an important bearing on the design of the 'organized' cancer system (Figure 15.1).

Systems designed to provide organized *treatment* services have the potential to impact mortality and other cancer-related outcomes but not incidence, and can influence the quality and safety of, and the satisfaction with, the treatment episode. Organized *care* will include all treatment, diagnostic, and supportive services, can impact cancer outcomes but not incidence, and can influence quality, safety and satisfaction with both treatment and continuity of care. Cancer *control* includes treatment and care; in addition, through prevention will affect incidence as well as mortality; addresses quality, safety, and satisfaction; and effects a cross-sectoral response (education, transportation, environment, health management, social services, and illness management) to enhancing both health and illness outcomes.

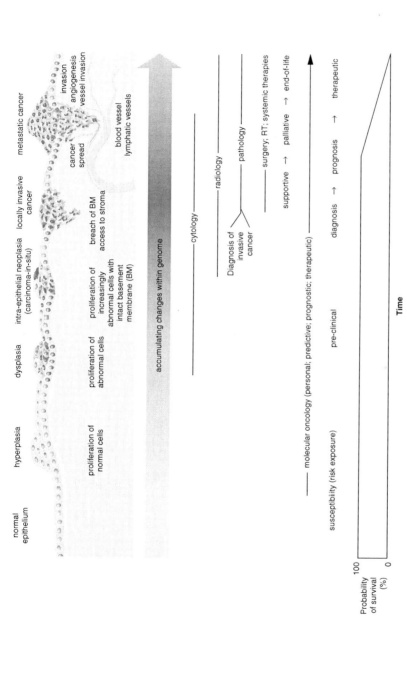

Fig. 15.1 Interventional services in relation to carcinogenesis and survival.

Cancer is a process ('carcinogenesis') through which the normal epithelium undergoes progressive change to acquire the characteristics of malignancy (invasion and metastasis). Survival is only impacted as local disease becomes advanced and/or metastatic. Conventional cytology has the ability to define cellular changes prior to the development of invasive cancer (dysplasia and carcinoma in situ). The majority of interventional services are relevant only to the diagnosis, definition of extent and therapy of invasive cancer. Molecular pathology offers the opportunity to examine carcinogenesis through pre-malignant and malignant phases, thus becoming relevant to primary prevention and high-risk screening (predictive and prognostic utility) as well as to the diagnosis, classification, staging, and selection of therapy for established cancer.

Population-based planning for cancer control

Population-based programme development for cancer control is a strategic activity, grounded in valid information about the burden of cancer both as an expression of impact (personal, family and community, society, and economy) and as a health and illness challenge to be controlled (volume, distribution by extent of disease, disparities, early detection, diagnostic, therapeutic, and care services) [6,8,9]

The design of a population-based programme must take many factors into account (Table 15.1):

- the needs of all members of the population from prevention to end-of-life care.
- the alignment of needs with capacity to provide services within defined parameters of access, timeliness, quality, and safety. Misalignment is characterized by queues, waiting times, disease progression whilst waiting for care, or lack or denial of care.
- the necessity for measures of outcome and output derived from valid data.
- prioritization of elements of the cancer control spectrum from primary care to end-of-life care according to needs and resources.
- addressing all aspects of the process of carcinogenesis from risk exposure, through pre-neoplasia to established cancer.
- the principles of quality and safety (including equity, equality, fairness, evidence, information and communication).
- integration to optimize coordination, efficiency, and effectiveness.
- alignment to principles and practices that enable and promote enhancements in other non-communicable disease control programmes (Figure 15.2).
- engagement of various sections of public to demonstrate adherence to principles, performance, and accountability.
- sustainability through ongoing secure resources.
- appropriate governance, and management of both the plan (strategy) to enhance cancer control as well as the demonstration of enhanced population-based outcomes deriving from the strategy (cancer control programme).

Certain themes underlie the design and implementation of a population-based cancer control programme. What is known to be beneficial (evidence-based interventions) must be applied to the population who stand to benefit – this applies to primary prevention through risk factor control, early detection through organized programmes, and diagnostic, therapeutic, and supportive interventions. This is commonly assisted by the use of practice guidelines, 'care paths', standards of practice and/or protocols through which inappropriate variations of care are minimized.

What is yet to be known, or has yet to be proven to be beneficial, should be the subject of research to enhance care through evidence of benefit [10]. Planning for an educated, skilled work force is required according to the current and projected capacity for interventional services defined in the cancer control plan.

Measures of outcome (such as incidence and mortality), process (such as accessibility and timeliness), quality, safety, and satisfaction need to be collected and reported periodically to all relevant stakeholders as a means of accountability and continuous programme development towards optimal outcomes. Finally, there must be measures of system effectiveness based on assessment of cost and benefit as a means of 'transparent' identification of priority and allocation, both within the cancer control programme and across broader health services.

Table 15.1 Population-based cancer control and the cancer control issues being addressed

Population-based cancer control – key principles	Population-based programme development – key elements	Cancer control issues being addressed
Control of process rather than a particular 'defining event/end point'	Comprehensive of all cancer control interventions – focused on measurable outputs and outcomes	Incidence, mortality, and quality of life Strategic focus directed to a quantified objective
Addresses the cancer control needs/expectations of the entire population	Identifies and plans for interventions according to evidence-based population need at a resource-appropriate level	A programme organized to be comprehensive to the spectrum of cancer control and the interventions necessary to address improving outcomes
Based on equity, 'fairness', evidence for benefit, and appropriate measures of quality and safety	Evidence-based standards of effectiveness, quality, and safety built into interventional programme structure	Disparities of outcome and mitigation of unnecessary variation of practice within the population Performance and accountability
Integration of interventions across institutions, health settings (community; tertiary, etc.) and socio-economic circumstances	Addressing the 'pathway of care', coordination and communication between care settings, and inter-relationship of health with socio-economic concerns, transportation (access), and education	Appropriate levels of care and care providers Evidence-based guidelines/pathways for cancer control Communication and coordination of services System linkage – within health; external to health Optimal use of resources; avoidance of fragmentation, exclusion and duplication
Focused on continuously enhancing cancer control outcomes	Interventions 'driven by' and 'linked to' application of valid knowledge from health research to clinical application	Knowledge transfer to achieve 'best' care Applying what is known to be beneficial to those who can benefit Engagement, awareness, and/or participation in knowledge generation through research
Patient, public, and political (societal) engagement in cancer control	Structural (organizational) and functional engagement of key stakeholders in programme content, priorities, and funding allocations	Accountability for use of public funds Transparent processes for prioritization and allocation of funds Establishment of understanding and trust between public, patients, providers and payors

It should be noted that the key principles, elements, and issues being addressed are not 'disease-specific', but can be applied to any health issue, communicable or non-communicable, affecting the population.

Outcomes of cancer control; measures of performance

The justification to commit current and incremental resources to a cancer control plan needs to be based in the ability to measure the performance, not only of the population-based strategy,

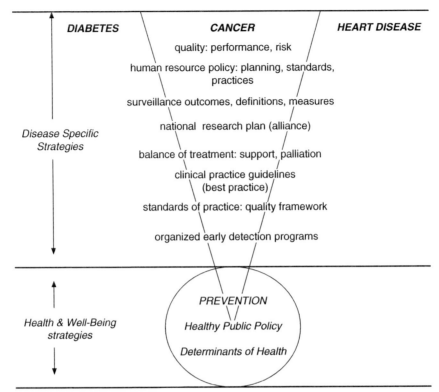

Fig. 15.2 Aligning the principles of cancer control and non-communicable disease strategies. The types of intervention to establish and maintain a quality population-based cancer control system range from primary prevention through organized early detection, treatment, research, human resource management, and quality/risk/performance management. These interventions are common to any population-based programme to control a chronic and non-communicable disease (NCD) (e.g. diabetes, heart disease, etc). Given that the majority of environmental risk factors are common for all NCDs, prevention strategies are largely disease non-specific. Specificity for disease becomes relevant as the type of intervention becomes aligned to the specific disease process, for example, early detection programme (common principles and process) aligns to cervical, breast, or colorectal cancer.

but also the outcomes of population-based cancer control. The measures used are important both to show the effectiveness of implementation of interventions, and to document the 'return on investment' in cancer control, as seen by the relevant stakeholder ('the observer proposition'). Thus, patients may place more importance upon quality of life, functionality, and lack of toxicity, compared to 'care providers' who may place more emphasis on effectiveness of care assessed, for example, by 5-year survival (measured from the date of diagnosis, not from the time of disease onset as experienced by the patient). System administration and politicians may place greatest importance on measures of cost effectiveness and cost-benefit (Table 15.2).

Table 15.2 presents outcome measures (indicators of performance) from system, population, patient, and disease control perspectives and illustrates the linkage between the measure and the attribute (outcome measures are also discussed in Chapter 18). In addition, within a publicly-funded system, there is an accountability to ensure that the cancer plan (strategy) delivers what it is funded to deliver over a period of time, and an accountability to ensure that population

Table 15.2 Cancer control outcomes in relation to attributes

Attribute(s) of relevance	Outcome measure
Cancer incidence and mortality	Age-standardized incidence rate (ASIR) Age-standardized mortality rate (ASMR) Potential years of life lost due to cancer (PYLL)
Treatment outcome	Survival rates – overall and cause specific mortality Remission rates; freedom from progression rates Effects on clinical and investigational outcomes, e.g. biochemical measures
Patient (person)-specific outcome measures (individual) Measures aggregated at population level	Effectiveness of treatment as experienced – effects on functionality, symptoms, physical and mental health, and quality of life; primary treatment effects and toxicity (short and long term) Perceived quality of, and satisfaction with, care Functionality Survivorship issues
Socio-economic outcomes	Person-years of life lost (PYLL); quality- and disability-adjusted life years (QALYs; DALYs) Return to employment (income, taxation, corporate profits) Functionality; disability (reliance on care system) Effects on families and carers Investment; return on investment in interventions (business case) Opportunity and missed opportunity costs and implications
Socio-political outcomes	Priorities and resource allocation (absolute, relative to other health demands, relative to non-health issues) Investment; return on investment in interventions (opportunity) Satisfaction and public opinion, and political priority and timeliness

health/cancer control outcome measures change in a favourable way as a consequence of implementing a population-based cancer plan. Aspects of this situation, whereby the implementation of a plan may be expected to have measures of performance that will subsequently give rise to favourable change in cancer control outcome measures, are depicted in Table 15.3. It will be apparent that the performance of the plan is a surrogate for performance of the system, the two being separable often by many years, but contingent upon sequential effective implementation.

Organizational planning for cancer control

The population includes individuals and groups who differ in terms of demographics, risk factor exposure profiles, geographic location and ease of access to services, socio-economic status and levels of education and health awareness. Within a population-based programme, the intent is to deliver services to all sub-groups in the population, to produce equitable benefits in cancer control to the degree possible based on evidence for benefit; that is, to overcome the disparities of outcome associated with inequalities of care resulting from, for example, heterogeneity of risk factor exposure and socio-economic circumstances within the population [9].

From a population perspective, this philosophy implies that the principles underlying the cancer control programme, the policies for interventional services, the priorities, and the allocation of resources will be common to the whole population, rather than discretionary to subsets of the population based on demographics, risk profile, geography, socio-economic status, or level of education. This whole-population philosophy has the objective of producing beneficial changes in cancer control in the whole population, and of reducing or removing inequities that may

Table 15.3 Performance of population-based cancer control 'programme' (strategy) and health system

Attribute	Performance of population-based cancer control programme (process measures)	Outcomes of population-based cancer control programme (outcome measures)
Organizational	Governance, corporate management Systems for enabling implementation	Cancer control outcomes (Table 15.2)
Implementation and service delivery	Performance according to 'targets' for implementation – on time and within budget	Quality, safety, and satisfaction measures 5-year survival rates by disease Disease stage 'shift' to earlier stages of disease Change in risk factor exposure
Financial and operational management	Performance to budget; variance Allocation	Comprehensiveness of programme across cancer control spectrum Accrual rates Allocation and priorities Sustainability
Stakeholder engagement	Linkage and integration within plan Leverage of resources Coherent relationships – alignment	Linkage and cross-constituency support Accountability to stakeholders Coherent messaging re population-based cancer control Meaningful public/patient engagement in priority setting
Oversight	Board (strategy 'governance' structure)	Multiple levels - designated providers/Boards - NGOs; foundations - patients and survivors - public
Accountability	Funders (including tax payers)	Public

currently exist. Achieving equity in outcomes, however, may demand planned and appropriate variation in the types of services offered to different individuals and groups and in the methods of service delivery. There is a practical reality to the degree that a population can be appropriately serviced through a single philosophic or geographic institutional entity. This necessitates the consideration of a cancer control system, with unified philosophy, principles and policies, distributed according to the geography of the population (as 'close to home as reasonably achievable') and enabled through common practices and infrastructure to function as one 'institutional', population-based programme.

The question of 'decentralization', or distribution of care 'as close to home as reasonably achievable', requires enunciation of the principles to be applied. In a publicly-funded system, the over-riding principle is that the quality of interventional care and its outcomes will be the same irrespective of location of care, i.e. quality of care does not differ according to the location of care.

To meet this principle requires consideration of:

◆ the facilities, personnel, skill-sets, and proficiencies necessary to provide cancer care at a certain level

◆ the availability of services and supports preceding or following the interventional element of care, for example, laboratory, pathology, and imaging capability as a pre-requisite for surgical services; diagnostic and surgical services to support early detection programmes

• the availability of services to support the conduct of cancer care, for example, imaging, pathology, pharmacy, nutrition, and patient support services

All this needs to function within a system that supports and continually develops evidence-based care [8,10,11] through various means: 'expert' practice groups, for example, tumour groups that bring together medical and other clinical staff who deal with a particular type of cancer; readily available and ongoing communication, informational and educational exchange methods, for example, teleconferencing, videoconferencing, tele-health, and clinico-pathological care conferences; the provision of enabling infrastructure, including clinical practice management guidelines, standards of practice, protocols, and pre-printed orders, preferably through a web-site or on-line access mechanism; and engagement of health care professionals in establishing policy and practice and ongoing information, educational, and human resource planning support.

The 'ideal' of a single system for cancer control for the population is complex beyond its philosophy, principles, and policies inasmuch as the cancer journey will cross many geographies, institutions, oncologists, health care providers, and possibly both public and private systems. This diversity may be addressed through a common approach to interventional care through guidelines, standards, and protocols, but with different 'effector' mechanisms depending upon whether interventional care is being delivered in a tertiary institutional setting or within the community (clinic or primary care). In the former, institutional policies and practices may be standardized through employment of professionals practicing within a dedicated cancer facility; in the latter, professionals are often working for other employers and in facilities or clinics serving multiple health purposes, giving less direct control. In this circumstance, the use of 'networks' may be a valuable mechanism to take evidence-based care guidelines or protocols from the tertiary institution setting to deployment across the community [12]. Networks are based in a common vision or purpose by a group of health professionals wishing to see enhanced outcomes, integration, and continuity of care, notwithstanding that they are in different employer/employee relationships, geographies, and health care settings. A single system for cancer control may, therefore, function at a population level through a variety of effector mechanisms: dedicated cancer facilities, employed cancer professionals providing population-based programmes in institutional settings, networks of health care professionals in various employment and facility settings providing care through common guidelines, protocols and standards according to mutually agreed intentions to enhance cancer control outcomes; all enabled through a commonly accessible infrastructure to provide instruction, direction, education, and communication to facilitate 'real time', evidence-based, best practice.

A further point of relevance is the alignment, or preparedness, of the health system to undertake population-based cancer control. The level of cancer control interventions, be they 'low tech' or 'high tech', needs to align with the anticipated outcome goals of the cancer control plan. In practical terms, this relates to the context in which cancer control can be effected based upon the type of health system (public, private, or mixed), and social, political, and economic circumstances. As represented in Figure 15.3, good population access with data capture through registries and/or surveys could support preventive, palliative, and supportive services impacting incidence, mortality, and quality of life, even without substantial infrastructure committed to treatment services. However, the intent to diagnose disease earlier in 'screened' populations, and to offer the interventional services to manage disease, requires not only investment in early detection (screening) services, but also the cytology, pathology, imaging, and treatment services necessary to manage detected disease. If the intent is to provide interventional services at a molecular level of understanding of disease and its response to therapy, the level of investment must be at the functional level of imaging, molecular pathology, and targeted therapeutics. Accordingly, the cancer control system can function appropriately, either at a low or high level of investment in infrastructure, provided the expected outcome measures of performance are aligned to the context and realities of the prevailing health care system.

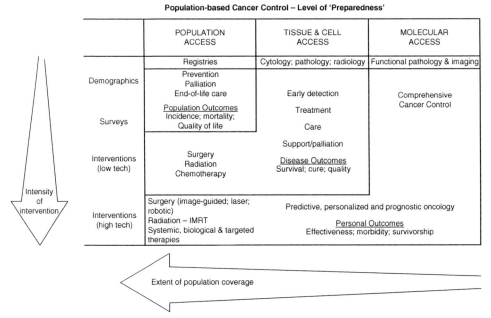

Fig. 15.3 Population-based cancer control plans – internal and external context.
The implementation of population-based cancer control requires alignment of context, here represented as level of intensity of intervention (a function of social, economic, and political realities) with the outputs/outcomes of the programme at a population, disease, and personal level. Population outcomes, expressed through incidence, mortality, and functionality (quality of life) can be approached by effective prevention, palliative and supportive care services without substantive investments in treatment services. Conversely, programmes designed to achieve 'personalized medicine' within a population framework require substantial investment in functional imaging, molecular pathology, and therapeutics.

Enhancing the efficiency and effectiveness of the cancer control system

Two concepts that relate to the efficiency and effectiveness of the cancer control system are '*continuity*' and '*integration*'. In considering continuity, the fundamental element is the individual requiring care, their experience of the episodes of care over the course of the disease, and their interpretation of the 'coherence and connectedness' of their interaction with the health system [13]. Continuity is seen from a different perspective by the provider. As expressed by Haggerty et al. for the provider, 'continuity' relates to the perception that they have sufficient knowledge and information about a patient to best apply their professional competence, and confidence that their care inputs will be recognized and pursued by others. For the patient, 'continuity' is the perception that providers know what has happened before, that different providers agree on the management plan, and that a provider who knows them will care for them in the future [13]. Common themes relating to continuity are informational continuity, management (clinical) continuity, and relational continuity (the linkage of past, present, and future).

Integrated service delivery refers to health services that are coordinated around the health needs of patients and communities [14]. Shortell et al. in their consideration of integrated health care delivery, refer to certain prevalent developments – that health care delivery value is created locally (greater decentralization and sharing of functional support services with, and within, local regions or units); blended models of centralization (strategy and direction) and decentralization (operations); greater emphasis on effective physician relationships; recognition of the complexity of integration and the necessity for focus on components for improvement; and the need for consideration of mixing 'vertical integration through ownership' with 'virtual' integration through contracting, alliances, partnerships, and out-sourcing [14]. Recognizing the common impediments – lack of aligned economic incentives, lack of coherent national policy, lack of a business case for quality or value, and a continuing focus on the 'bottom line' – they propose that 'five forces' will drive directionally towards integrated health care delivery: the aging population (greater volume and need for care), technology, empowered consumers, payment innovations, for example, pay for performance or outcomes, and the need for institutional partners to effect strategy [15]. From the 'system' perspective, common themes related to service integration arise – functional integration (common, core support services), clinical integration (patient service management), information (technology and management) and 'vertical' integration (joint ventures, multi-institutional alliances, and linkage across health and other public service sectors) [13–16].

From a cancer control system perspective, integration of cancer control ensures that programmes and services are coordinated around the health needs of public, patients, and communities at risk of or experiencing cancer. The relationship between the desired situation, the common reality, key enablers, and some key inhibitors for enhanced performance regarding continuity and integration is outlined in Table 15.4.

Vertical and virtual integration is explored by Shortell et al. in the context of the 'need to partner' within the traditional health sector and across sectors; the concepts of 'trading alliances' of an instrumental (intended for each partner to achieve its separate objectives) or symbiotic (intended to achieve a shared goal that neither can achieve alone) nature, and designed to involve the exchange of different resources and capabilities to create value [14]. From a cancer control perspective, this raises the questions of 'where and how does the cancer control activity fit within the broader health agenda at local, national, and global levels' and 'who does what to ensure coherent, effective implementation'? Figure 15.4 provides a simple illustration of 'fit' – at an institutional or state/province/country level, how does the cancer control plan relate to other health plans for communicable and non-communicable diseases; and within what context (resource setting for health and illness control), and with what priority, relative to other health and societal issues? How does a state/province/country cancer control plan 'fit', or relate, to cancer control plans for a nation (or another governed jurisdiction); how do national plans relate to cancer control for a 'health region', for example, Latin America and the Caribbean, or Europe, recognizing the heterogeneity of context and priority within differing countries within a region; and how do cancer control plans at institutional, national, or health region levels relate to the global endeavour in cancer control – the enabling of enhanced cancer control through knowledge sharing and collaboration amongst nations.

The roles of different constituencies in the provision of population-based cancer control are explored in Figure 15.5. Within the content and process of cancer control, knowledge generation through research, knowledge validation through derivation of evidence for benefit, and knowledge application (best practice) are the key steps in knowledge transfer from science to population application. The participants and their potential roles within and across the knowledge transfer framework are illustrated schematically.

The important point is that integration of all partners into a coherent representation and implementation of the cancer control plan is necessary – each has an important role and a relatively unique ability to influence the public/patient/provider/political spectrum necessary to effect and implement a population-based cancer control plan.

Table 15.4 Achieving continuity and integration of service delivery for cancer control

Perspectives	Desired situation	Reality	Key enablers	Inhibitors
Patient	Coherent and connected experience by the individual over time. Expectation that what has happened before is communicated in real-time, that different providers agree on the management plan, and that a provider who knows them will care for them in the future	Perception of fragmentation Poor continuity of prior knowledge, current health state, information transfer Breakdown between tertiary & community Illness management rather than whole person care Variable use of evidence	Information management/ technology (IM/IT) Electronic health record (EHR) Care-paths Clinical practice guidelines Standards of care Protocols Multidisciplinary team Networks (primary/community/ tertiary)	Jurisdictional competition Payment and reimbursement systems Provider and institutional role ambiguity Territoriality: geographic; professional; administrative
Health Provider	Providers have sufficient knowledge and current and past information about a patient to best apply their professional competence, and confidence that their care inputs will be recognized and pursued by other providers	Inadequate real-time access to current and past information about patients Currency of medical competence and decision-making through evidence/best practice Time/inclination to explore all appropriate options for care and healing	IM/IT EHR Multidisciplinary teams Evidence-based care Tumour groups Integrative care frameworks	Jurisdictional competition Payment systems Inter-professional rivalries Policy/frameworks for health and illness management
Health system/ administration	Modern, cost-effective system characterized by closer working relations across and between components of health care (hospitals) and other sector elements (long term care, primary care, home care, public health, social welfare, housing, schools, police, etc)	Mounting cost pressure Duplication of services Gaps in service provision Manage to 'budget' rather than better health	IM/IT EHR Intersectoral 'system' perspective Functional integration of care services Out-sourcing as appropriate	Segmented budgets Manage by 'budget performance' rather than health performance Policy frameworks

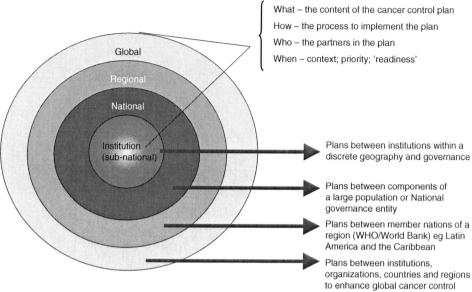

What – the content of the cancer control plan

How – the process to implement the plan

Who – the partners in the plan

When – context; priority; 'readiness'

Plans between institutions within a discrete geography and governance

Plans between components of a large population or National governance entity

Plans between member nations of a region (WHO/World Bank) eg Latin America and the Caribbean

Plans between institutions, organizations, countries and regions to enhance global cancer control

Fig 15.4 Population-based cancer control plans – a framework for partnership. Population-based cancer control plans do not exist in isolation of other health priorities. They have an alignment within institutional priorities (based on 'burden', referral practice, critical mass of expertise, strategic priorities, priorities of other institutions, etc.); within national cancer plans across regions, states, provinces etc. to 'benchmark', create critical mass, and 'add value' through collaboration and knowledge transfer; within regions, for example, North America, Latin America, the Caribbean, etc. and at a global level to effect knowledge sharing, mentorship, assistance at personnel, programme, or financial level and 'progress through partnership'.

Are organized, population-based disease control plans necessary? . . . effective?

Cancer is a process – the process of carcinogenesis – enacted at a cellular level, with impacts at an individual and population level. The opportunities to intervene in the process to achieve a more beneficial outcome range from primary prevention (often deriving from interventions impacting early life circumstances and choices) to end-of-life care. Accordingly, a cancer strategy needs to be directed to the multiple steps in the process in a manner related to context of population circumstances, resource-availability, and appropriateness of allocation. Thus, a strategy to control cancer is necessary . . . but, insufficient unless effectively implemented.

Implementation of the cancer strategy can be evaluated in a number of ways (Table 15.3); however, the ultimate question is whether 'implemented' plans favourably influence cancer control outcomes, and more specifically, outcomes determined to be beneficial as defined by the needs of the stakeholders and partners enacting the plan.

Rochester et al. in addressing the evaluation of comprehensive cancer control efforts draw attention to the challenges inherent in linking the plan to the outcomes [17] – aligning the evaluation, its process, rigour, and measures of benefit, to the needs of the stakeholders; the difficulties in attributing 'causality' between interventions and outcomes. In ideal circumstances interventions would clearly precede results, 'control populations' would be used, and there would be no

Population-based cancer control plans – a framework for partnership

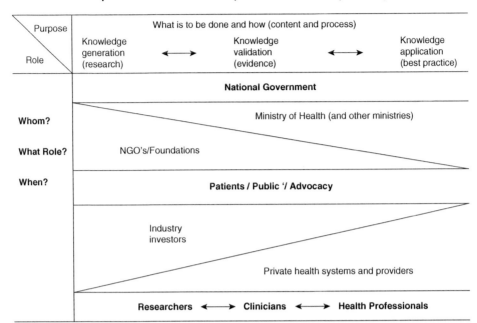

Fig 15.5 The relationship between the purpose of the population-based cancer control plan (what is to be done and how – the content and process of the plan) and the roles of the various constituencies (stakeholders) in effecting the plan.

The constituencies will have differing roles relative to the elements of the plan, for example, knowledge generation and the research community; patients, public, and NGOs, with respect to advocacy; provincial/state governments at knowledge application (best practice). All constituencies, however, have a role which needs to be understood in the context of 'value greater than the sum of the parts' rather than fragmented or competitive relationships between necessary partners.

variation of other factors affecting outcomes. In reality, it is often difficult to define the onset of interventions impacting outcomes, 'control populations' would imply denial of health interventions, and separating the effects of cancer control interventions from other relevant societal and health system interventions is impossible.

Thus, Rochester et al. conclude that 'causality can be approximated and can be discussed; it cannot be assured' [17]: noting the difficulty in defining the 'value add' of the strategy, i.e. the benefits attributable to the collaborative activity that could not be achieved by the partners functioning independently; the 'time lag' between interventions to control cancer and evidence of improved cancer control; and the lack of data underlying the ability to link intervention and effect, for example, nutritional intake, sun exposure, exercise, quality of life, and functionality.

Given the difficulties in providing evidence that cancer control strategies per se are effective, a reasonable approximation would be the demonstration that interventions can cause changes within components of the cancer control spectrum that may reasonably be expected to influence outcomes favourably. Suitable examples of this premise might include the following:

◆ Primary prevention – tobacco control; the reduction in tobacco smoking through various forms of intervention (legislation, taxation, social practice, etc) has resulted in serial reductions in age-standardized incidence rates of lung cancer, predominantly in males, in developed countries [18] (see also Chapter 2).

◆ Cervical screening – organized cervical cytology programmes have been demonstrated to be more effective than opportunistic activity in terms of age-adjusted incidence reduction and accrual rates within the target population [19–21], and a reversal of adverse trends in incidence and mortality has been shown following the introduction of organized, population screening [22] (see also Chapter 4).

◆ Screening mammography – notwithstanding controversy, there is general agreement that screening mammography has contributed to declining age-standardized mortality rates for breast cancer. The magnitude of the effect is more difficult to assess, given the introduction of systemic therapies in adjuvant settings (hormonal and chemotherapeutic), a refined role for adjuvant radiation therapy and greater use of, and compliance with, guidelines for optimal practice [23,24] (see also Chapter 4). An alternative determination of the beneficial impact of organized screening mammography lies in the domain of 'efficiency' of population-based interventions. Thus, in British Columbia, provincial expenditures on bilateral mammography have declined whilst the number of examinations has increased; this has been achieved by increasing the number of screens within the 'organized' programmes at a lower unit cost whilst decreasing the number of 'non-organized programmes/diagnostic' screens at higher unit cost. The effectiveness of screening mammography increased through interpretation by accredited radiologists within the programme, clear guidelines for eligibility, increasing participation, and a reduction in the inflation-adjusted budget for mammography services [25].

◆ Treatment/research – enrolment in clinical trials. Funding commitments through the National Cancer Research Institute in England have resulted in more than a doubling of the enrolment of cancer patients into clinical studies within a three-year time frame, to a 2006-07 enrolment of 11.2 per cent of incident cases (see also Chapter 14).

◆ Treatment/patient experience. Independent evaluations of the National Cancer Plan in England show progress in relation to improved cancer patient experiences, meeting targets for access to cancer services, reconfiguring services, increasing multidisciplinary care and improving staffing ratios and capital equipment/facilities. As yet, eight years into the initiative, the benefits of the plan in terms of survival of cancer patients remain to be established [26] (see also Chapter 14).

◆ Treatment – changes in 'standards' derived from practice audit. Mitry et al. described improvements in colorectal cancer survival among 5874 patients studied over a 24-year period between period 1976 to 1987 and 1988 to 1999 [27]. Factors associated with improvements in relative survival included a higher proportion of patients resected for cure, standardization of surgical technique (total meso-rectal excision), reduction in post-operative mortality, increased use of adjuvant chemotherapy for colon cancer and of surgery with radiation therapy for rectal cancer, and an increasing use of interdisciplinary consultation [28].

◆ Treatment – compliance with clinical practice guidelines. In March, 2001, the BC Cancer Agency implemented a policy recommending (and reimbursing) the use of CHOP (cyclophosphamide, adriamycin, vincristine, and prednisone) and rituximab for all newly diagnosed patients with advanced stage DLBCL (diffuse/large B-cell lymphoma), regardless of age, in the province of British Columbia (BC), Canada. Comparison of overall survival and progression-free survival rates for all patients in BC diagnosed in the 18-month periods before and after the introduction of rituximab showed a dramatic improvement in outcome, with an approximate doubling of overall and progression-free survival, with a median of 24 months of follow-up [30] (see also Chapter 10 and Figure 10.9).

◆ Similarly, in a study of the impact of guidelines on the consistency of adjuvant therapy for node-negative breast cancer, comparing British Columbia (with province-wide guidelines) and Ontario (with no province-wide guidelines), Sawka et al. observed that patterns of pathology reporting were consistent with awareness of the factors to define indications for adjuvant therapy in British Columbia, consistency of care was greater in British Columbia than Ontario by all diagnostic grouping systems, and that the observed patterns of practice in British Columbia corresponded to the BC guidelines [31].

The evidence to determine a favourable impact of population-based cancer plans on cancer outcomes is difficult to establish, other than in a 'piece-meal' fashion. The situation for other communicable and non-communicable diseases is more apparent, perhaps because the pathogen or attributable cause is easier to define, and hence, eradicate or mitigate, and the time course of the disease is shorter. The World Bank has put forward criteria by which it has proposed sixteen examples of diseases or health states that have been improved, or substantially eradicated, by population-based strategic interventions, largely of a public health nature [32]. The criteria include: implementation on a significant scale; address a major public health problem; lasted at least five consecutive years; cost effective (less than $100 US per disability-adjusted life year (DALY) averted); clear and measurable effect on health outcomes (i.e. not 'process', 'accrual', or 'coverage'); and variable interventional methods (e.g. products, services, behaviours, and risks).

The successful interventions identified have been directed to communicable diseases (Chagas disease, infectious diarrhoea, guinea-worm, measles, tuberculosis, hepatitis-B, onchocerciasis, polio, smallpox, trachoma, and HIV/AIDS), public health systems (salt fluoridation, salt iodination, and maternal health), life-style, and social policy (tobacco control; family planning, and financial incentives for health). Many of these examples, for example, smallpox, polio, and onchocerciasis, clearly indicate the principles of definition of a strategy to control a disease process, implementation of the strategy preceding results, and control or eradication of an attributable cause of population ill-health.

Conclusions

Are population-based cancer control programmes necessary to control cancer? This premise is supported in this chapter, given that cancer is an increasing burden for all populations; it is a process with an underlying genetic basis that arises in health and progresses through illness, reduced functionality, and death, if not reversed; multiple opportunities exist for intervention through prevention, early detection, treatment, and palliation/end-of-life care; and interventions can be demonstrably effective and directionally consistent with expectations of improved cancer control outcomes. The issue, however, is not whether population-based strategies are necessary; it is a question of whether, and to what degree, they are implemented that will ultimately determine their value in controlling cancer. The problem has less to do with the 'content' of population-based cancer control, but rather to the context, opportunity, and reality of implementing population-based interventions.

References

1 Hanahan D & Weinberg RA (2000). The hallmarks of cancer. *Cell*, **100**(1):57–70.

2 Jones LA, Chilton JA, Hajek RA, Iammarino NK, & Laufman L (2006). Between and within: international perspectives on cancer and health disparities. *J Clin Oncol*, **24**(14):2204–08.

3 Coleman MP, Quaresma M, Berrino F, et al (2008). Cancer survival in five continents: a worldwide population-based study (CONCORD). *Lancet Oncol*, **9**(8):730–56.

4 World Health Organization & International Agency for Research on Cancer (2003). *World cancer report*. IARC Press, Lyon.

5 Canadian Strategy for Cancer Control (2006). *The Canadian strategy for Cancer Control: A Cancer Plan for Canada*, 1–25. Available from: http://www.partnershipagainstcancer.ca/sites/default/files/documents/reports/CSCC_CancerPlan_2006.pdf

6 Given LS, Black B, Lowry G, Huang P, & Kerner JF (2005). Collaborating to conquer cancer: a comprehensive approach to cancer control. *Cancer Causes Control*, **16**(Suppl 1):3–14.

7 Caron L, De Civita M, & Law S (2008). Cancer control interventions in selected jurisdictions: design, governance, and implementation. 1–343. 1 May2008. Agence d'évaluation des technologies et des modes d'intervention en santé (AETMIS), Quebec.

8 True S, Kean T, Nolan PA, Haviland ES, & Hohman K (2005). In conclusion: The promise of comprehensive cancer control. *Cancer Causes Control*, **16**(Suppl 1):79–88.

9 Hayes N, Rollins R, Weinberg A, et al (2005). Cancer-related disparities: Weathering the perfect storm through comprehensive cancer control approaches. *Cancer Causes Control*, **1**(16 Suppl):41–50.

10 Kerner JF, Guirguis-Blake J, Hennessy KD, et al (2005). Translating research into improved outcomes in comprehensive cancer control. *Cancer Causes Control*, **16**(Suppl 1):27–40.

11 Grunfeld E, Zitzelsberger L, Evans WK, et al (2004). Better knowledge translation for effective cancer control: a priority for action. *Cancer Causes Control*, **15**(5):503–10.

12 Strack MN, Poole B, Lasser F, & Sutcliffe S (2005). Where there is a will, there is a way: Networks as a means of cancer control. *J Oncol Manag*, **14**(4):20–28.

13 Haggerty JL, Reid RJ, Freeman GK, Starfield BH, Adair CE, & McKendry R (2003). Continuity of care: a multidisciplinary review. *BMJ*, **327**(7425):1219–21.

14 Shortell SM (2000). Integrated health care and the community health care management system: Prospects for the future. *Remaking health care in America: the evolution of organized delivery systems*, 2nd ed, pp.247–295. Jossey-Bass, San Francisco.

15 Leatt P (2002). Health Transition Fund (Canada). Integrated service delivery. Minister of Public Works and Government Services Canada, Ottawa.

16 Conrad DA (1993). Coordinating patient care services in regional health systems: The challenge of clinical integration. *Hosp Health Serv Adm*, **38**(4):491–508.

17 Rochester P, Chapel T, Black B, Bucher J, & Housemann R (2005). The evaluation of comprehensive cancer control efforts: Useful techniques and unique requirements. *Cancer Causes Control*, **16**(Suppl 1):69–78.

18 Boyle P, Autier P, Bartelink H, et al (2003). European Code Against Cancer and scientific justification: Third version. *Ann Oncol*, **14**(7):973–1005.

19 Anttila A, Pukkala E, Soderman B, Kallio M, Nieminen P, & Hakama M (1999). Effect of organised screening on cervical cancer incidence and mortality in Finland, 1963–1995: Recent increase in cervical cancer incidence. *Int J Cancer*, **83**(1):59–65.

20 Nieminen P, Kallio M, Anttila A, & Hakama M (1999). Organised vs. spontaneous Pap-smear screening for cervical cancer: A case-control study. *Int J Cancer*, **83**(1):55–58.

21 Ronco G, Pilutti S, Patriarca S, et al (2005). Impact of the introduction of organised screening for cervical cancer in Turin, Italy: Cancer incidence by screening history 1992–98. *Br J Cancer*, **93**(3):376–78.

22 Peto J, Gilham C, Fletcher O, & Matthews FE (2004). The cervical cancer epidemic that screening has prevented in the UK. *Lancet*, **364**(9430):249–56.

23 Hakama M, Coleman MP, Alexe DM, & Auvinen A (2008). European Observatory on Health Systems and Policies. Cancer screening. In Coleman MP, Alexe DM, Albreht T, & McKee M (eds) *Responding to the challenge of cancer in Europe*, pp. 69–92. Institute of Public Health of the Republic of Slovenia, Ljubljana.

24 Haward R (2008). European Observatory on Health Systems and Policies. Organizing a comprehensive framework for cancer control. In Coleman MP, Alexe DM, Albreht T, & McKee M (eds) *Responding to the challenge of cancer in Europe*, pp. 113–33. Institute of Public Health of the Republic of Slovenia, Ljubljana.

25 Coldman AJ (2008). British Columbia breast cancer screening program. Personal communication.

26 National Audit Office, Department of Health (2009). The NHS Cancer Plan: A progress report. HC 343, 1–35. March 11 2005. The Stationery Office, London. May 25 2009.

27 Mitry E, Bouvier AM, Esteve J, & Faivre J (2005). Improvement in colorectal cancer survival: A population-based study. *Eur J Cancer*, **41**(15):2297–2303.

28 Phang PT, Strack M, & Poole B (2003). Proposal to improve rectal cancer outcomes in BC. *BCMJ*, **45**(7):330–35.

29 Murata A, Brown CJ, Raval M, & Phang PT (2008). Impact of short-course radiotherapy and low anterior resection on quality of life and bowel function in primary rectal cancer. *Am J Surg*, **195**(5):611–15.

30 Sehn LH, Donaldson J, Chhanabhai M, et al (2005). Introduction of combined CHOP plus rituximab therapy dramatically improved outcome of diffuse large B-cell lymphoma in British Columbia. *J Clin Oncol*, **23**(22):5027–33.

31 Sawka C, Olivotto I, Coldman A, Goel V, Holowaty E, & Hislop TG (1997). The association between population-based treatment guidelines and adjuvant therapy for node-negative breast cancer. British Columbia/Ontario Working Group. *Br J Cancer*, **75**(10):1534–42.

32 Jamison DT, Breman JG, Meashorn AR, et al. *Disease control priorities in developing countries*. 2nd ed. International Bank for Reconstruction and Development. The World Bank, Washington DC.

Chapter 16

Getting the public involved in cancer control – doing something besides worrying

Patricia Kelly, William Friedman, Tara Addis, Mark Elwood, Claire Neal, Mark Sarner, Simon Sutcliffe[1]

Public engagement refers to the public's involvement in determining how a society steers itself, makes decisions on major public policy issues, and delivers programmes for the benefit of people. It is closely linked to the concept of social cohesion and the building of shared values, reducing disparities in wealth and income, and enabling people to engage in a common enterprise and face shared challenges as members of a same community.

Public engagement is the continuum along which individuals move from a basis of awareness of an issue through understanding to personal involvement and informed action, as shown by the 'ladder of engagement' used by the Campaign to Control Cancer (Canada) organization (Figure 16.1). Basic awareness is the first step in the continuum and individual or collective informed action is the last and most desired step.

Cancer control – with its greater emphasis on prevention and information prior to a cancer diagnosis – benefits from employing a public engagement/social mobilization model in many ways. Public engagement:

◆ Accelerates collective momentum and social change

◆ Fosters inclusivity (shared goals, aspirations, language, and action)

◆ Engages highly motivated individuals as credible spokespersons

◆ Reduces stigma and isolation

◆ Increases effective management and allocation of resources and effort

◆ Enhances transparency and accountability

◆ Engages decision-makers and key influencers

◆ Mobilizes stakeholders and citizens to act

[1] Patricia Kelly, MA, Chief Executive Officer, Campaign to Control Cancer (C2CC), Toronto, Ontario Canada; William Friedman, PhD, Chief Operating Officer and Director of Public Engagement, Public Agenda, New York, NY, USA; Tara Addis, BSc., Chair, Stakeholder Relations, Campaign to Control Cancer (C2CC), Toronto, Canada; J. Mark Elwood, MD, DSc, FRCPC, FAFPHM, Vice-President, Family and Community Oncology, BC Cancer Agency, Vancouver, British Columbia, Canada; Claire Neal, MPH, CHES, Director of Education and Program Development, Lance Armstrong Foundation, Austin, Texas, USA; Mark Sarner, President/CEO, Manifest Communications, Toronto, Ontario, Canada; Simon B. Sutcliffe, MD, FRCP, FRCPC, FRCR, Board Chair, Canadian Partnership Against Cancer, Canada; Past President, BC Cancer Agency, Vancouver, British Columbia, Canada.

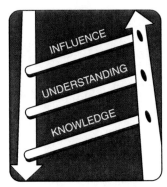

Fig. 16.1 Schema of public engagement.
Source: From Campaign to Control Cancer in Canada, reproduced with permission [3]. http://www. controlcancer.ca/en/know.

Cancer control represents a conceptual shift from concentrating on the individual patient who presents at a cancer clinic to a concern for the whole population, and lends itself well to the public engagement potential for accelerating change. The call to public engagement is shown in the approach of Lance Armstrong, champion cyclist, cancer survivor, and founder of the Lance Armstrong Foundation in the United States [1], dedicated to inspiring and empowering people affected by cancer (Figure 16.2): 'At the Lance Armstrong Foundation, we unite people to fight cancer believing that unity is strength, knowledge is power, and attitude is everything'.

> People are often surprised to learn that cycling is a team sport. The team is critical. It's everything. The images of a lone guy crossing the line on a mountain top betray an important reality–eight other teammates and a tireless crowd of support staffers got him there.
>
> Every good fight needs a good team. The fight to make cancer a global priority is no exception.
>
> I believe we must ensure that everyone benefits from what we know today about cancer prevention and detection. We must fully support scientific discovery, which is our best hope for improved screening and therapies and better understanding of prevention and metastases. We must ask ourselves what is at stake and recognize that it is our spouses, parents, children and friends.
>
> It is time to change the experiences and expectations of cancer. It is time to marshal our collective will, our passion, our outrage, our insistence and our voices.
>
> Significant accomplishments–winning a Tour de France, surviving cancer–almost always demand an active and engaged team. The fight against cancer is no exception.
>
> Millions of cancer survivors are counting on you. Their loved ones are counting on you. I'm counting on you.
>
> LIVESTRONG,
>
> *Lance Armstrong*

Fig. 16.2 A letter from the Lance Armstrong Foundation Founder and Chairman.
Source: From Lance Armstrong Foundation, reproduced with permission [1]. http://www.livestrong.org.

Increasing public capacity for cancer control

The approach to the public will emphasize messages such as these: in today's world, anyone can develop cancer, including world-class athletes and other people at low risk. Everyone will be touched by cancer – as a person living with a diagnosis, or a family member or a friend. Even though scientists understand many of the factors that put people at risk, these factors may only account for part of the disease. Over 40 per cent of the more than 7 million cancer deaths world wide could be prevented. The technology for screening, diagnosing, and treating is mature, and many further cases of cancer could be cured.

Understanding why we have been unable to convince the public that treating and preventing cancer is not only possible, but a wondrous thing is a first step in understanding the potential for a public engagement approach. Consider the following questions:

♦ How might an engaged and mobilized public and corporate sector accelerate increased compliance with screening programmes?

♦ How might public reporting of outcomes, access, and waiting times help to sustain public confidence and political commitment to quality cancer care, in a socially responsible context of competing healthcare needs?

♦ How might school-based programmes help impact risk factors such as tobacco use, sun exposure, unhealthy diet, and physical inactivity?

♦ Human papillomavirus (HPV) vaccines have the potential to prevent infection with strains of HPV that are responsible for the bulk of cases of cervical cancer (not to mention that HPV is also responsible for some cases of throat cancer and penile cancer), as discussed in Chapter 6. Logically, this should prevent most cases of cervical cancer. Yet acceptance of HPV vaccination involves many economic, cultural, social, and religious issues, and many teenaged girls and their parents may reject an HPV vaccine programme. How might public engagement strategies that include evidence-based messaging from diverse communities help address the issue?

Answering these questions should be a priority for cancer control professionals and health policy makers, because everywhere the problem of fatalism and failing to translate cancer progress into behaviour change appears alarming. Recent studies conducted in the United States have shown that almost half of the American public believes that 'it seems that almost everything causes cancer, about 1 in 4 feel there's not much one can do to lower the chances of getting cancer, and 3 out of 4 felt there were so many recommendations, it's hard to know which ones to follow [2]. This is evidence that there is widespread confusion and helplessness in the American adult population in terms of cancer prevention. Such fatalistic beliefs about cancer prevention are having a negative impact, and those who hold fatalistic beliefs about cancer prevention may be at greater risk of cancer because they are less likely to engage in various prevention behaviours such as exercising weekly, not smoking, and eating five or more fruits and vegetables daily.

Understanding the public's starting point suggests that insensitive approaches to cancer control communications will fail. The hallmark of some has been proselytizing: 'If we say everyone should have the vaccine, everyone should have the vaccine. Trust us'. That way of communicating – preaching rather than educating – just doesn't succeed any more; not in the age of 24-hour news channels, the Internet and instant messaging. It is not enough to tell people what to do because it's good for them: you have to make your case and make it well. That is particularly true when tackling sensitive topics such as sexual mores and gynaecological health – which will necessarily arise in a discussion of HPV.

Public engagement efforts that address social change and cancer can be a unique and bold experiment in citizen-led policy-making where, working alongside experts, practitioners, patients and survivors, everyday citizens can take account of cancer's effects and future. Convening authentic public engagement efforts communicates confidence in the capacity of people to understand complex issues and make good decisions. When given the information and the opportunity, the collective intelligence of citizens is a remarkable and powerful force for public action. The future of cancer is an issue public engagement processes can deal with constructively by raising awareness, generating a sense of purpose and urgency, and deepening a sense of shared responsibility for choices made.

To have sustainable impact, there remains a need to broaden our understanding of the key principles and practices that underlie successful public engagement in cancer control. This chapter draws attention to the importance of public engagement in sustainable cancer control policy, the continuum for engagement practices based upon intended outcomes, the principles and practices that guide successful efforts, and new trends and ideas for building organizational capacity. Practical action steps are recommended, indicating how diverse groups can support effective public engagement in cancer control efforts.

One illustration that has been used in Canadian cancer strategy developments shows the strategy (the CSCC, Canadian Strategy for Cancer Control [3,4] as dependent on maintaining the constants of collaboration and collective social capital (k), managing the five variables (p) of 'population, people, platform, profile, and politics', and raising the necessary funding (f) (Figure 16.3). The formula helps illustrate the emerging prominence and value of public engagement in supporting comprehensive cancer control.

Authentic engagement versus business as usual

In the past, one of the most common approaches to engaging the public in cancer control programmes – the expert panel – subjected a passive, glassy-eyed audience to the pontificating of a few knowledgeable individuals. This approach operates on the assumption that providing more information is the key to engaging people. Information has a place in the grand scheme, but it's easy for this approach to amount to little more than a data-dump. Public education campaigns based upon a static model of information dissemination have a role to play but ultimately it's up to individuals, communities, and governments to understand what's at stake and take action. Action planning requires time to build a knowledge base, engage in choice-making and determine priorities. By involving citizens in meaningful partnerships, people can help improve not only

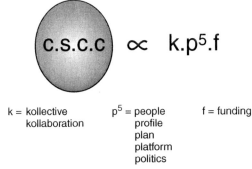

$$\text{c.s.c.c} \propto k.p^5.f$$

k = kollective p^5 = people   f = funding
         kollaboration   profile
                         plan
                         platform
                         politics

Fig. 16.3 A Theory of Relationships for successful implementation of the Canadian Strategy for Cancer Control.
Source: From National Cancer Leadership Forum, reproduced with permission [4]. http://www.controlcancer.ca/en/news/nclf-events.

Increasing level of public impact →

	Inform	Consult	Involve	Collaborate	Empower
Public participation goal	To provide the public with balanced and objective information to assist them in understanding the problem, alternatives, opportunities and/or solutions.	To obtain public feedback on analysis, alternatives and/or decisions.	To work directly with the public throughout the process to ensure that public concerns and aspirations are consistently understood and considered.	To partner with the public in each aspect of the decision including the development of alternatives and the indentification of the preferred solution.	To place final decision-makin in the hands of the public.
Promise to the public	We will keep you informed.	We will keep you informed, listen to and acknowledge concerns and aspirations, and provide feedback on how public input influenced the decision.	We will work with you to ensure that your concerns and aspirations are directly reflected in the alternatives developed and provide feedback on how public input influenced the decision.	We will look to you for advice and innovation in formulating solutions and incorporate your advice and recommendations into the decisions to the maximum extent possible.	We will implement what you decide
Example techniques	■ Fact sheets ■ Web sites ■ Open houses	■ Public comment ■ Focus groups ■ Surveys ■ Public meetings	■ Workshops ■ Deliberative polling	■ Citizen advisory committees ■ Consensus-building ■ Participatory decision-making	■ Citizen juries ■ Ballots ■ Delegated decision

Fig. 16.4 The spectrum of public engagement – continuum.
Source: From International Association for Public Participation, reproduced with permission [5].
http://www.iap2.org/associations/4748/files/spectrum.pdf.

individual health but also the health of neighbours, family, and friends. A spectrum of public engagement, moving from passive to active involvement, is shown in Figure 16.4 [5].

Finding ways of genuinely involving those directly affected by cancer will also help to strengthen public engagement in the long-run. Although it may take more time in the short term to attract a network of people affected by cancer, and to build leadership skills in cancer control, it is worth the investment.

Frameworks for public engagement

This framework can be applied to action at all levels: local, national, and international. These models have been used to guide the successful public engagement campaigns for implementation of comprehensive cancer control plans in developing and developed countries. This section draws on work by Dr. Will Friedman and his colleagues at the Center for Advances in Public Engagement at Public Agenda, especially on their document, 'Public Engagement: A Primer from Public Agenda' [6].

The framework can be used in many ways to plan public engagement work systematically, and allows participants to gain skills by learning and networking with others. These planning activities allow participants to deepen their understanding of engagement and build partnerships and alliances with other organizations.

There are a number of formats or structures available for conducting public participation. The format is selected based upon the desired outcomes. These formats can:

- Share information
- Bring people together to seek common ground
- Collect input and provide feedback

If we model sincerity, respect, and transparency in selecting and using the technique, we are more likely to achieve the aim of building relationships or social capital – trust, openness, and communication.

Techniques for sharing information

Techniques for sharing information are generally either part of an awareness campaign or an information/education programme.

Awareness campaigns are usually conducted along with a participatory process: the purpose is to make people aware of the opportunity to learn more or get involved. For example, a community initiating a long-range plan banning the use of cosmetic pesticides might start by conducting an awareness campaign to alert people to the project.

An information/education programme is designed to educate people on a particular topic. An example is a national campaign conducted by government to educate citizens about food and physical activity guides to promote healthy active living.

The difference between these techniques is that while awareness campaigns are geared to getting people's attention, they convey little information. Education programmes provide information intended to help influence behaviours and should be sensitive to the complexity and language used as well as how it is received.

Public engagement strategies

Various strategies can be employed to reach out to stakeholders, raise their awareness, gain their insights, and build common ground and active support for cancer control plans. Where one is more efficient, another leads to greater public buy-in, while yet another is better at gaining media attention. Specifically, we will discuss the following public engagement strategies:

- Focus groups and surveys
- Stakeholder dialogues
- Community forums

Focus groups

Focus groups – essentially, small-group research interviews – are a tool that can accomplish some, but not all, of the goals of public engagement. They are an efficient means to inform the planning team of the priorities and concerns of various stakeholders. Focus groups can help planners understand the public's starting point, frame the relevant issue, develop background materials, become aware of potential hot-button issues that can derail the dialogue, prepare moderator training materials, etc. Examples are given by the Public Agenda Engagement Resource Center [6,7] (www.publicagenda.org). But, while focus groups achieve some public engagement goals, they do not achieve them all. They provide a reading of people's state of mind, but do not, by themselves, help advance thinking. They can illuminate confusion but not constitute the communication needed to correct it. They can distinguish issues that the public are willing to delegate to professionals from those they want to have a say in, but do not help communities work through those differences to build the common ground and collaborations. Nor does focus group research provide the public vetting of a solution that helps legitimize it. Planners can always argue that they received good input from many stakeholders via focus groups, and that this was incorporated into the thinking and planning; but as focus groups are a controlled process, not a public one, the outputs from them can easily be questioned. The strengths of focus groups include:

◆ They are an efficient way to gain input from the community, to refine plans, communicate about them more effectively, and prepare for more ambitious public engagement.
◆ They are a relatively controlled process, in that the information can easily be managed by the planners.

Among the disadvantages are:

◆ Focus groups do not do much to legitimize the plans presented to them.
◆ People are unlikely to accept them as a democratic process.
◆ They require resources and expertise to do well.

Stakeholder dialogues

Focus groups keep control in the hands of those who organize and lead them. In focus groups, for example, people are often paid to attend. By contrast, stakeholder dialogues are by nature a less controlled process. Participants are not selected subjects; they are peers, citizens who are voluntarily contributing their time and ideas. Compared to focus group participants, they will feel less constrained about commenting to others – including, perhaps, the media, about what it is they have discussed.

These sessions can be with highly homogeneous groups such as patients only, or a wider group, as in the example of the UK-based all-party parliamentary group that organized an annual 'Britain Against Cancer' event [8] for patients, health professionals, and policy-makers (Box 16.1). In either case, the purpose is to engage people in productive dialogue about an issue of shared interest, to elicit their level of interest and ideas about how to make it work.

The strengths of stakeholder dialogues include:

◆ They allow the organizers, as with focus groups, to target specific groups that are most important to the work.
◆ They are inexpensive and require limited expertise.

Drawbacks, limitations, and challenges of stakeholder dialogues include:

◆ They require time and care to do well.
◆ They do not raise general awareness and engagement across the community as effectively as community forums will.

Community forums

These are opportunities to engage a broad cross-section of the community in dialogue, including both specific stakeholders and average citizens. A Canadian example is shown in Box 16.2 [9]. They include more of the public than the engagement strategies discussed so far, as these can be large-scale civic events to include all sectors of the community on the issue at hand. The basic principles for community dialogue are:

◆ Non-partisan sponsors and organizers
◆ Diverse cross-section of participants
◆ Small, diverse dialogue groups

Box 16.1 Example of a stakeholder dialogue: from the United Kingdom

Updating the national strategy for cancer

In the United Kingdom, the All Party Parliamentary Group on Cancer (APPGC) was founded in 1998 to keep cancer at the top of the political agenda, and to ensure that policy-making remains patient-centred. It brings together members of parliament and peers from across the political spectrum to debate key issues and campaign together to improve the national cancer plan and cancer services. APPGC organizes an annual event, Britain Against Cancer that for the past eight years has successfully brought together patients, health professionals, and policy-makers to look at the impact of public policy on cancer services and research.

According to Dr Ian Gibson MP, Chairman of APPGC in 2007, 'The original National Health System Cancer Plan, launched in 2000, led to improvements in front line cancer services. The cancer landscape has changed dramatically since then but health inequalities still persist. A new, holistic vision that creates patient entitlements to standards of care covering the whole patient pathway is needed'.

Early in 2007, APPGC launched its new vision for the future of cancer services. The vision focuses on bridging the gap between health and social care; educating professionals and the public; improving prevention, diagnosis and treatment; researching genetics, the causes of, and treatments for, cancer; and producing national standards and specifying entitlements that people with cancer can expect from health and social care services. A few months later, at the Britain Against Cancer event held in December 2007, the Government announced its commitment to an updated national strategy which will include, as top priorities, strengthening prevention and early detection, as well as reducing inequalities and improving cancer services for treatment, care and rehabilitation.

From: Britain Against Cancer, reproduced with permission [8]. http://www.macmillan.org.uk/Get_Involved/Campaigns/APPG/cancer_news_in_parliament.aspx.

♦ Non-partisan discussion materials that help participants weigh alternatives

♦ Trained moderators and recorders

♦ Forum follow-up

These elements will help create participative, productive, inclusive, and effective community forums.

The strengths of community forums are:

♦ They will tend to reach the largest number of people and to gain the broadest input.

♦ They can generate positive press coverage and raise general awareness.

♦ They bring new ideas, resources, and partners to your initiative.

Disadvantages of a public forum strategy are:

♦ They are labour intensive and require significant lead time to recruit participants.

♦ Organizers, if not already experienced in public forum work, will need technical assistance to create useful discussion materials, develop organizing strategies, train moderators and recorders, and form plans for moving from dialogue to action.

♦ They are not one-time affairs: organizers must be prepared to follow up.

Box 16.2 Example of a community forum from Canada

A successful nationwide advocacy campaign to control cancer

The Campaign to Control Cancer emerged from a forum of more than 70 leading cancer organizations of Canada. The campaign engaged the public, raised public awareness of cancer control nationwide through prominent media advertisements, and galvanized grassroots advocacy and media support.

The campaign was launched to educate political leaders about cancer statistics and the need for sustainable commitment of pan-Canadian cancer control efforts. Leadership training workshops were set up to train groups across the country in advocacy skills, to enable them to mobilize government support through an integrated strategic plan for stakeholder, government, and public relations. Workshop participants followed up by meeting with elected officials, wrote letters to the newspapers, circulated petitions, and engaged their organizations in the effort to fund and implement the Canadian Strategy for Cancer Control. At the same time, a national newspaper media campaign raised the profile of the cancer situation and engaged the public in knowing about the need for a national strategy. Once the media seized upon the topic, multiple stories began to unfold on national radio, newspaper, and television, gathering public responses through letters and calling political attention to the need for a national strategy.

These advocacy actions culminated in the government's commitment to fund the Canadian Partnership against Cancer. Two measures that may indicate success of the advocacy include the formal funding commitment in the federal budget, and the establishment of an independent structure to administer the funding and implementation of the strategy.

From: Campaign to Control Cancer in Canada, reproduced with permission [9]. http://www. controlcancer.ca.

Principles for public engagement

Many traditional leaders view cancer control and public policy decision-making as an expert-driven process: get the best information, bring trained minds to bear, make the best decision, and only then reach out to wider audiences to persuade them to sign on and change public health, individual behaviours, and communities. The wider public are rarely viewed as a vital resource. From this perspective, planning and decision-making are confined to a small circle to make progress quickly and minimize static. There is sometimes a nod towards gaining a degree of 'input' from 'patients/advocates/families/customers' or 'the public'. An advisory committee, perhaps, a questionnaire, or some form of public consultation might be put in play. In the best case, these minor measures add a small degree of useful input and lend some legitimacy to the planning process. More valid principles for public engagement are described here, based on the work of Friedman and colleagues [6,7].

A mutual struggle for solutions

Authentic engagement involves substantive give and take with those who have a vested interest in the decisions that are made. It involves communication aimed at prompting deliberation, dialogue, shared responsibility, and cooperative action. In the cancer control context, 'authentic' public engagement means involving many sectors of a community to build common ground that will benefit the public interest. It presupposes more collaborative relationships between cancer control leadership and various stakeholders and public than is typically the case. An authentic public engagement perspective assumes that many stakeholders can and should be involved, not in every technical detail of research and public policy, but in helping to set the broad directions and values from which policy proceeds. It assumes that many members of the community can play a vital role in making cancer control work.

To be clear, to promote public engagement, as this chapter does, is not to argue that all members of the community should have an equal say in every aspect, and that traditional cancer control leadership and professional expertise no longer count. Nor would we recommend ignoring more traditional communications efforts, which remain absolutely essential. But there can be an important place for well-designed public engagement.

Principles described here are intended to provide non-government organizations, advocates, public health professionals, and community leaders with a science base and practical guidelines for engaging the public in community decision-making and action for health promotion, health protection, and disease prevention. Engagement principles can be used by people in a range of roles, from the chief executive of an organization or programme funder who needs to know how to support community engagement, to the frontline health professional or community leader who needs hands-on, practical information on how to mobilize members of a community. In practice, engagement is a blend of science and art. The science comes from sociology, political science, cultural anthropology, organizational development, psychology, social work, and other disciplines with organizing concepts drawn from the literature on community participation, community mobilization, constituency building, community psychology, cultural influences, and other sources. The art comes from the leadership skills, understanding, skill, and sensitivity that are used to apply and adapt the science in ways that fit the community and the purposes of specific engagement efforts.

Engaging how? General principles and guidelines

We will set this next section as advice to cancer control leaders who want to engage a wider public successfully.

Bring people into the process early

If you are simply bringing people together to announce your intentions, you're likely to turn them into critics. If you bring them together to gain their perspectives as you are developing plans, you are more likely to turn them into allies. If you've fine-tuned your plan based on useful feedback, and given a good number of people a chance to weigh in and contribute, you'll be in a solid position to continue to engage stakeholders to help you figure out the best ways to implement the plan and keep things moving in the right direction.

Go beyond the usual suspects

While it's fine to consult with the most accessible community leaders (the 'village elders'), and it's inevitable that you'll be dealing with interest groups and civic activists, public engagement should always strive to reach beyond the usual suspects to include those not typically involved. In short, public engagement is more useful, and tends to be considerably more interesting and fun, if you can bring fresh faces, energy, and ideas to the table.

Listen more, talk less

While you will surely have some important things to say, public engagement is not well served by speechmaking. The idea is to set the stage for dialogue, and you will get more out of it if you listen more and talk less than anyone else.

Set a constructive, problem-solving tone

Avoid easy polarization, accusations, and stridency. Get beyond 'sounding the alarm' to create discussions that have forward momentum. This also means that you should look to engage people using their interests, concerns, and language – and avoid jargon completely.

Avoid overly technical discussions

Focus on broad policy directions and the values and trade-offs rather than technical details of policy. Avoid the data-dumps (giving too much technical information) that may work at a professional conference, but may make it impossible for regular citizens to participate effectively.

Offer choices for deliberation

Let people wrestle with alternatives, and point out the pros and cons. Doing so communicates that there are no easy answers and many points of view are essential and welcome. This technique (that Public Agenda calls 'choicework') [7] also helps people with very different levels of expertise engage both the issues and each other more effectively than a wide-open discussion with no structure. Based on Public Agenda's long experience with public engagement, this is one of the most important steps you can take – especially with average citizens as opposed to professionals and experts.

Expect obstacles and resistance

People are used to doing things in a familiar way and it's hard to grapple with new possibilities. It takes time, and repeated opportunities, for people to really work through problems, absorb information about the tradeoffs of different approaches, and build common ground.

Ongoing communication and follow up is critical

Once you've elicited people's interest and participation, it's extremely important to follow up with them. It means you need to take participation seriously, explain in what ways participation has affected your plans, how things are proceeding, and how they can stay involved over time. Dan Yankelovich's 'Coming to Public Judgment' [10] gives a fuller discussion of the seven stages people go through as they wrestle with issues.

New trends in public engagement and stakeholder relations

With increased scrutiny from a broader circle of stakeholders along with heightened expectations for transparency, accountability, and participatory decision-making, we are witnessing a new approach to stakeholder and public engagement. Today, engagement is a 'must-do practice' across sectors, regions, and disciplines. This traditional model of stakeholder 'management' is giving way to a more proactive, participatory, and collaborative model, one that is emergent, co-creative, and solution-centric in nature (Figure 16.5).

As a result the new approach to stakeholder engagement is:

- Collaborative
- Emergent and solution-centred
- Focused on building long-term, yet flexible, relationships
- Illustrative of mutual benefit, risk, and involved decision-making
- Inspired by values
- Driven by a commitment to a shared vision and mutual goals
- Built upon dialogue, listening, and two-way communication

Stakeholder management	Stakeholder network engagement
■ Unilateral or bilateral	■ Multilateral or system-wide
■ Inform & consult	■ Involve & empower
■ Reactive, compliant, & responsive	■ Proactive, engaged, & co-creative
■ Organization-centric	■ Solution-centric
■ Managed & controlled	■ Self-organizing around common issues
■ Independent, fragmented, & ad hoc	■ Interdependent, complex, & cross-boundary

Fig. 16.5 Trends in stakeholder engagement
Source: From Addis & Associates, reproduced with permission.

◆ Includes a level of trust

◆ Fosters innovation and collective action

Fostering a collective understanding of a vision for wide-spread cancer control amongst key stakeholders from the outset is essential to ensure the successful realization of the goals. Introducing community leaders and decision-makers to the concept of cancer control, cultivating receptivity and support amongst health professionals, advocates, survivors, corporations, schools and community groups, enabling key stakeholders to be champions, and involving the broader community are factors critical to success. Consultation, informed dialogue and decision-making, and joint action are essential to realize meaningful engagement.

A good example of a multi-faceted community engagement campaign is the US programme on childhood cancer built around the TV film 'A lion in the house' (http://mylion.org). With many partners and advisers, including the Independent Television Service, the Public Broadcasting Service, the American Cancer Society and many other cancer groups, and the National Cancer Institute, it aims to inform and educate the public about childhood cancer, empower survivors and assist their families, and encourage community volunteer activities. The methods include discussion materials based on the film, fact sheets, video modules, newsletters, a blog, a community service kit for teenagers and their leaders, and awards certificates for new activities registered on its website.

What is a stakeholder?

A stakeholder is anyone who is affected or can affect the outcome of the initiative and has an interest or a stake in cancer control. Those who have been touched by cancer, those who care for people living with cancer, those who set cancer care policy, or those who financially support control efforts are just some of the stakeholders to be engaged.

Steps to Engaging Key Stakeholders:

◆ Identify key stakeholders, assess common ground, and encourage ideas.

◆ Develop a shared vision and mutually defined goals.

◆ Learn together and plan together.

◆ Act together.

Strengthening organizational capacity for public engagement through applications of technology

As use of the internet continues to grow, innovative technologies are creating new ways of engaging and maintaining the public's involvement in cancer control. Advances in technology have opened the door to reaching new constituencies, creating spaces for sharing ideas and taking action, and offering opportunities for increased communication. Public engagement can be significantly advanced through the use of online surveys, internet forums, blogs, social networking and virtual communities, and group communication tools.

Online surveys

Online surveys provide a mechanism for connecting with the public and learning more about their knowledge, attitudes, and behaviours related to cancer control. A number of online survey tools, such as surveymonkey.com and zoomerang.com, offer the ability to survey, analyze, and share results. With the increase in the number of people using the internet, more people can now be reached through online methods.

Online surveys offer an inexpensive way to tap into the interests and perceptions of the public. Surveys can be generated to evaluate many different aspects of work, including but not limited to: people's awareness of certain initiatives, the public's engagement in activities, public priorities, and public responses to certain proposals. Prior to surveying members of the public, there should be a commitment to use the survey results in decision-making. If the public's opinions are sought but not acted on, it can create distrust and reluctance to engage in related activities in the future. However, engaging the public in this way can have many benefits.

The strengths of online surveys include:

- They are inexpensive and easy to create.
- They provide an easy pathway for engagement by the public, as responding is usually easy and requires a very brief time commitment.
- They facilitate the use of survey results in the decision-making processes by providing tools for analysis and the ability to share the results with others.
- They can build commitment to decisions, as more people have the ability to have their voices heard.
- They can help to illuminate difficult issues, as people often feel free to express sentiments they would not express in a public meeting.

Drawbacks, limitations, and challenges of online surveys include:

- To get the information needed, skilled personnel may be needed to help formulate the questions appropriately.
- If people can respond anonymously, it will be challenging to follow-up with anyone on their comments and responses.
- Online survey respondents may represent only a segment of the population, which may not be representative.

Internet forums

Internet forums are an online place where people have discussions over time on particular topics. They are generally organized by category or topic and may also be referred to as message boards, web forums, discussion boards, discussion forums, discussion groups, or bulletin boards. Forums can be open to the public or password protected for members only.

Internet forums can enhance communication and support the open flow of ideas. They can be used to spark discussion on certain elements of cancer control, to share best practices and lessons learned, and to raise awareness around priority topics. They provide an easy access point for the public to engage in the discussion as all that is necessary for the user is a computer and internet access. While internet forums can help generate discussion and provide guideposts, an important limitation is that the ideas expressed in the forums may not be representative of the larger population.

The strengths of internet forums include:

◆ They can create a sense of community.

◆ They can give people a reason to return to the website and stay engaged.

◆ The interactive nature of forums makes the subject area both interesting and informative and can attract new people to participate.

◆ They can expand the exchange of ideas by attracting people beyond the usual suspects.

Drawbacks, limitations, and challenges of internet forums include:

◆ They require an investment of resources, time, and energy in creating, moderating, and ensuring the forum is both engaging and up to standard.

◆ The organizers will have less control over the messages or what is said about a particular aspect of the cancer control efforts. Because these are public forums, the views expressed may not represent those of the organizers. While the goal is to encourage the expression of multiple viewpoints, if the views expressed are volatile or irrational, this can reflect negatively on the host organization. Despite disclaimers that may be in place, perception can be reality in the public domain, and the organizers may find themselves having to defend the opinions of people whose views are significantly outside the mainstream.

◆ Public forums may be dominated by vocal minorities. Because of the anonymous nature of the internet, certain users can create drama and cause problems. Forums must be moderated not only for personal attacks, but for accuracy of information presented, and conflicts between product marketing and actual communication. Careful moderation of public forums is critical.

◆ Organizations can choose whether to host their own forums or participate in existing ones. Hosting a forum on the organization's website provides the added benefit of drawing people to the website again and again. However, existing internet forums can provide a good venue to promote discussion around areas of cancer control that are relevant to the developing plans. The task with this strategy is to find a forum that fits with the area of interest and to introduce discussion topics as appropriate.

Blogs

Blog is short for 'web log'. Blogs are interactive in nature in that they allow readers to post comments. Increasingly, individuals use blogs to share information, provide commentary, or provide updates on new events. There are multiple ways in which blogs can be used to engage the public in cancer control. Organizers may:

◆ Create each blog entry themselves.

◆ Create the blog and invite others to post guest blogs.

◆ Encourage those who are engaged to blog independently.

Which strategy is chosen will depend on the resources and staff time available, as well as the interest of the community. For the greatest level of public engagement, members of the public can be invited to post guest blogs and encourage all others to respond in the comments section. Reader comments are a critical component of blogging. Comments can point the way towards elements of planning that may be controversial, unsupported, or require more dialogue. Organizers can also use the comments to their blog in helping identify where to focus future efforts in public engagement.

As with internet forums, it is important to remember that those who participate in reading and responding to the blog do not represent the totality of the public. While internet access is increasing, those who are willing and able to participate in blog posting may be just a small segment of those who are interested in participating in cancer control planning overall.

The strengths of blogs are:

• Blogs are inexpensive to create, operate, and maintain.

• Blogs provide a way of speaking to the public in a direct, conversational tone that can help increase involvement and better inform those who might not otherwise participate.

• Because blogs are personal in nature, they allow organizers to build long-term relationships with readers that foster trust.

• Blogs can link to multiple sites allowing people to learn about efforts across the cancer control spectrum. Because comprehensive cancer control often involves multiple stakeholders engaged in a myriad of activities, the interactive and 'linked' nature of blogs allows people to access information on multiple levels.

Drawbacks of blogs include:

• Blogs should be updated frequently, requiring ample time and content.

• Reader comments require moderation to ensure they are appropriate and directed to the goals.

• Those who write and respond represent a small portion of the public.

Social networking and virtual communities

Social networking sites connect individuals online in an interactive way. They generally offer a space for blogs, user profiles (a profile that a person creates that tells others about themselves), forums, chat groups (a mechanism for people to discuss a topic in real time online), and photos. Social networking groups can be used to connect people from diverse areas who are interested in similar aspects of cancer control. They provide a fun, social environment to engage people in the fight against cancer. If a call to action does not exist, blogs or internet forums can be considered as a substitute.

For example, the Lance Armstrong Foundation uses social networking groups as a tool for groups of advocates in specific geographical regions to connect with each other, share information about events, and draw in new participants [1]. Advocate teams each create their own sites and then invite members of the public to get involved with their efforts.

The strengths of social networking and virtual communities include:

• Online communities allow people to stay closely connected.

• They enable people in distant locations to stay connected without travel or oddly timed phone calls.

• They increase awareness and aid in recruitment by providing an easy way to spread the word and get others to join in.

• Many people who are comfortable with this medium have existing online networks from which they can draw.

Drawbacks, limitations, and challenges of social networking and virtual communities include:

• They do not have universal appeal.

• It is important to balance the time and resources devoted to these strategies with the reach they have in the community being engaged.

• Content is user-generated so there is no control over what is said.

Group communications tools

Group communications tools are a way to manage information and activities of a group. Examples of group communications tools include web conferencing, bulletin boards, list servers, the Wiki Wiki Web system, which is a set of Web pages where anybody can modify the contents using standard Web browsers and mailing list management systems. Many group communications tools offer free list-management, emailing services, calendar tools and mini-database services. Recent improvements in group communications tools allow people to network, hold meetings and discussions, make decisions, revise documents, send newsletters, and schedule tasks.

For example, www.cancerplan.org provides tools for cancer control planners to share resources in order to effectively develop, implement, and evaluate comprehensive cancer control plans. Guests can use the site to see what is happening in cancer control planning in their state in the United States, find local resources, or participate in the message board.

Online group communications tools provide a simple and easy way to keep people informed, sign up new members, and manage projects. They can be particularly useful as a way to allow work groups to continue to plan strategies between in-person meetings. They can be set up to give anyone access to the tools or to allow certain work groups access to certain tools.

The strengths of group communications tools include:

- They allow people to participate in ways that are meaningful to them. As people are engaged in the process, they will be able to choose how to participate. Some people may choose to stay informed by reading a newsletter, some will share tools and exchange stories, while others will join work groups.

- Group communications tools can foster a sense of shared purpose. If all members of the group are given access to the tools, people can clearly see who else is involved in the effort, how they are providing support, and how their individual efforts connect to the greater whole.

- They allow people to continue to connect despite great distances.

  Drawbacks, limitations, and challenges of group communications tools include:

- Group communications tools can be costly to host, create, and monitor.

- Because the tools are internet based, there will be limitations on the number of people who can participate.

Developing influential public and private sector cancer control leadership skills

Whether you are a cancer care professional, patient, policy maker, a staff member of a cancer hospital or charity – or just a person who wants to make a difference – you probably wish you had more influence over people. Most of us stop trying to make change happen because we believe it is too difficult. We develop complicated strategies when we should be learning the tools and techniques for effective influence. Behavioural scientists and business leaders offer robust strategies for making change happen, and cancer control can benefit from learning how to:

- Identify a handful of high-leverage behaviours that can lead to rapid change.

- Apply strategies for changing thoughts and actions.

- Marshal sources of influence to make change inevitable.

For example, in developed countries unhealthy diet, obesity, and inactivity are major factors in the increase in cancer incidence and mortality. But there is good news that shows that if we make good eating and active living choices a little easier and bad ones a little harder, we can make a substantial impact on individual choices (see also Chapters 2 and 3 in this book).

As an example of a 'Best Practice' school-based approach, the 'Gimme 5 intervention' in US high schools involved (www.gimme5.org; www.gimme5.ca):

◆ A mass media campaign in schools

◆ Five 55-minute workshops per year about healthy living knowledge, attitudes, and skills

◆ More fruits and vegetables in the cafeteria

◆ Mailings to parents with recipes, calendars, tips, and information brochures

As a result of the three-year high school programme, students increased their consumption of fruits and vegetables by over 2.5 servings per day on average [11].

Leadership in cancer control doesn't always require clinical expertise or expense. Corporate and public sector employers can help create working environments that promote healthy living [12]; an example is given in Box 16.3.

'Best Practices' in workplace cancer control include the following efforts:

1 Develop a corporate culture that values and supports healthy eating, physical activity, and employee wellness.

2 Audit the workplace to assess available food choices, and opportunities for physical activity.

3 Plan 'Health Days': quarterly events that focus on aspects of healthy weights and healthy living.

4 Implement strategies to help people be more physically active at work, such as:

   ◆ Building a task team to identify ways to increase physical activity opportunities

   ◆ Allowing employees time to be physically active during the day

   ◆ Adjusting working hours to allow parents to walk their children to school

   ◆ Providing physical activity facilities, programmes, and incentives

5 Identify and implement strategies to promote healthy eating at work, such as ensuring vending machines and cafeterias offer healthy choices.

6 Develop a policy to support women returning to work to continue breastfeeding.

Box 16.3 Example of best practices in workplace cancer control: the CEO Roundtable

The CEO Roundtable on Cancer was founded in 2001 to enable executives from diverse industries to engage in the fight against cancer. Members from workplaces across the United States collaborate to develop and implement initiatives that reduce the risk of cancer, enable early diagnosis, facilitate better access to best-available treatments, and hasten the discovery of novel and more effective diagnostic tools and anti-cancer therapies.

As part of this initiative, the CEO Cancer Gold Standard™ was created to help establish a roadmap that companies can use to help prevent cancer, detect it early and ensure access to the best available treatment for those who are diagnosed. The CEO Cancer Gold Standard allows companies to affirm their commitment to fighting cancer, to easily assess their own readiness to implement recommended strategies, and to become accredited.

From: CEO Roundtable on Cancer Control, reproduced with permission [12]. http://www. ceoroundtableoncancer.org/.

Conclusions

Complex public health campaigns such as those required in cancer control should never be undertaken without first doing the necessary groundwork, including public engagement and developing a twenty-first century communications plan. As an example, the Indonesian cancer control programme illustrates the synergistic role of government, non-government organizations, cancer patients and their carers and supporters, and health professionals in developing and implementing a comprehensive programme [13] (Box 16.4). This is an example that is matched by many other functioning or developing programmes.

Box 16.4 Community involvement in comprehensive cancer control in Indonesia

The Integrated Comprehensive Cancer Control Programme was established in 1993 by the Indonesia Minister of Health and was adopted by Jakarta province in 1996. One of the basic components of this programme is the Population-Based Cancer Control programme which aims at improving people's knowledge through education, focusing on prevention, and early detection of the most important cancers.

The Indonesian Cancer Foundation (ICF) was established as a non-governmental organization to assist the Government of Indonesia in cancer control by promoting awareness, early detection, public and professional education, research, and giving aid to needy cancer patients to reduce their suffering. The foundation works mainly through community participation and in cooperation with other cancer-related institutions.

The ICF Population-Based Cancer Control programme is meant for the people, is carried out by the people, and serves the people. It involves large numbers of volunteers who come from all sectors and disciplines in the communities, such as health-care providers, government officers, social workers, private employees, self-employed persons, and housewives. PKK includes women from the smallest communities at village level up to the provincial level, whose aim is to increase the welfare and health of their communities. The PKK cadres and the primary health centres in villages help to select other volunteers. The criteria for selection are spare time and willingness to teach and help others.

The volunteers are informed about the 10 most common cancers in Indonesia: the risks; general treatments and rehabilitation; and the primary and secondary prevention. They are also trained in how to motivate other people.

Home Palliative Care Programme helps terminally staged and incurable patients, in their own homes to improve the quality of their lives. Training is done by specialists, psychologists, the Population-Based Cancer Control team and others. After the training, the volunteers are called Population-Based Cancer Control teachers if they can demonstrate their ability to teach or inform other people about public health aspects of cancer. The Population-Based Cancer Control programme has support and receives funds from the Governor of Jakarta (mostly) and foreign foundations and institutions.

From: Indonesian Cancer Foundation, reproduced with permission [13]. http://2006.confex.com/uicc/uicc/techprogram/P10602.HTM.

References

1 Lance Armstrong Foundation (2008). *LIVESTRONG™ Army Grassroots Field Manual*. Available from: http://www.livestrong.org.

2 Niederdeppe J & Levy AG (2007). Fatalistic beliefs about cancer prevention and three prevention behaviors. *Cancer Epidemiol Biomarkers Prev*, **16**(5):998–1003.

3 Campaign to Control Cancer (Canada) (2008). Available from: http://www.controlcancer.ca/en/know.

4 National Cancer Leadership Forum (2006). *NCLF Theory of Relationships*. Available from: http://www. controlcancer.ca/en/news/nclf-events.

5 International Association for Public Participation (2007). *IAP2 Spectrum of public engagement*. Available from: http://www.iap2.org/associations/4748/files/spectrum.pdf.

6 Public Agenda Engagement Resource Center (2008). *Public Engagement: A Primer from Public Agenda*. Available from: http://www.publicagenda.org/files/pdf/public_engagement_primer_0.pdf.

7 Public Agenda Engagement Resource Center (2008). *Choicework*. Available from: http://www. publicagenda.org/public-engagement-materials/citizen-choicework-technical-assistance.

8 Britain Against Cancer (2007). *Updating the national strategy for cancer*. Available from: http://www. macmillan.org.uk/Get_Involved/Campaigns/APPG/cancer_news_in_parliament.aspx. Also cited on page 9 of http://www.who.int/cancer/FINAL-Advocacy-Module%206.pdf.

9 Canadian Strategy for Cancer Control (2008). *A successful nationwide advocacy campaign to control cancer*. Available from: http://www.controlcancer.ca.

10 Yankelovich D (1991). *Coming to public judgement: Making democracy work in a complex world*. Syracuse University Press, Syracuse, New York.

11 Baranowski T, Davis M, Resnicow K, et al (2000). Gimme 5 fruit, juice, and vegetables for fun and health: outcome evaluation. *Health Educ Behav*, **27**(1):96–111.

12 CEO Roundtable on Cancer (2008). *Cancer Gold Standard*. URL:http://www.cancergoldstandard.org

13 Indonesian Cancer Foundation (2006). *Community involvement in cancer control in Indonesia*. Available from: http://2006.confex.com/uicc/uicc/techprogram/P10602.HTM.

Additional resources

Public engagement

Barber B (1984). *Strong Democracy: Participatory Politics for a New Age*. University of California Press, Berkeley and Los Angeles.

Coleman, S & Gøtze, J (2001). 'Bowling Together: Online Public Engagement in Policy Deliberation'. Hansard Society. Available from: http://www.bowlingtogether.net/references.html.

DialogueCircles (Ascentum). Available from: http://www.ascentum.ca/dialoguecircles.

Gauvin, F & Abelson, J (2006). Primer on Public Involvement (prepared for the Health Council of Canada). *CPRN*. Available from: http://www.cprn.org/en/doc.cfm?doc=1519.

Gastil, J & Peter L (eds). Strategies for effective civic engagement in the 21st century. *The Deliberative Democracy Handbook*. Jossey-Bass Publishers, San Francisco. In particular see Chapter 19 'Future Directions for Public Deliberation' by Levine, Peter, Archon Fung, & John Gastil.

Goldman, J & Lars HT (2004). Approaches to public engagement in the US. *AmericaSpeaks*. Available from: http://www.americaspeaks.org/.

Gutmann, A & Thomson, D (2004). *Why Deliberative Democracy?* Princeton University Press, Princeton, New Jersey.

Matthews, D & McAfee, N (1997). *Making Choices Together: The Power of Public Deliberation*. Charles F. Kettering Foundation, Dayton, Ohio.

Phillips, S & Orsini, M (2002). Mapping the links: citizen involvement in policy processes. *CPRN*. Available from: http://www.cprn.org/en/doc.cfm?doc=169.

Public Agenda – Center for Advances in Public Engagement. http://www.publicagenda.org/cape.

Royal Roads University e-dialogues for sustainable development. http://e-dialogues.royalroads.ca/.

Yankelovich, D (1991). *Coming to Public Judgement*. University of Syracuse Press, New York.

How-To-Guides for public involvement

Building Democratic Governance: Tools and Structures for Engaging Citizens (2005). National League of Cities. Available from: http://www.nlc.org/ASSETS/6B83BE044C544D4AA963D48B884434FF/demgov.pdf.

Core Values of Public Participation; Public Participation Toolbox: Techniques to Share Information. International Association for Public Participation. Available from: http://www.iap2.org/associations/4748/files/toolbox.pdf.

Creighton, JL (2005). *The Public Participation Handbook: Making Better Decisions through Citizen Involvement*. Jossey-Bass Publishers, San Francisco.

Harrison, O (1997). *Open Space Technology: A User's Guide*. 2nd ed. Berret-Koehler Publishers, Inc., San Francisco.

Lukensmeyer, CJ & Lars HT (2006). Public Deliberation: A Manager's Guide to Citizen Engagement. *AmericaSpeaks*. IBM Center for The Business of Government. Available from: http://www.businessofgovernment.org/pdfs/LukensmeyerReport.pdf.

Chapter 17

Organizational structures for cancer control

Lorraine Caron[1]

In the past, governments at all levels have viewed cancer as a disease to fight through treatment and care. Over the years, a more global approach to fighting cancer has emerged, supported by evidence that cancer could be prevented. Indeed, it has been estimated that about one third of cancers worldwide could be prevented with the implementation of existing knowledge and strategies in health promotion, prevention, and screening [1]. When cancer cannot be prevented, a treatment programme is implemented that usually combines supportive care, and in less fortunate circumstances, palliative care for terminally ill patients. If treatment is successful, cancer management generally evolves towards rehabilitation, including regular check-ups and promotion of a healthy lifestyle to prevent recurrence of the cancer or the development of a new cancer [2].

Cancer control and the management of chronic conditions both challenge health care systems, wherein the primary focus is to respond to acute problems. A more adapted response to individuals with complex and chronic conditions requires making a paradigm shift in the way that health care systems operate and interact [3]. Such a shift has direct implications for patients, families, health care workers, as well as organizations, communities, and health policy makers.

The complexity and chronic nature of many cancers has called for a comprehensive approach that is defined as cancer control. Cancer control is a systematic and evidence-based approach that seeks to encompass the continuum of cancer care [4], as well as health professional and public education, research, and epidemiological surveillance. Cancer control involves 'the identification, development, promotion, diffusion, and delivery of effective and ethical cancer prevention, screening, and care services and programmes for individuals and groups, always with their active participation' [5],(p. 1141).

Table 17.1 illustrates this conceptual evolution towards a cancer control perspective, highlighting the salient features of that progression that bear upon health care systems, namely: (1) the target populations; (2) the structural features related to service delivery; (3) the level of integration related to service provision; and (4) the management focus [6]. Hence, moving from cancer treatment to cancer care and to cancer control entails an ever more embracing approach that requires significant changes in health system configuration and practices: from a hospital-based to a system-based delivery setting; from a focus on discrete episodes of care to the notion of continuum of care; from providing treatment to promoting health and preventing disease; from caring for individual patients to ensuring healthy populations; and from working in silos to linking systems. To address this ongoing challenge, comprehensive cancer control initiatives guided by well known frameworks [3,7] are being established through concerted stakeholders' collaborations that include government, non-governmental organizations, as well as public/patient representatives [8].

[1] Lorraine Caron, PhD, Consulting Researcher, Agence d'évaluation des technologies et des modes d'intervention en santé (AETMIS), Montréal, Québec, Canada.

Table 17.1 From cancer treatment to cancer control: requirements for health care systems

Approach	Cancer treatment	Cancer care	Cancer control
Target populations	Patients diagnosed with cancer	Patients diagnosed with cancer and individuals suspected of having cancer	Multiple populations: healthy, at-risk, suspected of cancer, diagnosed with cancer, in remission, at the end-of-life
Structural features related to service delivery	Facilities: centres and hospitals	Multidisciplinary teams Patient navigators Networks of providers within and across regions Integrated care programmes at local, regional, national levels	Inter-sectoral (e.g. health and education) and intra-sectoral (e.g. public health and health care system) collaborations Systemic approach to knowledge formation, exchange, transfer, and application Participatory decision-making for patients and the public
Level of integration in service provision	Integrated care protocols (care episode)	Seamless trajectory of care across services and places (continuum of services)	Linkages among public health, health care delivery system, and community services (health system)
Management focus	Institutional (silo)	Continuity and coordination of health care services (transitions between services and places)	Health system performance (sustainable, responsive, and efficient health system)

Table adapted from [6]

Learning from international comparisons

The present chapter reports on the experiences of a number of jurisdictions in planning and organizing cancer control strategies, plans, and programmes at the national and provincial levels. It is based on a comparative study conducted between 2003 and 2007 for the Québec Ministry of Health and Social services that examined four countries (Canada, England, France, and New Zealand) and five Canadian provinces (Alberta, British Columbia, Nova Scotia, Ontario, and Québec) [6,9]. The study sought to provide a broad understanding of cancer control strategies, plans, and programmes in terms of how those initiatives came into being (development history) what they intended to achieve (design), how they were managed (governance), what they achieved and how (implementation), and what contextual factors may have been shaping and influencing them.

The study compared the selected jurisdictions according to elements of an integrated framework that was specifically built from existing frameworks related to cancer control and the management of chronic conditions [6]. Sources of information included scientific literature, key informant interviews and grey literature, such as government documents, newsletters, reports, and experts' presentations. The different points along which the selected countries and provinces rested in terms of planning and implementation, as well as the differences in their social and political context called for a descriptive inquiry. Comparative analysis consisted in using a bottom-up approach based on the juxtaposition of detailed information about similar initiatives in the selected jurisdictions. Given the type and scope of data considered, no assessment of strategy/programme effectiveness was conducted. However, documented achievements regarding cancer services organization reforms were used as the basis on which to draw lessons for improving cancer control strategy implementation [9].

This chapter highlights the central features of this comparative study. It first examines the influence of critical events in policy development and then describes organizational means that have been put in place by the jurisdictions to implement the current strategies, plans, or programmes. Focusing on the differences and commonalities as regards to main governing models and levers for change, the chapter offers some insights on the strengths and challenges of the various organizational models and on key ingredients for successful implementation.

Features of policy development*

All jurisdictions examined have an interesting history regarding the development of their cancer control policy. Though taking place in different contexts, such development features have a number of common threads which are worth highlighting. First, policy development is a cyclical and iterative process, with more or less successful attempts. Second, successful policy planning and implementation of resulting plans and strategies require that cancer control be considered a top priority at the highest levels of government.

For example, the development of the 2002 Canadian Strategy for Cancer Control (CSCC) [10] was preceded by the Cancer 2000 Report, published ten years before [11] and never implemented. The CSCC planning and consultation process involved over 700 Canadians from the health and allied professions, academia, the voluntary sector, all levels of government, and cancer patients/survivors. Despite such consensus, tremendous efforts had to be deployed by the CSCC council as well as advocacy and support groups[2] to keep the national strategy on the political agenda. In 2006, the newly elected federal government committed substantial funds over five years for the implementation of the CSCC. The Canadian Partnership against Cancer (CPAC), a new governing organization, was also formed to lead the implementation.

In New Zealand (NZ), work to develop a broad level framework for cancer control dates back to 1996, but this initiative was slowed down by changes in government and health system governance reforms. At the end of 1999, a new government was elected, and cancer became one of 13 priorities of the NZ Health Strategy [12]. A Cancer Control Trust was established in 2001 as a partnership between the Ministry of Health, the Cancer Society of New Zealand, and other non-governmental organizations. Later that year, a cancer control steering group was set up, along with a number of expert working groups, to establish priorities following the Canadian model. One important goal of the strategy would be to improve access and care for the Māori and Pacific populations that had the worst health outcomes. After a public consultation, the NZ Cancer Control Strategy [13] was launched by the Minister of Health in 2003. Later that year, a national workshop was held to begin planning for its implementation. A Cancer Control Taskforce was set up to produce an action plan [14] that was released in 2005. A Cancer Control Council was appointed by the Minister of Health to monitor implementation of the strategy, and a principal advisor (now named national clinical director, cancer control) was appointed by the director-general of health to drive the implementation from within the ministry. In 2006, a cancer control work programme steering group was formed by the Ministry of Health to begin implementation. The group is under the leadership of the national clinical director, and comprises representatives from the district health boards, the Cancer Control Council, and the Cancer Society of New Zealand as well as oncology experts and other stakeholders.

---

* See list of acronyms at the end of the chapter for the specific names of the organizations.

2 These included the National Cancer Leadership Forum, the Canadian Cancer Society (CCS), and the Cancer Advocacy Coalition of Canada.

In France, a turning point can be traced back to the signing by President Chirac of the Paris Charter, a founding text that recognizes the fight against cancer as an international priority, during the 'World summit against cancer for the new millennium', hosted by UNESCO in Paris in 2000. This momentum came after a series of public reports depicting the failure of prior policy initiatives and the unmet needs of patients [15–18]. A *programme national de lutte contre le cancer 2000–2005* had been published by the Minister of Health [19], but it was not implemented due to lack of funding and leadership. Significant progress began when President Chirac declared that cancer control would be a top priority following his re-election in 2002. A first step was the setting up of a *Commission d'orientation sur le cancer* to document the situation. The Commission benefited from the input of many groups, including patients, health care professionals, and associations involved in the field. It noted that France had the worst cancer premature mortality rate across Europe, and that research efforts were not sufficient. The Commission's report [20] formed the basis for the drafting, by the Minister of Health and the Minister of Research, of a five-year action plan [21] that was launched by President Chirac in 2003. Implementation began right away under the governance of a *Mission interministérielle de lutte contre le cancer* appointed by the Prime Minister until the newly created *Institut national du cancer* took over in 2005.

In England and Wales, landmark efforts at a concerted policy approach to improve cancer care began with the Calman-Hine report [22] that recommended a fundamental restructuring of cancer services in England and in Wales, including the creation of cancer services networks. Impetus for reform in England was largely linked to results from the EUROCARE study, examining five-year cancer survival rates in European countries that demonstrated that England was faring well below (by 5 per cent) the European average for all common cancers (lung, breast, colorectal, and prostate) [23]. In 1999, following a specific meeting on cancer with the Prime Minister and a group of experts (Ten Downing Street cancer summit) [24] important steps were taken to improve the pace of reform: (1) a target was set of a maximum two-week wait between an urgent referral from a general physician and a hospital clinic appointment for breast cancer [25]; (2) a national cancer director was appointed to develop and implement a national cancer programme for England; (3) the National Cancer Action Team was mandated to support the national cancer director, in addition to overseeing the implementation of the cancer networks; and (4) a Cancer Services Collaborative was established to support the National Health and Social Care Service (NHS) in England and its partner organizations in the task of redesigning more efficient services and improving experiences and outcomes for patients. In 2000, the Department of Health launched the NHS cancer plan for England [26]. A Cancer Taskforce was formed to lead national implementation of the plan, supported by a substantial financial commitment by the government. Implementation progress was closely monitored. In 2006, the Secretary of State mandated the national cancer director to head a reform strategy board to develop the next strategy for cancer services. The Cancer Reform Strategy (2008–2012) was launched in December 2007 [27].

As seen already in the stories described, another important characteristic is that the political willingness to develop and implement a global and concerted approach to cancer control is triggered by the need to take action on the following problems:

◆ Higher cancer incidence and/or mortality rates and/or lower survival rates compared with other jurisdictions

◆ Inequalities among social and/or ethnic groups, and/or among regions, whether in health status or in access to and provision of cancer services

◆ Problems in the quality of cancer care delivered as well as its lack of continuity and coordination

Experiences of several Canadian provinces

Canada is a federation that comprises ten provinces and three territories. The health care sector is of provincial jurisdiction and the majority of funding for health care is provided by the provinces through taxation. The federal level provides the general legal framework governing the provincial health care systems (Canada Health Act) and is responsible for the licensing of drugs. It is also involved in some public health activities and in the provision of health care to aboriginal people residing on federal reserves.

In Ontario, initiatives to improve cancer services date back to the early 1990s amidst a crisis related to long delays for radiotherapy. A public consultation process initiated by the Minister of Health in 1993 highlighted a number of problems including the lack of service coordination, lack of clinical practice standards, variations in access to care, and the lack of the patient perspective in cancer policy planning. The resulting report [28], which can be considered as the first provincial cancer control strategy, recommended the development of a provincial framework to be implemented through regional cancer networks. In 1997, a provincial cancer agency (Cancer Care Ontario, CCO) was launched by the Ontario Premier with the mandate to integrate and coordinate all cancer services in the province. In 1999, however, another crisis occurred regarding radiotherapy waiting times, which led to the transfer of many patients to the United States for their treatment. The government formed a cancer services implementation committee to conduct a thorough review of cancer services delivery throughout the province. The committee recommended important changes to the mandate of the cancer agency [29]. CCO would no longer be responsible for the direct delivery of care through its regional cancer centers; it would instead be responsible for planning and coordinating all cancer services across the province in addition to becoming the advisory body on cancer to the Ministry of Health. In 2002 the Cancer Quality Council of Ontario (CQCO) was created to serve as the major driver for cancer control performance monitoring, managing, and reporting. From 2002 to 2004, CCO published an assessment of the quality of cancer services in Ontario [30] as well as a number of strategic plans, including Cancer 2020, an action plan for cancer prevention and early detection prepared jointly with the Canadian Cancer Society [31]. In 2004, CCO published the Ontario Cancer Plan 2005–2008 [32]. The development of this plan involved more than 3000 people across the continuum of care. The plan was informed by a regional planning process, a corporate planning process, and it also underwent a formal review by international experts. Significant funding was committed by the government for implementation of reforms. Building on these new foundations, CCO recently launched its next cancer plan (2008–2011) [33].

In Nova Scotia, serious concerns were raised during the 1990s regarding access to, and quality of, oncology services [34]. At that time, the province had among the highest rates of cancer incidence and mortality in Canada. In 1995, the Department of Health established the Nova Scotia Cancer Action Committee to develop an action plan for a coordinated and systematic approach to cancer care. The committee's report was submitted to the Deputy Minister of Health in 1996 [35]. This first comprehensive strategy came amidst an important reform in the governance of cancer services that was marked by the abolition, in 1996, of the provincial organization dedicated to cancer treatment, surveillance, and research (Cancer Treatment and Research Foundation of Nova Scotia), and its fusion with the Queen Elizabeth II Health Sciences Centre [36]. In 1998, a provincial programme called Cancer Care Nova Scotia (CCNS) was established within the Department of Health and a commissioner was appointed to lead the development of this programme. In 2006, the Department of Health commissioned a provincial health services operational review that included an assessment of the CCNS programme. The review indicated that, over the eight years since CCNS had been created, the programme had made significant accomplishments in cancer control by developing ambitious programmes and initiatives related to prevention, coordination of services, clinical practice guidelines, professional education, and research. However, the review noted a lack of support from the Department of Health (financial resources and delegation of proper authority) that would have enabled CCNS to enforce the implementation of its programmes, and to adequately assume its monitoring and evaluation mandate [37]. The year 2006 was also marked by two important events: the CCNS commissioner resigned; and an epidemiological survey showed that cancer incidence and mortality rates remained high [38]. In 2007, the improvement of cancer services was among the four priorities of the Acute and Tertiary Care branch of the Department of Health [39], with most recent initiatives focusing on cancer screening and on reducing waiting times for treatments [40].

Québec's comprehensive cancer control strategy was adopted in 1998. Involving the collaboration of more than a hundred stakeholders, the *programme québécois de lutte contre le cancer* was the product of the *Comité consultatif sur le cancer* [41], established in 1993 by the Minister of Health and Social Services. In 2003, a progress report noted that, despite existing efforts, important changes were still needed to occur to reduce the cancer burden [42]. Indeed, by the year 2000, cancer had become the first cause of death in Québec [43]. These findings gave support to the *Coalition priorité cancer au Québec*, a group of voluntary, community, and professional organizations, created in 2001 to mobilize all stakeholders and the government in advancing cancer control. Since its creation, the Coalition has asked the Québec government to make cancer control a priority, to set up a more coherent leadership and management, and to provide the necessary means to implement the existing programme [44]. In 2003, the newly elected Minister of Health established cancer as one of his top priorities. The previous cancer governing bodies were replaced by a *Direction de la lutte contre le cancer* (DLCC), and the 1998 *programme* was reaffirmed. In 2007, the Direction released its five-year action plan [45].

While the experiences of the countries mentioned earlier and Canadian provinces are related to establishing and implementing their first comprehensive and coordinated strategy on the prevention and management of cancer, in the Canadian provinces of Alberta and British Columbia, recent policy development is mostly intended to enhance a longstanding provincial cancer programme.

In Alberta, the Alberta Cancer Board (ACB), a provincial health council created in 1967, is mandated by the Albertan government to coordinate cancer control research, prevention, and treatment for the entire province. In 1999, ACB established the Alberta Coordinating Council for Cancer Control (ACCCC) to foster collaboration among ACB, the health authorities, the Canadian Cancer Society (CCS), and the Ministry of Health in planning cancer control activities. ACCCC took the lead in 2002, to develop a provincial cancer control plan. The 2004 Alberta Cancer Control Plan [46] provides a global and concerted vision for provincial cancer control that builds on existing cancer control programmes in Alberta, the priorities of the Canadian Strategy for Cancer Control, and on the recommendations from the Premier's advisory council on health report [47]. In 2006, the Alberta government committed a 500 million dollar endowment for research, screening, and prevention through the Alberta Cancer Prevention Legacy Act [48].

British Columbia (BC) is viewed as a Canadian pioneer in cancer control. For example, it launched Canada's first cervical screening programme in 1949, which included many components of an organized screening programme [49]. In 1974, existing organizations involved in cancer treatment and in research, prevention, education, and epidemiology, were amalgamated under the Cancer Control Agency of British Columbia (now called BC Cancer Agency or BCCA), through a tripartite agreement of the provincial government, the BC Cancer Treatment and Research Foundation (which had been created in the 1930s), and the Cancer Control Agency of

British Columbia [50]. The BCCA is mandated to develop and manage a cancer control programme for the entire province. In 1996, BCCA established population-based provincial programmes that are regionally delivered [51]. In 2001, BCCA was put under the governance of the Provincial Health Services Authority (PHSA), along with many other existing provincial health services agencies. In addition to developing its own strategic plan in 2003 [50], BCCA collaborated to several regional and provincial initiatives to improve cancer control in the province, including: (1) the setting up in 2004 of a BC and Yukon council for the CSCC, jointly financed by the BCCA, the PHSA, and the CCS, to develop a BC and Yukon cancer control strategy based on the CSCC; and (2) the production, in collaboration with the Northern Health Authority, of a strategic proposal for cancer control in the Northern British Columbia region [52]. This latter initiative was part of the BC Premier's consultation on improved cancer care in Northern British Columbia that took place in 2005-06. The consultation aimed to design a comprehensive and integrated cancer care programme that would best meet the unique needs of the people of Northern British Columbia. While British Columbia has the lowest cancer incidence and mortality rates in Canada, the people of Northern British Columbia have the highest mortality rates in the province for all forms of cancer [53]. The Premier's consultation final report's recommendations are now being implemented [54].

A final characteristic worth noting regarding cancer policy development is that non-governmental organizations (NGOs) play an important role in cancer control policy initiation, development, and implementation in all jurisdictions examined. At the initiation and development phases, NGOs might be involved in producing relevant data on the cancer burden and cancer services, creating a sense of urgency, mobilizing action, achieving political commitment, and/or promoting the patient and public perspective through their knowledge of community issues. In New Zealand, for example, the Cancer Society of New Zealand and the Child Cancer Foundation formed a partnership with the Ministry of Health (Cancer Control Trust) and financed a good part of the groundwork for developing the NZ cancer control strategy. The Cancer Society of New Zealand is also involved in the cancer control work programme, contributing to several projects related to the implementation of the NZ action plan. In Canada, the Canadian Cancer Society and its research arm, the National Cancer Institute of Canada, were among the founders of the CSCC. As previously described, the Canadian Cancer Society played a substantial role in advocating for its implementation. Its provincial divisions are also involved in advocacy, policy planning, prevention, research, as well as in patient support and information.

This overview of several jurisdictions' experiences in cancer control policy development suggests there are a number of essential ingredients or critical events that act as drivers and success factors for policy development. The recognition by policy makers of important problems regarding the cancer burden, the organization and management of cancer services, and a perceived crisis situation usually amplified by the media can become strong incentives for change. In any case, however, the most important factor for success remains the unequivocal commitment of government officials at the highest political levels in making cancer control a top priority.

Features of strategy implementation

Establishing priorities for action

Developing a comprehensive cancer control strategy is the first step that provides the foundation on which to transform the health care system in order to lessen the cancer burden and improve the patient journey. Such a strategy sets out the vision, values, and key directions to improve the situation. It usually follows from a review of existing cancer control activities that have identified major gaps and formulated recommendations. It may or may not straightaway include the plan that sets out priorities for action, including specific objectives, targets, or milestones that are required to realize the vision. For example, some jurisdictions (Canada, New Zealand, and Québec) have first developed a strategy and then its associated action plan, with more or less time between those steps. Others (England, France, and Ontario) have put forth an action plan.

In the remaining jurisdictions (Alberta, British Columbia, and Nova Scotia) the situation is a bit different. The Alberta cancer control action plan (2004) does not have a timeline, but the planned steps to meet the priorities have been included in ACB annual business plans. A similar approach is taken by the BCCA that has developed a strategic plan in 2003 and whose operational planning is included in the PHSA annual service plans. Nova Scotia's programmatic approach rests on a report to the Deputy Minister of Health [35], and while CCNS might produce strategic operational plans, the only publicly available document establishing priorities for action with clear timeline in relation to the cancer system is the Department of Health annual business plan.

Governing cancer control reforms

The concept of 'governing' refers to purposeful actions to guide, steer, control, and manage public policy [55]. These actions include: the setting of policy visions, goals, and priorities; the creation of structures and mandates; the allocation of resources; the management of programmes; the organization of services; the setting of benchmarks and desired outcomes; the monitoring of progress; and the assessment of results [56].

The jurisdictions reviewed herein have developed varying governing approaches to drive and manage their cancer control strategies, plans, and programmes. These differences are observed by examining the public sector actors involved in cancer control management, their roles and responsibilities, as well as their links of accountability [9]. This section will focus on the varying ties between the selected jurisdictions' Departments or Ministries of Health and the cancer dedicated organizations that were created to manage the implementation of the cancer strategy or programme.

Dedicated versus general approaches

Jurisdictions first differ by whether cancer control services are planned, organized, and managed according to a 'dedicated' (disease specific) approach within the health care system or whether cancer services are viewed more generally, as any other health care service. For example, Alberta, British Columbia, and Ontario can be considered as having developed a strongly dedicated approach to cancer control, namely because these jurisdictions' provincial governments decided to view cancer as a specific health problem that required particular management. Such a dedicated approach, analogous to 'disease management' at the level of the health care system, involved the creation of a dedicated cancer agency that would be responsible for the planning, organization, management, and delivery of cancer services throughout the province. It also involved the creation of provincial and/or regional cancer programmes, organized around tertiary or comprehensive cancer centres, as well as other specific structures and infrastructure for the management of cancer services. One important difference between Alberta and British Columbia on the one hand and Ontario on the other is the recent change in the mandate of Ontario's cancer agency. Since 2001, service delivery is no longer part of the mandate of Cancer Care Ontario, but the agency assumes a purchaser role, by directing and overseeing substantial funding to hospitals and other cancer care providers. In contrast, Québec can be considered as having favoured a more general approach, where service organization reflects the general configuration advocated for all primary, secondary, and tertiary health care, and hence where most cancer services are delivered in many hospitals throughout the province instead of being concentrated in a few specially designated cancer centres.

Centralization versus decentralization of authority

Jurisdictions also differ in the ways power is shared between the central command within the Ministry of Health and the various actors involved in cancer strategy management and implementation, be it at the national/provincial, regional, and local levels. Highly centralized approaches mean that most if not all of the governance functions (such as setting goals and indicators of outcome, resource allocation, monitoring of strategy implementation, programme management, service organization, system performance evaluation, etc.) are concentrated within a central administration [57], usually the Ministry of Health or a national/provincial organization to which the Ministry has delegated such authority. The latter organization is usually an autonomous entity with its own legal identity that remains, however, accountable to the government.

In contrast, a highly decentralized approach means that a significant part of the governing authority is delegated to regional and local entities [58]. While not always concordant, the sharing of governing functions usually goes hand in hand with the decentralization of responsibilities. However, this is not always the case, since a decentralization of responsibilities is always possible without adequate decentralization (delegation) of governing authority.

If there is no example of a strongly decentralized approach in the jurisdictions reviewed, some elements of decentralization are more apparent in some jurisdictions than others. For example, in England, there is a significant element of decentralization of governing powers towards the 34 cancer networks, each covering a territory comprising a population of about 1 to 2 million. Such delegation of powers is attributed to the networks' management teams and governing boards, and relates to the planning, commissioning, organization, management, and delivery of cancer services. Nevertheless, the Department of Health still holds very important governing authority at the national level, namely as regards strategic planning, the financing of NHS Trusts, national service frameworks (such as the cancer plan), and other national programmes (screening, research, palliative care, etc.) as well as the setting of milestones and indicators of outcomes. Moreover, the Department of Health has developed a sophisticated system of performance measurement and monitoring for the NHS that includes clinical governance activities and service quality improvement programmes specifically designed for oncology.

In France, cancer control governance is mainly centralized under the Ministry of Health that is responsible for the planning, financing, organization, and management of cancer control activities. However, the Ministry shares some of its powers and responsibilities with a number of national health agencies under its administrative supervision, namely the *Institut national du cancer* (INCa), but also with the *Institut national de veille sanitaire* (INVS), and the *Institut national de prévention et d'éducation à la santé* (INPES). At the regional level, the *Agences régionales d'hospitalisation* (ARH) are responsible for translating the Ministry of Health's requirements regarding service organization into regional schemes, in addition to being responsible for the planning and financing of health care services. Finally, the regional cancer networks are responsible for implementing cancer plan measures related to service provision, including service coordination and quality management. While INCa, an autonomous organization, holds significant responsibilities in all aspects of the cancer control continuum (prevention, care, and research), the Ministry of Health has full authority on health services. Hence, cancer plan measures related to service organization and quality cannot take place without a congruent action that involves the Ministry of Health, INCa, and other mandated organizations. For example, the publication in 2007 by the Prime Minister of a statutory order related to authorizing cancer practice for health care facilities was an essential pre-requisite for the implementation of the accreditation standards that had been prepared by INCa.

In New Zealand, cancer control governance is centralized under the Ministry of Health. A cancer team within the Ministry, led by a national clinical director for cancer control and including representatives from the District Health Boards, has formed a steering group that is jointly managing a structured cancer control work programme to implement actions identified by the New Zealand cancer control strategy action plan 2005–10. The cancer control work programme also includes representatives from other key cancer control stakeholders, such as the New Zealand cancer treatment working party and its workgroups, the Cancer Control Council, the Cancer Society of New Zealand, as well as consumer groups. The Ministry of Health shares some of its authority with the Cancer Control Council, an independent advisory body appointed by the Minister of Health to monitor and review implementation of the strategy, to foster collaboration and cooperation in cancer control (providing opportunities for non-government involvement) and to provide independent strategic advice.

Main governing models

Based on previous detailed analyses of governing arrangements [6,9], and as exemplified by some of the governing features described in the previous sections, the jurisdictions examined can be classified according to three main governing models (Table 17.2):

◆ Model 1: Authority for governance is *delegated* to an organization, distinct from the Department or Ministry of Health, and dedicated to cancer control: Alberta, British Columbia, and Ontario.

◆ Model 2: Authority for governance is *shared* between the Department or Ministry of Health and distinct national, and/or local, governmental organizations dedicated to cancer control: England, France, and New Zealand.

◆ Model 3: Authority for governance is *distributed* among branches of the Department or Ministry of Health, including organizations dedicated to cancer control: Nova Scotia and Québec.

The Canadian federal level has not been included in Table 17.2 because it does not have jurisdiction over the organization, management, and delivery of health services. Yet, it favours a dedicated approach to cancer control, with a somewhat different philosophy as regards the content of its strategy (focus on information gathering, identification of best practices, and knowledge transfer along the cancer control continuum). It also chose a unique approach for the composition and power arrangements of its cancer governing organization. From 2002 to 2006, the CSCC Council served as the first board of directors for the CSCC, which was established as an independent coalition of major cancer control organizations, appointed by, and accountable to, a forum of stakeholder groups outside the mandate of the government. This model was said to promote collective responsibility, inclusiveness, and an evidence-based decision-making process [53]. These arrangements evolved as a closer relationship to the government was formed when the Council was replaced by the Canadian Partnership against Cancer (CPAC). While remaining an autonomous not-for-profit organization, the CPAC now operates at arm's length from the government, and it is accountable to the federal Minister of Health for the funds it receives.

Strengths and challenges of the main governing models

An unquestionable advantage of governing model 1 is that it confers a single organization with the ability to plan, manage, and coordinate cancer services as well as cancer surveillance and research for an entire jurisdiction. In addition, it confers substantial authority over the volume and quality of a significant number of cancer services. This model's main challenge is to exert influence on, and ensure the collaboration of, health service providers that are 'outside' the cancer agency's centres or direct authority (e.g. cancer surgeons, primary care providers involved in

Table 17.2 Main governing models

Governing model	Model 1			Model 2			Model 3	
	Alberta	**British columbia**	**Ontario**	**England**	**France**	**New zealand**	**Nova scotia**	**Québec**
Approach to the cancer problem	Strongly dedicated	Strongly dedicated	Strongly dedicated	Rather dedicated than general	Rather dedicated than general	Rather dedicated than general	Rather general than dedicated	General
Authority	**Delegated** to a provincial cancer agency	**Delegated** to a provincial cancer agency	**Delegated** to a provincial cancer agency that shares authority as regards the management of service delivery	**Shared** between the Department of Health (its cancer dedicated entities) and managed cancer networks	**Shared** between the Ministry of Health, its national health agencies, and a dedicated cancer institute	**Shared** between the Ministry of Health (its cancer team), District Health Boards, and a Cancer Control Council	**Distributed** within the Department of Health, including a dedicated cancer programme	**Distributed** within the Ministry of Health, including a dedicated cancer division

Table adapted from [9]

prevention efforts, physicians, and other providers involved in cancer screening activities or palliative care, etc.).

An important point to make regarding the jurisdictions that embraced a governing approach along the lines of model 1 relates to the conditions that must be in place for successful implementation of this model. Some insights on these conditions can be drawn from the experiences of Alberta and British Columbia (thriving cancer agencies responsible for provincial delivery of cancer services), the less successful experience of Nova Scotia in the 1990s (replacement of a provincial cancer agency that was responsible for service delivery by a programme within the Department of Health), and the recent experience of Ontario (removing the delivery of cancer services function from the mandate of the provincial cancer agency, but enabling it to drive quality and accountability of service provision) [9]. Three elements can be drawn from analyzing these experiences. First, it seems obvious that a provincial agency entrusted with such a huge mandate (to develop a cancer control system for an entire jurisdiction) must have the necessary powers to fully fulfil its mandate, and accordingly, must have the unequivocal support of the Ministry of Health. Second, the establishment of a strongly dedicated and highly centralized approach, and subsequent development of a cancer sub-system, must fit well with the overall configuration of the jurisdiction's health care system. Third, forces (leadership support, commitment, etc.) must be in place to defend and maintain such an approach in the midst of ongoing health system reforms that touch upon the governance and organization of health services, especially if these reforms are not congruent with the model advocated in cancer control.

A strong point in favour of governing model 2 is its ability to take all existing cancer services and initiatives at one point in time (once a nation-wide cancer strategy or plan is launched) and organize them into a coherent system (using a step-wise integration process that usually takes a couple of years and whose pace will depend on various levers to be discussed later on in this chapter). This is in contrast to a cancer system that would have been progressively built over many years, on the basis of an existing core programme, as it is the case in Alberta or British Columbia. An important point to make regarding the jurisdictions that embraced a governing approach along the lines of model 2 is the need for clear lines of accountability, and effective coordination among the various mandated players. This was a significant challenge in England, and may well be in New Zealand as its four regional managed cancer control networks develop. England's past experience showed the need for strong collaborations between members of the cancer networks and support from their associated NHS primary care trusts and Strategic Health Authority (SHA), as well as clear lines of accountability between all the players to ensure effective coordination of efforts for the implementation of the NHS cancer plan measures [59]. In spite of this challenge, substantial progress was achieved, greatly facilitated by a successful network development programme and the performance measuring and reporting system developed by the Department of Health [59,60].

In governing model 3 there are three main challenges as illustrated by the experiences of both Québec and Nova Scotia. The first challenge (mostly apparent in Québec) relates to the dispersion of the management and governance of cancer control activities, with some responsibilities (implementation of the cancer control strategy, clinical practice guidelines, establishment of a provincial registry, and palliative care) being held by the dedicated ministerial division (DLCC), with others (prevention and screening) being held by the public health branch, and still others (like the planning and management of research) not considered as a central ministerial responsibility. The second challenge (mostly apparent in Nova Scotia) relates to the disconnect between the scale of the responsibilities attributed to a provincial departmental programme (CCNS) and the extent of departmental support provided in terms of appropriate delegation of authority and resources to ensure the fulfilling of all of the components of the programme's mandate. The third challenge for these dedicated organizations (DLCC or CCNS) is trying to promote a cancer control vision in a health system configuration that is not already inclined to a disease-specific approach. This last challenge could, however, be seen as a strong point, as a general approach is likely to enhance the system's ability to answer cancer patients' needs that are not cancer related.

Varying abilities of cancer-dedicated organizations to manage the cancer continuum

As briefly alluded to in the previous section, existing provincial and national organizations dedicated to overseeing cancer control strategy implementation do not have the same powers when it comes to coordinating actions within the health system to ensure best possible service delivery along the cancer control continuum. Indeed, a comparative overview of each organization's governing functions along the cancer control continuum (Table 17.3) shows that in addition to having more suitable structures for coordinated actions, the provincial cancer agencies of Alberta, British Columbia, and Ontario have a larger mandate for cancer control involvement and greater room to manoeuvre.

In France, INCa plays a substantial role also but has significantly less powers in service organization and delivery than the Canadian provincial cancer agencies. In the other jurisdictions, to achieve such coordinating power requires close collaboration between the Department or Ministry of Health and the dedicated organization, whether inside or outside the Ministry. In England, while the national cancer control director and its cancer action team and taskforce (which are sitting inside the Department of Health) do not hold the strings as regards the financing, organization, and delivery of cancer control services, they, however, have the authority to oversee the implementation of the cancer plan measures, which include several outcome indicators for cancer networks and NHS primary care trusts to meet. The development and management of efforts to ensure an optimal patient journey is under the responsibility and authority of the cancer control networks. Each network is headed by a management team that includes representatives from the NHS primary care trusts and the strategic health authority that serve the geographic area covered by the network.

In Nova Scotia, CCNS is involved in all aspects of the cancer control continuum, but with varying authority. CCNS mandate is to enhance service coordination, support best practices through education, clinical practice guidelines and standard setting, as well as to foster research. It is also mandated with evaluating the various cancer control programmes and initiatives being developed. Like the other provincial cancer agencies included in this study, CCNS manages the provincial cancer registry. It also manages the cervical cancer screening programme, while the breast screening programme is governed by a distinct group within the acute and tertiary care branch of the Department of Health. As regards services, CCNS' main role has been to develop programmes and to set standards, while their implementation has been undertaken by the Department of Health and its District Health Authorities. As a result, CCNS authority has remained largely derived from health professional training and education.

In Québec, the cancer control division within the Ministry of Health (DLCC) is mandated to ensuring the quality and organization of cancer care services. The influence of the DLCC on the other dimensions of the cancer control spectrum is drawn from its ability to establish effective collaborations with the relevant ministry divisions and other stakeholder organizations outside the Ministry of Health. For example, the public health branch, which is not dedicated to cancer, is responsible for general prevention activities, the organized breast cancer screening programme and a tumour file (*fichier des tumeurs*). An important ongoing project led by the DLCC, but requiring the active participation of the public health branch, is the upgrade of the tumour file in order to develop a full-fledged provincial cancer registry.

Table 17.3 Authority of national and provincial dedicated cancer organizations

	ACB (Alberta)	BCCA (British Columbia)	CCO (Ontario)	DoH cancer taskforce and NCAT (England)	INCA (France)	MoH cancer team and Cancer Control Council (New Zealand)	CCNS (Nova Scotia)	DLCC (Québec)
Prevention	M, P	M, P	M, P	M	M, P	M	M, P	---
Screening	M, P	M, P	M	M	M	M	M	M
Treatment	D, F, M, P	D, F, M, P	D, M	M	M	M	M	D, M
Support and palliative care	D, F, M, P	D, F, M, P	D, M	M	M, P (patient support)	M	M, P (patient support)	D, M
Research	D, F, M, P	D, F, M, P	D, M, P	M	D, M,	M	M, P	---
Surveillance	D, M, P	D, M, P	D, M, P	M	M, P	M	D, M, P	M
	Model 1			**Model 2**			**Model 3**	

Table adapted from [9]

Legend (adapted from [57]): **D**: Decision-making authority; **F**: Financing: the capacity to obtain the necessary financial resources for the functioning of the organization. In most cases, financing is done by the government (as well as health insurance in France). Cancer dedicated organizations finance some of their activities through fundraising or revenues external to the basic budget they receive from the Ministry of Health; **M**: Management: to implement Department or Ministry of Health decisions, to allocate the necessary funds to conduct planned activities; to coordinate actors and development efforts for existing and new initiatives, to monitor progress; **P**: Production of health care services or research or epidemiological surveillance.

Essential powers remaining within the Department or Ministry of Health

Notwithstanding the governing model being embraced, it should be noted that health promotion and prevention programmes are governed by the Department or Ministry of Health, while the cancer treatment and care component is the focus of the cancer dedicated organization. The governance of organized cancer screening programmes is less homogeneous, with some jurisdictions having delegated the management of those programmes to their central cancer dedicated organization (Alberta, British Columbia, Ontario, and France), while others have those programmes located within the core business of the Ministry or Department of Health (England, New Zealand, Nova Scotia, and Québec).

In all jurisdictions examined, Departments and Ministries of Health still keep important powers that mainly relate to sustaining and enhancing the capacity of the cancer control system to deal with increasing demand for services. These powers are related to: financing of dedicated organizations and other structures such as the construction of new cancer centres, capital equipment acquisition, human resources management, as well as the establishment of information management infrastructures; and decision-making, namely for establishing organized screening programmes and for developing prevention initiatives such as tobacco control and healthy eating and living strategies.

Another important feature regarding the authority of the Department or Ministry of Health is in the setting of targets and indicators of outcome. While cancer dedicated organizations may well develop such targets or indicators, and propose them to the Ministry, it usually remains the prerogative of the Ministry to decide when, how, and what targets will be put forth.

In this context, the transfer of authority from the Ministry of Health to dedicated cancer agencies (governing model 1) does not mean a complete delegation of powers and responsibilities. Dedicated agencies still depend on the support given by the Ministry of Health for ensuring the agency's adequate capacity to respond to emerging needs. Hence, even when there is a deliberate choice to concentrate authority within a specific organization, the priority given to cancer control by high level government officials remains a pivotal element for advancing cancer control.

Leveraging change to improve cancer services

Implementing cancer control strategies, programmes, and plans to ultimately improve cancer control systems and ensure optimal care pathways is a Herculean task that not only requires coordinated action but, most importantly, an effective mix of leadership, strategy, and tools for enabling change on the ground. Cancer control key informants questioned about the barriers and facilitators of implementing reform noted the importance of achieving political commitment, securing adequate resources, ensuring strong leadership, promoting participation (clinician and user involvement), establishing implementation strategies, and providing incentives to promote change [6].

Levers provide the governing organizations with the necessary powers and incentives to drive all those actors responsible for implementing the planned reforms. A previous study of available levers within selected jurisdictions [9] revealed that jurisdictions are both developing cancer-specific levers as well as harnessing existing health system levers. Cancer-dedicated (or otherwise relevant) levers that were examined have been mapped to the following three categories:

1 *Attributes of, and powers available to, the organizations that are responsible for the implementation.* In addition to the governing features of the cancer dedicated organizations described in the previous sections of this chapter, these levers include: laws and regulations, accountability structures, management agreements, and financial and human resources dedicated to implementing cancer control reforms.

2 *Service quality assurance and improvement systems.* These levers bring together tools and mechanisms such as clinical practice guidelines, service organization guidance, quality standards, as well as processes such as peer-review visits, audits, and accreditation.

3 *Mechanisms for monitoring progress and for evaluation of the cancer system, programme, or plan.* These levers relate to the various tools available (cancer registries and other clinical databases, progress reports, patients' surveys, programme assessments, etc.) to inform the governing organization (as well as all cancer control actors and the public alike) about main accomplishments, progress towards achieving planned actions, as well as impact of reforms on services quality, and ultimately, on health outcomes.

By examining jurisdictions' progress on service organization reforms, the study mentioned earlier showed that, in addition to government's strong commitment, and financial support, the most important levers for driving change included clear accountability lines, information gathering and management systems, and performance measurement systems [9]. Moreover, the study suggested that the key to success resided in the coordinated implementation of these levers. Table 17.4 compares the jurisdictions examined herein along a selected number of levers to illustrate some of the jurisdictions' assets.

Critical factors for successful implementation of organizational change

In sum, based on results obtained from previous comparative studies [6,9], as well as expert opinions in the field of cancer control [51,60–62], we propose the following list of factors that we believe are critical for successful implementation of organizational change:

1 Recognizing the need for change and making cancer control a top priority
2 Obtaining clear commitment from high level government officials
3 Promoting active participation of all stakeholders in the planning phase
4 Setting clear priorities for action with timeline, as well as targets and indicators of outcome
5 Securing strong leadership and creating cancer dedicated organization(s)
6 Reaching consensus (obtaining buy-in from actors) on the plan's goals and means
7 Securing dedicated financial and human resources
8 Establishing performance and management agreements between key players
9 Planning for the implementation phase
10 Organizing the implementation process – sharing and coordinating responsibilities
11 Providing incentives to actors on the ground
12 Developing information gathering and management systems to build capacity for progress monitoring and evaluation
13 Developing performance measurement initiatives to improve the quality of services delivered
14 Monitoring progress and performing assessments that entail public reporting

Conclusion

Cancer control strategies involve multiple objectives and activities seeking to improve jurisdictions' cancer burden through health promotion, cancer prevention, and early detection, as well as

Table 17.4 Selected levers available for driving change towards better cancer control

Jurisdictions	Canada	Alberta	British Columbia	Ontario	England	France	New Zealand	Nova Scotia	Québec
Governing model	Dedicated cancer agencies			DoH/MoH with external dedicated bodies				Dedicated divisions in MoH	
Priorities for action with timeline	CSCC. 2006–2010 business plan for the CSCC [53]	ACB. Business plan 2005–06 [63]	PHSA. Service plan 2007/08–2009/10 [64] (includes BCCA planned activities)	CCO. Ontario cancer plan 2008–2012 [33] and Ontario cancer plan 2005–2008 [32]	DoH. Cancer reform strategy 2008–2012 [27] and NHS cancer plan (2000–2010) [26]	MoH. Cancer plan (2003–2007) [21]	Cancer Control Taskforce. NZ Cancer control strategy action plan 2005–2010 [14]	NS DoH. Business plan 2008-09 [40]	DLCC. Orientations prioritaires 2007–2012 du PQLC [45]
Website	http://www.partnershipagainstcancer.ca/	http://www.cancerboard.ab.ca/ http://www.albertahealthservices.ca/	http://www.phsa.ca/ http://www.bccancer.bc.ca	http://www.cancercare.on.ca/	http://www.dh.gov.uk/en/Healthcare/NationalServiceFrameworks/Cancer/	http://www.e-cancer.fr/	http://www.moh.govt.nz/cancercontrol http://www.cancercontrol-council.govt.nz/	http://www.gov.ns.ca/health/ http://www.cancercare.ns.ca/	http://www.msss.gouv.qc.ca/sujets/prob_sante/cancer/
Dedicated or relevant legislations and regulations	Tobacco law (1997)	Cancer programs Act (2000) Smoke-free places Act (2005) Alberta Cancer prevention legacy Act (2006)	Society Act (created BCCA in 1972) Tobacco control Act (2006, amenced 2007)	Cancer Act (1990) Smoke-free Ontario Act (2006)	Health Bill. Part 1: Smoke-free premises, places and vehicles (2006) Health services circulars (1999/205; 2000/021; 2001/012; 2002/005)	Tobacco law (1991, amended 2006) Palliative care law (1999) Public health law (2004) Statutory orders on cancer care (2007) Circulars on cancer services organization (1998, 2005) and palliative care (2002)	Smoke-free environments amendment Act (2003) NZ health and disability Act (section 11 created NZ Cancer Control Council in 2005)	Cancer treatment and research foundation Act (1989, repealed 1996) Smoke-free places Act (2002, amended 2006)	Tobacco law (1998, amended 2005, 2006)

(Continued)

Table 17.4 (Continued) Selected levers available for driving change towards better cancer control*

Jurisdictions	Canada	Alberta	British Columbia	Ontario	England	France	New Zealand	Nova Scotia	Québec
Governing model	Dedicated cancer agencies		DoH/MoH with external dedicated bodies					Dedicated divisions in MoH	
Accountability links and management agreements	CPAC board is accountable to the federal minister of health	ACB board is accountable to the minister of health. Multi-year performance agreements between MoH and ACB and MoH and regional authorities. ACB annual reports	BCCA President is accountable to the minister of health. PHSA CEO and PHSA board. PHSA board is accountable to the minister of health services. Performance agreements between MoH and PHSA; MoH and regional authorities; and regional authorities and hospitals. PHSA annual reports include BCCA's activities	CCO board is accountable to the minister of health. Memorandum of understanding between MoH and CCO. Accountability agreements between MoH and local authorities and local authorities and hospitals. Accountability agreements between CCO and hospitals. Clinical accountability framework between CCO and service providers. CCO annual progress reports	NCD is accountable to the Department of Health board. The DoH board is accountable to secretary of state for health. Cancer taskforce and cancer action team accountable to NCD. Strategic health authorities (SHAs) accountable to NHS chief executive, who is accountable to secretary of state for health. Primary care trusts (PCTs) accountable to SHAs for performance and to NHS for financing. Cancer services networks accountable to PCTs and to their governing board, that is accountable to SHA. DNC produces progress reports	INCa, and ARH(s) are under administrative supervision (sous-tutelle) by the MoH. INCa produces progress reports	Cancer Control Council is accountable to the minister of health. NCD is accountable to director-general of health. Ministry cancer control team accountable to NCD. DHB boards responsible to the minister of health. Operation policy framework by MoH for DHBs and DHBs' performance are measured by MoH. Regional cancer networks accountable to their governance group and produce progress reports to DHBs	CCNS board chair is accountable to minister of health. CCNS reports to the deputy minister of health (since resignation of commissioner, CCNS COO reports to a director of the acute and tertiary care branch). District health boards are part of the DoH and must produce regular reports. CCNS produces reports to the community	DLCC director is accountable to the minister of health through the director of the DGSSMU branch. Performance and management agreements between MoH and regional agencies and regional agencies and local authorities. DLCC produces annual report to MoH

| Independent evaluation of entire national or provincial system, strategy, plan or programme | Not found | Not found | Not found | Arm's length approach with Cancer System Quality Index (since 2005) National Audit Office [65–67] | Cour des comptes [68] Haut conseil de santé publique [69] | Cancer Control Council of NZ [70] | External evaluation teams [37,71] | Not found |

the cancer patients' journey through the best possible provision of health services along the care continuum.

All jurisdictions recognize the need to improve their cancer burden through a comprehensive cancer control approach, though they differ in the means that they make available to bring out the planned reforms. One important difference lies in the more or less extensive use of cancer-dedicated structures and infrastructures to tackle this complex health problem. While all jurisdictions have some form of structures dedicated to cancer, such as interdisciplinary cancer teams, jurisdictions show various degree of a dedicated approach. Alberta, British Columbia, and Ontario can be viewed as having built the most extreme versions of that approach, a 'cancer system' within the more general health care system.

Three main governing models could be identified when examining the relationship between the Department or the Ministry of Health and dedicated cancer organizations as regards the degree of authority sharing. Moreover, the varying abilities demonstrated by these cancer governing organizations to manage the various activities comprising the cancer control spectrum are generally mapped to the three main governing models identified. However, irrespective of governing models, functional governing arrangements should ensure that cancer dedicated organizations have sufficient authority and adequate means to carry out their mandate.

The most important lesson is that a clear commitment from the highest government authority needs to be obtained. In addition to this crucial element, significant progress in implementing organizational change is likely to be obtained when all actors responsible: (1) have the appropriate means to properly plan the implementation, (2) have or develop together a functional governing organization, (3) have available the most important levers to sustain change and coordinate actions, and (4) are provided with the means to assess progress and publicly report on that progress. Hence, not only is it important to sketch out where to go and how, it is equally important to be able to know what was accomplished, what remains to be done, and what is the impact of the efforts and resources that have been committed. This is the single most difficult challenge awaiting Departments or Ministries of Health and their cancer dedicated organizations.

References

1 World Health Organization (WHO) (2003). Global cancer rates could increase by 50% to 15 million by 2020. World Cancer Report provides clear evidence that action on smoking, diet and infections can prevent one third of cancers, another third can be cured. Available from: http://www.who.int/mediacentre/news/releases/2003/pr27/en/.

2 Zapka JG, Taplin SH, Solberg LI, & Manos MM (2003). A framework for improving the quality of cancer care: The case of breast and cervical cancer screening. *Cancer Epidemiol Biomarkers Prev*, Jan;12(1):4–13.

3 World Health Organization (WHO) (2002). National cancer control programmes: Policies and managerial guidelines. WHO, Geneva.

4 Hewitt ME & Simone JV (1999). *Ensuring quality cancer care*. National Academy Press, Washington, DC.

5 Bridging research to action: A framework and decision-making process for cancer control (1994). Advisory Committee on Cancer Control, National Cancer Institute of Canada. *CMAJ*, Oct 15;151(8): 1141–46.

6 Agence d'évaluation des technologies et des modes d'intervention en santé (AETMIS), Caron L, De Civita M, Law S, & Brault I. (2008) Cancer control interventions in selected jurisdictions: design, governance, and implementation Montréal: *AETMIS*, Report No. 07–08a.

7 Abed J, Reilley B, Butler MO, Kean T, Wong F, & Hohman K (2000). Developing a framework for comprehensive cancer prevention and control in the United States: An initiative of the Centers for Disease Control and Prevention. *J Public Health Manag Pract*, Mar;6(2):67–78.

8 Given LS, Black B, Lowry G, Huang P, & Kerner JF (2005). Collaborating to conquer cancer: A comprehensive approach to cancer control. *Cancer Causes Control*, Oct;**16** (Suppl 1):3–14.

9 Agence d'évaluation des technologies et des modes d'intervention en santé (AETMIS), Caron L, De Civita M, Law S, & Brault I (2007). Aperçu comparatif des stratégies de lutte contre le cancer dans quelques pays et provinces canadiennes. Montréal. *AETMIS*, Report No. 07–08.

10 Canadian Strategy for Cancer Control (CSCC) (2002). Canadian Strategy for Cancer Control, Ottawa, ON. *CSCC*.

11 Cancer 2000: Strategies for cancer control in Canada. The proceedings of cancer 2000. A report on the work of a national task force. Cancer 2000 Task Force, Toronto, ON. 1992.

12 New Zealand Ministry of Health (NZMoH) (2000). The New Zealand health strategy. NZMoH, Wellington, NZ.

13 New Zealand Ministry of Health (NZMoH) (2003). The New Zealand cancer control strategy. NZMoH and the NZ Cancer Control Trust, Wellington, NZ.

14 Cancer Control Taskforce (2005). The New Zealand cancer control strategy: Action plan 2005–2010. Ministry of Health, Wellington, NZ. Available from: http://www.moh.govt.nz/cancercontrol.

15 Cour des comptes (2000). *La mise en œuvre de la politique de santé: l'exemple de la lutte contre le cancer*. Cour des comptes, Paris, France.

16 Ligue nationale contre le cancer (1999). *Les malades prennent la parole. Le livre blanc des 1ers États généraux des malades du cancer*. Ramsay, Paris, France.

17 Neuwirth L (2001). Rapport d'information fait au nom de la commission des Affaires sociales par la mission d'information sur la politique de lutte contre le cancer. Sénat; Paris, France.

18 Oudin J (1998). Le financement et l'organisation de la politique de lutte contre le cancer: rapport d'information. Sénat, Paris, France.

19 Secrétariat d'État à la santé et à l'action sociale (2000). Programme national de lutte contre le cancer (2000–2005). *Secrétariat d'État à la santé et à l'action sociale*, Paris, France.

20 Commission d'orientation sur le cancer (2003). Rapport de la Commission d'orientation sur le cancer. Ministère de la santé, Paris, France.

21 Ministère de la santé, de la famille et des personnes handicapées (2003). Cancer: une mobilisation nationale, tous ensemble. Ministère de la santé, de la famille et des personnes handicapées, Paris, France. Available from: http://www.e-cancer.fr/.

22 Department of Health (DoH) (1995). A policy framework for commissioning cancer services: A report by the Expert Advisory Group on Cancer to the Chief Medical Officers of England and Wales. London, England: DoH.

23 Berrino F, Sant M, Verdecchia A, Capocaccia R, Hakulinen T, & Esteve J (1995). Survival of cancer patients in Europe: The EUROCARE Study. World Health Organization, International Agency for Research on Cancer, Lyon, France.

24 Department of Health (DoH) (1999). Prime Minister announces 10 year cancer action plan to save 60,000 lives. Available from: http://www.dh.gov.uk/en/Publicationsandstatistics/Pressreleases/DH_4025536.

25 Department of Health (DoH) (1999). Health Service Circular 1999/205: Cancer waiting times achieving the two week target, DoH, London, England.

26 Department of Health (DoH) (2000). The NHS cancer plan: A plan for investment, a plan for reform. DoH, London, England. Available from: http://www.dh.gov.uk/en/Healthcare/NationalServiceFrameworks/Cancer/.

27 Department of Health (DoH) (2007). Cancer reform strategy. DoH, London, England. Available from: http://www.dh.gov.uk/en/Healthcare/NationalServiceFrameworks/Cancer/.

28 Ontario Ministry of Health (1994). Life to gain: A cancer strategy for Ontario. Ministry of Health, Toronto, ON.

29 Cancer Services Implementation Committee (2001). Report of the Cancer Services Implementation Committee (Alan R. Hudson, Chair). Ministry of Health and Long-Term Care (MOHLTC), Toronto, ON.

30 Sullivan T, Evans W, Angus H, & Hudson A (2003). *Strengthening the quality of cancer services in Ontario.* Canadian Healthcare Association Press, Ottawa, ON.

31 Cancer Care Ontario (CCO), Canadian Cancer Society (CCS) (2003). Targeting cancer: An action plan for cancer prevention and early detection. Cancer 2020: Background report. CCO; CCS, Toronto, ON.

32 Cancer Care Ontario (CCO) (2004). Ontario cancer plan 2005–2008. CCO, Toronto, ON. Available from: http://www.cancercare.on.ca/.

33 Cancer Care Ontario (CCO) (2008). Ontario cancer plan 2008–2011. CCO, Toronto, ON. Available from: http://www.cancercare.on.ca/.

34 Metropolitan Hospital Advisory Committee (MHAC) (1993). Oncology services: A strategy for comprehensive cancer control in Nova Scotia. MHAC, Halifax, NS.

35 Cancer Action Committee (1996). Cancer Care Nova Scotia: A plan for action. The comprehensive, integrated, accountable cancer management strategy. Department of Health, Halifax, NS.

36 Government of Nova Scotia (1996). Queen Elizabeth II Health Sciences Centre Act, S.N.S. 1995-96, c.15. Available from: http://www.canlii.org/ns/laws/sta/1995-96c.15/20080616/whole.html.

37 Corpus Sanchez International Consultancy (2007). Changing Nova Scotia's healthcare system: Creating sustainability through transformation. System-level findings and overall directions for change from the provincial health services operational review. Nova Scotia Department of Health, Halifax, NS.

38 Cancer Care Nova Scotia (CCNS) (2006). Understanding cancer in Nova Scotia: A statistical report by Cancer Care Nova Scotia with a focus on 2000–2004. CCNS, Halifax, NS. Available from: http://www.cancercare.ns.ca/.

39 Nova Scotia Department of Health (NSDoH) (2007). 2007-2008 business plan. NSDoH, Halifax, NS.

40 Nova Scotia Department of Health (NSDoH) 2008). Business plan 2008-09. NSDoH Halifax, NS. Available from: http://www.gov.ns.ca/health/.

41 Comité consultatif sur le cancer (1998). Programme québécois de lutte contre le cancer. Pour lutter efficacement contre le cancer, formons équipe. Ministère de la Santé et des Services sociaux (MSSS) Québec, QC.

42 Centre de coordination de la lutte contre le cancer au Québec (CCLCQ) (2003). La lutte contre le cancer dans les régions du Québec: un premier bilan. Ministère de la Santé et des Services sociaux (MSSS), Québec, QC.

43 Institut national de santé publique du Québec (INSPQ) (2006), Ministère de la Santé et des Services sociaux (MSSS). Portrait de santé du Québec et de ses régions 2006: les analyses. Deuxième rapport national sur l'état de santé de la population du Québec. Gouvernement du Québec, Québec, QC.

44 Coalition Priorité Cancer au Québec. Available from: http://www.coalitioncancer.com/nos-actions.php.

45 Direction de la lutte contre le cancer. Orientations prioritaires 2007–2012 du programme québécois de lutte contre le cancer (2007). Ministère de la Santé et des Services sociaux du Québec, Québec, QC. Available from: http://www.msss.gouv.qc.ca/sujets/prob_sante/cancer/.

46 Alberta Cancer Board (ACB) (2004). Alberta cancer control action plan. ACB, Edmonton, AB.

47 Premier's Advisory Council on Health (Mazankowski D. Chair) (2001). A framework for reform. Report of the Premier's Advisory Council on Health. Government of Alberta, Edmonton, AB.

48 Government of Alberta (2006). Alberta Cancer Prevention Legacy Act, S.A. 2006, c. A-14.2. Alberta Queen's printer, Edmonton, AB.

49 Canadian Cancer Society (CCS), National Cancer Institute of Canada (NCIC) (2006). Canadian cancer statistics 2006. CCS, Toronto, ON.

50 BC Cancer Agency (BCCA) (2003). BC Cancer Agency strategic plan. BCCA, Victoria, BC. Available from: http://www.bccancer.bc.ca.

51 Carlow DR (2000). The British Columbia Cancer Agency: A comprehensive and integrated system of cancer control. *Hosp Q*, Spring;**3**(3):31–45.

52 BC Cancer Agency (BCCA), Northern Health Authority (2005). Northern cancer control strategy: Final report. BCCA, Victoria, BC.

53 Canadian Strategy for Cancer Control (CSCC) (2006). 2006–2010 business plan for the Canadian Strategy for Cancer Control. CSCC, Ottawa, ON. Available from: http://www.partnershipagainstcancer.ca/

54 Premier's Consultation for Improved Cancer Care in Northern BC (2006). Final report: Premier's Consultation for Improved Cancer Care in Northern BC. Government of BC, Victoria, BC.

55 Lemieux V (2000). Government roles in governance processes. *Modernizing governance: A preliminary exploration*, pp. 117–45. Canadian Center for Management Development, Ottawa, ON.

56 Prince MJ (2001). Governing in an integrated fashion: Lessons from the disability domain. Canadian Policy Research Networks (CPRN), Ottawa, ON.

57 Turgeon J & Lemieux V (1999). La décentralisation: panacée ou boîte de Pandore ? In: Bégin C, Bergeron P, Forest P-G, & Lemieux V (eds) *Le système de santé québécois: un modèle en transformation*, pp. 173–94. Presses de l'Université de Montréal, Montréal.

58 Mills A, Vaughan JP, Smith DL, & Tabibzadeh I (1990). Health systems decentralization: Concepts, issues and country experience. WHO, Geneva.

59 Richards MA (2006). Implementing cancer networks in England. Cancer Networks Seminar; 2006; New Zealand, Wellington.

60 Richards MA (2005). The cancer control programme in England. 1st International Cancer Control Congress 2005; Canada, Vancouver.

61 Richards MA (2003). The politics of change in healthcare – The example of cancer in England. 2003; University of Sydney, Australia.

62 Sullivan T, Dobrow M, Thompson L, & Hudson A (2004). Reconstructing cancer services in Ontario. *Healthc Pap*, **5**(1):69–80; discussion 96–99.

63 Alberta Cancer Board (ACB) (2005). Business plan 2005-2006. ACB, Edmonton, AB. Available from: http://www.cancerboard.ab.ca/; http://www.albertahealthservices.ca/.

64 Provincial Health Services Authority (PHSA) (2007). Service plan 2007/08-2009/10. PHSA, Victoria, BC. Available from: http://www.phsa.ca/.

65 National Audit Office (NAO) (2004). Tackling cancer in England: Saving more lives. Report by the Comptroller and Auditor general. The Stationary Office, London, England.

66 National Audit Office (NAO) (2005). Tackling cancer: Improving the patient journey. Report by the Comptroller and Auditor general. The Stationary Office, London, England.

67 National Audit Office (NAO) (2005). The NHS cancer plan: A progress report. Report by the Comptroller and Auditor general. The Stationary Office, London, England.

68 Cour des comptes (2008). Rapport public thématique: la mise en oeuvre du plan cancer. Cour des comptes, Paris, France.

69 Haut conseil de la santé publique (2008). Évaluation du plan cancer. Rapport d'étape 1. Les objectifs de la loi de santé publique de 2004 relatifs à la prévention et au dépistage des cancers. Ministère de la santé, de la jeunesse, des sports et de la vie associative, Paris, France.

70 Cancer Control Council of New Zealand (CCCNZ) (2007). Mapping progress: The first two years of the cancer control strategy action plan 2005–2010. CCCNZ, Wellington, NZ. Available from: http://www.cancercontrolcouncil.govt.nz/.

71 Smith ER, McCutcheon D, & Schmidt B (2001). Evaluation of Cancer Care Nova Scotia. CCNS, Halifax, NS.

Acronyms

ACB	Alberta Cancer Board
ACCCC	Alberta Coordinating Council for Cancer Control
BC	British Columbia
BCCA	British Columbia Cancer Agency
CCNS	Cancer Care Nova Scotia
CCO	Cancer Care Ontario
CCS	Canadian Cancer Society
CPAC	Canadian Partnership Against Cancer
CQCO	Cancer Quality Council of Ontario
CSCC	Canadian strategy for cancer control
DGSSMU	Direction générale des services de santé et médecine universitaire, MSSS (Québec)
DoH	Department of Health (England, Nova Scotia)
DHA	District Health Authority (Nova Scotia)
DHB	District Health Board (New Zealand)
DLCC	Direction de la lutte contre le cancer (Québec)
INCa	Institut national du cancer (France)
MoH	Ministry of Health
MHLTC	Ministry of Health and Long Term Care (Ontario)
MHS	Ministry of Health Services (British Columbia)
MSSS	Ministère de la Santé et des Services sociaux (Québec)
NCAT	National Cancer Action Team (England)
NCD	National Cancer Director (England, New Zealand)
NGO	Non-governmental organization
NHS	National Health and Social Services (England)
NS	Nova Scotia
NZ	New Zealand
PCT	Primary Care Trust (England)
PHSA	Provincial Health Services Authority (British Columbia)
PQLC	Programme québécois de lutte contre le cancer
SHA	Strategic Health Authority (England)
UNESCO	United Nations Educational Scientific and Cultural Organization

Chapter 18

Evaluating the outcomes of cancer control

Andrea Micheli, Paolo Baili, Roberta Ciampichini, Arduino Verdecchia[1]

In the developed world, cancer is the second cause of death (about 26 per cent of all deaths for 2001) after heart diseases, while it is the third cause of death in the developing world (10 per cent of all deaths), preceded by diarrhoeal diseases [1,2]. There are a number of reasons why cancer has become a major public health issue in developed countries. With few exceptions over the world, the incidence of cancer has been increasing since the 1950s when the first cancer statistics became available, partly because the prevalence of cancer risk factors was already increasing and partly because the life expectancy at birth has increased and cancer is mainly a disease of older age [3]. The life expectancy at birth of countries undergoing rapid economic development (China, India, Brazil, etc.) is now increasing rapidly, and these countries are expected to experience a cancer epidemic in the near future, as has already happened in the developed world. It has been estimated that over six million people died from cancer worldwide in 2002; this figure will be 50 per cent higher in 2020 [4].

Awareness of the importance of cancer control plans has consequently increased since the end of the last century. A cancer control plan can include policies for cancer prevention, and for diagnosis and treatment, to improve survival and quality of life for cancer patients. The choice of appropriate policies depends on availability of resources, health systems, social and cultural conditions, political systems, evaluation of past policies, new scientific knowledge, international experience, etc. Each of these factors can influence cancer control. Thus effective cancer control is a continuous process in which a fundamental role is played by the evaluation of the outcomes and the identification of priorities.

This is possible only when cancer information systems work on population-based data. The main sources are the population-based cancer registries through which we are aware of the cancer incidence increase. They also inform us that in developed countries, the survival of cancer patients has increased markedly in recent years and mortality is decreasing [5,6]. Cancer prevalence (the proportion of subjects living in the population at a given date with past diagnosis of cancer) is therefore increasing. Using these cancer indicators, the present chapter synthesizes the epidemiological situation that cancer control planners have to face both in defining new plans and in evaluating past ones. The chapter covers the main characteristics and indicators necessary

[1] Andrea Micheli, PhD, Paolo Baili, PhD, Roberta Ciampichini, PhD, Descriptive Studies and Health Planning Unit, Fondazione IRCCS Istituto Nazionale dei Tumori, Milan, Italy; Arduino Verdecchia, PhD, National Centre of Epidemiology, Health Surveillance and Promotion, Istituto Superiore di Sanità, Rome, Italy.

to implement a well-functioning cancer information system, and the up to date situation for the main cancer outcome indicators in various world geographical areas, and discusses them in relation to the implementation of the cancer control process.

Cancer information systems: the role of population-based cancer registries

Cancer control plans should stick to reality. The main purpose of the cancer information system is to bridge the gap between cancer research and cancer control activities. The prerequisites for achieving this goal are:

◆ Availability of population-based data

◆ Completeness of data collection in all the countries or region

◆ Standardization of data-collection methods to allow comparisons (comparisons make data intelligible)

◆ Ability to adapt information systems to changing circumstances

These characteristics are largely achieved by the population-based cancer registries (CRs) established in the majority of developed countries. CRs collect data on all new cases of cancer occurring in a well-defined population. Data refer to the entire population covered, and are frequently sent from different units (e.g. pathology departments, medical records, radiotherapy databases, cancer centres, hospices, private hospitals, screening registries, other CRs, primary care facilities, nursing homes, and death certificates) within a single institution or several institutions [7].

Population-level patient data are becoming more and more useful for several purposes:

◆ Measuring the burden and the public health impact of cancer – nowadays the minimal role of any cancer registry is the provision of timely and robust data on cancer mortality, incidence, survival (following up incident cases for a given time after diagnosis) and prevalence

◆ Evaluating the impact of environmental and social factors on cancer risk and outcomes, and supporting investigations into the causes of cancer – for instance, thanks to cancer registration we know that mesothelioma is caused by exposure to asbestos; lymphoma and oral cancer rates are higher in ethnic minorities; cancer survival for patients living in poor areas is lower than for those living in rich areas

◆ Evaluating the quality of cancer care by providing comparative data about treatment patterns and outcomes, access to treatment between social groups, etc. – to perform these studies additional data to the minimum, such as details on treatment, quality of life, hospitalization, or cost per case need to be collected usually in ad hoc studies on representative samples of registered cases

◆ Contributing to the evaluation of screening programmes – a number of cancer registries already contribute to the efficient evaluation of screening programmes

Cancer registries use well-established quality criteria to measure cancer incidence. The International Agency on Research on Cancer (IARC) regularly publishes the book 'Cancer Incidence in Five Continents' [8] which includes observed cancer incidence data from all world CRs satisfying specific data quality criteria (e.g. internal consistency; histological verification of cancer diagnosis; percentage of cases registered by 'Death Certificate Only', with unspecified sites, or with age unknown) [8]. Table 18.1 shows the percentage of population covered by CRs included in 'Cancer Incidence in Five Continents – Volume IX'; coverage is higher in developed areas with a maximum of 80 per cent in North America.

Table 18.1 Percentage of population covered by cancer registries by geographical region [8]

	Percentage of coverage
Africa	1
Asia	4
South and Central America	4
Europe	33
Oceania	73
North America	80

Cancer information system in detail: cancer outcome indicators

The long tradition of population-based cancer registries in the majority of developed countries allows the use of standardized methodologies and facilitates international projects and networks for the collection of four main outcome indicators, shown in Table 18.2.

- *Incidence* (Table 18.2 A): the main epidemiological measurement of cancer occurrence. This indicator describes the frequency with which new cases of cancer occur in a population. Cancer incidence is the main indicator to define the priorities for cancer control by primary prevention and, for some cancer sites, by early diagnosis.

- *Mortality* (Table 18.2 B): it is the final indicator of the cancer impact in the population. Cancer mortality gives information on the social burden of the disease, and it is useful to measure the ultimate impact at population level of effective curative approaches, and to define surveillance policies and also priorities in early diagnosis.

- *Relative survival* (Table 18.2. C): together with the number of new cases (incidence) and deaths (mortality), information on the survival of all patients after a cancer diagnosis is a key indicator of cancer control. It measures the outcome of curative approaches (mainly surgery, chemotherapy, radiotherapy, and in the future diet therapy and genetic therapy), at population level. Relative survival will also depend on the efficiency of diagnosis and the stage distribution of cancer.

- *Prevalence* (Table 18.2 D): by estimating the total number of the present population who experience cancer, calculates the total cancer burden in the population and is a useful indicator for planning and allocation of resources.

These four indicators give a descriptive vision of cancer epidemiology in various populations. In developed countries, discussions in recent years have aimed to define other cancer outcome indicators able to show aspects of the quality of cancer care and treatment. For instance, in Europe, the European Commission subsidized the EUROCHIP project to define a list of cancer health indicators to be collected in all European Union Member States [9,10]. Table 18.3 shows the list of the indicators proposed by EUROCHIP-1 lying within various cancer domains – prevention, epidemiology and cancer registration, screening, cancer treatment and clinical aspects, macro-social, and economic variables. The sources of information may be cancer registries, health surveys, cancer screening programmes, and other international databases.

For the indicators on the performance of cancer care and treatment, EUROCHIP underlined firstly that these indicators must be at population level to be useful for cancer control. Consequently, the sources of these indicators can be population-based cancer registries collecting information

Table 18.2 Key parameters to describe the burden of cancer

A. Cancer incidence rate

Generic definition	Number of new cases diagnosed in a time interval/Person years at risk in the interval
Rationale	Main epidemiological measurement of cancer occurrence
Utility	Basic measure of cancer burden and cancer occurrence
Caveat	Dependent on accuracy of diagnosis and documentation. Affected by screening activities and quality of cancer registration
Main source of information	Population-based cancer registries (CRs), which collect information of all cancer cases diagnosed in the population covered by them
International projects	International Agency on Research of Cancer (IARC) reports periodically centralized data for 'Cancer Incidence in 5 Continents' [8]. The last volume IX covered cancers diagnosed in 1998–2002. GLOBOCAN [11,12,13] gives *estimates* of cancer incidence in 1998, 2000, & 2002

B. Cancer mortality rate

Generic definition	Number of cancer deaths in a period / Person-years at risk during the same period
Rationale	Main epidemiological measurement of cancer deaths
Utility	Basic measure of cancer burden and outcome
Caveat	Dependent on accuracy of the assigned cause of mortality and completeness of documentation
Main source of information	National statistical offices
international projects	WHO make available mortality data for all major causes of death. IARC has produced a web-based databank (http://www-dep.iarc.fr) from which cancer mortality rates are downloadable by population, cancer site, age, calendar year, etc.

C. Cancer relative survival rate

Generic definition	Ratio of the observed survival rate from time of diagnosis in the group of cancer patients to the expected survival rate in a demographically comparable subset of the general population
Rationale	Reflects the survival experience of cancer patients, after removing the effects of non-cancer causes of death. It is recommended for geographical and temporal comparisons of survival
Utility	Basic epidemiological and clinically relevant measure of cancer burden
Caveat	Dependent on quality and timing of diagnosis and completeness of follow up and data linkage; may be not directly understandable by patients
Main source of information	Population-based cancer registries linked to vital statistical systems
International projects	EUROCARE [5,14], CONCORD [15]

D. Cancer prevalence proportion

Generic definition	*Total prevalence* is the proportion of subjects living in the population at a given date with past diagnosis of cancer. Prevalence can be also decomposed by disease duration (i.e. 1-, 2-, 5-, and 10-year prevalence)
Rationale	Indicates how many people show potential medical, physical, psychological, or social problems as a consequence of their cancer
Utility	Epidemiological measure for cancer burden description
Caveat	Total prevalence includes also cancer cured patients; dependent on completeness of data linkage
Main source of information	Population-based cancer registries linked to vital statistical systems
international projects	GLOBOCAN [9,12,13] gave the *estimates* of 5-year prevalence

E. Stage at diagnosis: percentage of cases with early diagnosis

Generic definition	Proportion of cases classified as 'localized' with the condensed-TNM staging system. (Cancer is stated using the TNM classification. The 'Condensed-TNM' grouped various stages in 'Localized' or 'Advanced' stage)
Rationale	Indicator of early diagnosis
Utility	Determinant of treatment and prognosis; indicator of health education and/or diagnosis processes
Caveat	The expected value of this percentage is cancer site-dependent, but comparisons among countries are still informative
Main source of information	Population-based cancer registries linked to hospital data (or clinical data). However, the majority of CRs are not routinely linked with these data. In this case, data can be collected by ad hoc studies

F. Delay of cancer treatment

Generic definition	Time between date of diagnosis (or date of first clinical contact) and date of first treatment
Rationale	Treatment delay could be related to: (a) individual condition of the patient; (b) biological condition of the patient; (c) health system deficiencies
Utility	Measure of health care processes in patient assessment and in service provision
Caveat	Comparison between countries has to be done carefully as the validity of this information may vary in the different health systems in various countries
Main source of information	Population-based cancer registries linked to hospital data (or clinical data). However, the majority of CRs are not routinely linked with these data. In this case, they can be collected by ad hoc studies

G. Organized screening coverage

Generic definition	Proportion of the national population that is covered by an organized screening programme in a given period by site (i.e. has the opportunity to participate in an organized programme)
Rationale	'Organized' screening is recognized as more effective than spontaneous 'opportunistic' screening
Utility	Measure of service provision related to cancer burden and outcomes
Caveat	Organized screening coverage is a very approximate measure of screening participation
Main source of information	Population-based organized cancer screening registries

Table 18.3. List of indicators proposed by EUROCHIP-1 by domain [9,10]

Prevention	Epidemiology & cancer registration	Screening	Treatment & clinical aspects	Macro-social and economic variables
Lifestyle	2.1. Population covered by high-quality cancer registries	**Screening examinations**	**Health system delay**	**Social indicators**
1.1. Consumption of fruit and vegetables	2.2. Cancer-incidence rates, trends and projections	3.1. % of women that have undergone mammography (breast cancer)	4.1. Delay of cancer treatment	5.1. Educational level attained
1.2. Consumption of alcohol	2.3. Cancer relative survival-rates, trends and projections	3.2. % of women that have undergone cervical cytology examination (cervical cancer)	**Resources**	5.2. Gini index
1.3. Body mass index (BMI) distribution in the population	2.4. Cancer prevalence proportions, trends and projections	3.3. % of persons that have undergone a CRC screening test	4.2. % of radiation systems in the population	**Macro-economic indicators**
1.4. Physical activity attitude	2.5. Cancer mortality rates, trends, projections and person-years of life lost due to cancer	**National evaluation of organized mass-screening process indicators**	4.3. %of diagnostic CT scanners in the population	5.3. GDP
1.5. Tobacco survey: prevalence of	2.6. Stage at diagnosis – % of cases with:	3.4a. Organized screening coverage	4.4. % of positron emission tomographies (PETs) in population (for future)	5.4. Total social expenditure
a. tobacco smokers among adults	a. early diagnosis	3.4b. Screening recall rate	4.5. % of magnetic resonances in population (for future)	5.5. Total national expenditure on health
b. tobacco smokers among 10–14 year olds	b. metastases	3.4c. Screening detection rate	**Treatment**	5.6. Total public expenditure on health
c. ex-smokers		3.4d. Screening localized cancers	4.6. Compliance with best oncology practice	5.7. Anti-tobacco regulations
Environment & occupational risk		3.4e. Screening positive predictive value	**Palliative care**	5.8a. Public expenditure for cancer prevention on anti-tobacco activity
d. exposure to environmental tobacco smoke (ETS)		3.4f. Screening benign/malignant biopsy ratio	4.7. Use of morphine in cancer patients	5.8b. Total expenditure for population-based cancer registries
1.6. Exposure to sun radiation		3.4g. Screening interval cancers	4.8. % of patients receiving palliative radiotherapy	5.8c. Total expenditure for organized cancer-screening programmes
1.7. PM10 emissions		3.4h. Screening specificity		5.8d. Public expenditure for cancer drugs
1.8. Indoor exposure to radon				5.8e. Total expenditure for cancer research
1.9. Prevalence of occupational exposure to carcinogens				5.8f. Estimated cost for one cancer patient
1.10. Exposure to asbestos: mesothelioma incidence and mortality trends				**Demographic indicators**
Medicaments				5.9. Age distribution in 2010, 2020, & 2030
1.11. Prevalence of use of hormone replacement therapy drugs				5.10. Life-table indicators

on the patients' cancer histories and collecting data on organized screening programmes. The main indicators suggested by EUROCHIP were, as shown in Table 18.2:

- *Stage at diagnosis* (Table 18.2 E): percentage of cases with early diagnosis. This indicator is a proxy for diagnostic awareness and the effectiveness of diagnostic services.

- *Delay in cancer treatment* (Table 18.2 F): average time between the date of cancer diagnosis and the date of first treatment.

- *Organized screening coverage* (Table 18.2 G): proportion of population resident in areas where population-based organized screening is implemented, divided by the national population in the comparable age/sex group.

Collection of these indicators or similar ones has been performed in some regions, while in others discussions are still ongoing at country or continental levels – in Europe, for example, specific pilot studies were organized to study the feasibility of collecting these indicators [10]. It is desirable that intercontinental comparisons will be possible in the future allowing incidence, survival, and prevalence be compared all over the world, as we will show in the next paragraphs.

Cancer incidence and primary prevention

Historically cancer is a disease of richer countries. In fact, Figure 18.1 shows that cancer incidence risk increases when gross domestic product (GDP) increases both for men and women. Applying these cancer incidence risks to the populations in 2007, the American Cancer Society estimated there were 12.3 million new cancer cases all over the world in 2007 subdivided as: 0.8 million in Africa, 5.6 million in Asia, 1.0 million in Central and South America, 3.0 million in Europe, 0.1 million in Oceania, and 1.8 million in North America [2]. The ageing of population foreseen in countries like China, Brazil, and India will dramatically increase the number of cancer cases in next decades.

Incidence specific by cancer site can be used to evaluate cancer control activities aimed to reduce the number of cancer cases (i.e. primary prevention and screening programmes to diagnose pre-cancerous disease). In this evaluation we have to consider that the cancer incidence

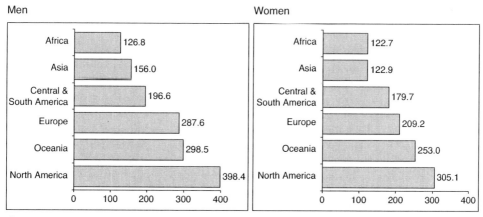

Fig. 18.1 Age-standardized incidence rates per 100,000 (world standard) by world regions 2002. Geographical areas are ordered by increasing gross domestic product (US $ per capita purchasing power parity) in 2006; Africa 2493$, Asia 4978$, South and Central America 9495$, Europe 23212$, Oceania 25423$, Northern America 43377$. (International Monetary Fund data). Source: GLOBOCAN [13].

indicator can be influenced by both the past prevalence of various risk factors and by new and improved diagnostic tests, as for the years after their full implementation they bring occurrence forward by detecting early invasive cancers (specifically for those cancer sites for which diagnostic tests successfully detect early diagnosis cancers and not only pre-cancerous diseases).

According to GLOBOCAN [13] the cancer sites with the highest incidence rates across the world are lung, prostate, stomach, and colorectal cancers for males, and breast, cervix uteri, color-ectal, lung, and stomach cancers for females. Figure 18.2 shows the contribution of these main cancer sites to overall cancer incidence in six world geographical areas. The analysis of these data in connection with information on risk factor prevalence and the diffusion of early diagnosis tests gives a picture of cancer control evaluation and priorities.

Historically tobacco smoking was one of the first risk factors defined in oncology, for lung cancer [16]. So, a first set of cancer control actions refers to tobacco control strategies (cigarette price increases, restrictions on advertising, smoking bans, etc). Ecological analysis in the United States demonstrates that state tobacco control efforts reduce state-wide lung cancer incidence rates in younger adults [17]. Current patterns of lung cancer incidence closely follow smoking

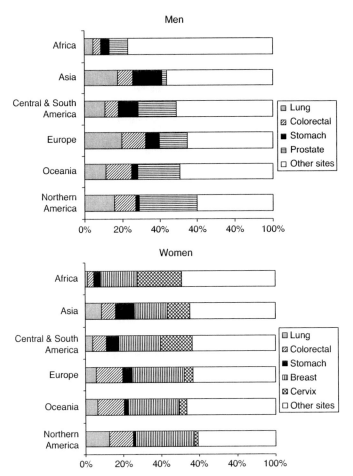

Fig. 18.2 Distribution of all cancer: numbers of cases by cancer site in 2002. Geographical areas are ordered by increasing gross domestic product.
Source: GLOBOCAN.

prevalence trends, directly linked with tobacco prevention activities [18]: a reduction (or increase) of smoking prevalence means a reduction (or increase) of lung cancer incidence after 20 to 30 years. So current lung cancer incidence rates measure the effects of policies performed 20 to 30 years ago, while current smoking prevalence gives us information on future cancer outcomes. Figure 18.2 shows that the influence of lung cancer on total cancer incidence for 2002 is highest in the developed world but almost as high in Asia. The prevalence of tobacco use is increasing in the developing countries, and tobacco control must be one of the main primary prevention cancer control strategies in the majority of countries. The WHO Tobacco Atlas shows that while consumption is levelling off and even decreasing in some countries, worldwide more people are smoking; by 2030 there will be at least two billion smoking people in the world. Even if prevalence rates fall, the absolute number of smokers will increase; the expected continuing decrease in male smoking prevalence in developed countries will be offset by the increase in female smoking rates [19]. According to the WHO Global Youth Tobacco Survey (GYTS) at the beginning of the twenty-first century, tobacco use among young people is unfortunately already well established in many parts of the world. Nearly 20 per cent of 13 to 15 year olds use some type of tobacco product, and among those who smoke cigarettes, nearly 25 per cent smoked their first cigarette before the age of 10 years [20].

Stomach and colorectal cancers have different impacts on overall incidence in various world areas. In Asia and Central and South America stomach cancer is more common than colorectal cancer, while in Europe, Oceania, and North America the contrary applies. Stomach cancer remains a primary prevention cancer control priority in Asia and Central and South America although incidence rates are universally decreasing [21], principally thanks to changes in food preservation and storage (refrigeration and consequently decreasing use of salt- and smoke-based food preservation methods), and to decreasing Helicobacter Pylori infection due to improved sanitation [18]. Major prevention strategies to reduce stomach cancer incidence include improved sanitation, higher intake of fresh fruits and vegetables, food preservation methods that are not salt- or smoke-based, avoidance of tobacco products, and maintenance of a normal body weight [18].

Colorectal cancer, on the contrary, is becoming a cancer control priority in Europe, Oceania, and North America. The World Cancer Research Fund (WCRF) [22] recently performed a meta-analysis on relationships between dietary habits and physical activity and various cancer sites; they concluded that physical activity protects against colorectal cancer (the main evidence is for colon rather than for rectal cancer) and that red meat, processed meat, body fatness, and abdominal fatness are causes of colorectal cancer. So, major colorectal cancer control strategies for primary prevention include the promotion of a healthy diet and physical activity aimed to contain the obesity and overweight epidemic that the developed world is experiencing [23].

Prostate cancer is becoming the most common cancer diagnosed in men in the Americas, Oceania, and Europe. During the last decades, prostate cancer incidence rates have shown an artefactual increase in all parts of the world thanks to an early diagnosis test (prostate-specific antigen [PSA] testing), mainly diffused outside organized screening programmes. This led to a rapid increase in the recorded incidence of early diagnosed cases. Diet has been implicated in the aetiology of prostate cancer, but convincing aetiologic evidence is lacking [22]. For this reason no specific primary prevention strategies are yet recommended.

Breast cancer is the most common cancer diagnosed in women in the world. It is hormone related, and the factors that modify the risk of this cancer when diagnosed pre-menopausally and when diagnosed (much more commonly) post-menopausally, have different roles. Risk factors for breast cancer in women include the events of reproductive life, and lifestyle factors (diet, alcohol, etc.) that modify endogenous levels of sex hormones [24]. Physical activity probably protects against breast cancer in post-menopause, and there is limited evidence suggesting that it also protects against this cancer diagnosed in pre-menopause. The evidence that alcoholic drinks are a cause of breast cancer at all ages is convincing. The evidence that the factors that lead to greater adult attained height, or its consequences, are a cause of post-menopausal breast cancer is convincing, and these are probably also a cause of breast cancer diagnosed pre-menopausally [22].

Differences existing in cervical cancer incidence across the world are one of the major examples of the unrealized potential of cancer control. Cervical cancer is probably the unique type of cancer which could be totally overcome because we know its cause (human papilloma virus [HPV] infection is a sine qua non condition of cervical cancer) and we know the method to diagnose the disease in a pre-cancerous stage (through the Pap smear test) [25]. But, as Figure 18.2 shows, cervical cancer is still one of the major cancer types diagnosed in developing populations. Low incidence rates in the developed world have been attributed to the extensive organized screening programmes based on the Pap smear test. This is one of the major results coming from the evaluation of cancer outcomes: at the international level we know that cervical cancer organized screening programs are effective and should be considered everywhere.

Cancer survival and cancer care

Information necessary for planning cancer control includes population-based survival (proportion of incident cases alive at a given time after diagnosis). Population-based survival is usually lower than survival calculated from hospital series or clinical trials because it includes all patients, including those who do not have access to adequate treatment or who are not eligible for trials. In Europe, population-based age-standardized, and cancer site-standardized, relative survival for all cancers has been shown to be a proxy indicator for monitoring countries' performance in cancer control [26]; by regression analysis of macro-economic variables in 19 countries it emerged as closely related to a country's wealth and also its overall investment in health.

Cancer survival is known to vary somewhat between the regions of the United States covered by the Surveillance, Epidemiology and End Results (SEER) Program [6] but the international range of survival showed by EUROCARE in Europe is much wider [5,14]. Comparisons of cancer survival between Europe and the United States since 2000 have identified wide differences, with survival usually higher in the United States [27]. Recently, the CONCORD study provided systematic comparisons of cancer relative survival between Europe, North America, Australia, and Japan for cancer patients diagnosed between 1990 and 1994 and followed up to 31st December 1999, for four cancers of substantial cancer control importance: breast cancer in women, and cancers of the colon, rectum, and prostate [15]. Five-year relative survival for these cancer sites was generally highest in the United States and lowest in Eastern Europe (Figure 18.3). If population-based survival in one country is substantially lower than that in other countries, especially those of similar wealth, the health system is probably not functioning as it should [14]. Various evaluating studies can be performed to find the reasons for this problem and to suggest remedies. One of the basic strategies to evaluate whether the higher survival rates observed in some populations are due to better therapy or to earlier diagnosis has been to collect standardized information on disease stage at diagnosis. If survival differences disappear once they are stratified or adjusted for stage at diagnosis (and for relevant variations in the use of staging techniques and tests), they can be assumed to be mainly due to earlier diagnosis. On the other hand, differences in stage-specific survival comparisons strongly suggest an important effect of treatment. Understanding the role of these two components in determining survival differences between populations over time is important for evaluating and planning cancer control strategies [28]. These types of studies are called by EUROCARE 'high resolution survival studies' because they require specific

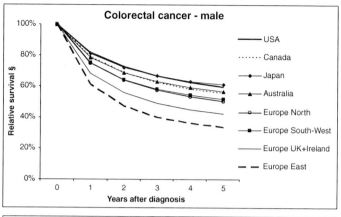

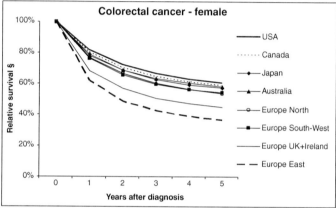

Fig. 18.3 Age-standardized§ relative survival up to 5 years after diagnosis by cancer site and area.
§ Standardization with Corraziari's method [37]
Notes: Data are derived from cancer registries in each country, as follows:
Australia. Cancer registries of Australian Capital Territory, New South Wales, Northern Territory, Queensland, South Australia, Tasmania, Victoria, Western Australia
Canada. Cancer registries of British Columbia, Manitoba, Nova Scotia, Ontario, Saskatchewan
Europe South-West. Cancer registries of Austria: Tyrol; France: Bas-Rhin, Calvados, Cote-dOr, Isère; Germany: Saarland; Italy: Ferrara, Genoa, Latina, Macerata, Modena, Parma, Ragusa, Romagna, Sassari, Turin, Tuscany, Varese, Veneto; Malta; Netherlands: Amsterdam, Northern Netherlands, Southern Netherlands; Portugal: Southern Portugal; Spain: Basque Country, Granada, Mallorca, Murcia, Navarra, Tarragona; Switzerland: Basel, Geneva, Graubunden-Glarus, St. Gall-Appenzell, Valais
Europe East. Cancer registries of Czech Republic: West Bohemia; Estonia; Poland: Cracow, Warsaw; Slovakia; Slovenia
Europe North. Cancer registries of Denmark; Finland; Iceland; Norway; Sweden
Europe UK+Ireland. Cancer registries of Ireland; England; Northern Ireland, Scotland, Wales
Japan. Cancer registries of Fukui, Osaka, Yamagata
USA. Cancer registries of Atlanta (Georgia), California, Colorado, Connecticut, Florida, Hawaii, Idaho, Iowa, Louisiana, Michigan, Nebraska, New Jersey, New Mexico, New York, Rhode Island, Seattle (Washington), Utah, Wyoming
Source: CONCORD [15].

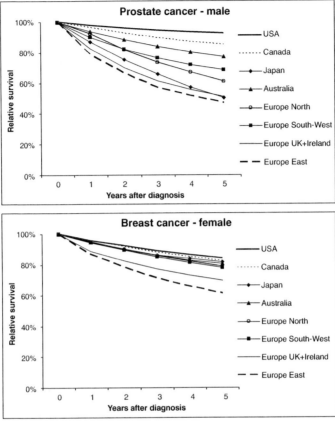

Fig. 18.3 (Continued)

information from patients' histories from diagnosis to treatment. They can be performed by population-based cancer registries with further ad-hoc data collection on samples of patients. High resolution studies performed on European and US cancer patient databases showed the explanatory effect of clinical variables such as stage at diagnosis, investigative approach, anatomic site and morphology on colorectal cancer [29,30] and breast cancer survival differences between United States and Europe [31].

The evaluation of these studies should consider the following possible biases [28]:

◆ *'Stage migration' phenomenon*: The evolution of diagnostic technology has increased the sensitivity of detecting loco-regional extension of tumours and silent distant metastases. Stage-specific survival, therefore, may increase just because a fraction of tumours that previously would have been labelled as localized can now be recognized as advanced, thus increasing the survival of both the localized set (because they are more localized) and the advanced stage set (because they also include the less advanced cases that in the absence of modern staging procedures would have been diagnosed as localized). The availability of information on relevant staging procedures may allow the control of the stage migration phenomenon in statistical analysis.

◆ *'Lead-time bias'*: Diagnosis at an earlier stage can increase survival (which is measured from date of diagnosis) by simply anticipating the date of diagnosis without postponing the date of death. In this case, longer survival associated to a more favourable stage distribution is not an advantage for the assessed population. This bias can be studied through the analysis of the trends by means of models that provide estimates of the proportions of patients who are cured (defined as those with the same survival as the general population of the same age) and of the life expectancy for fatal cases (those patients who die from the disease). Lead-time bias can just result in a longer survival time of fatal cases without an increase in the cured patient proportion [32].

♦ Possible inclusion in the patient population of a number of 'pseudo-cancers', that is, of incidentally found cancers that would never have progressed to give clinical signs. A certain proportion of cancers detected during screening fall into this category. If the frequency of these pseudo-cancers is variable between populations, or is increasing over time, the consequent difference in survival will be entirely reflected in the proportion of cured. Cure survival models are therefore not able to detect this bias, unless they are applied to stage-specific subgroups of patients. It is reasonable to assume that pseudo-cancers will all belong to the lowest stage category. Differences in the proportion of cured in stage-specific subgroups other than the lowest stage group can therefore be interpreted as genuine survival gain.

In conclusion, the application of cure models to high resolution studies can theoretically provide a complete conceptual framework for a meaningful evaluation of survival differences. However, the interpretation of survival trends should always take into account the contemporary trends in incidence and mortality rates, as well as in care practices.

Other evaluation studies correlate cancer survival with macro-economic variables. Figure 18.4 shows the relationship in Europe between age- and cancer site-standardized relative survival (ASRS) for all cancers at five years after diagnosis, for patients diagnosed in 1990 to 1994 and followed up to 31st December 1999, and an index of technological financial investment in cancer care (CTS/TNEH: the ratio between investment in computer tomography scanners and total national expenditure on health). European countries in Figure 18.4 are ordered by TNEH. The figure shows a clearer relation of ASRS to TNEH for the less rich countries – in the lower portions of the graphs – compared to rich countries. ASRS was lower than expected in Denmark, England, Wales, and Poland, that is countries with lower investment in technology for cancer (low CTS/TNEH), compared to other countries with comparable total health expenditure. Moreover, high ASRS for Austria, Sweden, Italy, and Finland can be explained in terms of high CTS/TNEH, corresponding to greater investment in technology for cancer than in other countries with similar total health expenditure. This ecological study in Europe showed that improving cancer care principally requires greater wealth: the most direct way for poorer European countries to close the 15 percentage point survival gap [33] between them and the richest countries would be to get richer [26]!

Other international ecological studies have examined cancer survival in comparison to socioeconomic indicators. In the United States, cancer registry-derived relative survival for individual cancer sites was used in models with socio-economic indicators to estimate survival in areas not covered by cancer registration. This study showed that breast, prostate, and, to a lesser degree, colorectal cancer survival were strongly associated with demographic and socioeconomic indicators (including percentage unemployed, median family income, percentage with high school diploma, etc.) at the county level [34]. The ELDCARE project (Europe) studied between country differences in cancer survival in the elderly, taking account of socioeconomic conditions and the characteristics, finding that cancer survival for various cancer sites in the elderly was strongly related with GDP, total national expenditure on health (TNEH) and distribution of computed tomography scanners in population (CTS) [35,36].

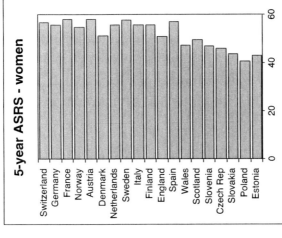
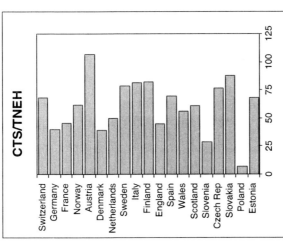
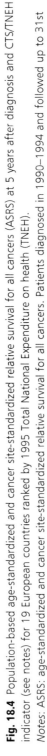

Fig. 18.4 Population-based age-standardized and cancer site-standardized relative survival for all cancers (ASRS) at 5 years after diagnosis and CTS/TNEH indicator (see notes) for 19 European countries ranked by 1995 Total National Expenditure on health (TNEH).

Notes: ASRS: age-standardized and cancer site-standardized relative survival for all cancers. Patients diagnosed in 1990–1994 and followed up to 31st December 1999. Source: EUROCARE-3 [26,33]

CTS: computer tomography scanners per person in 1995. Sources: Organization for Economic Co-operation and Development (OECD), ELDCARE [35]

TNEH: total national expenditure on health expressed in US dollars ($) per capita adjusted for purchasing power parity (PPP) in 1995. Sources: Organization for Economic Co-operation and Development (OECD), ELDCARE [35]

CTS/TNEH: ratio between CTS and TNEH by 10^{10}

Cancer mortality

Mortality is the final indicator of cancer's impact in the population. Figure 18.5 shows that cancer mortality risk increases when gross domestic product (GDP) increases, with the exception of Europe for men, and Africa for women that had in 2002 a higher mortality rate than other geographical areas with similar GDP. Applying these risks to the populations, the American Cancer Society estimated 7.6 million cancer deaths all over the world in 2007 subdivided as: 0.6 million in Africa, 3.9 million in Asia, 0.5 million in Central and South America, 1.8 million in Europe, 0.06 million in Oceania, and 0.7 million in North America [2].

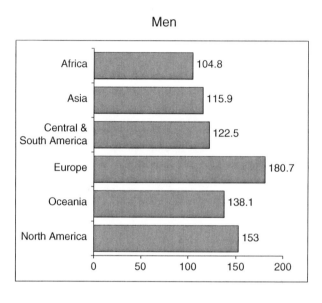

Men

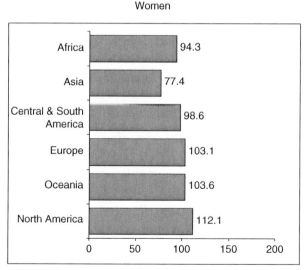

Women

Fig. 18.5 Age-standardized mortality rates per 100,000 (world standard) 2002. Geographical areas are ordered by increasing GDP.
Source: GLOBOCAN [13].

Cancer mortality gives information on the social burden of the disease. In the evaluation of cancer mortality trends it is important to underline that they depend on (a) previous incidence trends and (b) survival trends. So the analysis of cancer mortality rates to evaluate past cancer control activities needs awareness as, for example, a reduction of mortality could depend on a primary prevention activity that reduced the risk factor prevalence in the population, or on a new treatment that increased survival, or on both.

Cancer mortality is one of the outcome indicators used to evaluate the efficacy of organized screening programmes. It is usually used in clinical trials performed to study the usefulness of specific diagnostic tests in screening programmes [38], but population-based cancer mortality can also be used in ecological studies to test the efficacy of organized screening programmes in the population after their implementation.

For breast cancer, the effectiveness of mammography screening has been evaluated in screening trials showing consistent mortality reductions of 20 to 35 per cent amongst women in the age range 50 to 69 years [38]. Moreover, several ecological studies have evaluated the service screening programmes showing statistically significant reductions in breast cancer mortality following the introduction of mammography screening [39,40,41]. For colorectal cancer a recent meta-analysis of the clinical trials estimated the pooled reduction in mortality to be 15 per cent for biennial screening, with a 25 per cent effect amongst screening attenders [42]. The objective of cervical cancer screening is to reduce both cervical cancer incidence and mortality. The value of the Pap smear in reducing the risk of invasive cancer and mortality has been firmly established, and it is estimated that regular screening reduces the risk of cancer by 80 per cent [43].

For other cancer sites, mortality reductions emerged from some clinical trials of specific screening tests for oral cancer [44] and for liver cancer (among hepatitis B virus-infected populations) [45], while no international consensus is yet achieved on screening tests for lung cancer (among smokers), or for prostate cancer using PSA tests. Several ecological studies and time series analyses have been published correlating the frequency of PSA testing (or the incidence of prostate cancer, as a surrogate for PSA testing) with prostate cancer mortality; the results have been inconsistent [38].

Cancer prevalence

Cancer prevalence, the measure of live persons with a past cancer diagnosis, calculates the total cancer burden in a population and is a useful indicator for planning and allocation of resources. It grows with incidence and with the percentage of patients surviving. Table 18.4 shows the huge

Table 18.4. Five-year all cancer prevalent cases in 2002 by geographical area

	M	F	M+F
Africa	443,813	566,341	1,010,154
Asia	4,239,349	4,859,232	9,098,581
Central & South America	694,205	991,823	1,686,028
Europe	3,364,950	3,916,640	7,281,590
Oceania	157,448	155,119	312,567
Northern America	2,647,700	2,533,495	5,181,195
World	**11,547,465**	**13,022,650**	**24,570,115**

Source: GLOBOCAN [13].

number of 5-year all cancer prevalent cases by geographical area in the world for 2002 according to the GLOBOCAN estimates [13]. These data represent the number of living subjects in 2002 who were diagnosed with cancer during the prior 5 years (i.e. they are a subset of the total prevalent cases). In Europe the ratio of 5-year prevalence to total prevalence is estimated as around 40 per cent [46,47]. Under the hypothesis that this percentage is applicable in other developed areas, we can estimate nearly 18 million prevalent cases in 2002 for Europe, 0.8 million in Oceania, and 13 million in North America.

Cancer prevalence is expected to dramatically increase in the developed world thanks to the increase of the number of new cases (because of population growth, the increase of life expectancy and because people are still exposed to cancer risk factors) and the increase in survival rate.

Cancer prevalence figures include various groups of cancer survivors with very different rehabilitation needs (e.g. clinical, psychological, psychiatric, nutritional, and social needs). Identifying these groups and meeting their needs is becoming a cancer control priority, but evaluation studies on the rehabilitation needs of prevalent cancer cases are still rare at the population level.

Time from diagnosis is a major criterion for categorizing people with cancer, since care and surveillance requirements vary with time. In the first few months after diagnosis, care generally consists of primary and adjuvant treatment. Subsequently, patients require follow-up to monitor recurrences or for the recognition and treatment of side-effects. A subset of cases will require treatment for recurrences, or palliation for persistent symptoms such as pain; thus, presence or absence of recurrence is another useful criterion for subdividing the prevalent population according to the intensity of care required. For the purposes of planning health resource allocation, it is useful to be able to estimate the prevalence of cancer patients who continue to need treatment, and those who will require follow-up and possible treatment for their cancer, and to exclude those who will survive for a long time after diagnosis and can be considered cured.

Following this approach, using a population-based cancer registry sample of colorectal cancer patients, a recent study classified prevalent cases as: (1) cases that will be cured (cured prevalence), that is patients with the same life expectancy as individuals in the general population of the same age; (2) cases with disease progression, that is with metastases at diagnosis, or whose disease recurred shortly after primary treatment (morbid prevalence); (3) cases with recurrence, that is who are clinically free of cancer after primary treatment, but later develop recurrence (premorbid prevalence) [48]. To estimate the health demand over time of cancer patients other studies used prevalence by stage at diagnosis [49,50] under the hypothesis that different stages have different needs and treatments. Another study in the United States introduced a different definition of prevalence: care prevalence that is the numbers of patients under care [51]. Care prevalence was estimated by phases of care defined as initial diagnosis (treated with curative intent), post-diagnostic monitoring, treatment for recurrent/metastatic disease or second primaries, and terminal care. In this case care prevalence includes also part of the cured patient fraction, those who still have some types of care. The findings indicated that for colorectal cancer several years after diagnosis (also after 5 years post-diagnosis, the time that most colorectal cancer survivors are considered 'cured') many patients were still receiving care for their cancer or its sequelae. All these studies were performed for a specific cancer site (colorectal cancer) and using ad-hoc collection of clinical follow-up data of cancer registry patient samples.

One direction for future prevalence studies would be to use increasingly available information such as prescription data, hospital and outpatient admissions, and pharmaceutical company databases to provide more refined breakdowns of the care needs of patients with cancer diagnoses.

Conclusions

Probably in a few years cancer will be the leading cause of death in developed countries and tens of millions of people will live with a past diagnosis. With increasing cancer prevalence, the demand for resources to follow-up cancer patients and identify and treat cancer recurrences increases. While this is happening, new knowledge is being acquired by genetic research which is tending to change the understanding of cancer from a limited number of major killer diseases to a long list of distinct rare diseases, each requiring a different treatment [52].

We have considered the major objectives of cancer control in the developed world in terms of short, medium, and long term objectives [52].

Short-term objectives

- *Cancer patient needs:* achieve full knowledge of the variation in demand for health services as a function of cancer type, patient age, and rehabilitation requirements, to address with adequate investments the problem of increasing prevalent cancer cases (e.g. increased needs of the elderly in richer countries).
- *Early diagnosis:* implement organized screening programmes and invest in modern diagnostic and treatment technologies to eliminate inequalities in access to diagnosis and treatment facilities in those developed countries with worst survival rate.

Medium and long term objectives

- *Reduce incidence:* address primary prevention as a main priority, sustaining collaboration between national health authorities, private sectors, research organizations, and stakeholders to put into effect policies that can achieve a substantial reduction in cancer incidence over the next 10 to 20 years.
- *Diffusion of best practice:* support the spread of best practice and use pressure to raise consistently poor standards. Give the best possible treatment and care to cancer patients, exchanging information on best practices for diagnosis, treatment, rehabilitation, and palliative care.

Long-term objectives

Guidelines for cancer research: research on the molecular bases of cancer offers new therapeutic possibilities everyday and has transformed cancer from being one disease into many rare diseases, requiring each a different treatment. Cancer control should also address the escalation of cancer costs, which even rich countries may soon be unable to meet.

Thus cancer control short, medium, and long term objectives should be defined in collaboration between health authorities, research organizations, stakeholders, and patients.

Acknowledgments

We are grateful for the support from EUROCHIP-3 (European Cancer Health Indicator Project), funded by the Health and Consumer Protection Directorate-General of the European Commission (contract No. 2007 121) and from the CONCORD project.

References

1 Lopez AD, Mathers CD, Ezzati M, Jamison DT, & Murray CJ (2006). Global and regional burden of disease and risk factors, 2001. Systematic analysis of population health data. *Lancet*, **367**:1747–57.

2 Garcia M, Jemal A, Ward EM, et al (2007). *Global Cancer Facts & Figures 2007*. American Cancer Society, Atlanta, GA. Available from: http://www.cancer.org/downloads/STT/Global_Cancer_Facts_and_Figures_2007_rev.pdf (accessed 7 October 2009).

3 Micheli A, Baili P, Quinn M, et al (2003). Life expectancy and cancer survival in the EUROCARE-3 cancer registry areas. *Ann Oncol*, **14**(Suppl 5):v28–v40.

4 WHO, UICC (2005). *Global Action Against Cancer – Updated version*. Available from: http://www.who.int/cancer/media/en/GlobalActionCancerEnglfull.pdf (accessed 7 October 2009).

5 Verdecchia A, Francisci S, Brenner H, et al (2007). Recent cancer survival in Europe: a 2000–02 period analysis of EUROCARE-4 data. *Lancet Oncol*, **8**(9):784–96.

6 Ries LAG, Melbert D, Krapcho M, et al (2008). *Statistics Review based on November 2007 SEER data submission, 1975–2005*. National Cancer Institute, Bethesda, MD. Available from: http://seer.cancer.gov/csr/1975_2005/ (accessed 7 October 2009).

7 Zanetti R & Primic-Zakelj M (2007). *Cancer registration*. EU Portuguese Presidency conference on Health Strategies in Europe, 12–13 July 2007, Strategies on specific issues, parallel session on cancer. Available from: http://www.acs.min-saude.pt/wp-content/uploads/2007/12/15h45robertozanettilisbon meeting_new.pdf (accessed 7 October 2009).

8 Curado MP, Edwards B, Shin HR, et al (2007). *Cancer Incidence in Five Continents, Vol. IX*. IARC Scientific Publications No. 160. IARC, Lyon, France.

9 Micheli A, Capocaccia R, Martinez C, et al (2003). Cancer control in Europe: a proposed set of European cancer health indicators. *Eur J Public Health*, **13**(Suppl 3):116–18.

10 EUROCHIP. Available from: http://www.tumori.net/eurochip (accessed 7 October 2009).

11 Ferlay J, Parkin DM, & Pisani P (1998). *GLOBOCAN: Cancer Incidence and Mortality Worldwide*. IARC CancerBase No. 3. IARC, Lyon, France.

12 Parkin DM, Bray F, Ferlay J, & Pisani P (2001). Estimating the world cancer burden: Globocan 2000. *Int J Cancer*, **94**(2):153–56.

13 Ferlay J, Bray F, Pisani P, & Parkin DM (2004). *GLOBOCAN 2002: Cancer Incidence, Mortality and Prevalence Worldwide*. IARC CancerBase No. 5. version 2.0. IARC, Lyon, France.

14 Berrino F, De Angelis R, Sant M, et al (2007). Survival for eight major cancers and all cancers combined for European adults diagnosed in 1995–99: results of the EUROCARE-4 study. *Lancet Oncol*, **8**(9):773–83.

15 Coleman MP, Quaresma M, Berrino F, et al (2008). Cancer survival in five continents: a worldwide population-based study (CONCORD). *Lancet Oncol*, **9**(8):730–56.

16 Doll R & Hill AB (1950). Smoking and carcinoma of the lung; preliminary report. *Br Med J*, **2**:739–48.

17 Polednak AP (2008). Tobacco control indicators and lung cancer rates in young adults by state in the United States. *Tob Control*, **17**(1):66–69.

18 Kamangar F, Dores GM, & Anderson WF (2006). Patterns of cancer incidence, mortality, and prevalence across five continents: defining priorities to reduce cancer disparities in different geographic regions of the world. *J Clin Oncol*, **24**(14):2137–50.

19 Mackay J & Eriksen M (2002). *The tobacco atlas*. WHO, Geneva, Switzerland. Available fromt: http://www.who.int/tobacco/statistics/tobacco_atlas/en/ (accessed 7 October 2009).

20 Global Youth Tabacco Survey Collaborative Group (2002). Tobacco use among youth: a cross country comparison. *Tob Control*, **11**(3):252–70.

21 Parkin DM, Bray FI, Devesa SS (2001). Cancer burden in the year 2000. The global picture. *Eur J Cancer*, **37** (Suppl 8):S4–66.

22 World Cancer Research Fund, American Institute for Cancer Research (2007). *Food, Nutrition, Physical Activity, and the Prevention of Cancer: a Global Perspective*. AICR, Washington, DC.

23 WHO. *Obesity and overweight*. Available from: http://www.who.int/mediacentre/factsheets/fs311/en/index.html (accessed 7 October 2009).

24 Key T, Appleby P, Barnes I, Reeves G, & Endogenous Hormones and Breast Cancer Collaborative Group (2002). Endogenous sex hormones and breast cancer in postmenopausal women. Reanalysis of nine prospective studies. *J Natl Cancer Inst*, **94**:606–16.

25 Stewart BW & Kleihues P (2003). *World Cancer Report*. IARC, Lyon, France.

26 Verdecchia A, Baili P, Quaglia A, et al (2008). Patient survival for all cancers combined as indicator of cancer control in Europe. *Eur J Public Health*, **18**(5):527–32.

27 Gatta G, Capocaccia R, Coleman MP, et al (2000). Toward a comparison of survival in American and European cancer patients. *Cancer*, **89**(4):893–900.

28 Berrino F (2003). The EUROCARE Study: strengths, limitations and perspectives of population-based, comparative survival studies. *Ann Oncol*, **14**(Suppl 5):v9–13.

29 Gatta G, Ciccolallo L, Capocaccia R, et al (2003). Differences in colorectal cancer survival between European and US populations: the importance of sub-site and morphology. *Eur J Cancer*, **39**(15):2214–22.

30 Ciccolallo L, Capocaccia R, Coleman MP, et al (2005). Survival differences between European and US patients with colorectal cancer: role of stage at diagnosis and surgery. *Gut*, **54**(2):268–73.

31 Sant M, Allemani C, Berrino F, et al (2004). Breast carcinoma survival in Europe and the USA: a population-based study. *Cancer*, **100**:715–22.

32 Verdecchia A, De Angelis R, Capocaccia R, et al (1998). The cure for colon cancer: results from the EUROCARE study. *Int J Cancer*, **77**(3):322–29.

33 Sant M, Aareleid T, Berrino F, et al (2003). EUROCARE-3: survival of cancer patients diagnosed 1990–94–results and commentary. *Ann Oncol*, **14**(Suppl 5), V61–V118.

34 Mariotto A, Capocaccia R, Verdecchia A, et al (2002). Projecting SEER cancer survival rates to the US: an ecological regression approach. *Cancer Causes and Control*, **13**:101–11.

35 Quaglia A, Vercelli M, Lillini R, et al (2005). ELDCARE working group. Socioeconomic factors and health care system characteristics related to cancer survival in the elderly. A population-based analysis in 16 European countries (ELDCARE project). *Crit Rev Oncol/Hematol*, **54**:117–28.

36 Vercelli M, Lillini R, Capocaccia R, et al (2006). Cancer survival in the elderly: effects of socio-economic factors and health care system features (ELDCARE project). *Eur J Cancer*, **42**:234–42.

37 Corazziari I, Quinn M, & Capocaccia R (2004). Standard cancer patient population for age standardising survival ratios. *Eur J Cancer*, **40**:2307–16.

38 Hakama M, Coleman MP, Alexe DM, & Auvinen A (2008). Cancer screening: Evidence and practice in Europe. *Eur J Cancer*, **44**(10):1404–13.

39 Otto SJ, Fracheboud J, Looman CW, et al (2003). Initiation of population-based mammography screening in Dutch municipalities and effect on breast-cancer mortality. *Lancet*, **361**:1411–17.

40 Duffy SW, Tabar L, Chen HH, et al (2002). The impact of organized mammography service screening on breast carcinoma mortality in seven Swedish counties. *Cancer*, **95**:458–69.

41 Blanks RG, Moss SM, McGahan CE, Quinn MJ, & Babb PJ (2000). Effect of NHS breast screening programme on mortality from breast cancer in England and Wales, 1990–98: comparison of observed with predicted mortality. *Br Med J*, **321**:665–69.

42 Hewitson P, Glasziou P, Irwig L, Towler B, & Watson E (2007). Screening for colorectal cancer using the faecal occult blood test, Hemoccult. *Cochrane Database Syst Rev*, **1**:CD001216.

43 Laara E, Day NE, Hakama M (1987). Trends in mortality from cervical cancer in the Nordic countries. *Lancet*, **1**:1247–49.

44 Sankaranarayanan R, Ramadas K, Thomas G, et al (2005). Effect of screening on oral cancer mortality in Kerala, India: a cluster-randomized controlled trial. *Lancet*, **365**:1927–33.

45 Zhang BH, Yang BH, Tang ZY (2004). Randomized controlled trial of screening for hepatocellular carcinoma. *J Cancer Res Clin Oncol*, **131**:417–22.

46 Micheli A, Mugno E, Krogh V, et al (2002). Cancer prevalence in European registry areas. *Ann Oncol*, **13**(6):840–65.

47 De Angelis R, Grande E, Inghelmann R, et al (2007). Cancer prevalence estimates in Italy from 1970 to 2010.*Tumori*, **93**(4):392–97.

48 Gatta G, Capocaccia R, Berrino F, Ruzza MR, Contiero P, & EUROPREVAL Working Group (2004). Colon cancer prevalence and estimation of differing care needs of colon cancer patients. *Ann Oncol*, **15**(7):1136–42.

49 Colonna M, Grosclaude P, Launoy G, et al (2001). Estimation of colorectal cancer prevalence in France. *Eur J Cancer*, **37**:93–96.

50 Benhamiche-Bouvier AM, Clinard F, Phelip JM, Rassiat E, & Faivre J (2000). Colorectal cancer prevalence in France. *Eur J Cancer Prev*, **9**:303–07.

51 Mariotto A, Warren JL, Knopf KB, & Feuer EJ (2003). The prevalence of patients with colorectal carcinoma under care in the US. *Cancer*, **98**:1253–61.

52 Micheli A, Berrino F, Paci E, Verdecchia A, & Pierotti MA (2007). Strategies for cancer control in Italy. *Tumori*, **93**(4):329–36.

Chapter 19

Priority setting methods and cancer control

Stuart Peacock, Lindsay Hedden, Craig Mitton[1]

Priority setting involves policy-makers, managers, and clinicians making decisions about competing claims – for alternative amounts and types of health care – on their limited budgets [1,2]. Choices have to be made about what health services to fund and what not to fund, and the extent to which services will or will not be funded. No additional influx of resources will alleviate the fundamental need to make such choices. The reason is straightforward: the needs and demands of the community will always exceed the resources available.

As a result, many countries have introduced legislation requiring that health service agencies employ effective priority setting methods to best meet the health needs of their community. However, evidence has shown that decision-makers often lack appropriate guidance on priority setting methods, training in the technical skills required, and the resources to seek out appropriate evidence [3,4,5,6]. The challenge for both the wider health sector and for cancer control is global: how do we develop robust, evidence-based, scientific methods for priority setting, whilst building managerial capacity in those methods through better guidance and training?

The purpose of this chapter is to introduce some fundamental principles of priority setting, critique the main priority setting approaches in the health sector, and describe some case studies which illustrate how alternative approaches have been employed. The chapter is laid out as follows. First, we provide a brief description of the burden and cost of cancer. We then introduce two fundamental principles of priority setting. Third, we critique the main approaches to priority setting and present a readily adaptable way forward for this type of planning activity. We conclude with a discussion of the need to balance economics and ethics when addressing the challenge of setting priorities in cancer control.

The burden and cost of cancer

In 2005, cancer accounted for 7.6 million or 12.5 per cent of all deaths worldwide [7]. More than 70 per cent of these deaths occurred in low- and middle-income countries, where access to prevention, screening, diagnosis, and treatment programmes may be limited. World Health Organization projections suggest that cancer deaths will increase 45 per cent between 2007 and 2030 (to 11.4 million deaths) and that incidence will rise from 11.3 to 15.5 million cases per year [7]. The steady increase in incidence is caused by an aging population, changes to

---

[1] Stuart J. Peacock, DPhil, Co-Director, (Canadian) National Centre for Health Economics, Services, Policy and Ethics in Cancer; Senior Scientist, British Columbia Cancer Agency; Associate Professor, University of British Columbia, Vancouver, British Columbia, Canada; Lindsay Hedden, MSc, Research Scientist, National Centre for Health Economics, Services, Policy and Ethics in Cancer; Research Scientist, British Columbia Cancer Agency, Vancouver, British Columbia, Canada; Craig Mitton, PhD , Associate Professor, University of British Columbia, Canada.

genetic susceptibility, and lifestyle factors (increased smoking prevalence among females, lower rates of reproduction, etc.) [8]. Cancer is also a source of substantial morbidity worldwide, accounting for nearly 10 million Disability Adjusted Life Years (DALYs) lost in Europe and more than 5.7 million lost in North America, representing 16.7 per cent and 12.5 per cent of total DALYs lost respectively in 2002 [8].

The direct costs of cancer care accounted for between 4.1 and 9.3 per cent of total health care spending in OECD countries in 2006 [9]. This corresponds to a spending of approximately € 57 billion or € 125 per capita (approximately $77 billion or $169 US dollars, respectively, with a €1 = $1.35 exchange rate, May 19, 2009). Despite substantial increases in the costs of cancer pharmaceuticals, inpatient care continues to dominate the cost of cancer care, accounting for approximately 70 per cent of the total cost (see Table 19.2) [9]. Spending on cancer care is also increasing with improved survival: patients are using more courses of chemotherapy and radiotherapy, and survivors of the disease frequently suffer long-term disability that requires continued therapy or monitoring [10].

Against this backdrop, cancer control faces many challenges: the rising costs of innovation and technology (equipment, drugs, and diagnostics); allocating resources across the spectrum of interventions; a lack of incremental funding despite growth in incidence and prevalence; growth in all cancer control programmes and the need for new programmes with no defined funding; and rising community expectations and demand. Short of unprecedented treatment 'breakthroughs', cancer control and care is incapable of significantly reducing the burden of cancer. In 2005, this led Canadian Strategy for Council Control to conclude that 'a systematic approach to organising the limited resources in cancer control and care is urgently needed to respond to these challenges' [11].

Economic principles of priority setting

Two fundamental economic concepts are central to priority setting: opportunity cost and marginal analysis. The principle of opportunity cost arises from the economic problem: resources for health services are scarce, and are insufficient to provide all health services that may provide benefits to society. Decision-makers – managers and clinicians – therefore have to address a series of questions: how, when, where, and what health services should be provided, and for whom? This involves deciding which services to provide, and which not to provide, recognizing either implicitly or explicitly that providing one service may result in an alternative service not being provided due to resource scarcity. The benefit forgone from not providing the alternative service is the 'opportunity cost'. This has an important implication for priority setting. If the aim of health services is to maximize the well-being of the community (e.g. through programmes that seek to improve patient outcomes and population health) then decision-makers must consider the costs and benefits of different health services.

The second fundamental concept is that of the margin, which refers to the next unit of benefit gained (or lost) or the next unit of resources invested (or disinvested). Thinking and acting 'at the margin' typically involves shifting resources from areas of low health gain per dollar spent to areas of higher health gain per dollar spent in order to improve benefit to the population as a whole. This can be illustrated with a simple example. If a cancer hospital was given $100,000 of 'additional money' and had to decide how best to allocate it, this money should be allocated to programmes which resulted in the greatest possible improvement in health gain for patients. Similarly, if a $100,000 budget cut was imposed on the hospital, the resources should be taken from places in which the detrimental impact on health gain would be minimal. Now, it then follows that if the overall budget is to stay the same, and the question is asked as to whether the

Table 19.1 Direct costs for cancer care in selected countries in 2004

	Direct costs for cancer (€ million)	Direct costs for cancer per capita (€)	Cancer costs as % of total health care costs	Total health care expenditure	Population (2004)
Austria	1247	153	6.6	18,897	8,175,000
Belgium	1543	148	6.6	23,375	10,399,000
Czech Republic	514	50	5.0	10,287	10,211,000
Denmark	760	141	6.6	11,516	5,401,000
Finland	571	109	6.6	8648	5,228,000
France	7458	124	5.3	140,714	60,200,000
Germany	12,108	147	6.6	183,455	82,491,000
Greece	1168	106	6.6	17,698	11,060,000
Hungary	495	49	5.0	9897	10,107,000
Ireland	513	127	6.6	7769	4,044,000
Italy	6725	117	6.6	101,888	57,553,000
Netherlands	1502	92	4.1	36,643	16,275,000
Norway	890	194	6.6	13,478	4,592,000
Poland	1138	30	5.0	22,758	38,180,000
Portugal	930	89	6.6	14,098	10,509,000
Spain	4367	102	6.6	66,169	42,692,000
Sweden	1316	146	7.0	18,802	8,994,000
Switzerland	1471	199	6.6	22,294	7,391,000
UK	5634	94	5.0	112,719	59,778,000
Europe	55,664	125	6.4	841,105	453,280,000
United States	62,321	212	4.7	1,325,988	293,655,000
Canada	5013	157	6.7	74818	31,946,000
Japan	19,750	155	9.3	212,370	127,687,000
Australia	2199	109	5.2	42,298	20,111,000
New Zealand	413	102	6.6	6261	4,061,000
South Africa	ND	ND	ND	12,586	42,769,000

Notes: 1. Cost data based on purchasing power parity (PPP); ND = no data;
2. Reproduced with permission from [8]
3. €1 = $1.35US exchange rate, May 19, 2009

current pattern of resources is 'correct', one might think about shifting resources from one area (i.e. the area which is producing the least health gain per dollar spent) to another (i.e. where the most health gain per dollar is expected to result). In economic terminology, the process of real-locating resources should continue until the ratios of marginal benefit to marginal cost across all programmes are equal. At this point, health gains are maximized.

Table 19.2 Breakdown of direct cancer health care costs (percentage of total direct costs)

	Inpatient care	Ambulatory care	Drugs
Germany (2002)	67% + 9% other	16%	8%
Sweden (2002)	73% (hospital)	15% (including home care)	10%
France (1998)	83%	7% + 6% transport costs	4%
Netherlands (1994)	60% + 11% non-hospital institutional care	18%	11%
Canada (1998)	75%	17% (physician care + direct costs)	9%
United States (1990)	65%	31%	4%
Australia (1993/1994)	71% (including nursinghomes)	26%	3%
Spain (1998, 1 region)	77%	7%	16%

Note: Reproduced with permission from [8]

Approaches to priority setting

The health policy literature contains numerous examples of different approaches to priority setting. These include historical allocation, needs assessment, core services, economic evaluation, and quality adjusted life year (QALY) league tables. In what follows, we provide a critique of each of these approaches illustrated with case studies, before discussing a potential way forward for priority setting in cancer control.

Historical allocation

To date, the most commonly used approach to priority setting, in cancer control and other areas of health services, has been historical allocation. Simply put, this means basing funding decisions on historical expenditure patterns, typically with crude adjustments for new growth monies (in years of budget surpluses) or budget cuts (in years of deficits) and/or for demographics. However, historical allocation methods provide no systematic mechanism for maximizing health gain from a given budget, because the approach fails to recognize the fundamental principle of opportunity cost [1,12]. Additionally, historical allocation fails to consider the costs and outcomes of alternative health services and the budget constraints faced by decision-makers [13]. Evidence has also shown that health service decision-makers are often dissatisfied with this approach to priority setting [4]. Since historical expenditure patterns are unlikely to maximize benefit to the population, many authors have suggested that a more systematic and explicit approach to priority setting is needed if this (and other) health sector goals are to be successfully pursued.

Needs assessment

Broadly speaking, needs assessment asks whether a need exists and whether programmes and services are in place to address that need [14]. A needs assessment exercise typically consists of a systematic appraisal and characterization of an unmet need, the characteristics (and in some cases preferences) of the population in need, and the nature and scope of existing services directed towards this target group [14,15]. Typically, attempts are made to define need at either the individual or population level, and then set a minimum standard of care (or set of services) to meet that need [16].

In practice, this is often a very difficult task because the definition of need itself is value based and is thus dependent on who is trying to define it, which can result in a multitude of definitions taken from different perspectives [1,16]. More importantly, attempting to set a minimum standard ignores the reality that there may not be enough resources available (i.e. the opportunity cost is too great) to meet the minimum standard, nor does it explicitly address the target population's capacity to benefit from the proposed intervention [1]. This then suggests that some sort of additional priority setting activity is still required [16].

A related approach that is sometimes used in lobbying for more resources for a particular condition is that of cost-of-illness studies. In such studies the overall cost of a particular disease is presented and compared to the overall cost of other conditions. In making such a comparison it is implied that if one condition imposes a greater economic burden on society than its comparators, more resources should be spent on that condition. However, shifting resources based on such quantifications will not necessarily lead to an improvement in benefit to the population overall, nor will efficiency necessarily be improved [17]. In essence, without explicit consideration of opportunity costs, and changes to services at the margin, maximizing benefit for the population as a whole may occur only by chance.

Core services

The core services approach involves developing guidelines to attempt to define a set of 'medically necessary' core services to be funded and provided under a given health plan (most often a publicly funded health system) [1]. This involves making clear distinctions between those programmes and services that are medically necessary and those that are not.

This approach has been the subject of much debate in the literature. New Zealand and the Netherlands have provided notable examples of attempts to put the core services approach into practice. They did so by developing guidelines for the inclusion of various programmes and services based on explicit criteria, such as: effectiveness, efficiency, necessity, fair use of public money, and involvement of public values (see Application 19.1) [18–20].

In practice, however, both of these countries have had difficulty rationing services in this manner. A major problem has been in deciding which treatments are necessary, and which treatments individual patients and families should be responsible for [21]. Similar to the problems of defining need, the concept of 'medically necessary' is difficult to characterize and operationalize [1].

More importantly, the core services approach lacks the flexibility to shift resources at the margin: even though some patients may benefit from services that are not included in the 'core', funds cannot be reallocated to such services once they are deemed not to be medically necessary [1]. For example, a particular service may not be included within the core services offered, yet for some potential consumers it may provide more benefit per dollar spent than for some consumers of services that are considered to be core. However, as those services that are not included are 'out', a shifting of resources from those services that are 'in' to those that are 'out' is unlikely to be possible. Without the flexibility to shift resources at the margin, improvement in benefit to the population overall will be unlikely. Overall, the core services approach has had a limited effect on policy making internationally, perhaps in part because of the lack of attention to the margin [1].

Economic evaluation

There are several economic approaches to priority setting that warrant discussion. The most common 'economic approach' is that of economic evaluation, which is defined as the comparative analysis of alternative courses of action in terms of both their costs and consequences [23]. Economic evaluations provide technical comparisons of two or more interventions or services on

Application 19.1 Core services: health care rationing policy in New Zealand

New Zealand adopted a core services approach to health care financing in 1991. The Core Services Committee (CSC) was tasked with defining a set of core services: a restricted set of services that purchasers would be responsible for, or a full service complement that a restricted population might access. The predominant view was that the Committee should seek to retain 'universal entitlement and access', seen to be a tradition in New Zealand. Thus, the Committee elected to define a set of core services that the full population would be able to access, based upon four criteria: effectiveness; value for money; fairness; and consistency with public values.

Those services falling outside of this 'core' basket would fall to the responsibility of private citizens. However, defining the gamut of services that fell within the boundaries of the core proved to be an impossible task, largely due to the political climate [19]. Unequivocal political support would have been necessary in order to implement any definition of core services, but no politician at the time was willing to deny 'the voting public access to health care'. Even if a final definition of core services had been agreed upon Gauld argues that 'few health professionals and administrators would have denied services to unfunded patients' [19].

As a result, the CSC abandoned the core services approach and shifted to providing two types of clinical guidelines, one that provided a synthesized source of research evidence to health professionals, and the other that focused on when care can be withheld. Adherence to these guidelines remains a matter of professional preference, an approach which is now common to many countries. Thus the plan for defining a core set of services, at least at the national level, failed. It was also recognized that guidelines do not necessarily promote efficiency or equity, and that a pragmatic, economic approach to priority setting would still be required at the local, regional, or national levels [22].

the basis of costs and benefits, most often using cost-effectiveness, cost-utility, or cost-benefit analysis methods. This type of economic approach suggests that priority setting is a relatively straightforward optimization problem: decision-makers should seek to maximize health-related benefits for their population subject to the constraint of scarce resources. As a result, much of the health economics literature has focussed on developing technical methods for the appraisal of the costs and benefits of health services. Economic evaluation approaches have often been applied at the national level, such as guidance issued from the 'one-off' health technology appraisals of the National Institute of Health and Clinical Excellence (United Kingdom) (see Application 19.2), the Pharmaceutical Benefits Scheme (Australia), and the Canadian Agency for Drugs and Technologies in Health.

The primary strengths of using economic evaluation methods are that both costs and benefits are being considered, and that two or more interventions are directly compared against each other providing incremental results. However, a major limitation of this approach is the time and cost involved in each study, meaning that such evaluations are not feasible for all relevant questions [24]. A single economic evaluation will rarely take account of all the options a decision-maker is faced with when setting priorities [25] and economic evaluation often fails to properly consider the budget constraints faced by local decision-makers [26]. This has been, at least in part, due to the failure of these approaches to adequately capture the complex and multifaceted

Application 19.2 Economic evaluation: National Institute of Health and Clinical Excellence (NICE) in England and Wales

The guidelines programme of NICE, arguably the largest of its type in the world, publishes guidelines based on clinical- and cost-effectiveness of interventions in the areas of public health, health technology, and clinical practice. Guidelines are developed by a Guideline Development Group (GDG), which includes health professionals, content experts, and members of the general public, following the stages outlined as under [28]:

- *Recruit and train GDG Chair and Clinical Advisor.*

- *Prepare the scope*   Identify key clinical issues and undertake a scoping literature review. Define the parameters of the guideline after consultation with relevant stakeholder groups.

- *Select GDG members*   GDGs consist of health professionals and other individuals familiar with patient and carer issues.

- *Formulate review questions*   Identify and formulate review questions based on scoping results, and identified patient experiences.

- *Identify and review evidence*   Using systematic methods, search relevant databases and consider stakeholder submissions of evidence. Assess quality of selected studies for clinical- and cost-effectiveness. Evidence requirements include quantification of clinical effectiveness, impact on quality of life, and estimation of the technology's resource impact in terms of physical and monetary units. Should an independent economic evaluation not exist, the GCG will produce one, assessing cost-effectiveness using an NHS perspective.

- *Develop guidelines*   GCGs interpret evidence, identify key issues for implementation, and formulate research recommendations, all of which form the basis of clinical or cost-effectiveness guidelines.

- *Prepare implementation support*   GCGs develop tools for costing and other issues to support implementation of new guidelines.

- *Revise guidelines*   Guidelines are revised in light of consultations and stakeholder comments.

- *Prepare and publish guidelines.*

NICE's guideline development process is iterative and ongoing; guidelines are revised on a case-by-case basis, typically when new evidence as to effectiveness or cost-effectiveness becomes available [28].

Since its inception, NICE has published more than 33 appraisals for drugs that treat cancer. [30]. The highest cost per QALY accepted as 'cost-effective' – imatinib for treating chronic myeloid leukemia – was estimated to be US$77,760. In total, 26 condition-treatment pairs have been deemed to be cost-effective, with 3 condition-treatment pairs deemed to be 'cost-ineffective' (fludarabine – as a single agent for chronic lymphocytic leukaemia; and bevacizumab and cetuximab – both for metastatic colorectal cancer. Very few technologies with ICERs mentioned earlier – US$48,600 (or £30,000) per QALY – are accepted by NICE, although, there is currently no empirical basis for the implementation of a threshold of cost-effectiveness in health care.

nature of both objectives and constraints in health service decision-making [2]. As such, results from individual economic evaluations most likely still need to fit into a broader priority setting framework.

A common output of economic evaluation studies is the incremental cost-effectiveness ratio (ICER). The ICER quantifies the incremental cost required to obtain a given unit of benefit. Study authors often state that a given treatment is 'cost-effective' because of the 'favourable' cost per unit of benefit derivation expressed through a particular ICER [e.g. 27]. In stating results in this manner explicit consideration is not being given to opportunity costs. That is, as the ICER by definition relates to additional costs to produce the stated health gain, the question of where those additional resources will come from necessarily arises. Of course, the additional resources must come from elsewhere in the health care budget, usually at the expense of some other treatment or service, thereby resulting in an opportunity cost. Only further examination, comparing the given treatment option with other options, can provide information as to whether the stated treatment is 'cost-effective'. Again, the question of the margin arises, as it is through shifting of resources, from one option to another, that maximization of benefit is achieved, not necessarily through funding an option with a low ICER.

Cost-per-QALY league tables

In an effort to move away from the type of one-off technology appraisals described herein, cost-per-QALY league tables has been used to compare the costs and outcomes of multiple technologies. Interventions are ranked against each other based on cost-per-QALY ratios and those with lower ratios are ranked better than those with higher ratios [23]. The most notable example of this type of approach was the 'Oregon experiment' of the 1990s, in which the Health Services Commission in Oregon State attempted to apply a league table approach to limit spending. A description of their approach is presented in Application 19.3.

Cost-per-QALY league tables are also problematic from an economic perspective. Most importantly, each entry in the league table uses a different baseline comparator. Because cost-per-QALY figures are incremental, an intervention's position on the league table depends on the presence, absence, or choice of a pre-existing intervention as a comparator, and the cost and benefit of said intervention [23,29]. A given intervention may appear higher in the league table ranking because of its apparent efficiency relative to a given comparator, but whether resources should be invested in that way can only be determined through explicit consideration of opportunity cost relative to a much wider range of alternative uses of those resources. An additional limitation is the inability to account for the quality or strength of research evidence within the context of the league table [1]. Finally, the margin is again ignored in this approach, as per the core services and economic evaluation discussions in the preceding paragraphs [1].

Programme budgeting and marginal analysis

The above discussion has criticized so-called 'non-economic' and 'economic' approaches alike, based on their lack of adherence to the fundamental principles of priority setting. It should also be mentioned that the way forward is not about simply advocating that more resources be allocated to the health system, because scarcity will always exist, independently of how much is in the total pot. As such, a framework is required which adheres to the principles outlined earlier but is pragmatic enough to deal with the complexities of health care decision-making in a timely and evidence-based manner. One approach which does adhere to the economic principles and has been used extensively in health care over the past 25 years is Programme Budgeting and Marginal

Analysis (PBMA). To date, over 100 PBMA studies have been reported in countries such as Australia, Canada, New Zealand, and the United Kingdom.

PBMA is an economic framework specifically designed to aid local, regional, or national decision-makers in setting priorities. The intent of PBMA is to provide assistance to decision-makers in directing resources to maximize benefits from health services. In doing so, PBMA makes explicit uses of the principles of opportunity cost and marginal analysis. Most importantly, the focus of PBMA is helping decision-makers who are budget-holders; those individuals who are responsible for the real-world implementation of resource allocation decisions. It is these decision-makers – whether they are based in government ministries, health authorities, health maintenance organizations, primary care trusts, or hospitals – that have to bear the opportunity cost of resource allocation decisions elsewhere in their budgets.

Application 19.3 Cost-per-QALY league tables: Oregon State

In 1987 the Oregon State Legislature sought to develop a method for allocating resources that was both efficient and accountable. Their strategy was to move away from rationing by excluding people from coverage. Instead, when budget limits were required, specified health services would be eliminated from coverage based on an explicit set of priorities and a systematic evaluation methodology (DiPrete and Coffman 2007). Based on this strategy, a Health Services Commission was created, and was charged with developing a prioritized list of health services that would determine the minimum acceptable benefit for Oregonians.

A cost-per-QALY league table approach was chosen. With help from clinical experts, the Commission gauged the relative effectiveness of condition/treatment (CT) pairs and then ranked them in a league table according to relative effectiveness. However, the approach was largely unsuccessful because league table rankings frequently conflicted with the judgment of both physician and non-physician members of the Commission. The problem was that very effective but very expensive treatments for less severe conditions (such as malocclusion due to thumb sucking) ranked better than moderately effective, moderately expensive treatments for very severe conditions. The Commission concluded that while such a league table approach may effectively gauge the cost of treating a particular condition, it cannot address the relative importance of treating that condition in the first place.

As a result, the Commission abandoned the league table approach and instead classified investments based on seventeen categories of treatment. Within these ranked categories, services were prioritized based on cost and effectiveness. Before decisions were finalized, Commission members moved CT pairs manually, ensuring that the final ranking was an accurate reflection of their best personal judgment.

In an evaluation of this method, DiPrete and Coffman (2007) conclude that the prioritized list has successfully guided resources allocations on the basis of clinical evidence and judgment in a manner that is explicit and accountable. However, they admit that the list has not successfully shifted responses to budgetary constraints to explicit reductions in benefits. They claim that the United States Federal Government has been reluctant to reduce benefits, 'forcing the state to make adjustments in eligibility and in payment levels to keep within budget'. This political constraint has 'prevented the full exploration of the effectiveness of the prioritization of services in meeting budget limits while maintaining commitment to cover all those in need and the commitment to pay providers at levels sufficient to cover the cost of care' (DiPrete and Coffman 2007).

In its simplest form PBMA addresses three questions:

1 For budget increases: how should the extra dollars be allocated between health services to maximize benefits?

2 For budget reductions: how should service reductions be made to minimize the impact on benefits?

3 For a given budget: how do we allocate dollars between services so that benefits are maximized?

A PBMA study can be broken down into the seven stages shown in Table 19.3, which are designed to provide a systematic and explicit framework for priority setting [1,2,31]. PBMA asks decision-makers to construct a programme budget (a map of how resources are currently spent) and then assists them in making recommendations for changing existing allocations of resources to services using marginal analysis. This type of priority setting activity can take place both within health programmes at the micro level or across programmes at the macro level.

The advisory panel plays a central role in any PBMA study, and is typically made up of 8 to 30 stakeholders from relevant clinical and non-clinical disciplines [1]. Relevant stakeholders may include those directly involved in the programmes being considered (e.g. clinicians, managers, and patient/consumer representatives) and those indirectly involved (collaborating/inter-related

Table 19.3 Stages in a PBMA priority setting exercise

1 Determine the aim and scope of the priority setting exercise
Determine whether programme budgeting and marginal analysis will be used to examine changes in services within a given programme (micro/within programme study design) or between programmes (macro/between programme study design).

2 Compile a 'programme budget'
The resources and costs of programmes may need to be identified and quantified, which, when combined activity information, is the programme budget.

3 Form a 'marginal analysis' advisory panel
The panel is made up of key stakeholders (managers, clinicians, consumers, etc.) in the priority setting process.

4 Identify options for (a) service growth (b) resource release from gains in operational efficiency (c) resource release from scaling back or ceasing some services
The programme budget, along with information on decision-making objectives, evidence on benefits from service, changes in local health care needs, and policy guidance, are used highlight options for investment and disinvestment.

5 Determine locally relevant decision-making criteria
To be elicited from the advisory panel (e.g. maximizing benefits, improving access and equity, reducing waiting times, etc.), with reference to national, regional, and local objectives, and specified objectives of the health system and the community.

6 Evaluate investments and disinvestments
Evaluate in terms of costs and benefits and make recommendations for (a) funding growth areas with new resources, (b) moving resources from 4 (b) and 4 (c) to 4 (a).

7 Validate results and reallocate resources
Re-examine and validate evidence and judgments used in the process and reallocate resources according to cost-benefit ratios and other decision-making criteria.

providers, policy-makers, finance/information personnel, ethicists, organizational behaviourists, health economists, health services researchers, and community representatives). Community stakeholders can play an integral part in the process, including defining appropriate criteria for decision-making based on community values and ensuring the needs of specific groups within the community are addressed. The advisory panel is responsible for: determining locally relevant decision-making criteria; identifying service options for investment and disinvestment; evaluating those options by considering decision-making criteria, available evidence and local data; and making recommendations for resource allocation.

Options for investment and disinvestment are generated from data gathered in constructing the programme budget, along with information on decision-making objectives, evidence on the benefits of existing and potential new services, changes in local health care needs, and policy guidance [32]. This may include identifying services that can potentially be provided as effectively using fewer resources, as well as identifying services that should receive fewer resources because they may provide less benefit per dollar than one or more of the investments.

Investments and disinvestments are then evaluated in terms of both their costs and benefits, where benefits may be expressed in effectiveness, utility, or monetary terms. Published evidence on the benefits from services can be used (where available). Where published evidence is unavailable, expert opinion can be used to estimate benefits using decision-analytic techniques [33]. If the principle of maximizing benefits from scarce resources is being followed, resources should be reallocated from services with lowest ratios of benefit to cost to those services with the highest ratios of benefit to cost. Importantly, the implications of changes in the configuration of services in terms of other decision-making criteria (e.g. access, equity, waiting times, etc.), in addition to costs and benefits, should be assessed. Defining these criteria is also useful when no evidence exists; so expert opinion can be used to inform judgments about the performance of investment and disinvestment options.

Recommendations for resource allocation are based on the evaluation of investments and disinvestments described earlier. The process can then be repeated over a period of time so that services which are more difficult to evaluate, or change, are progressively assessed. By sequentially repeating the process, the emphasis of PBMA is gradually to move towards the goal of maximizing benefits for a given level of resources. In this way, use of the PBMA framework is relevant regardless of the total amount of resources available.

A major limitation of many PBMA studies has been the lack of high quality effectiveness evidence available for use in marginal analysis. Such studies have often relied on experts' subjective estimates of effectiveness where data is not available. However, two recent programmes of research in cancer control have sought to address this limitation. The first, based in Australia, employed systematic reviews and meta-analyses of effectiveness evidence in conjunction with Disability Adjusted Life Years (DALYs) as outcome measures to set priorities across a wide range of cancer control programmes (see Application 19.4) [34,35]. The second research programme is based in British Columbia, Canada, and is using methods drawn from health technology assessment in conjunction with Life Years and QALYs gained as outcome measures to set cancer control priorities (see Application 19.5).

The way forward – balancing economics and ethics

Recent developments in the health policy literature have highlighted the need for an interdisciplinary approach to priority setting. In particular, a number of authors have argued that the search for a rational set of decision-making rules in no longer adequate; and that researchers and decision-makers also need to focus their attention on the priority setting process itself [1,36,37].

Application 19.4 PBMA: cancer control in Australia (DALYs)

The Cancer Strategy Group (CSG) of the National Health Priorities Committee in Australia trialed a PBMA approach that incorporated the use of Disability-Adjusted Life Years (DALYs) as a measure of health outcomes in order to inform the development of the National Cancer Strategy [40]. Characteristics of the PBMA method adopted included a strong focus on the marginal analysis component of PBMA, the incorporation of an evidence-based approach, and the adoption of a two-stage approach to the assessment of benefit involving both 'technical' aspects (cost-per-DALY recovered; level of evidence) and 'judgment' aspects (equity; size of the problem; acceptability to stakeholders; and feasibility of implementation) [40].

Eight options for change, involving both investments (additional expenditure) and disinvestments (reduced expenditure) were evaluated and ranked (separately) according to their cost-per-DALY results (see Table A1). Options evaluated included primary prevention, early detection, treatment, rehabilitation, and palliation programs. All options were compared in terms of DALYs recovered or lost; that is, the extent to which investments reduced the DALY burden of cancer, or disinvestments increased the DALY burden, in the Australian population.

All investment options were considered suitable for inclusion within the National Cancer Strategy, with the lowest ranked option (colorectal cancer screening) having a net cost-per-DALY recovered of $10,300. Of the two disinvestment options evaluated, one (extending the interval for cervical cancer screening from two to three years) was considered suitable for implementation.

There was general agreement amongst the members of the CSG that PBMA represented a significant step forward in cancer control decision-making methods. In particular, the incorporation of the best-available evidence was strongly supported. The CSG concluded that although there were elements of the PBMA process that could be improved upon, the process had the potential to play a valuable role in cancer control planning in Australia.

Table A1 Ranking of Australian PBMA investment options

Programme	Gross costs of new programme $AU millions	Net cost after health cost savings $AUmillions	DALYs recovered	Cost per DALY (based on gross costs) $AUD
Reduce prevalence of smoking by coordinated strategies	8.95	Savings of 39.1	10,559	Dominant
Reduce skin cancer by national coordinated SunSmart campaign	2.53	Savings of 37.4	9,965	Dominant
Increase consumption of fruit and vegetables by coordinated campaign	2.46	Savings of 12.2	3,626	Dominant
Improve psychosocial care for breast cancer patients by providing breast care nurses	4.85	Not assessed	5,186	935
Improve psychosocial care for cancer patients by providing psychologists in cancer centres	25.70	Not assessed	4,849	5,300
Introduce a national colorectal screening program at ages 55–69	53.30	38.1	3,187	16,724

> **Application 19.4 PBMA: cancer control in Australia (DALYs)** *(continued)*
>
> The three prevention programmes shown were estimated to produce health gains with net cost savings, as the reductions in health costs exceeded the costs of implementation; hence the result is 'dominant'. Several other interventions were also considered, including the effects of some decrements in services, such as increasing the screening interval for cervix cancer [41].

Any priority setting process inevitably raises a range of ethical questions. Ethical questions relate to the need for any priority setting process to be fair, accountable, and transparent. That is, irrespective of the final resource allocation recommendations, importance may be placed on whether the process itself is fair [38]. One approach to examining fairness in decision-making processes is the ethical framework of accountability for reasonableness or A4R [39]. Within the A4R framework, a priority setting process is considered to be fair if it satisfies the four conditions required to demonstrate accountability for reasonableness. These conditions relate to publicity, relevance, appeals, and enforcement (see Table 19.4).

In order to ensure publicity of priority setting processes, decisions and their rationales should be communicated to internal and external stakeholders (health service staff, patients, the general public, and so on) in a transparent manner. Information exchange is a two-way process, focusing on building a shared understanding of the need for priority setting, goals of the process, decision-making criteria, how the process will work, and resulting decisions. Focus groups or individual

> # Application 19.5 PBMA: cancer control in British Columbia, Canada (QALYs)
>
> The British Columbia Cancer Agency (BCCA) is developing a novel, modified PBMA approach to help decision-makers set cancer control priorities in British Columbia. Innovations to the PBMA framework include the incorporation of local cost and outcomes data, and published QALY evidence to conduct health technology assessments using Markov models. The study is guided by a steering committee of BCCA senior management, tumour group leaders, surgeons, nurse managers, finance/administration staff, and academics.
>
> In the first year of the study, three pilot programme areas were identified for analysis: (1) the use of an expensive drug, trastuzumab (Herceptin) as an adjuvant breast cancer treatment; (2) increasing the frequency of screening mammography for women with high mammographic density (who may be at increased risk of breast cancer); and (3) the use of PET/CT scans in non-small cell lung cancer (these investigations are expensive but may give better information about the cancer and avoid some unnecessary treatment). Advisory panels, consisting of clinicians, decision-makers, data experts, and researchers, were formed for each of these programme areas. The panels were charged with identifying decision-making criteria and assisting the research team in constructing Markov models to undertake cost-effectiveness analyses. Models were built using high-quality clinical and BCCA administrative datasets to yield economic evidence to assist in informing decision-making in each program area. Economic evidence was generated in each programme area, with incremental cost-effectiveness ratios ranging from $35,000/QALY to $120,000/QALY, and results have been used to inform resource allocation decisions at the provincial level.

Table 19.4 Checklist for ethical considerations in priority setting processes

---

1 Ensure publicity of priority setting processes
Priority setting processes and decisions, and the rationales for those processes and decisions, should be made accessible to managers, doctors, patients, and the public

2 Ensure relevance of priority setting processes
The rationales for priority setting processes and decisions should be based on principles, reasons, and evidence that managers, doctors, patients, and the public can agree are relevant to deciding how to meet the diverse needs of the community given resource constraints

3 Establish an appeals mechanism
An appeals mechanism should be established for challenge and dispute resolution regarding priority setting decisions, including the opportunity for revising decisions in light of further evidence or arguments

4 Establish an enforcement mechanism
Voluntary or public regulation mechanisms should be established for the priority setting process to ensure that the first three conditions are met

---

meetings with stakeholders can be used to exchange ideas and information concerning values, needs, and opportunities for service improvements. Newsletters to health service staff and 'town hall' meetings can also be effective mechanisms for communication.

Ensuring relevance of the processes involves developing a rationale for priority setting decisions and relevant decision-making criteria. Documents describing the organization's mission, vision, and values provide a useful starting point, but as discussed hereunder, eliciting criteria requires careful consideration of a wide range of potentially conflicting viewpoints. An advisory panel of key stakeholders should then review the best available evidence on the services being appraised, and evaluate their performance against chosen decision-making criteria. It is important to recognize that decision-making will typically be based on multiple criteria by stakeholders from multidisciplinary backgrounds. Stakeholders should understand the process, be allowed to present their views, express conflicts of interest, and be receptive to external advice when needed. Roles and responsibilities of stakeholders should be outlined clearly at the outset, by developing and discussing terms of reference.

Establishing a transparent appeals (or revision) mechanism entails developing a formal decision-review process based on explicit decision-review criteria. Decision review ensures that decisions are 'reasonable' based on available evidence and local circumstances. Decisions may be reviewed in order to improve quality for a number of reasons, for example, if procedural rules are violated, if new trial data is published, or other new evidence comes to light.

In establishing an enforcement mechanism, leadership by senior managers and executives is critical. Experience from both the PBMA and A4R literature suggests that senior management has considerable influence over whether other actors engage in fair play or not. Facilitating group and organizational learning can also reduce the extent to which actors seek to game the system. However, priority setting is iterative. Monitoring the process and enforcing rules should be an ongoing process which seeks to evaluate what has happened in the past, what is happening in the present, and then refines the process for the future.

A primary aim of A4R in this context is to ensure the process is credible to relevant stakeholders and to reduce the impact of barriers to making effective priority setting decisions. This requires that the process is perceived to be fair and legitimate so that stakeholders commit to it, its rationale, and the resulting decisions. Fairness and transparency in the process may help to mitigate practical problems potentially arising due to resources being shifted from one service to another. In recent years, researchers have increasingly aligned the implementation of PBMA with the conditions of A4R. The added value of A4R lies in its explicit framework for pursuing fairness and legitimacy in the priority setting process, rather than leaving fairness considerations largely 'to chance'.

All of these 'lessons learned' can be applied in the cancer control context. Whether at the level of an entire cancer agency, or within specific programmes, moving away from historical and/or political resource allocation processes to an explicit, evidence driven approach that is based upon both economics and ethics should serve to improve value for money and increase the perceived legitimacy of the decision-making process itself. Decision-makers who have used PBMA and A4R across a range of contexts, including cancer, have commented specifically on improvements in the use of evidence, greater accountability and defensibility, and, ultimately, better decisions being made.

Conclusion

The recognition that claims on resources will always outstrip the resources available indicates a need to set priorities, and to allocate resources according to agreed upon principles and rules. Many approaches to priority setting have failed to incorporate the fundamental economic principles of opportunity cost and the margin. As a result, decision-makers are often left with 'sub-optimal' programmes and growing budgetary pressures. This certainly is the case in cancer control programmes.

Priority setting requires multi-professional and interdisciplinary research, recognizing that the challenges that decision-makers face are 'real-life' challenges which transcend academic boundaries. The added value of an approach like PBMA is in making the priority setting process more explicit and systematic. Such a process can be thought of as a vehicle for drawing evidence into the decision-making process in cancer control, and combining evidence with the values of the key stakeholders, which include clinicians, managers, researchers, cancer patients, survivors and the community. Most importantly, whilst achieving the above, PBMA is based explicitly on the premise of having to make difficult choices amongst competing claims on scarce resources.

It is important to recognize that we are not proposing an 'all-encompassing' economic, political, and social model of decision-making processes in cancer control. Constructing such a model would be intractable. Decision-making processes are complex, sometimes idiosyncratic, and subject to unpredictable influences. Instead, we have described some tools drawn from economics and ethics which can be used to address the challenge of setting priorities in cancer control. We are proposing a move towards an interdisciplinary and pragmatic framework for priority setting, recognizing that economists' methods provide only one of several sets of tools needed to inform priority setting decisions.

Acknowledgements

Stuart Peacock and Craig Mitton are Michael Smith Foundation for Health Research Scholars. Craig Mitton also holds a Canada Research Chair (Tier 2) in Health Care Priority Setting. Research was funded by Canadian Institutes of Health Research grant no. 162964. We would like to thank the editors for their useful comments on earlier drafts of this chapter. The views expressed in this chapter are those of the authors, not of the funding agencies.

References

1 Mitton C & Donaldson C (2004). *Priority setting toolkit: a guide to the use of economics in healthcare decision making*. BMJ Books, London.

2 Peacock S, Ruta D, Mitton C, Donaldson C, Bate A, & Murtagh M (2006). Using economics to set pragmatic and ethical priorities. *BMJ*, Feb 25;**332**(7539):482–85.

3 Lomas J, Veenstra G, & Woods J (1997). Devolving authority for health care in Canada's provinces: 2. Backgrounds, resources and activities of board members. *CMAJ*, Feb 15;**156**(4):513–20.

4 Mitton C & Donaldson C (2002). Setting priorities in Canadian regional health authorities: a survey of key decision makers. *Health Policy*, **60**(1):39–58.

5 Smith J, Mays N, Dixon J, et al (2004). *A review of the effectiveness of primary care-led commissioning and its place in the NHS*. The Health Foundation, London.

6 MacDonald R (2002). *Using health economics in health services: rationing rationally?* Open University Press, Houston.

7 World Health Organization (2005). *Preventing chronic diseases: a vital investment*. World Health Organization, Geneva.

8 Jönsson B & Wilking N (2007). The burden and cost of cancer. *Ann Oncol*, Apr;**18**(Suppl 3):iii8–22.

9 World Health Organization (2006). *Global burden of disease and risk factors*. World Health Organization, Geneva.

10 Bosanquet N & Sikora K (2004). The economics of cancer care in the UK. *Lancet Oncol*, Sep;**5**(9): 568–74.

11 Canadian Strategy for Cancer Control (2005). Establishing the strategic framework for the Canadian strategy for cancer control. Available at http://www.cancer.ca/canada-wide/how%20you%20can%20 help/take%20action/advocacy%20what%20were%20doing/cancer%20control.aspx?sc_lang=en

12 Birch S & Chambers S (1993). To each according to need: a community-based approach to allocating health care resources. *CMAJ*, Sep 1;**149**(5):607–12.

13 Mitton C & Donaldson C (2003). Tools of the trade: a comparative analysis of approaches to priority setting in health care. *Health Serv Manage Res*,**16**(2):96–105.

14 Fitzpatrick JL, Sanders JR, & Worthen BR (2004). *Program evaluation: alternative approaches and practical guidelines*. 3rd ed. Pearson Education Inc, Boston.

15 Myers A (1999). *Program evaluation for exercise leaders*. Human Kinetics, Waterloo.

16 Mooney G, Russell E, & Weir R (1986). *Choices for health care: a practical introduction to the economics of health provision*. Macmillan, London.

17 Shiell A, Gerard K, & Donaldson C (1987). Cost of illness studies: an aid to decision making? *Health Policy*, **8**:317–23.

18 National Health Committee (1995). *Fourth annual report*. National Health Committee, Wellington.

19 Gauld R (2004). Health care rationing policy in New Zealand: development and lessons. *Soc Policy Society*, **3**(3):235–42.

20 Sabik L & Lie R (2008). Priority setting in health care: lessons from the experiences of eight countries. *Int J Equity Health*, **7**(1):4.

21 Maynard A & Bloor K (1998). *Our certain fate: rationing in health care*. Office of Health Economics, London.

22 Ashton T, Cumming J, & Devlin N (2000). Priority-setting in New Zealand: translating principles into practice. *J Health Serv Res Po*, **5**(3):170–75.

23 Drummond M, Sculpher M, Torrance G, O'Brien B, & Stoddart G (2005). *Methods for the economic evaluation of health care programs*. 3rd ed. Oxford Medical Publications, Oxford.

24 Donaldson C & Mooney G (1991). Needs assessment, priority setting, and contracts for health care: an economic view. *BMJ*, **303**:1529–30.

25 Peacock S (1997). *Program budgeting and marginal analysis: options for health sector reform*. Centre for Health Program Evaluation, Melbourne.

26 Gafni A & Birch S (2006). Incremental cost-effectiveness ratios (ICERs): the silence of the lambda. *Soc Sci Med*, **62**(9):2091–2100.

27 Freedberg KA, Losina E, Weinstein MC, et al (2001). The cost effectiveness of combination antiretroviral therapy for HIV disease. *N Engl J Med*, **344**(11):824–31.

28 National Institute for Health and Clinical Excellence (2009). *The guidelines manual* (Internet). National Institute for Health and Clinical Excellence, London (cited 2009 Jun 1). Available from: www.nice.org.uk.

29 Birch S & Gafni A (1992). Cost-effectiveness ratios: in a league of their own. *Health Policy*, **28**(2): 133–41.

30 Rawlins, M (2007). Paying for modern cancer care – a global perspective. *Lancet Oncol*, Sep;**8**(9): 749–51.

31 Ruta D, Mitton C, Bate A, & Donaldson C (2005). Program budgeting and marginal analysis: bridging the divide between doctors and managers. *BMJ*, **330**:1501–3.

32 Ruta DA, Donaldson C, & Gilray I (1996). Economics, public health and health care purchasing: the Tayside experience of program budgeting and marginal analysis. *J Health Serv Res Po*, **1**(4):185–93.

33 Peacock SJ, Richardson JRJ, Carter R, & Edwards D (2007). Priority setting in health care using multi-attribute utility theory and program budgeting and marginal analysis (PBMA). *Soc Sci Med*, **64**(4):897–910.

34 Carter R, Stone C, Vos T, et al (2000). Trial of program budgeting and marginal analysis (PBMA) to assist cancer control planning in Australia. Centre for Health Program Evaluation, Melbourne. Monash University. Research Report 19. *PBMA* Series No. 5.

35 Carter R, Vos T, Moodie M, Haby M, Magnus A, & Mihalopoulos C (2008). Priority setting in health: origins, description and application of the assessing cost effectiveness (ACE) initiative. *Expert Rev Pharmacoecon Outcomes Res*, **8**(6):593–617.

36 Holm S (1998). Goodbye to the simple solutions: the second phase of priority setting in health care. *BMJ*, **317**(7164):1000–07.

37 Peacock S, Donaldson C, Mitton C, Bate A, & McCoy B (2009). Overcoming barriers to priority setting using interdisciplinary methods. *Health Policy*, Epub 2009 Apr 5.

38 Ham C & Coulter A (2001). Explicit and implicit rationing: taking responsibility and avoiding blame for health care choices. *J Health Serv Res Po*, **6**(3):163–9.

39 Daniels N & Sabin J (1998). The ethics of accountability in managed care reform. *Health Affair*, Sep 1;**17**(5):50–64.

40 DiPrete B & Coffman D (2007). A brief history of health services prioritization in Oregon. Health Services Commission, State of Oregon, Oregon.

41 Cancer Strategies Group. Priorities for action in cancer control 2001–2003. Canberra: Commonwealth Department of Health and Ageing; 2001.

Chapter 20

Ethics and the idea of cancer control

Lisa Schwartz[1]

The term 'cancer control' raises ethical concerns just on first reading. Really the idea of control is what engenders this attention. Control of what? Control of whom? How will this affect the lives of individuals?

Most ethics literature related to cancer is dominated by concerns about individuals: individual patients, and health care providers. Topics tend to focus mostly upon the needs and challenges associated with consent, disclosure, and decision-making. The history of ethics in health care is dominated by this type of individual focused question about patients and their care providers, and the moral challenges they face – even create – in the attempt to provide compassionate, dignified, quality care. The principles of respect for autonomy, beneficence, and non-maleficence, as well as the virtues of a good practitioner, have for a long time held the spotlight and focused our interest when health ethics was being discussed.

With the idea of 'cancer-control' the field broadens. Cancer control is not only directed at specific individuals, but directs our attention to wider issues, issues of public health, health policy and other elements of wider interest. This is not to say that cancer control will not have an effect on individual people, in fact some programmes are explicit about aiming at the health and well being of individuals and their families, but the process of responding to individual needs is recognized as being part of something wider [1]. Cancer control programmes are attempts at creating a fully embracing system that is designed to engage at multiple levels. What this tends to mean is that decisions related to cancer control will have impact on the lives of multiple individuals and are directed at overall community benefit.

Ethics in health care has taken a similar turn in interests. An emerging literature in ethics is directed at policy and organizational issues, recognizing that the experience of individual care occurs within the wider context of politics and policy, institutions, and environmental and social patterns. Ethics of health policy and organizational ethics are growing fields of enquiry and are especially relevant to the idea of cancer control.

The chief concerns of ethics of health policy and of organizational ethics are first, ethical process in decision-making, and second, attention to the values and substantive claims that will inform the decisions. Emphasis on fair process is the interest of procedural ethics. Here critical analysis is applied to the ways in which public policy decisions ought to be made, who will be involved, what steps need to be taken to plan, inform, and implement decisions, and how will appeals be attended to. In the first part of this chapter, I will examine how proposed cancer control programmes can include ethical procedures and explore the value in their so doing. In part two of the chapter, I will look more closely at the kinds of decisions that need to be made and

[1] Lisa Schwartz, PhD, Arnold L. Johnson Chair in Health Care Ethics, Department of Clinical Epidemiology and Biostatistics, McMaster University, Hamilton, Ontario, Canada.

at the ethical values and principles that can be applied to the decision-making processes. So part one is about how decisions are made, and part two is about what decisions are made.

Part I: Procedural ethics and cancer control

To have an ethical procedure promotes justice by helping to ensure fair process. Regardless of the outcomes, if the process is fair the overall results will be, to some extent, justifiable and the results more trustworthy. Legal theory demonstrates exactly that. The legal system would not be just without fair, reliable processes which are predictable and stable. If this were not the case, the system would fail to give direction and fail to make us feel secure in the knowledge that we can assess and anticipate when we do something which is legally condoned and when we do not. There is something about the stability and predictability that makes it fair because everyone who knows about it can act accordingly without fearing surprise sanctions. This belies certain qualities of the process that make it just. In the first instance, it must be transparent so that everyone who may be subject to a given law will be able to find out what it requires, permits, or prohibits. It must be fairly applied, so that we can anticipate its application regardless of who is subject to it; also it must be somewhat stable so outcomes can be relied upon. This reliance on procedure is not of value only in law. What law offers is an illustration of the importance of fair and reliable process that makes a system just, but these qualities are relevant elsewhere as well, and in health care most certainly. Procedural ethics is valuable in and of itself, but it is also instrumental in fostering and securing trust and cooperation because it demonstrates fairness and reliability [2–4].

The many ethical questions that emerge from the very idea of cancer control are the sorts that can be resolved, at least in part, by appeal to fair processes. How ought control to be applied? Who ought to make policy decisions about cancer control? What if the decisions are not universally applicable? Can it incorporate an appeal process? All of these emphasize a core belief in procedural ethics, that integrity of process is at least as important as the outcome and sometimes more important [5].

Of the many proposals for a procedural ethics, the most frequently sighted and most relevant to cancer control are the following:

- Inclusiveness
- Stability
- Review mechanisms
- Right of appeal
- Transparency
- Pertinence to social values and relevant knowledge or evidence
- Timeliness and efficiency
- Collaboration

I will examine the relevance of these to formulating an ethical procedural framework for cancer control. The embracing of diversity and inclusiveness, the role of transparency, stability and collaboration, and the requirement of review and appeal, are all core to a programme for cancer control.

Inclusiveness

To engage the public and specific stakeholders in the process of decision-making is generally recognized as morally significant. Lawrence Solum [6] refers in legal scholarship to 'the Participatory Legitimacy Thesis: it is (usually) a condition for the fairness of a procedure that those who are to be finally bound shall have a reasonable opportunity to participate in the proceedings'. Solum states that the

> Participation Principle stipulates a minimum (and minimal) right of participation, in the form of notice and an opportunity to be heard, that must be satisfied (if feasible) in order for a procedure to be considered fair. (Brackets from the original) [6].

Inclusiveness by using some form of stakeholder consultation is clearly important to the process of developing cancer control policy. In the first instance, cancer control programmes will have implications for the entire community, even those who are fortunate enough never to be touched by cancer in their lives, because the resulting decisions regarding funding, accessibility, and available choices will affect everyone. Within the constraints of budgets and other resources, the decision to fund cancer control, prevention, care, etc. necessarily means a depletion of generally available resources. This may be believed justifiable, but it necessarily entails that some health opportunities will be impeded by under-funding while others thrive. As a result of their far reaching impact, decisions about funding cancer control programmes ought to be made with information about preferences, challenges, and concerns of those who will live with the outcomes.

So the stakeholders in cancer control include the broad community to some extent. This may be the case for some sorts of wide decision-making, but not necessarily for all, and for more precise decisions we will do better to consult specific stakeholders. Identification of relevant stakeholders will be based upon expertise and experience and include those people who can shed light on and relevantly inform decisions. Inclusiveness ought to be broad in some cases, narrow in others.

Public consultations and surveys are therefore crucially linked to fair process. Mechanisms such as these are required for a variety of reasons – reasons that dictate the types of methodologies that ought to be employed. Attention needs to be paid to how public engagement methods work, and the different types of outcomes it can produce [7]. For example, if policy-makers want to learn about the specific health concerns affecting a population, they can engage in public consultation to elicit debate and conversation to create a ranking or consensus about generally approved priorities [8]. However, a different method is required if policy-makers want only to inform the public of decisions already made. The two types of approach are sufficiently different and it would be a mistake, even morally wrong, to do one when the other is required, because it would mislead the participants and give them a false idea of the kind of input and uptake they can expect their ideas to have. Misleading uses of public consultation could induce public opposition not because outcomes are believed to be unacceptable, but because the process was misleading and therefore not trustworthy [9]. Because cancer control programmes and developers rely on public trust to maintain effectiveness, the processes by which they engage with the public need to be chosen carefully and applied fairly.

Inclusiveness is relevant to every area of cancer control programmes. Research should be informed by, and to a certain extent guided by, public consultations or at least some form of collaboration with beneficiaries such as patients, families, and communities. This will help keep research relevant and help respond to needs that might otherwise go neglected because they are not within the grasp of researchers who do not live the experience of having cancer. Decisions about the areas of research that will be included ought also to be open to inclusiveness. Small groups of individuals suffering from rare forms of cancer could be excluded or ignored if they are not heard in the process. Decisions about priority setting can lack inclusiveness when they focus on majority interests and thereby marginalize minority interests.

The research agenda for cancer control has broad ranging impact and as such ought to include a broad range of interests and innovators. Wide consultation is necessary to ensure that the wider research agenda is set fairly. The research agenda is a broad term here meaning all the elements, agencies, resources and people who are part of determining what research will be done and who will receive funding to do it. In order to promote wide ranging, innovative research, it is necessary to involve the public and also to ensue that opportunities are made available for novel concepts to be included and supported by resources. The example of the relevance of viruses in both causes and treatments of cancer is an excellent example of how important it is to be able and willing to entertain even bizarre or apparently vague contributions to research. We cannot know when one of these will prove useful or even advance a new paradigm for the approach to cancer control.

Inclusiveness in policy development, research, system review, and improvement are all necessary parts of procedural ethics.

Stability and reviewability

Stability is desirable because it permits actors to expect and predict the process by which decisions will be made and applied. For example, there is a certain stability in the way decisions about funding of treatments or programmes will be made. As a result, drug manufacturers can estimate in advance how long it will take for a drug to go from research to approval for drug funding by a government. The long trajectory can be estimated and patients, hopeful and awaiting new treatments, can anticipate when they will have access, or funded access to a particular medication. If the rules were unstable they would be unpredictable and no one would be able to reliably navigate the systems that apply to, for example, access to care and treatment, or decisions about funding and prevention.

On its own, however, stability is not infallible. There is virtue in the rules remaining stable so that all players know the rules of the game. However, stability can cause its own problems. Stable rules can become outdated, new information and counter-examples can shed light on weaknesses and illuminate where changes need to be made. So stability needs to be tempered with review and be open to the possibility of change or response to special cases. No process is truly just if it is not subject to regular review. John Stuart Mill noted that rules become dogma if they are not subject to regular reconsideration and challenge [10]. A system for cancer control will need to be extremely agile in its review processes because the landscape of cancer prevention, research, treatment, and experience undergo such rapid change. To return to our example, historically the link between viruses and human cancer was generally rejected, but it has now become one of the most promising avenues of cancer prevention and treatment. As scientific paradigms change, so the rules (policies and treatments) that govern them need to be adjusted in response.

Appeals

Justice requires review of the processes used to make decisions. However, not all rules need to be changed and some only need to yield temporarily for the interests of a few. In addition to regular review, the process must also permit individuals to appeal general decisions, so that the broad decisions of cancer control programmes are sensitive to the differing needs of the different individuals they affect. An example of a useful appeal mechanism is where appeals are made through compassionate access mechanisms that ask the health care provider, patient, doctor, nurse, social worker, or other to make an appeal for access to a drug not yet approved or funded by a system. These mechanisms are essential elements of just and fair access for individual patients whose needs are not met within the established decisions of a cancer programme.

No matter their importance, there is a lingering injustice in the appeals mechanisms that ought to be attended to for the mechanisms to meet procedural ethics standards. Appeals need to be made and heard effectively. This may require that the system offer an advocate for the person or the group making the appeal. Otherwise they are left to navigate a potentially complex system and create a persuasive justification on their own. Most patients do not have the resources to accomplish this adequately. It leaves them vulnerable to a process that favours expertise. The process is unfair unless an advocate is available who is familiar with the system and who has the vulnerable party's interest at heart. It is the case that few health care providers are adequately trained to write effective appeals for their patients, many do not even realize the mechanisms exist until they require them and then find themselves having to write a letter that is sufficiently persuasive to successfully gain access to the care the patient is believed to require. It is incumbent upon our professional training schools that they at least draw students' attention to the existence of appeals mechanisms, and ideally provide training to ensure the best case is presented for patients relying on them. For example, preparing health care professionals with knowledge of the system, options, and examples of letters of special appeals, as well as opportunities to practice and receive feedback on appeal letters they write. Otherwise, like a person who confronting a complex legal system will stumble and possibly fail without a lawyer to advocate for them, so patients will suffer and miss out without an adequately trained representative to advocate for them in the complex maze of the health care system.

Thus appeals mechanisms themselves need to be sensitive to fair process. Not all patients can advocate for themselves, especially when they are fragile with illness and vulnerable to the complexities of the system they must navigate. It is worth noting that the existence of an appeal process does not mean that every appeal will be successful, it merely introduces an essential element of fairness. Here again, clarity of process, and stability of the rules to be followed are vital to just and fair application of an appeal process.

Transparency

Throughout this discussion there has been an implicit suggestion of the importance of transparency to fair process. Transparency permits scrutiny and helps build trust because observers feel there is nothing hidden in the process. It is a mechanism of support for the other elements of procedural ethics because it permits the public to be engaged in an informed way, not trying to guess at the reasons for decisions. It makes rules and outcomes clear and accessible, and thereby makes opportunities for review and appeal possible.

Transparency is a term we hear a great deal of and one that is sometimes embraced without consideration of how it ought to be best applied. Many see it as crucial without examining why it is important, and as a result we have seen examples of how it has run afoul. The classic example of this is the problems associated with merely posting surgical league tables without contextualizing the results. So the morbidity rates of a collection of surgeons might be posted with ranking for high morbidity and low. It may seem like useful information to patients in a position to select a surgeon, but it is not very helpful if it is not accompanied by freedom to choose or by more detail. Obviously the types of disease the surgeons specialize in will be relevant. Cardiac surgeons and brain surgeons may work with greater risks than those specializing in surgeries of the hand. In addition, the type of surgery the surgeon performs is relevant, surgeons who perform challenging procedures such as in utero techniques will also face challenges other surgeons do not. Also, experience and context will be relevant. Surgeons who work in communities that have high co-morbidities or with patients with more advanced stages of illness are also likely to see more deaths. This is not because they are less skilled than their colleagues, but may even be because they are more skilled and therefore relied upon to accept more difficult cases. Information must be contextualized to make a meaningful difference to those who rely on it.

Thus, transparency in and of itself is not always a helpful part of process. It is important, but information needs to be made relevant to those it is intended to inform. Otherwise it can even create confusion as information overloads the process causing delays while it is sorted through or even creating distracting impediments.

Pertinence to social values and relevant evidence

All decisions need to be made on the basis of information. A process that includes gathering and consideration or inclusion of relevant information is mandatory to fair process and to reliable outcomes. The concept of Evidence-based Practice is essential to and well respected in health care delivery. It is also at the foundation of sound development of good practice guidelines and health policy. An ethical procedural framework will incorporate research and evaluation of accepted practice to inform decisions about funding and priority setting. Mechanisms to incorporate both relevant research evidence and standard or innovative practices are a natural aspect of sound process. So a cancer control programme must involve schemes for incorporating published information and as far as possible even unpublished, inconclusive, or negative finding research (for example through clinical trials registration). Availability of information, development of new information through the fair funding of research, and the determined incorporation of empirical findings in decision-making are all part of ethical process.

Scientific evidence does not stand alone in its usefulness to fair decision-making processes. This sort of information is not isolated from context and so values, beliefs, and social norms have a role to play as well. The evidence of empirical research needs to be sorted through and understood within the context of the values and ideals of a community. Programmes in health care such as one for cancer control will sort out and impose priorities, and reject the relevance of certain proposals or findings. In a fair process, this will be done in a manner consistent with the values of the community in which they will be applied. So the evidence and knowledge must be considered and used to make decisions that reflect the known values of that community.

A community's values will not always be explicit or evident. Where they are not, time and effort must be given to working out what they are and validating them through general consultation with the community's members. In some places, however, these values are more explicit. Institutions often have vision statements to help clarify values. Countries, states, and provinces will make their statements in constitutions or public acts, such as the Canada Health Act [11]. These statements explicitly instantiate values which can be applied and inform fair process, such as accessibility of care, fair distribution, and commitments to high quality. Part II of this chapter will explore what these values might be; this section is only intended to emphasize that values are relevant information in the decision-making process and ought to be used to steer policy decisions in a programme for cancer control.

The combination of empirical, scientific data and the accepted values of the community need to be part of decision-making in health care. Neither can stand in isolation, but both must be used to inform and help interpret best processes and decisions. Decisions made in this way will be more easily justified and embraced by the people to whom they will apply.

Timeliness and efficiency

The value of a process that permits functional, inclusive, and accessible decisions in a timely manner is crucial to fair ethical process. Nowhere has this been more clear than in the area of cancer control. The lives of individuals depend on rapid generation of, and responses to, new knowledge and information. This does not mean rushing blindly into accepting every bit of new information to make hasty, unconsidered decisions. It does, however, mean dedication of mechanisms and resources for the creation of and response to new information. Whether this be the funding of promising new research or hearing the appeal from a group of patients with a rare form of cancer, a system needs to be in place to keep the process moving and not to impede it by leaving it under-resourced or overloaded. Shared information, processes, and other resources will ensure that the best use is made of scarce resources and will make efficient use of what resources are available. Given what is at stake, namely the suffering and deaths of patients, an ethical process will be one that is careful and attentive, but also rapid and efficient.

Collaboration

A procedural element common to the vision statements of cancer control programmes is collaborative process. This is relevant to the discussion in part II because it is a value in many contexts, but it is discussed here because collaboration is described as a functional mechanism for achieving the goals of cancer control.

Collaboration is applied to cancer control in more than one way. It is relevant to care of individual patients, where multidisciplinary approaches are advocated to give patients wide access to a variety of care to meet the complex experience of cancer. So a given patient will receive care from medical oncologists working with radiation oncologists, pathologists, and laboratory technicians who diagnose, cardiologists who monitor the long-term effects of chemotherapies, pharmacists who prepare and help monitor treatment, nurses who deliver therapies and nurses who provide supportive care, psychologists and social workers who help patients and their families cope, and so on. This multidisciplinary collaboration is a complex but highly worthy process that permits the patient to access expert and experienced care as it is needed. It is also a complex system that requires communication and a degree of focus, guidance, and advocacy to assist patients to make the most of what may be available to them.

Equally relevant to procedural ethics is collaboration at the level of policy, research, and agencies. It is clear that a partnership approach is the most productive and efficient means of providing cancer control. Value of coordinated efforts is seen in all the documents related to cancer control and there are good reasons for this. Collaborative mechanisms that assist and permit agencies to support one another and avoid unnecessary overlaps are extremely important. For example, readily accessible patient information through adequate communication and electronic health records can make the process of obtaining appropriate care more accessible.

In research, collaborative methods that incorporate the goals and needs of patients will promote relevancy and effectiveness. Not all research needs to be collaborative in this way, but many communities have found it illuminates directions and contributes to more successful outcomes to begin by taking account of the perceptions and experiences of the potential benefactors of the research.

Researchers ought also to be encouraged to share information at early stages. This is not just a requirement of academic freedom, important in its own right, but it will also contribute to rapid growth of research and progress towards successful findings. Secretiveness in research is unethical if it obstructs or delays productive outcomes. Pressures from private interest groups that aim to profit from protecting intellectual property and patent interests will no doubt take issue with certain forms of collaboration. They need to consider that the first goal of the research is to aid those in need, and the second goal to promote shareholder profits. New ethical models of business practice demonstrate that high ethical standards, even to the extent of a little self-sacrifice is actually good for business and can contribute to financial success by promoting public faith and approbation [12]. Collaboration of this sort is beneficial to all.

Collaborative practice and mechanisms that assist collaboration can also lead to better policy decisions. The aims of knowledge translation are to encourage communication and understanding along the continuum from bench to bedside to facilitate more efficient process. In between, experts in scientific knowledge need to be able to collaborate with policy-makers in order to inform decisions about priorities to set, legislation to apply, invoke, or change. For example, laboratory research and clinical trials outcomes produce information necessary for making drug-funding decisions. Collaboration between the various players, researchers, trialists, clinicians, patients, and policy-makers, make it possible for policies to be based on evidence and reflect the realities of care delivery and living with the outcomes.

Finally, the mission statements of various cancer control projects emphasize how collaboration promotes efficiency and eliminates unnecessary redundancy. This is valuable as long as it is tempered by the realization that efficiency is not the same as stretching resources beyond capacity.

The limitations of procedural ethics

Procedural ethics is useful for guiding how decisions ought to be made, and the elements outlined here are arguably relevant to the creation and sustenance of a programme in cancer control. Each of the elements is important to ensuring that fair process is applied across a cancer control programme, ensuring inclusion, review, appeals, transparency, relevance, timeliness, and collaboration in policies that will be applied in a cancer control programme. Nevertheless, we must not place too much stock in procedure alone. The rules that guide decisions are important, but they offer no substantive insights as to what those decisions ought to be. They tell how we ought to conduct ourselves fairly, but not what it will mean to do so. In isolation, pure dedication to rule-following can even be dangerous. It lacks grounding in moral values that guide the substance of our choices. Some say that emphasis on process implies some sort of neutrality, which may be highly valuable, but not if applied blindly without compassion and vision. Applied this way, procedures leave some people unfairly treated, alienated and marginalized. Neither can it account for the degree to which values, ideologies, and other commitments are consciously or unconsciously applied to the process [13]. Explicit acknowledgement of value preferences will enhance the process by making it more fair, as well as making transparent why decisions are being made in the way that they are.

Substantive questions about the values that will be embraced and prioritized in a cancer control programme must therefore be addressed. Otherwise they are in danger of being ignored in favour of mere rule-following. While the elements of procedural ethics discussed herein are all very important, they are just a structure of rules that need to be fleshed out with substantive claims that demonstrate ideals such as how we value equity, liberty, and compassion. Part II offers an examination of the issues and concerns that will help illuminate what values ought to be encouraged in a programme for cancer control.

Part II: Substantive directions for ethics of cancer control

The many cancer control projects emerging globally govern themselves according to expressed visions and value statements [1,14–17]. Statements are listed on websites, in reports and posted on walls and serve the useful purpose of reminding contributors to, and beneficiaries of cancer control of the intentions, directions, priorities, and in some cases the limitations, of a given programme. They are there to help guide the motivations and actions of the players and clarify expectations. They are also meant to be embodied in the specific actions of individual actors in the programmes, and to be called upon to help resolve conflicts and make difficult decisions. While each project will express these values differently and select them differently, there is bound to be some overlap between them because the common goals that drive each project also help to define the values they endorse.

What are the values cancer control ought to embrace? How can they be put into action in a given decision? Existing social values and political contexts will have a role in defining the values embraced by a programme. The realities of the health care context, systems of payment, accessibility, and portion of gross national product available for health care are all factors that will impact on how values are selected. But values are dependent as much on ideals and normative beliefs as they are on actualities and existing social norms. So while the set socio-political context will shape values, they will also be tempered by critical analysis of how a programme ought to shape itself. The difference between how things are and how things ought to be needs to be attended to in the process of deciding what vision and values will direct a programme in cancer control.

In this section, the ideals and values of a just health care system will be explored. The proposal offers a partial vision of how things ought to be in cancer control, and are guided by a normative preference for justice in health care. This inevitably invites discussion of health equity, which in turn raises problems associated with social determinants of health and how they impact upon equity and justice. The social determinants are a useful framework for bringing social and health issues together; however, they raise a lingering philosophical problem related to privacy and self-determination which needs to be attended to in order to balance potentially paternalistic health protection-oriented values with values of personal liberty. This vision and balance must be examined here in order to attend to the very idea of cancer control.

Values of a just health care system

Literature on the foundations of a just health care system describes certain fundamental elements. Allen Buchanan [18] proposed the following as values any health care system ought to embrace:

1 Universal access

2 Access to an 'adequate level of care'

3 Access without excessive burdens

4 Fair distribution of financial costs to ensure 1 and 2

5 Fair distribution of the burdens of rationing

6 Capacity for improvement towards a more just system

This list is simple and probably not exhaustive. It arises from its own context of the US health care system, so Buchanan makes explicit reference to financial costs. Nevertheless, the content is still generally applicable and ought to be considered in determining the values that will guide a programme for cancer control. Buchanan's list is similar to a de facto consensus emergent from the visions in various cancer control statements [1,14–17]. The variety of cancer control strategies worldwide tend to address the same points using different terminology, and can be summarized in three ways: first, they endorse health equity in terms of access and affordability; second, they address the social distribution of elements that contribute to health, good or ill; and third, they incorporate concern for individual and shared effects of illness. I will examine some of these, although no further examination will be given to the last point on Buchanan's list because it has already been addressed in Part I in relation to the stability, review, and appeals processes required for the system to be consistent with the goals of procedural ethics. It is sufficient to restate that review, potential for change in response to new information, and an appeals process are all fundamental to the just process of health care programming, and therefore appropriate to cancer control programmes.

Equity of access

Access is universally recognized as a priority for cancer control programmes. The Canadian Strategy for Cancer Control, for example, emphasizes accessibility of care with explicit concerns regarding 'gaps between supply of services and demand', as well as responses to wait times and geographic availability [14]. This illustrates that the challenges of health equity involve not just scientific and clinical elements, but are also touched by social issues. As Nobel Prize winning economist, Amartya Sen notes [19], 'In any discussion of social equity and justice, illness and health must figure as a major concern'. So it is no surprise that discussions about illness and health raise social issues in their turn. Thus attempts to address equity tend to be closely associated with access in health ethics and cancer, which raises complex challenges that require multidisciplinary responses from clinical as well as social science perspectives.

Fair share

Health equity and access challenge the existence of gaps in availability, and are social issues of a particular type, namely that of resource allocation. Priorities for just distribution of resources are relevant to cancer control in more than one arena. First, in a global context, cancer control is only one health-related priority worldwide. While cancer is acknowledged as having one of the highest burdens [20], the combined burdens originating from other diseases and disasters are significant as well, and unfortunately will compete for the same limited resources. Second, within cancer programmes themselves resource allocation challenges arise, at the level of patient care (micro issues), at the level of institutional practice and inter-agency collaboration (meso issues), and at the level of policy (macro issues). Fair distribution among competitors is one aim of equity.

Prioritizing how resources will be distributed is a persistent question in health care, and will likely remain so. It is often expressed that simple equality of distribution of resources is insufficient for assessing resource distribution in health care [2,3]. For the most part this is because equal distribution assumes equal need, but the needs of patients and communities are never equal. They may have equal merit to be considered, but it is clear that different elements will impact on need in different ways. Most obvious is that some diseases require more, or more costly, interventions per individual patient, while other types of diseases are more common and therefore require that resources must be distributed more widely. Cancer is both more common and is rapidly becoming more costly to treat [20], so it might appear to deserve a greater share of health-related resources worldwide. However, other diseases clearly impose significant impact, especially as they tend to affect people who live with a greater share of other burdens and needs, (as will be explored as follows in relation to the social determinants of health and equity). The obvious competitors for global health resources include HIV/AIDS, tuberculosis, and malaria, diseases that dominate health care resources in lower and middle income countries (LMICs). These are diseases that touch specific communities so greatly that they cannot be ignored and they tend to affect people who live with other burdens (health-related and not), so their claim to need is palpable. It is the unfortunate truth that the needs of the beneficiaries of a cancer control programme are in direct competition with others in equal or greater need. Put like this, it is almost difficult to ask for any more.

Of course, there is always merit to a need, and no health-related area can be said to be deserving of absolutely no share of resources. But given the competitive atmosphere created by the combination of need and limited resources, it will always be necessary to make a choice. This means that there is a strong role for advocacy to promote adequate share of resources available for cancer research, prevention, diagnosis, care, and treatment. And because the same competition exists between stakeholders for the limited resources available to cancer, advocacy is as relevant to ensure fair access to resources among cancer-related needs as it is among wider health-related needs. Collaborative mechanisms can be employed to help disarm some of this competition by making more efficient use of resources and share the burdens of illness.

Indeed, in relation to equity of accessibility, Buchanan's list implies another social value that requires a kind of collaboration, and as such deserves explicit mention. The list is founded on an implicit value that it is worthwhile to share the costs of illness and the burden illness has on individuals, their families and communities. Such a normative claim is borne out in the way statistics are reported about the burden of cancer on society. For instance, in 2008 the World Health Organization identified cancer as a leading cause of death worldwide [20]. To say this is to make a claim that cancer is a global problem and therefore everyone shares its burden whether we realize it or not. Because WHO describes cancer as a global problem they can then make assertions regarding the importance of integrated care, partnerships, and the need to 'facilitate broad networks of cancer control partners at global, regional, and national levels'. These partnerships imply shared burden, suggesting that it is the responsibility of all to respond, or at least not obstruct, a response.

There is little doubt about the relevance and urgency of a global collaborative approach towards cancer control. Equitable access to prevention and treatment for all people touched by cancer should be recognized as a value in the field, although it is far from being a reality. Costs of care make it impossible for some to obtain the care they need, and force others to make impossible choices between health (life?) and devastating financial losses. It is therefore a requirement of just cancer control within Buchanan's model that element 4 be respected so that the burden of financial costs is shared or contained.

Private interests

The costs of cancer drugs and treatments have grown rapidly over the past decade. Where the price of care doubles and triples even within the span of a single patient's life, there is a clear need to try to contain costs [21]. Private industry's interests in recuperating research and development costs of new medical treatments is understandable to an extent, but not to the point of exploiting public and private insurers and, even more problematically, uninsured patients who must cover the ever increasing costs of medicines. Controls and constraints of excessive pricing are reasonable when patients' suffering is ongoing and lives are at stake. Here again, private industry ought to be encouraged to adopt ethical business models and consider the successes of companies that employ them [22]. Responsible ethical practices have been profitable for some private companies and allow share holders to profit and still keep a clear conscience. The rewards of such ethical practices will come, though sometimes in less than obvious ways. One way is as goodwill marketing that generates interests and trust in a company brand, and could in the long run increase other benefits such as public willingness to aid in research and development by enrolling in studies and contributing to tissue banks.

Cost control is a type of cost-burden sharing that will protect against individual patients being forced to make the choice between their health interests and their financial interests, both of which are further connected to personal responsibilities such as family obligation. A parent with cancer should not have to choose to sell the family home in order to obtain care, nor to forgo treatment in order to feed children. It is because of such scenarios that discussion of equity of access and distribution of resources reveals other significant moral issues associated with cancer control, namely the influence of the social determinants of health.

Health equity and the social determinants of health

Pauline Braveman and Sofia Gruskin [23, 24] helpfully describe equity in health care as follows:

> 'For the purposes of measurement and operationalisation, equity in health is the absence of systematic disparities in health (or in the major social determinants of health) between groups with different

levels of underlying social advantage/disadvantage—that is, wealth, power, or prestige. Inequities in health systematically put groups of people who are already socially disadvantaged (for example, by virtue of being poor, female, and/or members of a disenfranchised racial, ethnic, or religious group) at further disadvantage with respect to their health; health is essential to wellbeing and to overcoming other effects of social disadvantage'. [23].

Braveman and Gruskin thus emphasize the social aspects of equity and associate just access to care with the elements often referred to as the social determinants of health. Furthermore, Sen asserts that equity of distribution and access to the resources of health care are insufficient for rectifying the injustices of inequity in health. Social determinants of health will of course include the health impact of financial and resource disparities, but they also include much more besides. Literature related to the social determinants of health argues that health is closely related to social circumstances. It demonstrates that certain social factors will impact health positively while others have the opposite effect. Thus, as Sen argues, equity in health is more than just access to resources of health care but requires attention to social and environmental determinants as well as the factors that interfere with capability for human flourishing. He states,

> An adequate policy approach to health has to take note not only of the influences that come from general social and economic factors, but also from a variety of other parameters, such as personal disabilities, individual proneness to illness, epidemiological hazards of particular regions, the influence of climatic variations, and so on. A proper theory of health equity has to give these factors their due within the discipline of health equity. [19].

Braveman and Gruskin advise that disparities are connected with wealth, power, and prestige so systems ought to be assessed to determine 'whether national and international policies are leading towards or away from greater social justice in health'. Their definition of health equity, mentioned earlier, offers a means of measuring and evaluating health programmes to determine their effectiveness at improving the disparities created by the social factors which enhance or diminish health.

Lung cancer is an excellent case in point. While estimated to cause 1.4 million deaths a year and have the highest level of morbidity worldwide of any cancer [20], lung cancer is also relatively low resourced. There are fewer alternatives for lung cancer patients, compared to other disease types of high impact, most notably breast and prostate cancers which are widespread but fortunately carry less morbidity. Indisputably, success rates for treatment are lower than for example, breast cancer; so while breast cancer success tends to be measured in terms of years or months of additional life, success in lung cancer is usually measured in additional weeks or days. Why this disparity? Could it be merely the complexities of the molecular differences between the diseases? We can speculate that lung cancer carries the highest social stigma of the three most common cancers. Lung cancer is causally linked to smoking and therefore implicitly described as a lifestyle-related cancer that is believed to be self-inflicted, the result of so-called lifestyle choice. This is a strange sort of double standard as it ignores numerous factors related to the determinants of health, social, and otherwise. It ignores the addictive nature of tobacco for one, and the extreme difficulty most smokers have of quitting. It ignores social factors, the pressure to take up the habit, and for some unbearable stresses associated with trying to quit. It ignores genetic factors; why some people smoke very little and still develop cancer while others smoke two or three packs of cigarettes a day and never develop cancer? It also ignores important environmental factors that may contribute to or cause lung cancer, and account for the number of people who develop the disease without smoking a day in their lives. We are aware of all of these factors, of its high global impact, and yet lung cancer is still a stigmatized condition. Even lobbyists and advocates tend to focus on lifestyle links and smoking. The risk of this, however, is that funders, researchers, and the general public will not find lung cancer a sympathetic cause because if its connection to smoking and the implied weakness of will and self-inflicted nature of the disease. The danger is that the stigma means that while there are special initiatives in breast and prostate cancer, there are few directed specifically at lung cancer [25, 26]. For example, there is nothing like the proliferation of campaigns for lung cancer as there are for breast and prostate cancer; relatively little is heard from lung cancer campaigners except in relation to the tobacco industry and smoking regulation. The associated stigma is an additional social determinant for the health of lung cancer sufferers. Sympathetic attitudes aside, given what we know about the social determinants of what starts and keeps people smoking, and of the environmental and genetic factors that effect lung cancer, an equitable response requires we provide help for those factors as well and ensure fair access to resources available for what accounts for the most illness and death worldwide each year.

The ideas associated with social determinants of health are well founded. A project of cancer control needs to be as attentive to these social issues, such as stigma for reasons described in the example of lung cancer, power such as the power to advocate for fair access or cost controls, environment such as protection from pollution and toxins in our food and air, geography in relation to access to appropriate levels and quality of treatment, and distribution such as of funding in research, to name a few. However, the effects of the social determinants on health do raise a significant moral concern. If social or other determinants hold so much sway over our health and our lives, to the extent that we need help to overcome them, then where does personal liberty fit? We tend to take for granted the ways in which such obvious or subtle determinants place coercive constraints on personal liberty and private choices, and the social determinants of health help explain these factors. So is it sufficient justification to override a person's liberty to say smoke, or work in a high risk area, because by interfering with their self-regarding action we are protecting them and practicing cancer control?

The value of tolerance and personal liberty

Privacy is widely discussed in health ethics, most often related to access to and protection of confidential information, such as the gathering of personal health information for the purposes of research. There is, however, a wider sense of privacy that is relevant to the concerns earlier expressed on the idea of control. This notion of privacy is rooted in personal liberty, and is concerned with tolerance and individual freedom to choose how to live, be treated, and die. If we value this notion of privacy, and most liberal-based democracies do, then the idea of cancer control will have to be able to accommodate individual choice-making. This may seem obvious, but it is less so than one might initially think. On the surface, we perhaps do not need to be reminded that people ought to be free to make the choice to do the things laboratory science and epidemiological research tell us are good for the prevention and treatment of cancer. We don't need to be reminded that people have the right to choose to drink alcohol or not, to eat the foods they choose, or decide whether or not to exercise regularly. The preference seems to be to educate people about these options and let them choose for themselves, even if their choices involve high risk behaviour [27].

The notion of privacy tends therefore to be used more broadly than just as a reference to personal information. It is often applied to the private sphere including personal life and the choices we make. The private sphere is contrasted with the public sphere, and while the borders are blurred on the subject of ongoing philosophical debate, there are certain things that can be said to help refine the distinction. Private life is what concerns oneself and one's family in a way that a claim can be made of non-interference from public or outside forces. What happens in the family home, in one's personal life, is protected by laws that prevent interference from others, such as neighbours, the government, etc. The private sphere is protected to provide space for individual liberty and flourishing. The public sphere, on the other hand is shared, and it arguably requires certain constraints upon individual liberty to ensure greater good, such as taxation which contributes to the benefits of shared community health resources. My home is private and I can decorate it any way I choose; the park is public and I have to work with others to determine how it will be composed.

This form of privacy is closely related then to personal liberty. We tend to value personal liberty greatly, though different social and political ideologies protect it to varying degrees. At its extreme, the only time liberty is compromised in strict liberal societies, is if the free exercise of one person's liberty infringes upon the liberty of others [10]. Then the social contract of a libertarian community will permit the overriding of one person's freedom to protect the liberty interest of others. Mandatory quarantine programmes are this sort of overriding. If an argument can be made that all people who carry a particular kind of infection must be quarantined to prevent spread and protect the public, then the liberty to make a personal, self-concerning choice not to comply with the quarantine will be overridden and justified by the interests of others.

Where cancer control, or any type of control, is considered, there is a clear blurring of the private and the public. If priorities are going to be planned, resources allocated and liberties restricted, then the programme is making a clear instantiation of a preference for overriding of certain individual liberties and restriction of personal privacy. This is not necessarily a bad thing. It is a decision that could be made, and has been made in the past, where community decision-makers have chosen to favour some values over others, for example to favour public interests and public health over individual interests and personal liberty. A good example of this is the banning of smoking in cars with child passengers. For the most part, parents are at liberty to make decisions for their children, unless the choices are not in the best interest of the child, in which case parental liberty is overridden. In addition, some liberties will be enhanced by compromising with certain limitations, for example paying taxes that contribute to social benefits such as public schools and hospitals.

In their book *Health Promotion: Models and Values*, Robin Downie, Carol Fyfe, and Andrew Tannahill [27] draw a helpful distinction between health protection on the one hand and prevention, promotion, and education on the other. The chief distinction between them is that while promotion, prevention, and education are seen as voluntary measures that can be offered to individuals, and in which they may choose to partake or not (e.g. campaigns on healthy eating, information on the preventive role of exercise in cancer control, and voluntary human papilloma virus [HPV] vaccination programmes),

> Health protection comprises legal or fiscal controls, other regulations and policies, and voluntary codes of practice, aimed at the enhancement of positive health and the prevention of ill health. [27, p. 51].

Health protection, in this sense, is meant 'to make healthy choices easier', such as workplace safety initiatives that legally enforce safety standards and devices. While they override a certain personal liberty to choose to take precautions or not, they also protect employees from feeling pressure to take risks that would compromise their health. To what extent health protection measures ought to be imposed is a challenge of balance between personal liberty to choose and protection via the kind of control which enhances health by decreasing the likelihood that individuals will

> encounter hazards in the environment, and that they will behave in an unhealthful manner, while increasing their chances of living in a positively healthful environment and having a lifestyle which promotes positive health. [27, p 51].

Sen has argued for a framework that promotes capabilities for achieving and maintaining human flourishing and includes health as one of the chief elements of this capabilities index [19]. It would be consistent with this that the sorts of restrictions described previously as health protective are justifiable because they promote the interests of good health and help to counter the potentially coercive or pervasive social and environmental forces that make ill health unavoidable. So while privacy and personal liberty are valued, they can be protected and enhanced by health protection measures. When these measures are aimed at external forces such as controlling pollution, the protection is more easily enforced. Control of more individual behaviours such as healthy eating is more obtrusive to individual privacy and is less desirable. Focus ought to be given to controlling external factors like pollution, and compromise internal factors only when it is certain to enhance future good and extend personal liberty.

For Sen [19] and Downie [27] and many others, the ability to achieve and maintain good health is in and of itself a value worthy of promotion. In some cases it may be just an instrumental value, not valued in its own right but because of its role in promoting human flourishing. However, more recently, the value of good health has taken on independent worth as a fundamental good to be promoted for its own sake. The extent to which personal liberty ought to be overridden to achieve good health, or promote the capabilities of achieving good health, is negotiable. But we probably ought to be cautious of too much overriding of personal choice and instead enhance opportunity for creating environments and systems which increase our capabilities to improve and sustain individual health. Thus control of cancer should not be confused with control of personal liberty.

Summary

In summary the following ethical concerns have been raised in this chapter. The exploration is not intended to be exhaustive but to enliven debate, and draw attention to ethically relevant considerations related to cancer control.

- A just approach to cancer control requires ethical procedures and appeal to certain moral values.
- Some elements of procedural ethics are proposed based on their relevance to cancer control or as they emerge from cancer control strategies.
- The limitations of procedural ethics demonstrate how process is not enough on its own to guide a just system.
- Also required are values, existing and normative, that will give substantive direction to a programme.
- Equity is a significant moral value in cancer control.
- Equity requires consideration of multiple aspects including resources, geography, accessibility, inclusion of rare as well as common diseases, and even at the level of research such as access to funding.
- Interests of private industry ought not to override or direct the priorities of cancer control.
- Social determinants of health include elements relevant to health equity problems beyond just financial distribution.
- Controlling some of these factors may be desirable and consistent with valuing health.
- However, control of cancer should not be confused with control of personal liberty.

References

1 Public Health Agency of Canada. *Centre for Chronic Disease Prevention and Control: Cancer.* Available from: http://www.phac-aspc.gc.ca/ccdpc-cpcmc/cancer/pub_e.html (accessed January 30, 2009).

2 Rawls J (1971). *A Theory of Justice.* Harvard University Press, Cambridge, Mass.

3 Rawls J (2001). *Justice as Fairness: A Restatement.* Harvard University Press, Cambridge, Mass.

4 Daniels N (2000). Accountability for reasonableness: Establishing a fair process for priority setting is easier than agreeing on principles. *BMJ*, **321**(7272):1300–01.

5 Harris MG (2005). *Managing Health Services*, p. 55. Elsevier, Australia, Available from: http://books. google.ca/books?id=yA2SR4DgU5wC&pg=PA54&lpg=PA54&dq=procedural+ethics&source= web&ots=bkmS0V3t8u&sig=7pF-WierqvLRRTjbn1lflgWAR8k&hl=en&sa=X&oi=book_ result&resnum=4&ct=result (accessed February 1, 2009).

6 Solum LB (2004). *Procedural Justice.* U San Diego Law & Econ Research Paper No. 04-02. Available from: http://ssrn.com/abstract=508282 or DOI: 10.2139/ssrn.508282 (accessed February 1, 2009).

7 Abelson J, Forest P-G, Eyles J, Smith P, Martin E & Gauvin F-P (2003). Deliberations about deliberative methods: issues in the design and evaluation of public participation processes. *Soc Sci Med*, **57**(2):239–51.

8 Romanow R (2002). *Building on Values: The Future of Health Care in Canada – Final Report.* Available from: http://healthcoalition.ca/romanow-report.pdf (accessed January 31, 2009).

9 Thompson P & Strauss S (2000). Research ethics for molecular silviculture. In S. Jain & C. Minocha (eds) *Molecular Biology of Woody Plants*, pp. 485–511. Kluwer Academic Publishers, Dordrecht, Netherlands.

10 Mill JS (1869). *On Liberty.* Longman, Roberts & Green, Bartleby.com, London. 1999. Available from: http://www.bartleby.com/130/ (accessed January 31, 2009).

11 Canada Health Act (R.S., 1985, c. C-6). Available from: http://laws.justice.gc.ca/en/showtdm/cs/C-6 (accessed January 31, 2009).

12 Gates BM (2008). Capitalism more creative. *TIME Magazine*, July 31, 2008. Available from: http://www.time.com/time/business/article/0,8599,1828069,00.html.

13 Sandel M (1998). *Democracy's Discontent.* Harvard University Press, Cambridge, MA.

14 Canadian Strategy for Cancer Control *Canadian Council for Cancer Control Governance Policies.* Available from: http://www.neutropenia.ca/community/cancer_control.html (accessed February 1, 2009).

15 Cancer Australia. Overview. Available from: http://www.canceraustralia.gov.au/about-us/overview.aspx (accessed February 1, 2009).

16 The NHS Cancer Plan: a plan for investment, a plan for reform 2000. Available from: http://www. dh.gov.uk/en/Publicationsandstatistics/Publications/PublicationsPolicyAndGuidance/Browsable/ DH_4098139 (accessed February 1, 2009).

17 Cancer Control P.L.A.N.E.T. Available from: http://cancercontrolplanet.cancer.gov/index.html (accessed February 1, 2009).

18 Buchanan A (1995). Privatization and just health care. *Bioethics*, **9**:220–39.

19 Sen A (2002). Why health equity? *Health Economics*, **11**(8):659–66.

20 World Health Organization. *Cancer.* Available from: http://www.who.int/topics/cancer/en/ (accessed February 1, 2009).

21 Sticker shock a side effect of cancer remedies: As chemo prices rise, doctors get first guidelines on discussing affordability, Associated Press March 24, 2008. Available from: http://www.msnbc.msn.com/ id/23783216/ (accessed January 31, 2009).

22 Cohen-Kohler JC, Forman L, & Lipkus N (2008). Addressing legal and political barriers to global pharmaceutical access: options for remedying the impact of the Agreement on Trade-Related Aspects of Intellectual Property Rights (TRIPS) and the imposition of TRIPS-plus standards. *Health Econ Policy Law*, **3**(Pt 3):229–56.

23 Braveman P & Gruskin S (2003). Defining equity in health. *J Epidemiol Community Health*, **57**:254–58.

24 Braveman P & Gruskin S (2003) Poverty, equity, human rights and health. *Bulletin of the World Health Organization*, **81**(7). Available from: http://www.scielosp.org/scielo.php?pid=S0042-96862003000700013&script=sci_arttext&tlng=en (accessed February 1, 2009).

25 Lung Cancer Alliance (2008). Lung cancer still lowest in federal funding. Available from: http://www.reuters.com/article/pressRelease/idUS213133+16-May-2008+PRN20080516 (accessed April 24, 2009).

26 Richardson H (2005). 'Toleration', *Internet Encyclopedia of Philosophy*. Available from: http://www.iep.utm.edu/t/tolerati.htm (accessed February 1, 2009).

27 Downie RS, Fyfe C, & Tannahill A (1990). *Health Promotion: Models and Values*. Oxford University Press, Oxford.

Chapter 21

Integrating cancer control with control of other non-communicable diseases

Robert Burton, Jerzy Leowski Jr, Maximilian de Courten[1]

The World Health Organization (WHO) estimates for 2005 indicated that 61 per cent of the 58 million deaths from all causes worldwide were due to chronic, non-communicable diseases (NCD), with cardio-vascular diseases (CVD) (17.5 million), cancer (7.6 million) and chronic obstructive pulmonary diseases (COPD) (4 million) accounting for half of all deaths (Figure 21.1).

The WHO has pointed out that 80 per cent of CVD and type 2 diabetes, and 40 per cent of cancer, could be avoided through effective prevention targeting their common behavioural risk factors: tobacco use, unhealthy nutrition, and physical inactivity leading to obesity [1]. Furthermore, about 20 per cent of cancer is caused by chronic infections and vaccines are currently available which could prevent almost half of these cancers, which are caused by the hepatitis B virus and strains 16 and 18 of the human papilloma virus (HPV) family (see Chapter 6).

In 2008, the WHO action plan for the Global Strategy for the Prevention and Control of NCD [2] was endorsed by more than 190 governments at the Sixty-first World Health Assembly [3]. This plan aims to guide and catalyze an intersectoral and multilevel response to NCD, with a particular focus on low and middle income countries and on vulnerable population groups. This action plan has six key objectives, each with actions requested of WHO, member states, and international partners. The objectives are, in summary:

1 To raise the priority accorded to NCD in development work, and to integrate their prevention and control into policies across government departments

2 To establish and strengthen national policies and plans for the prevention and control of NCD

3 To promote interventions to reduce the main shared modifiable risk factors for NCD: tobacco use, unhealthy diets, physical inactivity, and harmful use of alcohol

4 To promote research for the prevention and control of NCD

5 To promote partnerships for the prevention and control of NCD

6 To monitor NCD and their determinants and evaluate progress at the national, regional and global levels

[1] Robert C. Burton MD, PhD, FAFPHM, Professor, School of Public Health and Preventive Medicine, Monash University, Melbourne, Victoria, Australia; Jerzy Leowski Jr, MD, Regional Adviser, Non-communicable Diseases, World Health Organization, Regional Office for South-East Asia, New Delhi, India; Maximilian de Courten MD, MPH, Associate Professor of Clinical Epidemiology, School of Public Health and Preventive Medicine, Monash University, Melbourne, Victoria, Australia.

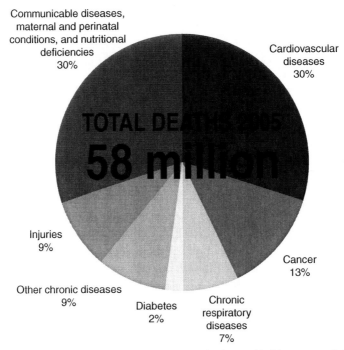

Fig. 21.1 Non-communicable diseases now cause most deaths worldwide; causes of death, worldwide.
Source: From World Health Organization (2005) [1, p. 38].

This generic direction applies across all the four major chronic NCD: CVD, cancer, COPD, and diabetes. This chapter binds this prescription more tightly to cancer and describes why the cancer control movement, while working for its specific objectives, may benefit from embracing integrated NCD prevention and control approaches in common areas, from addressing the causes of inequity to synergizing with the movement to renew primary health care. Certain important areas where cancer control could be better integrated with other major NCD programmes will be considered. These include those which focus on health promotion and on the equitable protection and maintenance of the health of entire populations: primordial and primary prevention; coordinated multisectoral actions which improve health; and health sector actions on early detection/screening, and in maintaining and supporting people with NCD in their communities. The proportion of cancer worldwide that can be prevented through actions which control chronic infections will not be considered (see Chapter 6). However, integration of some of these actions into immunization programmes and other strategies which target chronic infections like HIV/AIDS and tuberculosis requires further strengthening. Specific diagnostic technologies and treatments of the various cancers, CVD, COPD, and diabetes, and the infrastructure and skilled workforces needed, will not be considered outside of the context of the systems needed for early detection/screening and palliation of NCD. Therefore, in general, hospital- and specialist-based care of individual NCD will not be considered.

In the context of cancer specifically, the WHO and the International Union Against Cancer (UICC])estimated that in the year 2002 there were 10.9 million new cases of cancer (incidence]), 6.7 million cancer deaths (mortality), and 24.6 million people living with a diagnosis of cancer [4]. Therefore, the global mortality: incidence ratio was 0.66, indicating that most people who were diagnosed with cancer died of it, highlighting the global need for effective community-based palliative care. Of particular note [5], is that this ratio is highest for males in developing countries (e.g. Egypt – 0.85) and lowest for females in the most developed countries (e.g. 0.35 – United States and Australia). Without effective actions on cancer prevention and early detection/screening, the WHO and UICC estimate that there will be 16 million new cases of cancer and 10.3 million deaths in the year 2020, with two-thirds of this cancer burden falling on developing countries [4].

Alarmed by rising trends of cancer-risk factors and the growing burden of cancer worldwide, in particular in developing countries, the Fifty-eight World Health Assembly passed, in 2005, a resolution urging member states, amongst other things, to integrate National Cancer Control Plans (NCCP) into existing health systems, and to consider an approach in the planning, implementation, and evaluation phases of cancer control that involves all key stakeholders representing governmental, nongovernmental, and community-based organizations [6]. NCCP and related programmes have been developed in many countries throughout the world in line with policies and managerial guidelines proposed by the WHO [7]. The programmes are often maintained as vertical structures closely linked to, and directed and managed by, specialized oncology institutes and centres. The positive implication of this fact is that programmes are backed by highly qualified professionals and are based on existing physical infrastructure which promotes scientific soundness of programmes and their logistical sustainability. The other implication, however, is that cancer programmes are often more orientated to cancer treatment and research than to other population health needs. As a consequence cancer surveillance, health promotion, population-based primary and secondary prevention, and palliative care components are often underdeveloped. Cancer programmes themselves may be inadequately integrated within overall health systems, and fail to identify and involve important stakeholders in governmental sectors beyond health as well as potential partners located in the private sector and representing civil society.

It is desirable that cancer control be better integrated with other major NCD programmes in the areas which focus on health promotion and on the equitable protection and maintenance of health of entire populations. Cancer should be better addressed in a well-coordinated and comprehensive way by consideration of the shared social, economic, and physical environmental determinants and the common risk factors of all major NCD. To be effective and efficient cancer control needs to be founded on strong public health infrastructure and have operating mechanisms which ensure multisectoral and interdisciplinary coordination at national, regional, and local levels. For at least five billion of the estimated 6.4 billion humans of the planet (75+ per cent) whole population control of NCD in general, and cancer specifically, is limited largely to the prevention of exposure to risk factors for which governments can legislate and regulate, for example through taxation of tobacco and prohibition of advertising tobacco use, and to the provision of oral morphine for palliating chronic pain. Improvements in socio-economic status can be achieved by governments through long term infrastructure and workforce investments which address inequities.

The health care sector has a role in supporting these government actions and implementing palliative care initiatives. In addition, as primary health care becomes available at the whole population level, programmes of primary prevention, largely behavioural but increasingly 'medical', as through immunization and early detection and treatment of secondary risk factors like cervical dysplasia and hypertension become possible. Wealthier sectors of developing countries usually enjoy these improvements in NCD control first, and also have first access to the available curative and supportive treatment and control of the NCD themselves; this 'inequity transition' is discussed further later in this chapter. In this respect, their opportunities to avoid and be successfully treated for NCD are akin to populations of developed countries, and so they are included in the estimated 1.4 billion people mentioned earlier. These more fortunate individuals and populations are not the primary focus of this chapter. The scenarios described, and NCD control measures considered, are relevant to all, but the focus here is on developing countries and the challenges they face. However, some developing countries are better placed to confront the coming NCD epidemic in several regards than some developed countries, where the epidemic is now well established. For example, some developing countries have well developed medical and non-medical primary health care systems which have brought major improvements in maternal and child health to large populations. These services can be re-orientated quickly to begin population NCD primary and secondary risk factor prevention, identification, and treatment, particularly if falling birth rates in these countries free up resources. Successful population-based demonstration projects have been conducted in Indonesia, Iran, and Philippines, among others, to reorientate such services to the prevention of NCD. For palliation of NCD, and particularly cancer causing pain, well established and externally-funded community support systems for patients with advanced HIV/AIDS in certain developing countries, for example Tanzania, have the potential to be further developed to expand home-based palliative care also to cancer patients.

It is in this context that this chapter argues for better governance in the control of the environmental and social risk factors for NCD and social inequalities, and improvements in systems for preventing, diagnosing early and treating modifiable and intermediate NCD risk factors and NCD themselves (see Figure 21.2) and finally palliating NCD in their terminal phases. The government actions and systems needed are common to all major NCD, albeit, for example, that screening tests for different cancers are as different between themselves as they are from screening tests for other NCD.

Shared modifiable social, environmental, and behavioural determinants

A model of causation

There are two complementary models of causation of NCD that can be used to develop synergistic approaches to integrated intervention.

The WHO report on 'Preventing Chronic Disease: A Vital Investment' [1] proposed a model of causation that has gained wide currency (Figure 21.2).

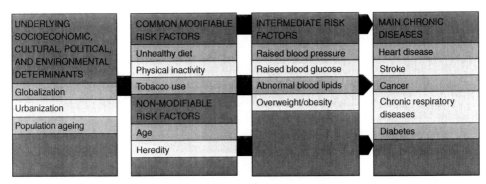

Fig. 21.2 The chain of causation of non-communicable diseases.
Source: From World Health Organization [1, p. 48].

The burden of NCD arises from exposure to behavioural and physiological risks modified by the effects of sex, age, and genes. The risky behaviours (tobacco smoking, unhealthy diet, physical inactivity, and the harmful use of alcohol) in turn arise out of personal choices facilitated or constrained by the policy, physical, cultural, and price environments within which people live. These environments have a micro- and a macro-dimension, for instance ranging at the micro-end from the price and choice of foods available to a community or household to the macro-effects of globalization, urbanization and demographic transition.

Evidence from the world of cancer and cardiovascular disease suggests that such a conventional model is extremely successful in explaining both the rise and, in some cases, the fall of these epidemics. The worldwide downward trend in gastric cancer incidence and mortality in many of the most developed countries began about 1950 when the widespread introduction of domestic refrigerators and improvements in animal slaughtering practices resulted in meat increasingly being stored fresh before eating; salting, drying, smoking, and other forms of meat preservation were no longer the norm [8]. This was a macro-consequence of industrialization and improved agriculture, not the result of a public health intervention. The classic curves of the rise and fall of male lung cancer in various developed countries' populations mirrored the rise and fall of tobacco smoking, albeit the peak of cancer mortality followed two decades or more after the peak male smoking prevalence [9]. This illustrates the powerful causal link between the two and the potential for primary prevention and the effectiveness of public (population) health actions. The IMPACT model [10] ascribed around 58 per cent of the decline in coronary heart disease in England and Wales to the downward trend in population risk factors, with similar results reported for other industrialized countries. While there is some controversy about the effectiveness of multiple risk factor interventions at community level [11,12], there is convincing evidence that population level interventions on specific risk factors such as tobacco and salt are both effective and cost-effective [13]. The conventional population-level risk factors explain about 75 per cent of new cases of coronary heart disease [14] and provide ample scope for effective primary prevention; a potential health improvement that would extend, through common risk factors, to many cancers.

The causation of inequity

Recently there has been intensified attention to the issue of inequity, and the relative burdens of disease. The WHO Commission on Social Determinants of Health has reported on a synthesis of the last decades of research on the social gradient in health [15]. This gradient is important for three reasons:

- *Human Rights Approach*: social gradients in health reflect unfairness in society where segments of the population are denied the right to the full enjoyment of health that is possible in their country

- *Direct Causation*: there is evidence that the social gradients themselves operate through various behavioural, psychological, and physiological mechanisms, and directly cause corresponding 'disease gradients' in society

- *Development Agenda*: in a global environment the development community is concerned primarily with economic development and poverty alleviation, and is fixed on a narrowly focused health agenda, to the extent that the Millennium Development Goals even exclude any overt NCD-related goals or targets [16]. The demonstration of disproportionate NCD burdens in poor populations is an important advocacy point to address this blind spot in policy, and to redress it.

The inequity transition

The issue of inequity in NCD is further complicated by what can be termed an 'inequity transition'. As a country develops economically, the first segments in society to suffer from the NCD epidemic are the newly affluent and the urban populations, those with higher socio-economic status. These groups are then the first ones to have better access to the means and the skills to control their own risk and are the first to experience improvements, whether through better prevention and/or better treatment. The poorer segments of society acquire these risks in turn and the familiar gradients prevalent in industrialized countries then result, leading to an 'inequity transition', a migration of NCD burden into poorer countries and disadvantaged communities. This pattern is witnessed in examples as different as the high rates of premature death in disadvantaged Russian men [17] or the high risk of diabetes in rural Cambodia [18]. These relative burdens are more difficult to address since they are compounded by the relative lack of access to health services and by poor income, poor neighbourhoods, poor childhood experience, and low levels of education among other constraints, all of which are beyond the control of the individual or the health sector to improve. In essence this transition suggests that focusing on a narrow range of diseases in developing countries may simply switch the dominant cause of premature mortality and preventable morbidity from infections now, to NCD later, without achieving a true improvement in overall adult population health. The NCD 'epidemic' now sweeping the world is in large part a result of the ageing of populations, which unlike the environmental, socio-economic, and behavioural determinants of health, cannot be directly addressed.

A synthesis

Each of the two models described in the earlier paragraphs, socio-economic/environmental and behavioural, has a set of points for intervention and, barring an ideological bias that favours one approach over the other, both need to be adopted via an integrated rationale for action to reduce the burden of cancer and other NCD and their inequitable distribution in society.

The WHO Commission on Social Determinants of Health, amongst other work, set up a series of Knowledge Networks that delved deeply into some aspects of the evidence for action on health inequities. One of the networks dealt with the 'Priority Public Health Conditions' and specifically considered the question of how vertical programmes (such as NCD prevention and control) would change if they adopted an equity lens. While the network did not formally study cancer control, this section will describe and adapt the model they used to tease out some of the cancer-related implications.

The network elaborated a cascade of causal influences that can be used in three ways: to describe and analyse inequity, to generate options for intervention, and to measure the differences and monitor progress of any programme of action. The determinants of health cascade through socio-economic position, exposure to risk, vulnerability to that exposure, to the health outcomes and their different consequences on the ability to function in society, on length of life, and on quality of life. These implications are briefly discussed with examples.

Differential socio-economic position

Social standing is a determinant of the risks to which groups are exposed and of the ability to protect themselves against their effects. Development policies, trade, education, and employment policies, among others, set the context for health. While they are outside the remit of the health sector, addressing these 'causes of the causes' [19] through intersectoral action and advocacy must be a foundation for work to reduce inequities.

Differential exposure

The broader contexts for health translate into more direct exposure to risk and protective factors. Trade, fiscal, and marketing policies set the levels of access to healthy foods and their prices. Employment and welfare policies affect the level to which groups have access to employment and occupational health and safety as well as access to support in unemployment. Urban planning policies determine the ease and safety of physical activity in different communities.

Differential vulnerability

The exposures to risk tend to cluster together in ways that are socially determined. The condition of being a single parent, in an insecure inner city, relatively isolated, with temporary or episodic employment, poorer quality housing, eating a cheap fast food diet, smoking and abusing alcohol, is not simply a stereotype but is a way of life for many groups in society. The ability to respond to such a set of risks is also socially determined. Higher social standing gives one the ability to control exposure to some risks, to predict other risks, to draw on material reserves to cushion periods of difficulty, and to connect with social networks with a larger number of strong and weak ties to sources of help.

Differential health outcome

The effects of these three sets of social influences are then seen in the plethora of reports of gradients in the incidence and burden of ill health. The clustering of risks is a structural influence leading to greater incidence of disease. The relative difficulties of accessing health care compound this effect by ensuring that disease presents to the health service later or not at all.

Differential consequences

All of this then impacts on the length and quality of life and of the person's potential for function-ing in society. Loss of earnings, loss of schooling, and catastrophic costs of health care, can lead to a downward spiral of negative influences on the individual and the household.

A shift in emphasis

Taking note of the burden of NCD, in aggregate terms and in the relative distribution across societies, it is valid to ask a classic question: 'So what?' The NCD epidemic is large and growing, and the burden is disproportionately affecting socially disadvantaged groups. Beyond serving as a frame for research and 'occupational therapy for epidemiologists' [14], what are the lessons that can be drawn for action? Most importantly, what lessons can be drawn that may be relevant to the health sector, within which most cancer control workers are located?

The World Health Report of 2008 [20] proposes that four shifts in emphasis (four 'reforms') are needed and they would be well-suited for consideration by the cancer control community:

1 *Reforms in favour of promoting equity*: the thrust here is to move to universal coverage and social health protection. A major barrier to equity is the barrier to access at least a basic package of primary preventive, curative, and palliative services at community level without incurring catastrophic financial consequences.

2 *Reforms in favour of people-centred care*: focusing health care at the primary level means focusing on the needs and expectations of people. This includes the delivery of care not simply as a set of discrete, evidence-based interventions, but more comprehensively as a coordinated service provided by a multidisciplinary team that is close to the community, with care that is organized around a person's needs rather than the separate stages of a given disease.

3 *Reforms in favour of more reliable health systems*: this is a management reform that steers away from totally centralized planning of health care yet not completely towards a laissez-faire model where health care access is totally market driven. The leadership of the health sector needs to be felt in ensuring that a coherent, evidence-based, socially just package of primary prevention and care is accessible by all through whatever public and private system is appropriate for the country.

4 *Reforms in policy*: this line of action requires the health sector and health advocates to take on the task of providing for the health of communities by addressing the policy environment, by linking primary care and public health activities, and by advocating for broader intersectoral actions ranging from school curricula through to a country's trade policies.

The rest of this chapter provides an illustration of the ways in which these models and reforms apply in the context of the cancer control movement as it makes its own journey from:

- A curative approach, to the a more risk-oriented public health and preventive approach
- A narrow cancer focus, to an integrated NCD focus based on a recognition of common risks
- A risk-oriented approach, to a wider social justice and equity-oriented approach
- A health sector-orientation to a broader involvement and advocacy for wider social change

Systems that improve health

The adoption of unhealthy behaviours by large segments of populations, resulting in the observed pandemic of CVD, cancer, COPD, diabetes and other common NCD is often argued to be a well-informed decision taken autonomously by individual members of the population. This plausible micro-perspective is being increasingly challenged from the public health point of view. The public health macro-standpoint claims that man-made socio-economic, psycho-social, cultural, political, and physical environments in which people live, work, and play limit the liberty of individuals to exercise true freedom in making informed behavioural choices and expose entire populations to multiple, powerful health-harming influences. From this perspective, people with NCD are seen as numerous, unlucky members of the society that, together with their families, bear direct, serious, often deadly consequences of the adoption of unhealthy social and behavioural norms by entire populations.

Focus on sick individuals and on those at very high risk of developing NCD, a prevailing strategy of contemporary health systems, results in prioritizing actions that address consequences rather than their underlying causes. This approach is inconsistent with public health paradigm based on principles of health promotion and population-based prevention. Since unhealthy human behaviours stem from specific milieu their modification through policy, social, economic, and environmental interventions is less expensive and more permanent than individual-level lifestyle change.

Efforts of health authorities to prevent and control NCD are often centred on identifying and managing individuals with a particular priority disease (e.g. cancer, CVD, COPD, etc.) or particular risk factor (tobacco consumption, high blood pressure, high cholesterol level, etc.). The coverage, hence public health impact, of applying such vertical strategies is limited. Various vertical NCD programmes compete for scarce health resources. They are heavily biased towards management of cases identified, despite all efforts, at rather advanced stage of disease, when effectiveness of intervention is limited even with engagement of highly specialized health workforce and sophisticated medical technology at high, hardly affordable cost. These programmes tend to be poorly coordinated, strongly entrenched within health services,and dominated by medical super-specialists and clinical researchers.

WHO's Framework Convention on Tobacco Control (FCTC) and the Global Strategy on Diet, Physical Activity and Health (DPAS) aim to guide integrated, multisectoral efforts to implement evidence-based interventions on common modifiable NCD risk factors and their determinants [21,22]. Involvement of health and non-health, public and private, stakeholders as well as civil society groups and international partners is seen as a basic prerequisite to generate efficiencies, minimize health inequities, and reduce disease burden.

The concept of multisectoral, multidisciplinary, and multilevel collaboration for integrated prevention and control of NCD is not new and is broadly accepted by the public health community. Application of integrated and well-coordinated approaches is expected to yield public health and economic benefits through avoidance of duplicative actions, minimizing rivalry for territories, pooling existing resources, improving chances to mobilize more resources, maximizing outcomes of high level advocacy, and identifying and addressing grey and border areas.

While establishing functional collaborative interfaces and modalities to involve other than health sectors in debate and coordinated action for population-based prevention of NCD, it is equally important to re-examine and strengthen intrasectoral (within health sector) collaboration. It is imperative to strengthen interaction between vertical disease or risk factor-specific NCD projects and programmes especially around advocacy, health policy development, surveillance, community and primary health care-based interventions, research and monitoring, and evaluation. Good coordination between vertical NCD programmes and with other health-related programmes such as health promotion, environmental and occupational health, nutrition, health information systems, child and adolescent health, reproductive health, immunization, etc. may result in better positioning of NCD prevention and control priorities within overall national health development plans.

As socio-economic, cultural, political, and other determinants of NCD reside largely outside the conventionally understood domain of health systems, the effective and efficient action to prevent these diseases requires a whole of government approach involving health and non-health sectors.

Collaboration with virtually all governmental sectors may bring efficiencies and smooth the progress in integrating the prevention of chronic diseases into an overall national socio-economic development policy/plan/agenda. The target sectors include amongst others finance, agriculture, food and other industry, trade and commerce, information and media, education, social welfare, transportation, infrastructure, sports and recreation, justice and law enforcement, internal affairs, and defence. In the process of establishing collaborative platforms, synergies in mandates and goals of potential partners need to be identified, existing legal and structural frames and mechanisms examined, and the capacity and capability of workforces to act together in addressing health objectives enhanced.

NCD prevention and control programmes require coordination with stakeholders beyond the government. Stakeholders from private sector and civil society add human and financial resources and bring valuable perspectives to the debate on priorities and the best ways to address them. International organizations and national civil society groups such as non-governmental organizations, professional and research community associations, and philanthropies are instrumental in the wide dissemination of information and in influencing behaviour of individuals. They lead grass-roots mobilization, organize campaigns and events that raise awareness, mobilize resources, plan and implement community-based activities, and contribute to improving health care delivery.

The private sector, such as the food industry and retailers, advertising and recreation businesses, pharmaceutical companies, the media, and others have an important role in promoting healthy behaviour. Assuming public health accountability by partners from the private sector, through developing and adopting health-enhancing self-regulation and other actions, could bring considerable health benefits to the people.

Recent reviews of evidence on cost-effective interventions for prevention and control of major NCD are available elsewhere [1,23,24]. It is beyond the scope of this chapter to systematically discuss the possible role of each sector and partner in implementing these interventions. Some examples related to application of *regulatory, fiscal, and marketing mechanisms* given hereunder illustrate the wide array of possible collaborative actions.

Legislative measures are more cost-effective than voluntary measures due to greater compliance [24]. At international level, the WHO FCTC is the only existing legal instrument specifically designed to target an important cause of chronic diseases [21]. This multilateral treaty, with more than 150 parties, presents a blueprint for countries to reduce both the supply and demand for tobacco. The International Health Regulations, which came into force in 2007, aim to help the international community prevent and respond to acute public health risks, but do not address health risks related to chronic diseases [25]. At the national level it is desirable to have the existing legislative and regulatory acts reviewed from the perspective of their impact on molding unhealthy environments. It is also important to examine and address the common problem of poor enforcement of existing tobacco, alcohol, and food-related legislation.

Taxation and other fiscal mechanisms are considered an effective tool in reducing demand and consumption of manufactured cigarettes, alcohol, and certain unhealthy food products. The significant reduction in coronary heart disease observed in Poland between 1991 and 2002 came from fiscal policy to reduce subsidies for butter and lard, which switched consumption from saturated to polyunsaturated fats [26]. Increasing the price of tobacco through higher taxes is the single most effective way to decrease consumption [27]. The health effects of fiscal policies aimed at improving health need to be closely monitored in order to put in place early warning mechanisms. For example in India, where handmade bidis and gutka taxed at a lower rate than machine-made tobacco products dominate the tobacco market, increase of taxes for manufactured cigarettes without concomitant taxation of other tobacco products led smokers to further shift to cheaper alternatives.

As developed countries have implemented successful tobacco control policies that led to declines in tobacco use, the tobacco industry, the main vector of the global tobacco epidemic, has shifted its attention to markets in developing countries. Its efforts to depict itself as a socially responsible partner via schemes aimed at improving labour practices and public philanthropy are clearly driven by corporate self-interest rather than social responsibility [28].

As a result of trade liberalization, diets throughout the world became increasingly similar. Large multinational companies, through global marketing of food products, control much of what people eat. It is not uncommon that contemporary populations consume more Coca Cola than milk [29]. The overarching aim of the food industry is to increase demand and sales of their products and generate profits. The convenience and availability of energy-dense foods offered globally has contributed to the epidemics of obesity [30]. In this context the food industry is taking progressive efforts to depict itself as a responsible stakeholder in multisectoral actions to prevent and control NCD.

In support of the WHO Global Strategy on Diet, Physical Activity, and Health (DPAS) the major international food and non-alcoholic beverage companies pledged to take steps to re-formulate existing products (e.g. altering composition by reducing salt and trans-fats), develop innovations that offer healthier options to consumers, and provide more and clearer information about the nutritional composition of products. They promised also to adopt voluntary measures on the marketing and advertising of food and beverages and promote healthier lifestyle in the workplace. These self-regulation actions seem to have so far rather limited coverage and scope.

Moreover, they do not involve small- and middle-sized food companies. The impact of these declarations is still to be demonstrated.

In view of pandemics of NCD, issues related to the commercial promotion of foods high in saturated fat, trans-fatty acids, sugars and salt, and of non-alcoholic beverages are receiving growing attention. Various civil society groups have proposed the development of an international code on marketing of food and non-alcoholic beverages to children. The WHO is in process of developing a set of recommendations in this regard.

The underlying economic, psycho-social, cultural, and political determinants of NCD, such as those related to rapid globalization and trade liberalization, uncontrolled urbanization, improved communication and technology, and population ageing are increasingly realized. With the imperative of applying a holistic, multisectoral, multidisciplinary, and multilevel perspective to address NCD, their risk factors and various determinants are well appreciated.

The proposed mechanisms to enable collaborative intersectoral action for health include joint planning and implementation of programmes, conducting joint situational analysis, generation of evidence, and assessing the outcomes and impact of interventions. It is proposed that the health sector should take the lead in establishing coordinating mechanisms, setting coordinating bodies and institutions, empowering the partners, and establishing channels for sharing and using information. However, there is limited evidence available demonstrating the effectiveness of structural interventions implemented by health and other sectors and directed at the social determinants of NCD [23]. The documentation of successful operationalization of integrated, multisectoral approaches and the empirical evidence on their feasibility and efficiency is still to be produced.

Health sector responses to non-communicable diseases

From a health systems perspective, interventions required for chronic disease management (control) and those recommended for preventing them have a large number of commonalities, even if there are some important differences. As we will argue in this section, both share the need to re-orient the acute-care practice approach to provide longitudinal care in a planned, proactive, and patient-oriented fashion [31].

Access to affordable and effective primary health care by whole populations is essential for the prevention and control of NCD. The concept and need of universally accessible and affordable primary health care was postulated in the 1978 Alma-Ata Declaration [32]. There is now good evidence that improved health outcomes, reduced health disparities, and lower costs of health care are related to health systems with well-functioning primary health care services [33]. Preventive interventions administered through the primary health care system together with evidence-based early treatment of NCD can often delay or replace more expensive specialist and tertiary care-based treatment of advanced illness and complications.

Such primary health care services for prevention and control of NCD need to be organized so that many essential interventions are delivered by trained non-physician health care workers. This certainly should occur under the supervision of a physician-led system – but the emphasis is that a large spectrum of prevention and control activities can be performed by trained non-physician health workers [34]. This is necessary for the efficient use of all the resources in a developing country, including the health care personnel resources, especially in view of the increasing rates of chronic diseases and their risk factors. Interestingly, such urgency to re-orient the chronic disease health care approach is being increasingly realized in highly resourced settings [35].

Historically, the gains in life-expectancy achieved through reducing childhood mortality from infectious diseases were based on the efforts of non-physician health care workers administering vaccinations and oral rehydration therapy. Hence the traditional physician-based treatment model in primary and secondary health care needs to be re-focused to addressing secondary and tertiary medical care of NCD in a referral-based system. Furthermore, the strengths of non-physician primary health care professionals in recognizing and maintaining health, and detecting and treating individuals at risk of or suffering from disease, need to be expanded from the traditional areas of ante-natal care, childbirth, and infant welfare to deal with NCD. This is already happening for women's health in some developing countries, where nurses and other trained non-medical health care workers help maintain the health of women and screen them for breast and cervical cancer. In India this role has been further developed in demonstration projects for the visual detection and immediate treatment of cervical dysplasia. Primary health care services can and should be provided by physicians in settings where patients with established NCD risk factors and NCD are being treated and supervised.

The key principles of universal primary health care envisioned in the Alma-Ata Declaration involved universal coverage of basic services such as education on methods of preventing and controlling common health problems; promotion of food security and healthy diets; basic sanitation; control of locally endemic diseases through appropriate treatment of common diseases and injuries; and provision of essential drugs. These are all essential to NCD prevention and control and point towards the need for an integrated multisectoral approach. In this context, the prime delivery of health services needs to change its focus from larger hospitals towards strengthening community-based services and promoting more balanced and cost-effective preventive and curative programmes. The reorientation of health services should be done by an intersectoral approach including the education, agricultural, non-governmental, and even religious sector where appropriate to extend service delivery. The community should be involved in planning and implementing its own health care services with non-physician health workers being trained under health sector leadership. For example, reducing harm from alcohol abuse, which is associated with cancers of the gastrointestinal system, breast cancer, hypertension, cardiovascular disease, and dementia, requires government and community action in many areas. These could include, for example, cultural change on the acceptability of drinking alcohol in public places, controls on excessive consumption in commercial settings through regulation, banning alcohol advertising, and school- and community-based education about alcohol abuse, changes in agricultural practices which otherwise would increase the availability of alcohol, taxation to reduce discretionary alcohol purchases, and restriction on sales to minors. Non-medical organizations and professionals contribute via counselling and providing other alcohol cessation services, and police action is important in a number of settings including drinking and driving. The health care sector has a number of roles in primary and secondary prevention through detection and management of problem drinking, early detection of disease caused by alcohol abuse, and management of patients with established alcohol-related NCD. Much of this is happening in some developed countries, and illustrates the cross-sectoral actions and responsibilities which characterize efforts to control NCD.

In summary, primary health care systems in many developing countries have to date made most progress in controlling infectious diseases, injuries, and maternal/child health issues, but have failed in providing continuing chronic disease prevention and care, together with the reliable system of accessible medical records needed for NCD prevention and control. Furthermore, many health care seekers in low and middle income countries bypass primary health care services and directly access secondary and tertiary centres because of the lack of competent staff and essential medicines at the local care level [36]. To increase the trust of community members in the benefits of primary health care for NCD prevention and control a number of steps need to be pursued: new and existing health care workers need to be up-skilled and provided with the tools to detect and manage NCD, including the use of proven low-cost pharmacological treatments where appropriate [37]. The training needs to include the maintenance of long-term follow-up and enhancement of treatment adherence assisted by simple medical record systems. This needs to be augmented by a transparent guideline-driven system of referral to hospitals for specialist care for those in need.

These observations also apply to a varying extent to general practitioner (GP)/physician-based primary health care attempts to detect and manage NCD risk factors and NCD in developed countries. In most countries this is opportunistic, and a population-based register of the NCD risk factor status is an exception. Songjiang, one of nine suburbs of Shanghai, with a resident population of 500,579 in 2005, is one notable exception (R. Burton, personal observations). The NCD risk factor and NCD management status of this population, 17 per cent of whom were over the age of 60 years in 2005, has been captured on an electronic health archives system linked to the community health care centres and hospitals. This ensures that population-based treatment and follow-up occurs. For example in 2005, of the 2963 cancer patients registered, 98 per cent were being followed up.

The role of self-care or self-management in the control of NCD is also regarded as critical, and an essential component to achieve long term beneficial change in NCD risk factor exposure and sustainable adherence to ongoing therapy [38,39]. As discussed by Clark and others [40,41] self-management or self-care in the context of chronic diseases involves a set of skilled behaviours to manage one's illness including engaging in activities that promote health, build physiologic reserve, and prevent adverse sequelae; interacting with health care providers and adhering to recommended treatment protocols; monitoring physical and emotional states and making appropriate management decisions on the basis of the results of self-monitoring; and managing the effects of illness on to function in important roles and on emotions, self-esteem, and relationships with others. In the context of cancer, relevant examples would be support for and administration of therapy to cancer sufferers in their community, where the patient and their immediate carers would learn to cope better with the side effects of treatment and manage pain relief in the home. The palliative care of cancer patients is largely community-based, but patients should have ongoing access to more specialized palliative care services as needed. The augmentation and partial reorientation of community palliative care services for HIV/AIDS so they can fulfil this role for cancer patients has been mentioned already, and illustrates the need to discover the breadth of community services available for chronic disease management before considering developing a new service.

We therefore prefer a more ecological view, which emphasizes how the individual and his or her self-care ability is related and dependent on the services and support they can access from carers and their social environment of family, friends, workplaces, community members and organizations, and the physical and policy environment represented by their neighbourhoods, communities, and governments as well as global issues. The ecological contextual view of chronic disease care and prevention (Figure 21.3) illustrates the different levels of influence on the individual and what aspects and functions in chronic disease care and prevention these levels assume, and the interplay of these levels that constrain and define available care.

This recognition of spheres of influence from the global context down to individual's choices and behaviour also reflects the previously introduced model of causation (Figure 21.2). It is therefore apparent that even the best-resourced interventions directed at only one level cannot achieve the necessary long-term sustainable changes needed for chronic disease control, but multilevel and comprehensive interventions are required. For example a review of various self-management interventions for diabetes control evaluating the success of different strategies directed solely at the individual could only identify the duration of the intervention as a significant predictor of

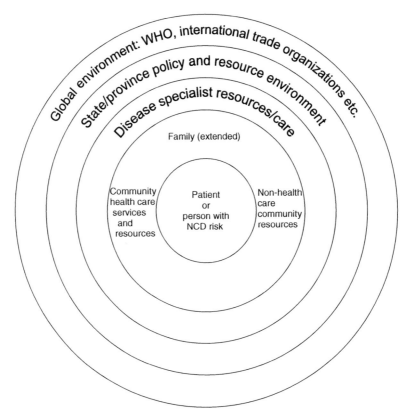

Fig. 21.3 Circles of influence in the prevention and management of NCD.

programmes' success, as none of them achieved long-term sustained benefits much beyond their timeline [42]. This illustrates that beneficial change can be achieved through focal intervention, but may not be sustained.

Although the patient with chronic disease or the person at risk for such disease is at the centre of our view, Figure 21.3 places next to the patient the most immediately accessible resources needed for care and prevention, and to support his or her ability to follow through with self-care. These are family members and volunteer carers; health centres and community health care resources; and the non-health care resources of the community impacting on chronic disease prevention (e.g. access to health information, healthy nutrition, clean environment and safe environments for undertaking physical activity). The next level of resources, specialist resources, and care facilities, refers to secondary and tertiary care for chronic disease prevention and control. Resource limitations in many countries make it mandatory that this level does not assume first-line involvement in chronic disease prevention and control. The disease specialist resources are in turn embedded in the national and regional policy and resource environment which can determine funding, access, pricing, and other resource distribution relevant factors. These in turn are surrounded by an even more remote level of influence, the global environment [43], which can set international guidelines and realities impacting both on the risk for chronic disease (e.g. international tobacco sales) and prevention and control of this risk factor and the NCD it causes, for example, the WHO Framework on Tobacco Control adopted by member countries and shown at the next circle of Figure 21.3.

This comprehensive view of chronic disease prevention and control also has implications for workforce and infrastructure planning. Without long-term commitments and supportive infrastructure, both within and outside the immediate health sector, there is little chance that effective systems can be created on a sustainable basis [44].

Conclusion

This chapter has argued strongly for an integrated approach to the prevention and control of NCD, where this offers advantages over a disease-specific approach. This is most obvious at the primordial and primary levels of prevention of NCD, which are dominated by government and NGO actions from sectors other than health. The health care sector does have crucial roles in advising and supporting government legislation and regulations which prevent NCD, and actively engaging in primary prevention actions as appropriate and necessary. These will, with the exception of immunization against infectious cancers of the liver and cervix which could be integrated into the childhood immunization system for infectious diseases, generally address the common behavioural risk factors for the major NCD. In early detection and screening for NCD the screening technologies will be specialized to the NCD; however, the systems for population education, recruitment of people, registration for follow-up, rescreening and referral for diagnostic tests and specialist management are the same for all NCD. The health care sector should advocate for an integrated approach where this is relevant. A population-based NCD risk factor register which would achieve this for early diagnosis/screening of particular NCD where early treatment gives better outcomes is possible, as Shanghai has shown. However, to date, a silo approach has dominated in most developing countries with Australia, for example, having separate cervical, breast, and colon cancer screening registers and no population registration of hypertension, obesity, or prediabetes/diabetes.

In contrast there are clearly areas of NCD prevention and control which demand specialized disease-specific approaches. Radiotherapy, which is mainly used with curative intent in developed countries, is the mainstay of hospital-based palliation in developing countries where most patients present with incurable disease. Although highly specialized, radiation oncologists should have a broad knowledge of cancer prevention and control, and as the first cancer specialists in some developing countries advocate to governments for cancer control actions that cover the spectrum from prevention to palliation, and advocate for integration into NCD control generally where this is appropriate. This concept is at the heart of the International Atomic Energy Agency (IAEA) Programme of Action for Cancer Therapy (PACT), which began in 2005 [45]. The balance between integrated and specific actions to control NCD will vary over time with a country's level of resources, system of government, strength of the health care and other relevant sectors, and changes in knowledge and technologies for the control of NCD. A country's Chronic Disease Control Strategy should be developed taking account of this. Pre-existing cancer and other NCD control plans should be acknowledged and revised in the light of this overall strategic approach; but separate NCD control plans will still be necessary for actions to control a particular NCD, for example immunization against infectious cancers and development of radiotherapy services.

Acknowledgement

We thank Dr Gauden Galea, MD, Coordinator, Primary Health Care, Health Promotion and Priority Public Health Conditions, World Health Organization, Geneva, Switzerland, for valuable input into this chapter.

References

1 World Health Organization (WHO) (2005). Preventing chronic diseases: a vital investment: WHO global report. WHO (cited 2009 Mar. 19);(1–182). Available from: Available from: http://www.who.int/chp/chronic_disease_report/full_report.pdf.

2 World Health Organization (WHO) (2000). Global Strategy for the prevention and control of noncommunicable diseases. WHO (cited 2008 Aug. 8);(1–6). Available from: http://ftp.who.int/gb/archive/pdf_files/WHA53/ea14.pdf.

3 World Health Organization (WHO) (2008). Prevention and control of noncommunicable diseases: implementation of the global strategy. WHO (cited 2008 Aug. 8);(1–21). Available from:http://www.who.int/gb/ebwha/pdf_files/A61/A61_8-en.pdf.

4 World Health Organization (WHO) (2005). International Union Against Cancer (UICC). Global action against cancer – Updated version. WHO (cited 2009 Mar. 19);(2nd):(1–24). Available from:http://www.who.int/cancer/media/GlobalActionCancerEnglfull.pdf.

5 Ferlay J, Bray F, Pisani P, & Parkin DM (2004). Globocan 2002: Cancer incidence, mortality and prevalence worldwide. *IARC CancerBase,* No. 5, version 2.0. IARC Press, Lyon.

6 World Health Organization (WHO) (2005). World Health Assembly resolution 58.22: Cancer prevention and control. WHO (cited 2008 Aug. 8);(103–107). Available from:http://www.who.int/gb/ebwha/pdf_files/WHA58/WHA58_22-en.pdf.

7 World Health Organization (WHO) (2002). National cancer control programmes: policies and managerial guidelines. WHO (cited 2008 Aug. 8);(2nd):(1–180). Available from: http://www.who.int/cancer/media/en/408.pdf.

8 Howson CP, Hiyama T, & Wynder EL (1986). The decline in gastric cancer: epidemiology of an unplanned triumph. *Epidemiol Rev,* **8**:1–27.

9 Peto R, Darby S, Deo H, Silcocks P, Whitley E, & Doll R (2000). Smoking, smoking cessation, and lung cancer in the UK since 1950: combination of national statistics with two case-control studies. *BMJ,* **321**(7257):323–29.

10 Unal B, Critchley JA, & Capewell S (2004). Explaining the decline in coronary heart disease mortality in England and Wales between 1981 and 2000. *Circulation,* **109**(9):1101–07.

11 Ebrahim S & Smith GD (2001). Exporting failure? Coronary heart disease and stroke in developing countries. *Int J Epidemiol,* **30**(2):201–05.

12 Puska P (2001). Coronary heart disease and stroke in developing countries: time to act. *Int J Epidemiol,* **30**(6):1493–94.

13 Asaria P, Chisholm D, Mathers C, Ezzati M, & Beaglehole R (2007). Chronic disease prevention: health effects and financial costs of strategies to reduce salt intake and control tobacco use. *Lancet,* **370**(9604):2044–53.

14 Beaglehole R & Magnus P (2002). The search for new risk factors for coronary heart disease: occupational therapy for epidemiologists? *Int J Epidemiol,* **31**(6):1117–22.

15 World Health Organization (WHO) (2008) Commission on Social Determinants of Health. Closing the gap in a generation: health equity through action on the social determinants of health. Final Report of the Commission on Social Determinants of Health. WHO (cited 2009 Apr. 2);(1–247). Available from: http://whqlibdoc.who.int/publications/2008/9789241563703_eng.pdf.

16 Fuster V, Voute J, Hunn M, & Smith SC, Jr (2007). Low priority of cardiovascular and chronic diseases on the global health agenda: a cause for concern. *Circulation,* **116**(17):1966–70.

17 McKee M & Shkolnikov V (2001). Understanding the toll of premature death among men in eastern Europe. *BMJ,* **323**(7320):1051–55.

18 King H, Keuky L, Seng S, Khun T, Roglic G, & Pinget M (2005). Diabetes and associated disorders in Cambodia: two epidemiological surveys. *Lancet,* **366**(9497):1633–39.

19 Marmot M (2005). Historical perspective: the social determinants of disease–some blossoms. *Epidemiol Perspect Innov,* **2**(4).

20 World Health Organization (WHO) (2008). The world health report 2008: Primary health care now more than ever. WHO (cited 2009 Apr. 2);(1–119). Available from: http://www.who.int/whr/2008/whr08_en.pdf.

21 World Health Organization (WHO) (2003). World Health Assembly resolution 56.1: WHO Framework Convention on Tobacco Control. WHO (cited 2009 Apr. 2). Available from: https://www.who.int/tobacco/framework/final_text/en/index.html.

22 World Health Organization (WHO) (2004). World Health Assembly resolution 57.17: Global strategy on diet, physical activity and health. WHO (cited 2009 Mar. 19);(38–55). Available from: http://www.who.int/gb/ebwha/pdf_files/WHA57/A57_R17-en.pdf.

23 Gaziano TA, Galea G, & Reddy KS (2007). Scaling up interventions for chronic disease prevention: the evidence. *Lancet*, **370**(9603):1939–46.

24 Suhrcke M, Nugent RA, Stuckler D, & Rocco L (2006). Chronic disease: an economic perspective. Oxford Health Alliance (cited 2009 Mar. 20);(1–59). Available from: http://www.oxha.org/knowledge/publications/oxha-chronic-disease-an-economic-perspective.pdf.

25 World Health Organization (WHO) (2005). World Health Assembly resolution 58.3: revision of the International Health Regulations. WHO (cited 2009 Mar. 19);(7–64). Available from: http://www.who.int/ipcs/publications/wha/ihr_resolution.pdf.

26 Zatonski WA & Willett W (2005). Changes in dietary fat and declining coronary heart disease in Poland: population based study. *BMJ*, **331**(7510):187–88.

27 World Health Organization (WHO) (2004). Building blocks for tobacco control: a handbook (Tools for advancing tobacco control in the 21st century). WHO (cited 2009 Mar. 19);(1–285). Available from: http://www.who.int/tobacco/resources/publications/general/HANDBOOK%20Lowres%20with%20cover.pdf.

28 MacKenzie R & Collin J (2008). Philanthropy, politics and promotion: Philip Morris' 'charitable contributions' in Thailand. *Tob Control*, **17**(4):284–85.

29 Jacobson MF (2005). Liquid candy: how soft drinks are harming Americans' health. Center for Science in the Public Interest (CSPI) (cited 2009 Mar. 20);(2nd):(1–35). Available from: http://cspi.cc/new/pdf/liquid_candy_final_w_new_supplement.pdf.

30 Chopra M & Darnton-Hill I (2004). Tobacco and obesity epidemics: not so different after all? *BMJ*, **328**(7455):1558–60.

31 Glasgow RE, Orleans CT, & Wagner EH (2001). Does the chronic care model serve also as a template for improving prevention? *Milbank Q*, **79**(4):579–612.

32 Declaration of Alma-Ata (1979). *Lancet*, **1**(8109):217–18.

33 Starfield B, Shi L, & Macinko J (2005). Contribution of primary care to health systems and health. *Milbank Q*, **83**(3):457–502.

34 Abegunde DO, Shengelia B, Luyten A, et al (2007). Can non-physician health-care workers assess and manage cardiovascular risk in primary care? *Bull World Health Organ*, **85**(6):432–40.

35 Fiscella K & Epstein RM (2008). So much to do, so little time: care for the socially disadvantaged and the 15-minute visit. *Arch Intern Med*, **168**(17):1843–52.

36 Hall JJ & Taylor R (2003). Health for all beyond 2000: the demise of the Alma-Ata Declaration and primary health care in developing countries. *Med J Aust*, **178**(1):17–20.

37 Joshi R, Jan S, Wu Y, & MacMahon S (2008). Global inequalities in access to cardiovascular health care: our greatest challenge. *J Am Coll Cardiol*, **52**(23):1817–25.

38 Bodenheimer T, Lorig K, Holman H, & Grumbach K (2002). Patient self-management of chronic disease in primary care. *JAMA*, **288**(19):2469–75.

39 Glasgow RE, Funnell MM, Bonomi AE, Davis C, Beckham V, & Wagner EH (2002). Self-management aspects of the improving chronic illness care breakthrough series: implementation with diabetes and heart failure teams. *Ann Behav Med*, **24**(2):80–87.

40 Clark NM & Gong M (2000). Management of chronic disease by practitioners and patients: are we teaching the wrong things? *BMJ*, **320**(7234):572–75.

41 Clark NM (2003). Management of chronic disease by patients. *Annu Rev Public Health*, **24**:289–313.

42 Norris SL, Engelgau MM, & Narayan KM (2001). Effectiveness of self-management training in type 2 diabetes: a systematic review of randomized controlled trials. *Diabetes Care,* **24**(3):561–87.

43 Beaglehole R (2005). Global partnerships for health. *Eur J Public Health,* **15**(2):113–14.

44 Yach D, Hawkes C, Gould CL, & Hofman KJ (2004). The global burden of chronic diseases: overcoming impediments to prevention and control. *JAMA*, **291**(21):2616–22.

45 International Atomic Energy Authority (IAEA) (2008). Building partnerships to fight the cancer epidemic: Programme of Action for Cancer Therapy (PACT). IAEA (cited 2009 Mar. 20);(1–24) Available from: http://www.iaea.org/Publications/Booklets/TreatingCancer/pact0808.pdf.

Chapter 22

Cancer control in developing countries

Ian Magrath[1]

The World Health Organization (WHO) recently projected that by approximately 2010, cancer would overtake ischemic heart disease as the leading cause of death in the world (Figure 22.1) [1,2]. Between 2005 (when some 7.6 million people died from cancer, accounting for 13 per cent of global deaths) and 2015, it is anticipated that 84 million people will die of cancer. In 2005, approximately 70 per cent of cancer deaths occurred in low and middle income countries where, although cancer has a lower incidence, survival rates are also much lower, largely because of delays in diagnosis leading to presentation with advanced disease. Because much of the cost of care must be borne 'out-of-pocket', and because of the low gross domestic product (GDP) of which only a few per cent is assigned to the provision of health services, poor patients often receive incomplete or sub-optimal therapy in overcrowded and unhygienic wards – or none at all. Those with incurable disease, or without financial support, are frequently sent home to die – without even the comfort of palliative care. Many patients (uncounted and uncountable) never reach a centre capable of providing treatment. This existing, though largely silent, catastrophe will soon become a crisis, since the global cancer burden is increasing rapidly in the developing countries, where populations continue to expand as communicable diseases are better controlled, resulting in longer life spans, ageing populations, and, consequently, higher cancer incidence. Unfortunately, death from infection is all too often replaced (or added to) by death from the non-communicable diseases (NCDs) caused by smoking or over-consumption of a diet lacking in fruits and vegetables and an increasingly sedentary life style; although in the low income countries, chronic infection is still an important cause of cancer. Tobacco and diet together account for up to 60 per cent of cancer in high income countries, but, at the present time, a much lower proportion in low and middle income countries, although they will take an increasing toll on the emerging middle class in developing countries, particularly in those undergoing rapid development, such as India and China. Even if the present constantly increasing smoking rates in developing countries are slowed or even reversed, a sufficient number of individuals have been smoking long enough to make an increase in tobacco-related cancers in the coming years inevitable [3–5]. The increase in cancer rates in developing countries will not be small; the International Agency for Research on Cancer (IARC) predicts that by 2030 there could be 27 million new cases and 17 million cancer deaths per year – an extra 10 million deaths compared to 2005 [6].

   This gloomy spectacle is not a reason for inaction. The reverse is the case. The high mortality rate from cancer in developing countries will improve only gradually, and determined largely by the resources available or identified, and efforts made to educate both health professionals and the public. While national cancer control planning based on an understanding of the problems and needs is essential, such plans will have no effect unless translated into action.

[1] Ian T. Magrath, DSc (Med), FRCP, FRCPath, President, International Network for Cancer Treatment and Research (INCTR), Brussels, Belgium.

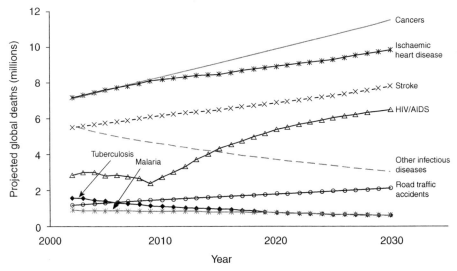

Fig. 22.1 Projected global deaths for selected causes of death, 2002–2030.
Large declines in mortality are projected to occur between 2002 and 2030 for all of the principal communicable, maternal, perinatal and nutritional causes, with the exception of HIV/AIDS. Although age-specific death rates for most non-communicable diseases are projected to decline, the ageing of the global population will result in significant increases in the total number of deaths caused by most non-communicable diseases over the next 30 years. Overall, non-communicable conditions will account for almost 70 per cent of all deaths in 2030 under the baseline scenario. Mortality rank order depends, of course, on how diseases are grouped together. If each cancer were considered a separate disease, ischaemic heart disease would remain the leading cause of death for the foreseeable future.
From: WHO Statistical Highlights 2007 [2].

Professional education should ideally be provided in a way that leads to immediate benefits to those who suffer from or could develop cancer, for example, through clinical studies that are relevant to the countries in which they are conducted, rather than being done for the economic benefit of technologically advanced countries. The problem of migration of health workers demands attention, and professional education, however delivered, must be adapted to the very different circumstances that apply in developing countries. Public education also needs different approaches in different cultures, where there may not only be a lack of knowledge, but incorrect beliefs about cancer. In such circumstances, methods need to be found to correct, or unlearn, messages that pervade the society. Solutions are most likely to be found through close collaboration between local health professionals and a variety of external organizations, institutions, and individuals that can offer specialized knowledge and training in appropriate skills.

Differences in the incidence and pattern of cancer worldwide

The incidence of cancer in less developed countries is several times lower than that in more developed countries (Table 22.1), even using rates adjusted to the age structure of the world population, which under-represent the absolute differences in incidence because of the younger age distribution in less developed countries. Age-adjusted data do, however, indicate what will happen in the coming years as the epidemiological transition from communicable to non-communicable diseases progresses, and populations age due to decreasing fertility rates and

Table 22.1 Incidence rate of cancer (all sites but skin) per 100,000 in selected global regions

Males	Incidence		Mortality		Females	Incidence		Mortality	
	Crude	ASR	Crude	ASR		Crude	ASR	Crude	ASR
North America	530	398	210	153		455	305	186	112
Western Europe	526	326	295	174		429	245	225	106
Middle Africa	78	142	66	121		76	122	62	99
South Central Asia	76	106	55	78		89	110	55	70

From: Globocan 2002 [1]. ASR = age-standardized rate (using World standard population).

increasing longevity. But already, the numbers of new cases and of deaths are higher in developing countries because together, they account for approximately 85 per cent of the world's population (Figure 22.2). Smoking and dietary factors are less important predisposing diseases and infectious diseases correspondingly more so in countries lower on the socio-economic ladder. In the poorest countries in equatorial Africa an infectious antecedent is likely to account for as much as 40 to 50 per cent of all cancer cases (compared to 8 per cent in high income countries) – demonstrating, remarkably, that if infection could be controlled in the absence of the introduction and expansion of risk factors currently prevalent in the highest income countries, the cancer incidence rate could decrease by almost half in the lowest income countries! Such a scenario is highly unlikely given present trends, but does indicate the need for the development of new programmes in cancer control even in the poorest countries, while continuing to address the major incapacity caused by chronic infections and intermittent epidemics.

Unfortunately, until very recently, cancer was not on the agenda of the major international agencies that deal with health – cancer, and NCDs in general, were not, for example, included in the Millennium Development Goals. Yet NCDs accounted for 60 per cent of global deaths in 2005 (35 million), with 80 per cent in low and middle income countries, and are projected to increase by a further 17 per cent in the next decade [7]. Such summary statistics, although important in the context of global decision making, are of limited use in developing national cancer control strategies, since variation in cancer patterns and resources can vary markedly from country to

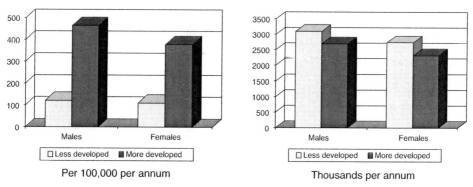

Per 100,000 per annum   Thousands per annum

Fig. 22.2 Incidence rates and incident cases in less and more developed countries. Although the incidence rates (crude) per annum are lower, the absolute number of cancer cases per year is higher in developing countries – because most people live in low and middle income countries.
Source: Data from Globocan 2002 [1].

country and even among different regions in the same country. The global distribution of cancers by type is shown in Figure 22.3.

The average age of patients with cancer in developing countries is much lower than in high income countries, and cancers in children, adolescents, and young adults comprise a much higher fraction of all cancers. This is in part due to the lower average age of the population and shorter duration of exposure to risk factors, such as smoking and potentially dietary factors, but in some

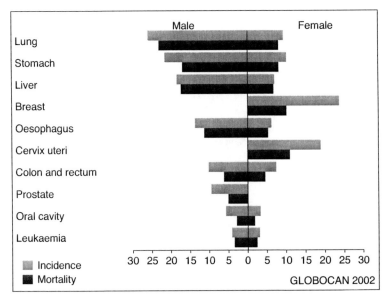

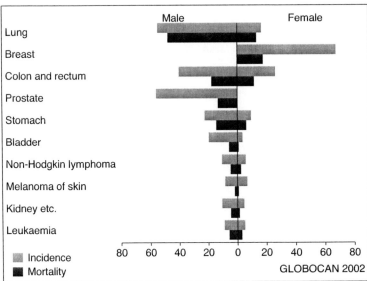

Fig. 22.3 Incidence and mortality rates (age-adjusted to the world population) per 100,000 of the top ten cancers in less (upper graph) and more developed countries (lower graph). Note that the horizontal scales are different.

Source: Data from Globocan 2002 [1].

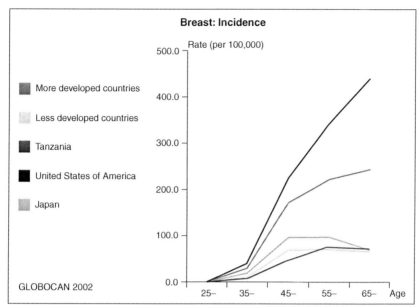

Fig. 22.4 Age-specific incidence rates for breast cancer in selected countries.
Source: Data from Globocan 2002 [1].

cancers this is an inadequate explanation since age-specific incidence curves indicate a lower incidence in older individuals. For example, the incidence of breast cancer increases throughout life in most high income countries, but peaks in incidence between the ages of 40 and 50 years in lower and middle income countries, as well as in Japan (Figure 22.4), suggesting differences in risk factors for pre- and post-menopausal breast cancer [1]. This is entirely consistent with the increasing proportion of estrogen-positive breast cancers with age.

The lower cancer risks do not mean that cancer is not an important health problem in the lower income countries. Indeed, unless cancer control measures are greatly augmented, the burden of cancer will create ever greater stress to health systems that are already overwhelmed, and as GDP increases, it will be necessary to ensure that health service improvements do not lag behind other aspects of development. This is important both from the perspective of human rights, and also from that of development, for the productivity of an unhealthy population can never equal that of a healthy population.

Resource limitations in developing countries

According to the World Bank, approximately 1.3 billion people live on less than a dollar a day, and almost half the world's population lives on less than 2 dollars a day [8]. While these numbers are somewhat arbitrary, as is the definition of 'poverty', they clearly indicate that the bulk of humanity is extremely poor. More than 75 per cent of the world's population (4.7 billion people) live in countries classified as low or low-middle income countries by the World Bank, that is, with an annual income of less than $3,705 in 2007 (Table 22.2). This contrasts with an average annual income of $39,177 for the 30 OECD (Organization for Economic Cooperation and Development) countries. Poverty at the level of individuals is associated with extremely limited public resources, such that even countries that give health and education a high priority have a drastically limited ability to provide for the needs of their populations. At the turn of the millennium, for example,

Table 22.2 World Bank Definitions of income categories (2007 Gross National Product per capita) in countries at different levels of socio-economic development, and population numbers. Note that least developed is also included in the low income category

Category	GNP per capita	Population size
Least developed	less than $496	800 million
Low income	less than $935	1.3 billion
Lower middle income	$936–$3,705	3.4 billion
Upper middle income	$3,706–$11,455	823 million
High income	$11,456 or more	1 billion

From: [8].

a billion people were unable to read or sign their name. According to UNICEF, some 11 million children die each year as a direct consequence of poverty, and the United Nations Development Program states that a million children a year die for want of clean water and adequate sanitation [8]. Poor health (malnutrition, anaemia, and common infectious diseases) also causes frequent interruptions in education, and reduces the ability to learn. Many children never go to school (which is rarely free), or have very little education. The lack of even a basic education condemns most to a life of perpetual poverty and potential catastrophe while markedly restricting the pool of young people who can undergo higher education and hence the number of trained professionals in all sectors of the economy. In this setting, natural disasters or inter-ethnic conflicts precipitate serious added health problems resulting from violence, epidemics, starvation, displacement from home, and lack of access to clean water, food, and medicine.

Clearly, difficult decisions must be made by governments regarding priorities for their limited budgets. In the poorer countries health expenditure is usually just a few per cent of total government spending – in absolute terms, sometimes hundreds of times less than is spent per capita in high income countries (Figure 22.5). Health workforces are correspondingly small and unable to cope with the burden of disease. The WHO, for example, reports that sub-Saharan Africa, with

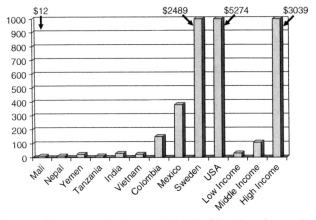

Figure 22.5 Health expenditure per capita (current US dollars) in selected countries. Source: Data from World Development Indicators, 2007.

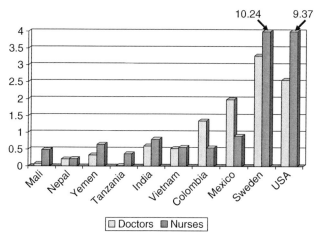

Figure 22.6 Number of physicians and nurses per 1000 in selected countries. This figure emphasizes the enormous differences between the richest and poorest countries.
Source: Data from World Health Report 2006 [45].

11 per cent of the world's population and 25 per cent of the global burden of disease, accounts for less than 1 per cent of global health expenditure. In contrast, the Americas, with 14 per cent of the world's population and 10 per cent of the global burden of disease, account for more than 50 per cent of the global health expenditure [8]. Comparisons of the numbers of doctors and nurses per 1000 of the population in selected countries are shown in Figure 22.6. Some populations in low income countries are considerably worse off than even these figures suggest, since the inadequate workforces are also mal-distributed (rural regions are particularly poorly provided for) and health services are poorly structured and managed. Some countries have fewer nurses than doctors such that nursing tasks, to the extent possible, must be performed by family members, or not at all – an unthinkable situation in high income countries. Health care providers are generally swamped with many more patients than they can adequately deal with; there is no time for continuing education (which is rarely a requirement for retaining a license to practice), except for a privileged few; and there is minimal incentive, knowledge or infrastructure for the collection of data relevant to measuring the impact of interventions in the local, resource-limited, context.

Resource limitations in the context of cancer

Although there are cancer registries in developing countries, much of the available data is institutional rather than population-based and of variable quality. Poorly organized health services and inadequate training of health workers often lead to delays in diagnosis, misdiagnosis, loss of clinical samples, inadequate investigations, poor record keeping and lack of communication within the health service, poor supportive care, and limited or no patient follow up. Professional education often leaves much to be desired – without continuing medical education, most senior health professionals are out-of-date and their large clinical workloads leave little time for teaching. Career choices are often governed more by the anticipated income than by interest or talent in a particular area of medicine. Too few doctors are likely to translate into even greater deficiencies in specialists. In many countries many specialties are not represented at all, so the vast majority of cancer patients who reach secondary or tertiary centres are cared for by non-cancer specialists.

The combination of factors that leads to advanced disease at presentation also leads to a fatalistic attitude to cancer, and hence an assumption that cancer is not important to diagnose or assess fully. Of course, there is much variation: some countries in the upper middle income category provide care and professional education that, at least in the best centres, can be equal or close to the level of high income countries, but in many rural regions, medical facilities are extremely limited. The inability to pay for care is not simply due to the cost of treatment, but also to the loss of income that occurs while away from home. Because in such circumstances the entire family will suffer, an unknown fraction of patients may never receive the care they need – even palliative care.

Resources for each of the three major modalities of cancer therapy are severely limited in low and lower middle income countries. Surgical oncologists, or even general surgeons with expertise in cancer surgery, are in short supply and like all other human, financial, and material resources, are more likely to be available in urban rather than rural regions. Radiation therapy, which evolved early in the twentieth century in Europe, has still not spread to all countries in the world, due both to the capital cost of equipment and the lack of radiation oncologists, medical physicists, and radiotherapy technicians. According to the International Atomic Energy Agency, half of the world's countries have 85 per cent of all radiation therapy machines – leaving 15 per cent for the other half. Barton et al. [9] have estimated that at the end of the 1990s there was a need for 842 megavoltage machines in Africa, 4936 in 12 low and middle income countries in the Asian Pacific region and 1530 in 23 selected Latin-American countries (see also Chapter 9). Limited maintenance and outdated cobalt sources compound the problem. In low income countries particularly, there are no medical oncologists and/or paediatric oncologists, and few have adequate numbers of other specialists, including oncology nurses.

Chemotherapy and hormonal therapy are available practically everywhere, although many countries purchase only 'essential' cytotoxic drugs based on the WHO Essential Drugs list [10]. Even so, deficiencies in procurement practices of these inexpensive, generic drugs often lead to intermittent supplies. Cost is also a major issue since much or all of the care, particularly drug costs, must frequently be paid for 'out-of-pocket'. Remarkably, sometimes only more expensive drugs are available in the absence of drugs with similar activity, for example, docitaxol versus paclitaxol in breast cancer [11]. These issues are discussed further in the following section.

These multiple deficiencies are compounded by the temptation faced by the few trained health workers (and those who aspire to become health workers) to emigrate in search of improved professional and financial rewards. Training fellowships given by high income countries (which may have been established with the intent of improving the workforces of low income countries) can significantly exacerbate this problem, but professionals are also actively recruited by some high income countries – or by commercial organizations, some of which may even train nurses in developing countries with the specific intent of arranging for them to work abroad. Such practices may overcome the government regulations established by some European countries to prohibit recruitment from countries with very limited numbers of health workers. Similarly, an increasing number of trained persons move partly or entirely into the for-profit health sector of their own country, leaving the poorer elements of the population with even less access to care. Some would argue that countries should simply train more doctors, nurses, or other health professionals than they themselves require, but this apparently simple solution pre-supposes a sufficient number of institutions of higher education, of teachers, and, as mentioned, of sufficiently qualified young people to receive higher education – that is, a higher level of socio-economic development than currently exists. Although emigration rates vary markedly from one country to another, and statistics can be difficult to compile, according to the Center for Global Development on average 40 per cent of African-born physicians work outside their country of birth, and for some countries the figure may be as high as 70 per cent [12].

Migrants are more likely to come from countries with better health systems (which some have, seemingly counter-intuitively, interpreted as indicating that migration of health workers benefits their country of origin. Although a small number of ex-patriots do assist in training or send money to family members in their countries of origin) this can compensate only to a very limited degree for the enormous limitations in human resources.

Approaches to cancer control in developing countries

Treatment has always been the primary approach to cancer control, in developing countries as in the rest of the world, as the immediate and obvious need is to care for sick patients. In contrast, the justification for prevention and early diagnosis programmes may need considerable development. Preventive strategies depend upon epidemiological research, which has been mainly conducted by investigators in, or from, high income countries, although there are a number of notable exceptions, particularly when a generally uncommon cancer occurs at high frequency in a particular population or has prominent clinical features that bring it to attention, such as do Bilharzia-related bladder cancer, nasopharyngeal cancer, and Burkitt lymphoma. In developing countries, the imbalance between the cancer burden and the health workforce leaves little time for clinical oncologists to think about epidemiology or public health, and epidemiologists are also grossly under-represented in the health professions in these countries. The relatively few health professionals who deal with population health in the poorest countries continue to be concerned almost exclusively with infectious diseases and nutrition, rather than NCDs.

Because in the past, cancer has accounted for a much smaller fraction of the disease burden, it has been under-emphasized or even omitted from educational programmes, such that primary care physicians and even specialists may not consider a diagnosis of cancer. Most oncologists do not see late diagnosis as an issue that falls within their purview – indeed, for the most part it is accepted as the 'usual' way in which cancer presents – which, in such countries, is, in fact, the case. This perception has become pervasive, so the emphasis on cancer as a public health problem is minimal. International bodies, until quite recently, have also focused on health issues that are much less expensive and easier to combat – thus providing no encouragement to governments to establish cancer control programmes. As a result, there have been few serious attempts to address cancer at the public health level, while cancer services have generally developed in a disorganized fashion, have often depended upon a small number of individuals who have, for one reason or another, been motivated to establish programmes – some of which have developed into major cancer institutes – or to persuade a state or national government to provide funds for the development of cancer services of some kind.

Recently, this attitude has undergone a welcome transformation; cancer has been recognized as an important health problem in developing countries. This is doubtless a consequence of the epidemiological transitions and inexorable increase in the cancer burden (see also Chapter 21) as well as greater control of communicable diseases. Sadly, this recognition has come at a time when cancer is about to become the leading cause of death in the world. Nonetheless, the World Health Assembly resolution, WHA58 22 (2005), has done much to ensure that governments, even those of the poorest countries, recognize that cancer is an important health problem [13].

Resolution WHA58 22 urges member states to implement 18 actions relating to cancer control, the first of which is:

'To collaborate with the Organization in developing and reinforcing comprehensive cancer control programmes tailored to the socio-economic context, and aimed at reducing cancer incidence and mortality and improving the quality of life of cancer patients and their families, specifically through the systematic, stepwise, and equitable implementation of evidence-based strategies for prevention, early detection, diagnosis, treatment, rehabilitation and palliative care, and to evaluate the impact of implementing such programmes'.

As stated in the WHA resolution, all aspects of cancer control are important for all countries, although priorities need to be adjusted to the available resources as well as the pattern of cancer. An important question is whether existing resources are being optimally used. Changes can often be made, at little cost, for example, to put a greater emphasis on cancer in the curricula of nurses, doctors and other health workers, and to introduce tobacco control measures and palliative care. Attention should also be given to improving communication within the health services and to the health service structure – which is particularly important in a disease which, if to be effectively dealt with, requires access and communication among many disciplines. Determining priorities in the context of available resources requires, as recommended in resolution WHA 58 22, the formation of a national cancer control committee, comprised of experts from all relevant disciplines, and the development of a national cancer control strategy.

Developing a national cancer control strategy

A number of steps need to be taken in the development of a national cancer control strategy. Of critical importance is an understanding of the cancer burden and the resources available to deal with it. Equally important is the political will to act on the plan, and to assign a budget to at least high priority elements of it (as also applies in developed countries, as discussed in Chapters 7 and 17). Coordination of the development of the plan will be required, and opportunities provided for expert input into relevant sections, as well as involving a broad range of stakeholders, for without their 'buy-in' and sense of joint ownership, cooperation will be limited. The initiative for the development of the plan may come from the government, the oncology community, or even civil society. Where the government is not the prime mover, steps should be taken to ensure that there is governmental support. Cancer survivors can often play an important role in lobbying politicians, participating in awareness raising campaigns and the development of non-governmental funding (see also Chapter 16).

Assessing the problem

The initial step in developing a national control strategy is an assessment of the national situation with respect to the cancer burden and the pattern of cancer – that is, the incidence and rank order of sub-types, the prevalence of risk factors, and the resources (particularly the quality and quantity of human resources) and infrastructure available to address each of the major elements of cancer control. This information is essential to the determination of priorities. Limited resources mean that good data, for example, from population-based cancer registries, is sparse; there were only 47 members of the International Association of Cancer Registries in Africa, for example, among the total of 449 members listed in 2006 [14]. While institutional-based registry information can give a sufficient idea of the pattern of cancer for priorities to be determined, population-based statistics are invaluable both to describe the existing pattern of cancer and to track trends in incidence and mortality. Population-based survival rates, if available, also give a truer picture of the national situation without distortion by the potentially unrepresentative results of a few major institutions. Even the best registries, however, cannot provide an estimate of access to care or the quality of diagnosis and treatment, while survival data, however valuable, is rarely collected because of the increased work load and generally poor follow-up which precludes accurate information. Registries could also collect information on available resources within the defined population they relate to, but in very low resource settings, where there is a great deal of heterogeneity (e.g., between urban and rural regions) such information may not be representative of the entire nation. Programmes conducted by non-governmental organizations are often hindered by lack of funds, while government statistics are limited, often out-of-date, and vary in accuracy. Information on the numbers of nurses, primary care physicians, and specialists is usually available, but the amount of time spent on dealing with cancer is difficult to calculate as much cancer diagnosis and care is delivered by persons without special training in cancer.

Setting priorities

Priority setting must derive from the situational analysis as described. The WHO has developed a set of brochures describing the process of cancer control planning, with guidance for determining the most appropriate actions in low, medium, and high resource settings [15,16] – a format that has been followed by others. It is often suggested that the highest priority in cancer control in the low and middle income countries is palliative care, since the immense burden of suffering can most immediately be relieved through effective symptom control, particularly pain, and attention to psycho-social problems. Prevention is also given a high priority, since this can be accomplished without major capacity building for the care of cancer patients. But while both are critically important, palliative care alone can only reduce morbidity, not mortality, while preventive measures, even if they meet all expectations, will, for the most part, not have an impact on cancer incidence rates for decades. Thus, even in the poorest countries, treatment must be afforded a significant place in the national cancer control strategy, with an emphasis on potentially curable patients. This means that there must be vigorous efforts to detect cancer earlier so that more patients present at a stage when treatment is less complex, toxic, and expensive and more likely to result in cure, even in the presence of severe resource limitations, assuming that at least some accessible facilities are able to provide competent care. International collaboration is likely to be extremely valuable in assisting countries to escape from the vicious cycles resulting from overloading of available resources with the effect this has on both access to and the efficiency of cancer treatment.

In broad terms, the highest priorities are relatively easy to identify, since they are universally necessary for any cancer control programme and cost little, although even these may face a variety of obstacles. They include full implementation of the Framework Convention on Tobacco Control (FCTC) [17], education of both the public and the health workforce about the early signs of cancer, ensuring efficient navigation through the health care system when cancer is suspected, so that prompt access to the available facilities for diagnosis and treatment is assured, and the provision of palliative care to all who need it. Important too, is the provision for accurate data collection (associated with contextually relevant research – see hereunder) both to provide evidence on which cancer control interventions can be based, and to permit evaluation of the interventions undertaken. Rehabilitation, including psychological rehabilitation, is important when patients have undergone mutilating surgery, or suffer from the late effects of chemotherapy or radiation. Where resources are totally lacking, there is no choice but to allow cancer control to continue in an unplanned way (as was the case, for example, in the technologically advanced countries for decades), although at a minimum, resource deficiencies can be identified such that attempts can be made by the government or civil society to fill the gaps. In the modern world much can be accomplished even with very limited funding, for example, through the development of international relationships with organizations or institutions able to provide both expertise and funding, and, in the context of training and education, through the use of free (open) resources for education available via the internet. Although broad-band internet access is constantly expanding, any form of internet access remains a problem in the poorest and most remote locations. Nonetheless, opportunities for supplementing available expertise, for example, in pathological and radiological diagnosis, via the 'commons' (i.e. resources owned by the global community rather than by individuals) and for other on-line interactions, such as international multidisciplinary meetings, are constantly increasing and can be used to supplement standard educational approaches, including basic, continuing, and specialist education, as well as providing accreditation by recognized authorities.

Challenges faced by developing countries in improving and implementing cancer control strategies

Cancer registration

Cancer registration can be considered part of 'assessment' since it provides incidence data at a population level, and, depending upon resources available, data on mortality and survival, and so is a valuable tool in developing a national cancer control strategy. Registration, however, can also be of great value in assessing the outcome of interventions. For example, a reduction in incidence could result from a preventive measure, and an increase in survival or decrease in mortality can result from earlier detection or improved treatment. In developing countries, however, survival data is often inaccurate because of poor follow up, and poor practice in completing death certificates may also lead to inaccurate mortality data. Even incidence data for some cancers may be unreliable because of misdiagnosis. In addition, although registries are inexpensive, because of the undeniable needs of patients and high cost of patient care, the support of a cancer registry may literally be at the expense of patient care – unless supported by outside funding. The next best thing to population-based information is the pooling of data collected from individual institutions, particularly those that serve large populations, or where (as for example, in former Soviet Union countries), each geographical division of the country has a cancer centre. At times this can be misleading because certain cancers may never reach tertiary referral centres (e.g. hepatoma) and their incidence therefore remains unknown in the absence of a population-based registry.

Prevention

Prevention, no less than treatment, is closely linked with business and politics and conflicts may arise because one sector's gain is sometimes another sector's loss. Effective tobacco control, for example, would result in a major 'restructuring' of the tobacco industry at the very least, while even vaccines are products which can deliver enormous profits, particularly if the target population for vaccination is large and suppliers few. Clearly, it is imperative that decisions are made on the basis of complete or at least balanced evidence, by persons without a conflict of interest. Governments, of course, are susceptible (and those in the poorest countries are often the most susceptible) to lobbying by industry representatives, and to the provision or withdrawal of donations, whether in the context of election campaigns or the consideration of specific legislation, such as that relating to tobacco control. While non-governmental organizations can influence governments and public opinion through their own lobbying, such organizations are relatively few and frequently weak compared to their counterparts in high income countries. Helping to build civil society in low income settings is an important role for organizations and influential individuals interested in cancer control.

Health care providers, particularly in primary care, have a critically important role to play in prevention. The decision of a high proportion of doctors in the United Kingdom to give up smoking, for example, had a major impact in reducing lung cancer rates [18] and advice on the part of a doctor to give up smoking has been shown to be effective in persuading smokers to quit. Advice on diet and other important health messages could be equally valuable, but unfortunately, health providers see their role largely as dealing with sick people rather than helping to keep them healthy. Basic medical and nursing training in most countries, and perhaps particularly in developing countries, includes little or no information on the importance of promoting a healthier lifestyle in their patients. This could easily be changed at minimal cost. Schools and universities provide excellent opportunities to give age- and culturally-sensitive information about cancer and its prevention; conversely, providing important health educational messages is more difficult when there is a high level of illiteracy – particularly in rural regions and females, who, in general, receive inferior educations. The Internet is rapidly becoming a major source of health information in high income countries, but lags far behind in poorer nations (the so-called digital divide), and, of course, requires literacy. Yet radio is almost universally available, television and video increasingly so, and mobile phones are available even in the most remote villages, even if owned by only a small number of the inhabitants. Maximal use of these tools and many others can make a major difference to the knowledge of the general public, of their health advisors, and of policy makers even in the poorest of countries.

Tobacco control

Tobacco control is of particular importance to low and middle income countries, whose smoking rates are rapidly increasing; as smoking decreases in high income countries, the tobacco industry is redoubling its efforts to increase smoking in developing countries. The measures recommended by the FCTC [17] should be considered a high priority in any national cancer control plan. As of February 2009, 162 countries had ratified or accepted the Convention (the United States is a prominent exception). Unfortunately, the tobacco industry is doing everything it can to prevent implementation of the recommendations. The governments of poor countries particularly, even if they have ratified the treaty, often succumb to the temptation of accepting funding from the tobacco industry in return for not implementing the FCTC as intended [4,19].

Because of the cost of smoking, the tobacco epidemic is at various stages of its development in countries at different levels of socio-economic development, being still at an early stage of development in the poorest countries, and well past its peak in the United States and many European countries (Figure 22.7). The introduction of anti-smoking legislation in the high income countries has been made easier by their decreasing smoking rates; in many high income countries only 20 to 33 per cent of people now smoke, compared to peak smoking rates of around 70 per cent in the 1960s and 70s (see The WHO Tobacco Atlas [20] and Chapter 2). By the same token, in countries where the rate of smoking is still, at least on average, quite low (e.g. many sub-Saharan African countries), a small and rapidly diminishing window of opportunity exists whereby anti-smoking legislation could be introduced and enforced by the government before there are sufficient smokers to make such legislation extremely unpopular. In many other countries, such as China [5], where the tobacco epidemic is advanced but still not at its peak, discouraging young people from starting to smoke is very important, but will have little impact prior to 2050 on tobacco-related cancer rates, whereas encouraging older adults to give up smoking will lead to a significant reduction in cancer rates (and deaths) in the first half of this century, and is a matter of the greatest urgency. Some progress in tobacco has been made in China, for example, the introduction of much higher tobacco taxes.

Many developing countries, particularly in South and South-East Asia, also face a significant frequency of use of smokeless tobacco – particularly chewing habits which are associated with oral cancer [21,22]. Chewing habits tend to be particularly common in poorer populations, which are more difficult to reach; users of smokeless tobacco are more likely to live in rural regions, while those who smoke manufactured cigarettes are more likely to live in urban regions. Behavioural modification may therefore need to be approached in different and culturally sensitive ways.

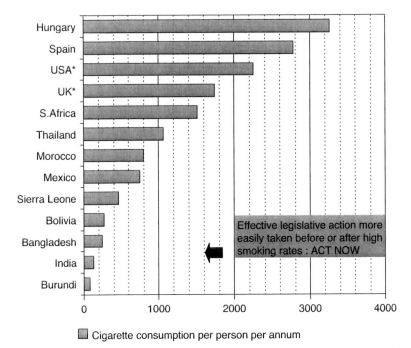

Cigarette consumption per person per annum

Fig. 22.7 Progression of the tobacco epidemic in various countries as measured in terms of cigarette consumption.
*Countries in which consumption has greatly diminished in recent years as a consequence of tobacco control measures.
Source: most recent data from WHO.

Diet

Fruits and vegetables generally comprise a higher fraction of the overall lower caloric intake in low income populations, where the majority of people lead anything but sedentary lifestyles, so that cancers associated with diet, such as colon cancer, tend to have a much lower incidence. However, in developing countries, the fraction of people who are overweight is steadily increasing – at least in the higher income strata. Unfortunately, there is such gross inequality between the richest and poorest segments of the populations in low and middle income countries that malnutrition often remains a serious problem while obesity is an increasing cause of NCDs.

HPV vaccines

An issue of particular importance to developing countries is the role of HPV vaccines in controlling cervical cancer (see also Chapter 6). Although an exciting advance, there remain a number of questions about the role of such vaccines in preventing cervical cancer in low and middle income countries, particularly the cost and the feasibility of vaccinating a sufficiently large number of girls and young women, and possibly boys, to make a difference. Cervical cancer affects some 500,000 women per year and causes approximately 300,000 annual deaths – a high proportion of which are likely to occur in hard–to-reach populations since the disease has a higher incidence in lower socio-economic groups. For various reasons it is clear that HPV vaccine cannot be the sole solution to the control of cervical cancer; screening programs will continue to be important for the foreseeable future. The crude incidence of cervical cancer varies greatly in different parts of the world, and the highest rates of around 80 per 100,000 occur in countries at low socio-economic levels. The cumulative risk up to the age of 64, however, of developing cervical cancer is only some 3 to 6 per cent even in high incidence regions, which means that a very large number of girls must be vaccinated in order to significantly reduce the incidence of cervical cancer; or, from a different perspective, a large majority of vaccinated individuals are not at risk for cervical cancer. Thus this vaccine differs markedly from most vaccines which are directed primarily at the prevention of a serious and highly prevalent (in the absence of vaccination) infectious disease. The financial cost of preventing cervical cancer at several hundred dollars for a course of vaccination (at the present time) compares poorly with, for example, measles prevention. According to the WHO, it costs less than one dollar to immunize a child against measles, a disease which affects 20 million children per year and results in almost 200,000 annual deaths. Also important is that the duration of protection with the available HPV vaccines remains unknown; if booster doses are required after several years, costs will be higher, and population coverage of sexually active women is likely to be lower. Screening for cervical cancer, unlike vaccination, also results in the detection of treatable benign diseases, such as infections and prolapsed uterus, which may cause considerable distress to women.

All of these considerations have implications for the toxicity profile of the vaccine, which, in view of the relatively small fraction of women who would benefit, must be, perhaps, even more favourable than those of vaccines used to prevent serious acute infectious diseases. These considerations may well be modified by the development of further vaccines and by likely cost reductions in the future, as discussed in Chapter 6. For the HPV vaccines, adverse events reported to date include vascular thrombosis, seizures, anaphylactic shock and possibly an increase in the incidence of grade 2 and 3 CIN lesions, as well as genital warts (at least with the quadrivalent vaccine) in women previously exposed to HPV. The FDA has stated that by July 2008 over 16 million doses of the quadrivalent vaccine, Gardasil, had been distributed in the United States (the number of people vaccinated – a critically important question – is not provided) and almost 10,000 adverse events reported; although more than 90 per cent of adverse events are reported to be 'not serious'; and many, possibly none of the deaths associated with vaccine administration (as this book goes to press, believed to be over 30) were caused by the vaccine [23]. However, given that there is little or no information on vaccine-related side-effects in girls and young women in developing countries, where the high prevalence of malnutrition, other infections, poor hygiene, and more limited health care could influence the pattern or outcome of adverse events, it would seem prudent to ensure that accurate data on toxicity is collected in these countries as vaccination programs proceed. In countries where the incidence of cervical cancer is low – even without screening (e.g. in many Middle-East countries), vaccination programs may not be indicated. These issues should be taken into consideration when deciding whether HPV vaccination will be incorporated into the national cancer plan.

Horizontal and vertical approaches

It is in the context of prevention in particular, that cross-cutting or horizontal approaches to disease control are of particular importance, since many risk factors are important to multiple diseases and cost-benefit ratios may be much more favourable in this context. For example, the control of infectious diseases that predispose to cancer in low and middle income countries, and for which treatment or vaccines are available, such as schistosomiasis, hepatitis B and C, and HIV/AIDS, although primarily undertaken because of the infectious disease itself, will also reduce the incidence of the associated cancers. It is, perhaps, important to note that cancer has become the commonest cause of death in HIV-infected individuals treated with highly active anti-retroviral therapy.

Many NCDs share risk factors – such as tobacco-related cardiac and pulmonary diseases and a broad range of conditions associated with overweight or obesity. Horizontal approaches, via the control of common risk factors, are often emphasized in the context of public health, as discussed in Chapter 21. Vertical measures, that is, the control of a disease through specific measures relevant only to the disease in question, are necessary, but have the danger in resource-poor settings that improved control of one disease may be achieved at the expense of worsening the situation in other areas of health, because the use of the limited available resources is distorted. It is worrisome that in 2007, of $2.5 billion in aid (in the health sector) to developing countries spent by governments, philanthropic organizations, and pharmaceutical companies, 80 per cent went to developing products for tuberculosis, malaria, and HIV infection [24]. A judicious mixture of horizontal and vertical approaches would seem to be the best prescription.

Early detection and screening programmes

The role of the primary care provider in cancer treatment is, in some respects, as important as that of the cancer specialist, since the best chance for cure is when the possibility of cancer is considered at an early time-point in the natural history of the disease. Perhaps the most important and widely applicable approaches to early diagnosis are education of the public and of the primary and secondary care providers so that care is sought at the earliest time, cancer is considered when warranted, and appropriate diagnostic steps are taken. It is essential to dispel the belief that cancer is always incurable. A focus on early detection of cancer is particularly important in developing countries where the majority of patients present with advanced disease, although early detection programmes must be linked to efficient diagnostic and treatment programmes.

While raising awareness about the early signs of cancer applies to all cancer, specific screening programmes for cancer are a different matter, since for some cancers at least, there is continuing controversy with respect to cost-benefit ratios and the ability of screening to lead to a reduction in mortality (see also Chapter 4). This applies to all countries, but takes on much greater significance when resources are limited – and particularly when treatment, even of early or in situ disease, may require significant human and other resources. In many cases trained personnel and equipment are not sufficient to permit large scale screening programmes (e.g. mammography for breast cancer and cytology for cervical cancer), while the detection of pre-symptomatic disease, a fraction of which will never develop into invasive cancer, may, arguably, be of secondary importance in populations in which there is a significant prevalence of un-diagnosed symptomatic disease. An important decision for the national cancer control committee is whether screening for any cancer can be justified. Even when simple, inexpensive techniques for screening have been developed and shown to be feasible and effective in developing countries, expanding such programmes to a national level may be difficult or impossible because of economic, logistic, or other reasons, including the lack of treatment facilities.

Some of the criteria relevant to the decision to screen for a particular cancer are its incidence (if unavailable, its rank order in hospital registries), attitudes and knowledge of the public, the technique to be used, its cost, required skill level and potential inconvenience or unwanted effects, the estimated number of patients in the target population (usually defined by age) who must be screened in order to detect a single early cancer (such information may not be available in the absence of population-based data), the availability and affordability of appropriate (definitive) diagnostic tests and of treatment, and the willingness of screen-positive individuals to undergo further diagnostic tests as well as the recommended therapy. Expensive screening techniques, such as mammography, cytology, endoscopy, the measurement of serum prostate-specific antigen and even magnetic resonance imaging are all used to a greater or lesser extent as screening tests in high income countries, but not only are these techniques generally beyond the reach of countries with limited resources, apart from the wealthier sectors of the population [25], but with the exception of screening for cervical and oral cancer, no screening techniques have, to date, been shown to lower the mortality rates, in low and middle income countries, of the cancers they are designed to detect in the low and middle income countries. The value of screening may vary over time and from one population to another, with factors such as the level of education of the public and the development of new treatment approaches potentially reducing its value. There is, for example, an ongoing debate on the value of screening by mammography and the measurement of prostate-specific antigen in technologically advanced countries [26,27], as discussed in Chapter 4.

Nevertheless, for two cancers, uterine cervical cancer [28,29] and oral cancer [30], screening for pre-malignant lesions has been shown to reduce mortality and to be cost-effective in research studies performed in developing countries. For cervical cancer, a disease in which 80 per cent of global deaths occur in developing countries, the techniques used have included direct visualization after painting the cervix with dilute acetic acid (VIA) or Lugol's iodine (VILI) [28], or, more recently, the detection of HPV in cervical mucus, which in India, was shown to be more effective than VIA in reducing incidence and mortality [29]. The recent availability of an inexpensive test for HPV requiring just three hours [31] suggests that HPV testing, which has the advantage of objectivity, may become the preferred screening test in developing countries. In both cervical and oral cancer, the therapy for lesions that have a high likelihood of transformation into invasive cancer is, in the vast majority of cases, simple, inexpensive, and can be carried out by trained nurses or even medical assistants. Indeed, detection (using direct visualization) and treatment (at least, of the majority of pre-malignant lesions detected) can be accomplished in a single visit in 'see and treat' programmes – thus avoiding the possibility that screen-positive women will fail to keep a subsequent appointment for therapy. Although this may result in some over-treatment, side-effects and long term consequences of treatment are minimal such that this should not be a reason to await a definitive diagnosis, for example, by biopsy.

In contrast, in early, pre-clinical breast cancer, whatever the method of screening used, treatment requires surgical intervention and often radiation therapy (for example, if breast conservation is envisaged) and some patients receive chemotherapy and hormonal therapy too. Even carcinoma in situ, and many benign breast lesions require surgical intervention, and radiation therapy is also sometimes recommended for carcinoma in situ. Clinical breast examination, designed to detect early breast lesions, but which, in unscreened populations in developing countries, will inevitably detect some advanced cancers, requires a relatively high degree of skill in the health workers (usually nurses, midwives, or doctors) who perform the screening. Moreover, to have an impact on cancer mortality, a high fraction of the female population must be screened (especially in countries where breast cancer, although important in rank order, still has an incidence 3 to 5 times lower than in technologically advanced countries). The diversion of significant numbers of health workers into screening programmes could lead to a negative impact on other health services.

A theoretically attractive alternative to clinical breast examination is breast self-examination (BSE). However, in two recent randomized studies (in Russia and China) this has not been shown to result in a reduction in mortality, although the frequency of biopsies for breast lumps (the majority were benign) was doubled in the self-screened groups – that is, there was a greater burden on the health system and more psychological stress for women [32–34]. While these studies can be criticized and their generalizability questioned, the fact remains that there is no evidence at present that BSE is effective in reducing mortality from breast cancer.

Any form of breast cancer screening will result in over-diagnosis, with some women being subject to potentially expensive and toxic treatment they do not need (as well as significant, unnecessary psychological trauma). This risk could be greater in countries with more limited diagnostic resources. In addition, resources dedicated to screening may be wasted since it has been reported that women screened for breast cancer often refuse diagnostic tests and/or treatment [35]. Other studies have shown that education alone can favourably alter the distribution of staging [36], such that at present it cannot be recommended that breast cancer screening be provided as a service in developing countries – it should only be undertaken in a research context. On the other hand, sensitization of both the public and primary health care providers to the potential significance of breast lumps could well significantly modify the present pattern of stage distribution such that a higher fraction of patients have early stage disease, resulting in decreased mortality from breast cancer even without significant changes being made to treatment, (assuming that reasonable care is available to the population in question) although simultaneous improvement of treatment, to the extent possible, is to be highly recommended.

Diagnosis

The vast majority of cancer patients require a tissue diagnosis, the remaining few (e.g. certain brain tumours) a radiological diagnosis. The quality of the diagnosis is important for many reasons, ranging from cancer registration (a major pillar of cancer public health) to cancer treatment (the goal of clinical medicine) and research. Unfortunately, as with other highly skilled health professionals, there is a dearth of well trained pathologists and radiologists in developing countries, and numerous other obstacles to good diagnosis must be overcome – including limited skills, paucity of imaging equipment, major delays in equipment maintenance and repair, limited or no access to reagents, and few and/or poorly trained technicians. There may be lengthy delays in tissues reaching pathologists, or in pathology reports reaching the treating physicians. Many of these problems could be overcome with limited expenditure, far less than the cost of treatment. Immunophenotyping is often available in a very limited number of institutions (mostly private) in the poorest countries, yet, assuming good technique, this can often greatly improve the accuracy of diagnosis and so potentially increase survival rates, at a lower overall cost. Similarly, testing for estrogen receptors in breast cancer, essential for the efficient use of hormonal therapy, is often not available, leading either to women who could benefit from hormonal therapy not receiving it, or women who will not benefit being subjected to oophorectomy or several years of hormonal therapy. Perhaps because cancer control is primarily seen as a public health issue, the quality of diagnosis is often overlooked or at least given inadequate attention. This needs to be rectified at all levels – training more pathologists, introducing at least basic immunophenotyping in addition to the standard haemotoxylin/eosin staining for histological diagnosis, and providing more access to consultation. Information technology permitting the national or international transmission of digital images (whether relating to pathology or radiology/nuclear medicine) of sufficient quality for diagnosis holds much promise for both training and consultation, and could also help speed up the time required to make a diagnosis when a patient is at a distant location – tissue could be processed by a technician or junior pathologist and transmitted to a larger centre for diagnosis. Other kinds of images could also be read at a central site. Maximal benefit from information technology will, of course, require good health services as well as well trained radiology and pathology technicians.

Treatment

Treatment is a critically important element of cancer control plans even in the lowest income countries, since patients suffering from cancer cannot be ignored. Moreover, no matter how limited resources may be, if treatment is not included in the national cancer control plan, a significantly higher fraction of patients who will develop cancer in the coming decades will die. At the very least, consideration should be given to improving the efficiency of existing treatment programmes particularly with regard to potentially curable cancers – associated, where possible, with programmes dedicated to earlier detection.

In high resource countries, as reported in the Eurocare-4 study [37] and by the US SEER programme [38] on average some 50 to 64 per cent of all cancer patients are alive at 5 years. Unfortunately, the proportion of cancers that are curable is significantly lower in developing countries, both because the cancers are generally advanced at the time of diagnosis and because treatment is frequently sub-optimal. As described, the limited resources for diagnosis and investigation into the extent of disease result in more frequent wrong or incomplete diagnoses, and a fraction of patients is likely to be under-staged – that is, have more advanced disease than is recognized, because of the lack or cost of modern imaging modalities. This, coupled to the high cost of treatment relative to the financial resources available, the lack of skilled cancer surgeons, poor access to radiation therapy, the lack, or sporadic availability of cytotoxic and other drugs, inadequate supportive care, limited specialized training, and inadequacies and overcrowding in treatment facilities, are some of the reasons that cancer mortality rates in developing countries – particularly low income countries – are much higher in proportion to the incidence of cancer, than those in technologically advanced countries.

National mortality rates reflect, of course, entire countries, which can be quite heterogeneous with respect to the provision of care. Cancer centres and major hospitals are few in number, and usually located in urban settings, whereas in the low income countries, the bulk of the population is in rural regions. As a result, patients often have to travel from their home and stay in or close to the treatment centre, for example, when adequate supportive care cannot be provided closer to home, or for radiation therapy. This may cause great hardship from loss of income or difficulties in caring for other family members. Developing an ability to provide basic supportive care and even straightforward chemotherapy close to home, for example, at a local or district hospital, after diagnosis, treatment planning and more complex treatment has been provided in a tertiary care setting, could significantly reduce the negative financial impact of serious disease.

It is difficult to obtain realistic estimates of survival rates, but where such data is available, or based on mortality data, there is no doubt that survival rates are substantially lower than in more developed countries. But, at least in paediatric cancer, there is evidence that countries with higher health expenditure and which are engaged in international programmes have improved outcomes for a given socio-economic level of development [39].

Capacity Building

To ameliorate deficiencies in diagnosis, staging and treatment in low resource settings, much more effort needs to be made to develop human capacity – firstly, by improving the skills and knowledge of existing experts, and secondly by expanding the number of health professionals. In the education of the current workforce in low resource countries, 'experts' from technologically advanced countries often have little understanding of the conditions in developing countries and assume that a discussion of the latest research findings and treatment approaches will somehow lead to improved treatment in the developing country. While such information has some educational value, it is usually not applicable to the day-to-day practice of oncologists in developing countries. Similarly, sending staff from developing countries for training programmes in Western centres – particularly those lasting for some years – may not only reduce further the local capacity, but lead to staff emigrating in search of better professional circumstances and a higher living standard. If such trained persons do return to their own country, whether or not they stay may depend greatly on professional and personal satisfaction, and much that they have learned abroad may not be applicable to their home circumstances. Occasionally, individuals trained abroad can help move things forward in their own country, but in general, training in the local context has the advantage that it brings immediate benefits to patients. Even when training abroad is not undertaken, oncologists in developing countries may try to emulate their colleagues in technologically advanced countries uncritically – that is, without careful consideration of cost benefit ratio, for example, the real extent of the difference that more sophisticated tests, or more expensive drugs will make to outcome. Often, for reasons of drug or radiation therapy availability, cost, toxicity, or 'personal preference' they introduce significant (un-evaluated and frequently on an individual basis) treatment modifications and because supportive care is often inadequate, the outcomes actually achieved are unlikely to match those obtained in the affluent setting. The high cost of new drugs and monoclonal antibody therapies raises considerable debate even in resource-rich countries (see Chapter 10) and a balance must be struck between making available standard therapy appropriate in the context of the local resources for a large number of patients, and providing more complex, expensive therapy for a small number of patients. This said, interventions such as high dose therapy with stem-cell rescue, which are available at a small number of centres in many middle income countries, will have a minor, even immeasurable, impact at a national level, but it may still be reasonable to establish a small number of such programmes at the leading institutions when resources allow, in part to provide for patients who can benefit from such programmes, and in part to improve professional morale and expertise and to be better prepared for the future. Indeed, one way of moving forward is to identify centres of excellence/competence, either in all aspects of cancer control, or for specific elements – for example, related to the treatment of a specific disease, or palliative care. Such centres can then provide focal points where others can be trained, such that satellite or even centres of equal competence can be developed in the same country or region. Such centres, particularly if 'comprehensive' cancer centres, should develop links with the community, to improve early detection and to collaborate in the provision of palliative care, and undertake patient care, professional education, and research (Figure 22.8).

The cost and quality of chemotherapeutic drugs

Many factors go into the cost of drugs required for cancer – sometimes differing, at least in degree, according to the class of drug (e.g. cytotoxic versus antibiotic or antiemetic). These include the costs of drug development, (higher prices can be commanded while the drug is on patent), manufacture, and formulation. Costs are generally much lower when drugs are manufactured in a developing country, particularly by a locally established company, but importation may give rise to a series of costs that are external to manufacture and packaging, including locally applied taxes and importation fees, shipping and delivery charges, as well as fees paid to local 'middle-men.' Drug procurement and shipping procedures are also relevant to drug cost, since drugs may be inactivated due to failure to maintain them within an appropriate temperature range, or supplies may be exhausted because orders were not placed in time. In this circumstance, national drug supplies may be affected, or, when public and private procurement is separate, drugs may remain available, but only from more expensive, private sources. Sometimes drugs are over-ordered, such that they exceed their expiration date and are thus wasted (although activity is often minimally decreased for months after the expiry date). For these and other reasons, including corrupt practices, even inexpensive drugs may not be available to patients in developing countries for lengthy periods – such that many patients may have significantly inferior treatment, or inordinate delays that have a negative impact on treatment outcome.

Drug quality in developing countries is also an important issue. When drugs are purchased from providers of generic drugs located in developing countries, quality and composition may differ from that of the original product, occasionally to the point of inactivity or even unanticipated toxicity, for example, from a contaminant. The WHO provides a broad range of guidelines

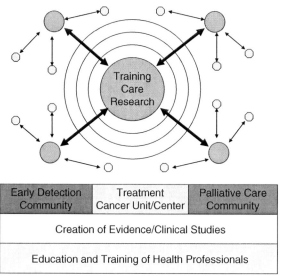

Early Detection Community	Treatment Cancer Unit/Center	Palliative Care Community
Creation of Evidence/Clinical Studies		
Education and Training of Health Professionals		

Fig. 22.8 A strategy for cancer control used by the International Network for Cancer Treatment and Research (INCTR). This strategy, which can be applied to essentially all cancer control projects is to develop a centre of excellence in care, education, and research which can help spawn centres of competence in other parts of the country or region. Training of a variety of professionals will be necessary in order to develop adequate early detection, clinical studies, standardized therapy, rehabilitation, and palliative care. This should be based on adequate evidence justifying the priorities identified and the interventions selected as well as support from the community, which may, along with the government, take a major role in promoting necessary legislation and public education, as well as patient support.

relating to the manufacture, quality control, and certification of medicines as well as the development and implementation of a national drug policy [40]. It also provides a list of essential medicines, which includes cytotoxic drugs [10]. These documents can be invaluable, given the necessary political will and financial means to implement recommendations at a national or regional level.

Paying for treatment and standardization of care

Most patients in high-income countries have health insurance, whether administered by the government as part of a national health service, provided by an employer, or by personal choice. This is not the case in developing countries, where the majority of patients pay out-of-pocket. In more than 167 countries, out-of-pocket expenses account for more than half of the total national health expenditure and in 87, more than 90 per cent [41]. Thus, the patient's (or their family's) ability to pay, or to take time off from work (generally unpaid), can make the difference between acceptance or rejection of treatment, or influence the type of treatment that is given. Some patients pay for only that part of a standard treatment regimen that they can afford, and abandon therapy when their funds are exhausted, thus significantly reducing the chance of successful therapy.

It is easy to see that standardization of treatment at institutional or national levels, taking into consideration a broad range of locally relevant issues, is important not only to cost-benefit ratios, but also to survival rates. Improved documentation of results achieved with standardized therapies can provide a good foundation on which to base future research – research which is tailored to the needs of the country or countries in question. Unfortunately, there is little standardization of therapy in developing countries – decisions are generally left to individual practitioners who may modify therapy or change it completely at a whim, and many practitioners work essentially in isolation; there may be only one specialist, for example, a medical oncologist, in an entire country (and sometimes, of course, none). Much may depend upon the referral route – most patients with cancer in developing countries still see a surgeon first (usually a general surgeon), who may perform surgery with no consultation with oncologists, and refer the patient for further therapy only in the case of recurrent disease – assuming that the patient returns for consultation. Multidisciplinary meetings to discuss pathology, staging studies, and the most appropriate treatment for individual patients are almost unknown in the poorest countries. Such meetings, particularly if conducted in concert with the input of outside experts (e.g. by videoconferencing) could be of great educational value to the range of health professionals present, as well as greatly increasing the likelihood that patients will receive appropriate care.

Rehabilitation

Rehabilitation of patients who have undergone therapy is an important issue from the twin perspectives of quality of life and an ability to re-enter the workforce (or, in the case of young people, continue their education). Those patients who are cured, however small a proportion, can have greatly increased quality of life through the use of prosthetic devices, many of which can be produced locally at greatly reduced cost compared to devices available in high-income countries. Similarly, re-training to overcome disabilities or permit cancer survivors to be gainfully employed in a different way can only benefit economies. Such programs, when they exist, are often carried out by NGOs in the poorer countries, largely because of the lack of government funding of such programmes.

Palliative care

Palliative care, as defined by the WHO, relates to the provision of medical and psycho-social care to patients with serious (potentially fatal) illness. In the context of cancer, most experts believe that palliative care should begin at the time of diagnosis and include a broad range of interventions relating to minimizing physical and psycho-social stress. This may, for example, include minimizing or avoiding pain during necessary procedures, such as biopsies, bone marrow examinations, or spinal taps, and ensuring that pain is effectively controlled post-operatively. In this regard, as well as in the context of patients with incurable disease, the level of palliative care increases as necessary according to the progression of symptoms. Moreover, much of palliative care can be considered preventive – that is, preventing the development of significant symptoms. Unfortunately, it is estimated that almost 60 per cent of people in the world each year who die require palliative care, yet only a small fraction receives it. This stems from a wide range of issues, the most important being that most deaths occur in developing countries (including most cancer deaths), where facilities and expertise in palliative care are rudimentary or patchy, and where many countries still do not have adequate legislation relating to the use of pain-killing medications, particularly opioids and other category C medications. Psychological and social support are, of course, essential components of palliative care, but significant physical suffering needs to be controlled, for the most part, before these issues can be adequately addressed, so that the most pressing need in palliative care is ensuring adequate access to good pain control.

If palliative care is to be accessible to a large number of patients in developing countries, their plight needs to be made clear to governments and other policy-makers (for long, for example, the International Narcotics Board has focused primarily upon preventing misuse of opioids rather than ensuring that patients who require these drugs have adequate access), so that necessary legislation regarding opioid availability is enacted and basic training in palliative care is provided as a standard element of the curriculum for all medical and nursing staff (and, where appropriate, other health workers). Because of strict anti-narcotic laws and sometimes cultural beliefs, some governments and health professionals minimize the use of opioids – sometimes to the point of refusing to prescribe them. Recently, a movement has emerged to label as 'torture' the deprivation of opioids from patients who clearly need them to control their pain. It sometimes takes a significant escalation of rhetoric of this kind to convince policy-makers that it is unethical to deprive patients of symptomatic relief – or of the prevention of pain and discomfort during procedures or after surgery. Ensuring opioid availability in developing countries, however, can be complex. It entails not only the provision of the drug or drugs themselves at an affordable price to the patient or family (dissolving morphine powder to create different strength solutions, preferably differently coloured, is very inexpensive, but slow release preparations are very expensive), but also ensuring that prescriptions provide medication for a sufficient time (in extreme cases, prescriptions can be given for only 24 hours), so that repeated journeys, that can be lengthy and extremely uncomfortable, to the nearest, but often distant hospital authorized to prescribe opioids, are avoided. Ideally, refills and dosage adjustments should be possible at a nearby health facility, where local doctors or even trained nurses are permitted to make adjustments in dosage as required.

Palliation may at times entail the use of specific anti-cancer therapy (e.g. radiation, chemotherapy, or even surgery). Indeed, incurable but relatively indolent cancers may be well controlled for many years by simple chemotherapy, while low dose radiation may be an effective way of controlling pain, for example arising from a bony metastasis. Unfortunately, cancers tend to be so advanced in some developing countries that by the time a patient reaches an institute capable of delivering care (assuming that they do), much of the practice of oncology is in the realm of palliative care. Ideally, palliative care should be introduced in a setting in which it is also made clear that many cancers are curable, particularly when detected early, for ultimately, the prevention or cure of cancer must be the goal – not simply the prevention of suffering from cancer, however important it may be.

Research

Cancer research should be a component of all national cancer control strategies. Although research conducted in other, mainly high income, countries should be used as the basis for interventions in developing countries to the extent possible, it is important to recognize that the research conducted in high income countries is directed to their own needs or circumstances and will often be irrelevant to cancer control in low and middle income countries. For example, already some valuable monoclonal antibodies have been developed that improve survival in cancers which express the relevant target molecule. However, such agents are prohibitively expensive for all but the wealthy in developing countries, and some of the presently available agents prolong life for only a matter of weeks to months. The high cost of such drugs while protected by patents is also a controversial issue in technologically advanced countries (it is justified by the manufacturers as necessary to recoup the cost of research required to develop new agents, including the many discarded because of minimal or no activity). In fact a high proportion of research throughout the world (in some high income countries, as much as 70 per cent, and in developing countries, more) is directed to drug development. And while this can result in real, if relatively small, degrees of progress, the problem of developing countries is primarily the lack of access to standard anticancer drugs (coupled to accurate diagnosis, staging, and care), rather than lack of access to new agents.

Where resources for research are limited, national needs rather than basic research should be emphasized (although basic research may realistically be accomplished in the context of international collaboration). Priority research projects should be drawn from a much broader research agenda encompassing all aspects of prevention, early detection and treatment (including all treatment modalities) adapted to the local context, or designed to determine whether resources can be spared in achieving a similar result. Research can address issues of diagnosis, staging, health service structure, and access to care, some of which will come under the heading of operational research; and can include surveys and situational analyses of topics such as attitudes and beliefs about cancer, the reasons for late presentation in particular cancers or populations, and the reasons for refusal of diagnostic tests or therapy. Such studies address the problems of the developing countries and can be rapidly translated into patient benefits. Clinical research can also be used as a focal point for professional training and education – including training in the collection of accurate data (which requires good follow up) and quality assurance – which should lead to more standardized approaches to diagnosis and treatment and introduce the idea of monitoring the degree of adherence to a planned study as well as the evaluation of results. Surveys and other forms of assessment can lead to the identification of potential deficiencies in health care delivery, including supportive care, which can make the difference between survival and death as well as preclude the identification of risk factors for survival because of a high rate of toxic deaths [42]. In the longer term, such studies result in the development of a foundation of evidence which can be built upon in a manner appropriate to the locally available resources and lead to improved national and international communication and learning from others who work in low-resource settings.

Finally, funding for research in developing countries is difficult to develop – much of the research in these countries is conducted by university staff from technologically advanced countries interested in epidemiological or other studies that often have no associated patient benefit, or, as described, by the pharmaceutical industry. To convince governments to invest in research, it is important that health authorities recognize that research conducted now can bring dividends both immediately and later, by increasing efficiency and knowledge. Civil society, both local and international, also has an important role in funding research, as have international inter-institutional collaborations, possibly as components of twinning or partnership programmes. Because of the sometimes unique research opportunities in developing countries, it is in the interest of the global community to develop ways of enhancing the infrastructure for research in these countries, and to develop research collaborations. Good research, regardless of where it is done, results in progress.

Research ethics

Research involving human subjects can only be conducted in an ethical environment in which the individual interests of the patient take precedence over those of society at large, and patients must be given information about the risks and benefits of the research elements of any study they agree to participate in. Clinical research in developing countries has special problems. Informed consent may be particularly difficult in a partially illiterate population with a limited, at best, understanding of cancer, and sometimes beliefs discordant with modern scientific medicine. However, this cannot be used as a reason to limit research in such countries (or, worse, to fail to obtain informed consent or assent), the argument being somewhat similar to the issue of research in vulnerable populations. In this respect, the Helsinki Declaration [43] states, in principle 17:

'Medical research involving a disadvantaged or vulnerable population or community is only justified if the research is responsive to the health needs and priorities of this population or community and if there is a reasonable likelihood that this population or community stands to benefit from the results of the research'.

Another issue is the increasing proportion of research – reflecting the funding available – that is related to product development. The pharmaceutical industry is rightly interested in reducing the cost of research and in bringing new drugs to the market as quickly as possible. Clearly, the large numbers of patients potentially eligible for research studies in developing countries could reduce the cost of such research. However, the most recent revision of the Declaration of Helsinki states that research subjects should benefit from the results of research (article 33). While not spelled out precisely, the implication, in conjunction with article 17, is that research should not be done in populations that cannot benefit from it. This has implications for the pricing of drugs in countries that participated in the development of a particular drug. Most new drugs cost many times the annual salary of participants in low and middle income countries – and sometimes, even in high income countries. There is room here for creative pricing. For example, methods could be developed to determine equivalent costs in different economies – similar to the use of purchasing power parity as a means of correcting GDP and other financial measures for differences in the cost of living in different countries. This is unlikely to be an issue when new drugs provide only minor patient benefits, but could become so as more effective targeted therapies are developed. Clearly, this is a complicated area and will require much thought and negotiation between governments, international organizations, and the pharmaceutical industry.

The Helsinki Declaration also requires that new interventions are tested against the best current proven intervention for the disease in question (principle 32) – although it does not specify whether this relates to the best available intervention in the context of the population from which research subjects will be drawn, or to the best available intervention on a global basis. This leaves open the complexities that may arise in determining the best therapy, which, in any event, may not be available in the country in question. Clarification of this principle would help to avoid inhibition of research that could greatly benefit the community. Apart from cost, the best available therapy in one country may not be optimal in another, for example, because of inadequate supportive care for a potentially toxic regimen. Indeed, in this circumstance, the 'best available therapy' defined in technologically advanced settings, could result in a higher death rate and give inferior results to less toxic regimens. It may be that the principle is intended to take local issues into consideration, but this is not clearly stated – presumably because the Declaration was revised with technologically advanced countries in mind.

Overcoming disciplinary and cultural divides and moving towards global cancer control

Cancer control (despite the broader definition used in this book) is often thought of as referring to prevention and early diagnosis and primarily involving epidemiologists and public health specialists. However, effective public education requires the active participation of care givers, who also play a critical role in early detection. Moreover, early detection has no value unless treatment can be immediately instituted. Treatment (including palliative care) is an essential element of cancer control in its own right – and the only way of controlling some cancers. Effective cancer control will entail collaboration among institutions and organizations, at both national and international levels, that have quite different cultures and often different goals, rendering effective communication and concerted action more difficult. Such divides must be overcome, since each element of the community has an important role to play. Supranational organizations provide information, guidance, and support to national governments which are responsible for the creation of relevant legislation, determining and regulating the structure of the health care system, and promoting (or endorsing) the creation and implementation of a national cancer control strategy. Academic institutions and cancer centres offer education and training to health professionals, while simultaneously providing health care and conducting the research needed to create and expand the evidence on which effective action depends. Industry is ultimately responsible for the manufacture of all the equipment and drugs needed for cancer control, and has an important role in the development of novel approaches and new technologies for diagnosis and treatment. Finally, civil society provides advocacy, funding, and information and may play an active role in professional and public education as well as participating directly in cancer control activities. As such, it plays an important role in helping to provide a connecting matrix among the range of involved institutions, for example in bringing silent disasters – such as the increasing cancer mortality rates – to the attention of those who are able to help, striving to create, in the process, a political climate of collective solidarity.

Overcoming the cultural divides that all too often separate countries and various elements of the community is essential to improving the control of cancer in developing countries. The term 'global cancer control' is frequently used today, but often has limited resonance, since there is little coordination at a genuine global level. A new trend, however, towards the development of regional cancer control plans – that is, plans that encompass each of the WHO regions – could create meaning to this term. Each region should have its own strategy based on the broad principles of cancer control articulated by WHO in Geneva, along with the efforts of other UN organizations, such as International Atomic Energy Agency (IAEA) Programme of Action in Cancer Treatment (PACT) [44], and civil society who can contribute by developing approaches in specific areas of cancer control that can be simultaneously tested or used in multiple countries at similar socio-economic levels. The regional approach can lead to much greater sharing of information and is likely to lead to rapid progress. Eventually, exchanges between or among regions will result in validation of the notion of global cancer control – and in the process, contributing to greater understanding and cooperation among countries throughout the entire spectrum of development.

References

1 Ferlay J, Bray F, Pisani P, & Parkin P (2004). Globocan 2002. Cancer incidence, mortality and prevalence worldwide. *IARC CancerBase*, No. 5, version 2.0. IARC Press, Lyon.

2 World Health Organization (WHO) (2007). Ten statistical highlights in global public health. In Pinchuk M (ed) *World Health Statistics*, 9–20, 3rd ed. WHO, Geneva.

3 Taha A & Ball K (1980). Smoking and Africa: the coming epidemic. *BMJ*, **280**(6219):991–93.

4 Sebrié E & Glantz SA (2006). The tobacco industry in developing countries. *BMJ*, **332**(7537):313–14.

5 Gu D, Kelly TN, Wu X, et al (2009). Mortality attributable to smoking in China. *N Engl J Med*, **360**(2):150–59.

6 World Health Organization, International Agency for Research on Cancer (2008). Boyle P & Levin B (eds). *World Cancer Report*, 1–510. International Agency for Research on Cancer, Lyon.

7 World Health Organization (WHO) (2008). 2008–2013 Action plan for the global strategy for the prevention and control of non-communicable diseases. WHO (cited 2009 June 8);1–33. Available from: http://www.who.int/nmh/en/.

8 United Nations Development Programme (UNDP) (2006). Human development report 2006. UNDP (cited 2009 June 8);1–422. Available from: http://hdr.undp.org/en/reports/global/hdr2006/.

9 Barton MB, Frommer M, & Shafiq J (2006). Role of radiotherapy in cancer control in low-income and middle-income countries. *Lancet Oncol*, **7**(7):584–95.

10 World Health Organization (WHO) (2007). WHO model list of essential medicines. WHO (cited 2009 June 8);(15th):(1–27). Available from: http://www.who.int/medicines/publications/08_ENGLISH_indexFINAL_EML15.pdf.

11 Sparano JA, Wang M, Martino S, et al (2008). Weekly paclitaxel in the adjuvant treatment of breast cancer. *N Engl J Med,* **358**(16):1663–71.

12 Clemens MA & Pettersson G (2008). New data on African health professionals abroad. *Hum Resour Health,* (cited 2009 June 10); **6**:1. Available from: http://www.human-resources-health.com/content/6/1/1.

13 World Health Organization (2005). World Health Assembly resolution 58.22: cancer prevention and control. World Health Organization (cited 2008 Aug. 8);103–107. Available from: http://www.who.int/gb/ebwha/pdf_files/WHA58/WHA58_22-en.pdf.

14 Parkin DM (2008). The cancer registry: its purpose and uses. *Network,* **8**:1–8.

15 World Health Organization (2007). The World Health Organization's fight against cancer: strategies that prevent, cure, and care. WHO, Geneva.

16 World Health Organization (2006). Cancer control: knowledge into action. WHO guide to effective programmes. Available from: http://www.who.int/cancer.

17 World Health Organization (WHO) (2009). WHO Framework Convention on Tobacco Control (FCTC). WHO FCTC (cited 2009 June 8). Available from: http://www.who.int/fctc/en/.

18 Doll R, Peto R, Wheatley K, Gray R, & Sutherland I (1994). Mortality in relation to smoking: 40 years' observations on male British doctors. *BMJ,* **309**(6959):901–11.

19 Sebrié EM & Glantz SA (2007). Attempts to undermine tobacco control: tobacco industry 'youth smoking prevention' programs to undermine meaningful tobacco control in Latin America. *Am J Public Health,* **97**(8):1357–67.

20 World Health Organization: The Tobacco Atlas. (http://www.who.int/tobacco/statistics/tobacco_atlas/en/)

21 Boffetta P, Hecht S, Gray N, Gupta P, & Straif K (2008). Smokeless tobacco and cancer. *Lancet Oncol,* **9**(7):667–75.

22 Zain RB, Ikeda N, Gupta PC, et al (1996). Oral mucosal lesions associated with betel quid, areca nut and tobacco chewing habits: consensus from a workshop held in Kuala Lumpur, Malaysia, November 25–27, 1996. *J Oral Pathol Med,* **28**(1):1–4.

23 Centers for Disease Control and Prevention (CDC) (1008). Information from FDA and CDC on Gardasil and its safety. CDC (cited 2009 June 8). Available from: http://www.cdc.gov/vaccinesafety/vaers/FDA_and_CDC_Statement.htm.

24 Grant B (2009). Spread the global health wealth. *The Scientist* (cited 2009 June 8); Available from: http://www.the-scientist.com/blog/display/55397/.

25 Arrossi S, Ramos S, Paolino M, & Sankaranarayanan R (2008). Social inequality in Pap smear coverage: identifying under-users of cervical cancer screening in Argentina. *Reprod Health Matters,* **16**(32):50–58.

26 Jorgensen KJ, Brodersen J, Nielsen M, Hartling OJ, & Gotzsche PC (2009). A cause for celebration, and caution. *BMJ,* **338**(b2126):1288.

27 Pienta KJ (2009). Critical appraisal of prostate-specific antigen in prostate cancer screening: 20 years later. *Urology,* **73**(5 Suppl):S11–S20.

28 Bhatla N, Gulati A, Mathur SR, et al (2009). Evaluation of cervical screening in rural North India. *Int J Gynaecol Obstet,* **105**(2):145–49.

29 Sankaranarayanan R, Nene BM, Shastri SS, et al (2009). HPV screening for cervical cancer in rural India. *N Engl J Med,* **360**(14):1385–94.

30 Subramanian S, Sankaranarayanan R, Bapat B, et al (2009). Cost-effectiveness of oral cancer screening: results from a cluster randomized controlled trial in India. *Bull World Health Organ,* **87**(3):200–06.

31 Qiao YL, Sellors JW, Eder PS, et al (2008). A new HPV-DNA test for cervical-cancer screening in developing regions: a cross-sectional study of clinical accuracy in rural China. *Lancet Oncol,* **9**(10):929–36.

32 Semiglazov VF, Moiseenko VM, Manikhas AG, et al (1999). Interim results of a prospective randomized study of self-examination for early detection of breast cancer. WHO, St.Petersburg, Russia. *Vopr Onkol,* **45**(3):265–71.

33 Thomas DB, Gao DL, Ray RM, et al (2002). Randomized trial of breast self-examination in Shanghai: final results. *J Natl Cancer Inst,* **94**(19):1445–57.

34 Kosters JP & Gotzsche PC (2008). Regular self-examination or clinical examination for early detection of breast cancer (review). *Cochrane Database Syst Rev.* (cited 2009 June 8);**3**:(CD003373). Available from: http://www.cochrane.dk/research/Regular%20self-examination,%20CD003373.pdf.

35 Pisani P, Parkin DM, Ngelangel C, et al (2006). Outcome of screening by clinical examination of the breast in a trial in the Philippines. *Int J Cancer,* **118**(1):149–54.

36 Devi BC, Tang TS, & Corbex M (2007). Reducing by half the percentage of late-stage presentation for breast and cervix cancer over 4 years: a pilot study of clinical downstaging in Sarawak, Malaysia. *Ann Oncol,* **18**(7):1172–76.

37 Verdecchia A, Francisci S, Brenner H, et al (2007). Recent cancer survival in Europe: a 2000–02 period analysis of EUROCARE-4 data. *Lancet Oncol,* **8**(9):784–96.

38 National Cancer Institute (NCI) (2009). Surveillance epidemiology and end results (SEER) stat fact sheets. NCI (cited 2009 June 8). Available from: http://seer.cancer.gov/statfacts/html/all.html.

39 Ribeiro RC, Steliarova-Foucher E, Magrath I, et al (2008). Baseline status of paediatric oncology care in ten low-income or mid-income countries receiving My Child Matters support: a descriptive study. *Lancet Oncol,* **9**(8):721–29.

40 World Health Organization (WHO) (2009). Essential medicines and pharmaceutical policies. WHO (cited 2009 June 8). Available from: http://www.who.int/medicines/en/.

41 World Health Organization (WHO) (2007). World health statistics 2007. WHO (cited 2009 June 8). 3rd, 1–86. Available from: http://www.who.int/whosis/whostat2007/en/index.html.

42 Magrath I, Shanta V, Advani S, et al (2005). Treatment of acute lymphoblastic leukaemia in countries with limited resources; lessons from use of a single protocol in India over a twenty year period. *Eur J Cancer,* **41**(11):1570–83.

43 World Medical Association (WMA) (2008). World Medical Association Declaration of Helsinki: ethical principles for medical research involving human subjects. WMA (cited 2009 June 8). 1–5. Available from: http://www.wma.net/e/policy/b3.htm.

44 International Atomic Energy Authority (IAEA) (2008). Building partnerships to fight the cancer epidemic: Programme of Action for Cancer Therapy (PACT). http://cancer iaea org/documents/PACT_2008_Small pdf. 1–24. Available from: http://cancer.iaea.org/documents/PACT_2008_Small.pdf.

45 World Health Organization (2008). The world health report 2006: working together for health. World Health Organization (cited 2009 Apr. 2). 1–237. Available from: http://www.who.int/whr/2006/whr06_en.pdf.

Chapter 23

Strengthening the global community for cancer control

Simon Sutcliffe, Mark Elwood[1]

The challenge

Cancer poses a major global health challenge – incidence, mortality, and prevalence are rising and will continue to do so with population growth and ageing, even though mortality rates in developed countries are now falling [1,2]. In all countries, even the richest and best resourced, evidence-based and carefully structured strategies are needed to extend effective cancer control interventions, including cancer treatment. For low and middle income countries, reliance on high cost solutions designed for other environments cannot be the way forward. So where is the light at the end of this tunnel?

Should one contemplate that population-based cancer control should be based on different principles for resource-challenged nations? Should there be different or 'lesser' standards for cancer control according to resource availability or priority?

We would argue against the premise of 'different principles for different peoples' – however, it is only realistic to accept different practices and priorities to address common principles applied within the context of different resource settings. We present some principles that underlie population cancer control in Table 23.1. They are based on premises that include an effective cancer control plan as an integral component of a population health plan; that health is not the absence of disease, but rather a 'resource for living' – the ability to realize aspirations and satisfy needs whilst changing and adjusting to change within a constantly evolving environment [3]; that improvements in cancer control derive through improvements to population development, population health, as well as through cancer-specific interventions [4,5]; that chronic diseases are the result of biological processes, driven by risk factors that have a commonality across diseases (tobacco, alcohol, nutrition, obesity, exercise, environment, behaviour, and choice); that health and the opportunity to be, and live, a healthy life is a 'human right' not a 'discretionary' response to social inequity; that disease control needs a plan that is based in evidence, standards of practice and care guidelines; and that differences of outcome across resource settings are much less based on biological differences than on socio-political, educational, and economic variables.

Accordingly, we defend the principles of population-based cancer control for all, but recognize that opportunities, priorities, and the real-life context will determine which policies and practices are pursued with what vigour, when, and how, to fulfil these principles.

[1] Simon B. Sutcliffe, MD, FRCP, FRCPC, FRCR Board Chair, Canadian Partnership Against Cancer, Canada, and Past President, BC Cancer Agency, Vancouver; and J. Mark Elwood, MD, DSc, FRCPC, FAFPHM, Vice-President, Family and Community Oncology, BC Cancer Agency, Vancouver, British Columbia, Canada.

Table 23.1 Principles of a population-based cancer control plan

Meets defined needs of the population to be serviced
Comprehensive to the spectrum of cancer control
Equitable, fair, reliable, and safe
Mitigates disparities of process and outcome
Based in evidence for benefit
Explicit standards of practice and clinical care guidelines
Integrated and coordinated (within and across diseases, professional groups, and health sectors)
Evaluable, evaluated, and reported
Sustainable
Appropriately governed and managed

Do we know enough about cancer to enhance outcomes across different resource settings?

What can be achieved in cancer control is a function of what is known and what is applied to the population who can benefit. A great deal about cancer and cancer control is known, but as shown in Chapter 5, some, but by no means all, of this knowledge has been successfully applied in some, but by no means all, jurisdictions, to achieve reductions in mortality and improvements in quality of life for those experiencing cancer.

Looking first at the strengths (what we know and what has been achieved), several major risk factors have been identified, quantified, and, at least to some extent, controlled. The key issues in cancer prevention are described by Colditz and Beers in Chapter 2 of this book as the control of nine key factors: tobacco, alcohol, body weight, diet and dietary supplementation, sun exposure, infections, environmental and occupational exposures, and medications. These are concordant with the prevention and screening goals of the European Code against Cancer [6], shown in Table 23.2.

Cancer shares many key risk factors with other chronic diseases. Dramatic reductions in cardiovascular mortality over the last 30 years have resulted from tobacco control, dietary interventions (polyunsaturated versus saturated fats; vegetable oils rather than animal fat; and increased vegetable to meat consumption), and the detection and control of increased blood pressure, blood glucose, and blood lipids [7–11], while being absent in countries where risk factors have not improved [12]. Physical inactivity and obesity have been identified as important linked risk factors; however, interventions, especially at the population level, have been less successful. While similar large decreases in total cancers have not been seen yet, smoking-related cancers in developed countries, particularly in men, have decreased rapidly as a result of tobacco control through legislation, regulation, taxation, awareness, communication, and social policy [13], as discussed in Chapter 2.

Cancer prevention has moved far beyond the simplistic concept of informing people of the hazards and expecting them to change their behaviour. Personal behaviour will change with the societal and environmental milieu, as discussed by Hill and Dixon in Chapter 3, leading to their 'Big Five' principles of behaviour change: motivation, modelling, capacity, remembering, and reinforcement.

Table 23.2 European Code against Cancer (http://www.cancercode.org/)

Many aspects of general health can be improved, and many cancer deaths prevented, if we adopt healthier lifestyles:

1 Do not smoke; if you smoke, stop doing so. If you fail to stop, do not smoke in the presence of non-smokers.

2 Avoid obesity.

3 Undertake some brisk, physical activity every day.

4 Increase your daily intake and variety of vegetables and fruits: eat at least five servings daily. Limit your intake of foods containing fats from animal sources.

5 If you drink alcohol, whether beer, wine, or spirits, moderate your consumption to two drinks per day if you are a man or one drink per day if you are a woman.

6 Care must be taken to avoid excessive sun exposure. It is specifically important to protect children and adolescents. For individuals who have a tendency to burn in the sun active protective measures must be taken throughout life.

7 Apply strictly regulations aimed at preventing any exposure to known cancer-causing substances. Follow all health and safety instructions on substances which may cause cancer. Follow advice of National Radiation Protection Offices.

There are public health programmes that could prevent cancers developing or increase the probability that a cancer may be cured:

8 Women from 25 years of age should participate in cervical screening. This should be within programmes with quality control procedures[a].

9 Women from 50 years of age should participate in breast screening. This should be within programmes with quality control procedures[a].

10 Men and women from 50 years of age should participate in colorectal screening. This should be within programmes with built-in quality assurance procedures.

11 Participate in vaccination programmes against hepatitis B virus and human papilloma virus[b], if available.

From: Third version [38], from Annals of Oncology 14: 973–1005, 2003, with permission of Oxford University Press. Slightly modified as shown:

[a]Original version refers to specific European quality control guidelines.

[b]Original version prepared in 2003: HPV added.

The impact of new knowledge on cancer causation is perhaps best shown by social trends in developed countries: from being an accepted behaviour of the majority, smoking is now a minority exposure and unacceptable in most social situations, workplaces, and even in recreational settings like bars and restaurants. Sun protection is an expected part of school programmes and even the architectural design of public areas in high risk regions. Almost everyone knows they should be active, eat well, and control their weight, even if the practice is harder than the intent. To question if a chemical is carcinogenic is a normal expectation rather than a rare situation. Indeed, anxiety about cancer risk can go too far, with perhaps unnecessary concern about many common exposures, from baby bottles to cell phones. In parallel with ongoing good research into potential hazards, better understanding and communication of the concept of risk and informed choice is needed [14]. Prevention also depends on new technologies and their application, as shown by the progress on immunization to reduce liver, cervical, and other cancers, as discussed in Chapter 6.

Are advances in diagnosis and treatment taking place?

Cancer mortality rates have been falling at about 1 per cent per year for adults over the past two decades in the developed world [15]. These trends show the success of prevention, early detection, and treatment. Early detection, including screening programmes, has certainly had a major effect on cervix and breast cancer, as discussed in Chapter 4, and earlier clinical detection has probably had a substantial effect on survival improvements in several other cancers.

One measure of improvements in care is increases in the 5-year relative survival rates, as discussed in Chapter 18. A long term perspective is shown by US data for patients diagnosed in 1999 to 2005 compared with fifty years earlier, 1950 to 54 (Figure 23.1). While this comparison is open to the problems of changes in diagnostic criteria and in data collection methods, it illustrates the huge improvement, with the all-cancer survival rate doubling from 35 to 69 per cent, and the survival in children with cancer increasing even further, from 20 to 82 per cent. So on this benchmark, survival rather than death has become the normative expectation. For individual

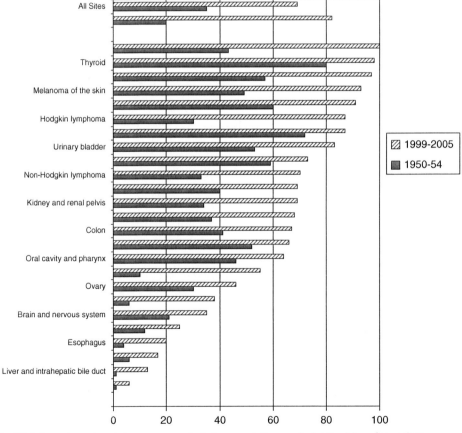

Fig. 23.1 Long term trends in cancer survival. 5-year relative survival, US whites, for patients diagnosed in 1950 to 1954 and in 1999 to 2005.
Source: Data from the US SEER system: http://seer.cancer.gov/csr/1975_2006/browse_csr.php?section=1&page=sect_01_table.03.html.

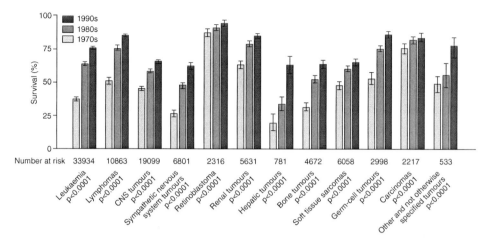

Fig. 23.2 Improvements in survival for children with cancer from the 1970s to 1990s in Europe. Vertical bars are 95 per cent confidence intervals; P values test equality over the three time periods. Source: Reprinted from (39), Steliatrova-Foucher et al., The Lancet, 364, 2097–2105, Copyright 2004, with permission from Elsevier.

cancer sites, the improvements have been generally very large, although the lack of progress for cancers of the lung, oesophagus, liver, and pancreas stands out.

The continuing gains in outcomes from advances in treatment for paediatric cancers is further shown by European data showing major improvements from the 1970s to the 1990s [16] (Figure 23.2). Undoubtedly, these are related to the high proportion of children with cancer who are treated in randomized trials or with evidence-based protocols and multidisciplinary teams – a much higher proportion than in adult cancers [17].

Medical imaging and pathology are both undergoing a transition from spatial and morphologic disciplines to integrated anatomic and functional modalities that impact upon predisposition, diagnosis, prognosis, and therapy selection in 'real time'. Molecular pathology (including biomarkers, micro-arrays, bio-banks, cytogenetics, and genomics) and advanced imaging (including functional imaging, co-registered images, image-guided interventions, and minimally invasive procedures) represent a shift from organ- and tissue-based practice to cellular- and molecular-based practice, with attendant implications for 'predictive, prognostic and personalized' medicine.

Surgery, radiation, and systemic therapy have all benefited by attention to quality and safety measures (for example, check-lists, standards of practice, practice guidelines, information management and technology, safety and quality protocols, and process review and improvement) as well as specific technical and procedural advances, for example, in surgery, minimally invasive surgery, robotics, and pre- and post-care enhancements; in radiation therapy, technical precision, 'target' definition and verification, image co-registration for beam localization, and interstitial techniques; and in systemic therapy, individually targeted therapies; protocols and pre-printed orders, pharmacy quality control, prescribing, and dispensing practices.

Is cancer care improving?

Just as important as, and in synergy with, advances in specific cancer therapies, have been improvements to the quality of care, discussed in Chapters 7 to 14. These are many: management by interdisciplinary teams; the development and adoption of evidence-based clinical practice guidelines; the definition and application of explicit standards of care associated with indicators and measures of performance; improved symptom control and pain management; expanded care models integrating community and facility-centred interventions; alternative service delivery models such as patient navigation and community nurse triage; increased enrolment in clinical trials, thereby increasing standardized care, therapeutic innovation and novel interventions in an ethical, evidence-based context; and an enhanced awareness of support, palliation, and survivorship considerations as fundamental requirements for compassion, dignity, comfort, and functionality [18–20].

Future progress

If all these improvements are real and evident, what is the problem? The difficulties are three-fold:

◆ The knowledge gain is not fast enough to offset the incidence and mortality consequences of an increasing and ageing population.

◆ The knowledge is not being transferred into application at a population level at an appropriate rate or with equitable uptake and distribution.

◆ The ability to access and implement valid knowledge about improving cancer control is unequal – the opportunities benefit the 10 per cent (the resource rich) rather than the 90 per cent (resource challenged) of the world's population.

So on the one hand, there is knowledge, 'light in the tunnel'; on the other, we are far from maximizing the benefits of that light, and making it available to everyone.

How might we mitigate unequal opportunities to benefit? Within developed countries, mal-distribution of the benefits reflects inequities in education and general socio-economic circumstances which impact how health services are used; inequities in the provision of health services, including those resulting from decisions about resource allocation, for example, between preventive, curative, and supportive services, and often, simply poorly designed and poorly managed services that are inefficient. Internationally, for lower resource countries, the solutions have to come from within, but with assistance from without, as has been shown by the successes against communicable diseases such as polio, smallpox, trachoma, and river blindness. In essence, in both developed and developing countries, collaboration and partnership are necessary – not just at the level of sharing information, protocols, guidelines, manuals, etc. – but collaborations based on a commitment to achieve mutually defined goals through establishment of joint, and jointly-resourced, capacity.

Looking now at the challenges and the opportunities of population-based cancer control, what are the directions to be pursued within the context of reality and collaborative relationships?

We suggest a number of key issues for current and future attention:

◆ The establishment and direction of a population-based health/illness/cancer control plan in each country or jurisdiction. The plan is about what should be done, how, by whom, and when; it is about a change in function, enabled by structural considerations, that 'adds value' to the existing contributions of the health system and renders the system more effective through direction, integration, coordination, and internal and external collaboration.

◆ Attention to leadership, 'followership', and sustained commitment. A plan to address incidence, prevalence, quality of life, and mortality of cancer, of necessity, requires a coalition of 'partners' or stakeholders. Government commitment is necessary, but not sufficient. A successful endeavour requires full engagement of funder, provider, and beneficiary – 'ownership' of the plan by civil society, on behalf of civil society.

◆ Identification and establishment of funding 'alliances' – collaboration and direction of funds to achieve cancer control (or wider disease control) goals. The needs of a population-based plan encompasses clinical service, research, and education (capacity, quality, and performance); capital and operating resources; inter-institutional and national linkages; and international collaborations, partnerships, and alliances. Plans that address population need go beyond institutional and regional/national geographic boundaries. Collaboration to enhance population outcomes will need collaborations of funders to achieve those goals – governments, charities and foundations, private sector, industry, and public philanthropy.

◆ Establishment of methods for measuring, monitoring, evaluating, and reporting process and outcome, from public and privately funded interventions, both within the population-based programme and relative to contextually relevant external comparators.

◆ The definition of 'targets', deliverables, and collaborations/partnerships. These relate to both the execution of the plan as well as the expected impact of the plan on longer-term population outcomes, including incidence, mortality, prevalence, quality of life, and economic indicators. Collaborations and partnerships may encompass system integration and coordination, research alignment with practice, relationships within cancer control, and relationships between non-communicable diseases and cancer, as elements of an integrated risk factor control and chronic disease management strategy.

◆ Clarification and communication of the compelling reasons for investment in a cancer control (chronic disease) plan and the anticipated 'return on investment' from health outcome, societal, and economic perspectives. Context will be particularly relevant with respect to 'returns' within cancer control, across diseases/health states, and relative to other expenditures for public services.

◆ A principled and flexible approach to addressing the mismatch between 'need for service' and 'capacity to deliver service'. Elements for consideration include alternative service delivery models, for example, medical or public/population health models for service delivery [21], nurse triage and navigation, integrated early detection and health awareness programmes, home-based palliative care linked to education and community-based interventions; the use of technology to address issues of distance, critical mass, expertise, education, and mentorship; and socially responsible recruitment, training, and human resource development practices and policies to advance capacity and capability in more resource-challenged environments.

The contribution of international strategic approaches

Over the past decade, valuable global strategies to prevent and control non-communicable diseases have been produced by the World Health Organization, being the international body of government health agencies, building their four pillars of cancer control [22] (see Table 23.3). In parallel, the International Union against Cancer (UICC), as the international linkage of non-government bodies, has given us the World Cancer Declaration [23] (Table 23.4).

Several other key WHO documents (some described in Chapter 21) include Preventing chronic disease: a vital investment [24]; Global action against cancer [25]; Closing the gap in a generation: health equity through action on the social determinants of health [26]; the Framework Convention

Table 23.3 The World Health Organization's four pillars of cancer control

---

◆ Prevent those cancers that can be prevented

◆ Treat those cancers that can be treated

◆ Cure those cancers that can be cured

◆ Palliate whenever palliation is needed

From: [22].

on Tobacco Control [27]; Primary health care now more than ever [28]; Diet, physical activity, and health [29]; and the World Cancer Report [22]. The reports on Food, nutrition, physical activity and the prevention of cancer [30], and Policy and action for cancer prevention [31] from the World Cancer Research Fund and the American Institute for Cancer Research are also very valuable. Amongst many others are the International Atomic Energy Agency's 'building partnerships to fight the cancer epidemic' [32]. Also, the strategic documents of national organizations such as the American Cancer Society and the British National Health Service are of great value to other countries, for example The Cancer Atlas 2006 [33], which had input from many organizations. The US Institute of Medicine report on cancer control in low and middle income countries [34] is also valuable. All these have shaped the definition of the cancer-chronic disease burden and the directions for response.

Table 23.4 Targets for cancer control to 2020, set by the International Union Against Cancer, linked to the World Cancer Declaration, 2008

◆ Sustainable delivery systems will be in place to ensure that effective cancer control programmes are available in all countries.

◆ The measurement of the global cancer burden and the impact of cancer control interventions will have improved significantly.

◆ Global tobacco consumption, obesity, and alcohol intake levels will have fallen significantly.

◆ Populations in the areas affected by HPV and HBV will be covered by universal vaccination programmes.

◆ Public attitude towards cancer will improve and damaging myths and misconceptions about the disease will be dispelled.

◆ Many more cancers will be diagnosed when still localized through the provision of screening and early detection programmes and high levels of public and professional awareness about important cancer warning signs.

◆ Access to accurate cancer diagnosis, appropriate cancer treatments, supportive care, rehabilitation services, and palliative care will have improved for all patients worldwide.

◆ Effective pain control measures will be available universally to all cancer patients in pain.

◆ The number of training opportunities available for health professionals in different aspects of cancer control will have improved significantly.

◆ Emigration of health workers with specialist training in cancer control will have reduced dramatically.

◆ There will be major improvements in cancer survival rates in all countries.

From: [23]

There are many valuable websites with international relevance, including those of governments and major international organizations, easy to find by search engines. Some perhaps less obvious ones include:

1 European Union cancer activities http://ec.europa.eu/health-eu/health_problems/cancer/index_en.htm

2 Canadian Partnership Against Cancer http://www.partnershipagainstcancer.ca/index.html

3 Cancer Control P.L.A.N.E.T. (Plan, Link, Act Network with Evidence-based Tools) http://cancercontrolplanet.cancer.gov/

4 NCRI ONIX – National Cancer Research Institute Oncology Information Exchange http://www.ncri-onix.org.uk

5 OERC-MERLOT – Open Educational Resources for Cancer Multimedia Educational Resource for Learning and Online Teaching http://voices.merlot.org/group/oercancer

6 International Observatory on End of Life Care http://www.eolc-observatory.net/

The International Cancer Control Congresses (the third was held in Cernobbio, Italy, in 2009) have been influential in promoting international links on cancer control issues, and indeed in stimulating the writing of this book (http://www.meet-ics.com/cancercontrol2009/).

Research has always been in essence international and collaborative, largely due to the ethical scientific imperative of publishing results openly. Having comparable world-wide data on cancer incidence is now accepted as routine, but this needed a great deal of effort, starting in the 1950s, to establish standards for cancer registries to give world-wide data on cancer incidence; 'Cancer Incidence in Five Continents' is now in its ninth edition, the first being in 1966 [35]. Now we are moving towards having world-wide data on cancer survival, which has already shown great value [36,37]. Large scale international collaborative clinical trials, and also large epidemiological studies, have been of immense value in advancing cancer knowledge. The logistic requirements for clinical trials to assess important but modest improvements in treatment, and to assess the effectiveness of screening and preventive interventions, are huge and challenging; the era of the single-centre study is all but gone, except for hypothesis-generating and preliminary studies, and in many cancer areas even single country studies are likely to be too limited. Yet getting support for such work is a major challenge. While much research is funded, there is as yet little progress on the best strategy for research – how do we get maximum value out of research investments, how do we answer key questions in good time, when can we decide that some questions need action, not more research?

The future

Much progress has been made. But more can be achieved – not by establishing more organizations, but by enhancing the effectiveness of existing organizations, by leveraging the capacity to collaborate at strategic, operational, and resource development levels through relationships between nations (alliances), organizations (twinning), teams (interdisciplinary work), and individual leaders. Whilst intuitively sensible and conceptually simple, collaboration is easily impeded by the weaknesses and challenges of leading, resourcing, and sustaining change within diverse health systems over protracted time.

The burden of cancer is great and the task of cancer control daunting. Recognition that cancer is a process with many elements amenable to interventions from health to end-of-life, and that there are many precedents for meaningful, favourable change within each of the elements, provides encouragement and incentive to achieve more. Achieving more necessitates a broader collaboration amongst partners at policy, health service, and civil society levels – the strengthening of the 'global communities of practice' and a renewed understanding of the relationships and resourcing necessary to effect the common purpose in advancing global cancer control.

References

1 Jemal A, Thun MJ, Ries LA, et al (2008). Annual report to the nation on the status of cancer, 1975–2005, featuring trends in lung cancer, tobacco use, and tobacco control. *J Natl Cancer Inst*, **100**(23):1672–94.

2 Bosetti C, Bertuccio P, Levi F, Lucchini F, Negri E, & La Vecchia C (2008). Cancer mortality in the European Union, 1970–2003, with a joinpoint analysis. *Ann Oncol*, **19**(4):631–40.

3 Young TK (2004). *Population Health: concepts and methods*. 2nd ed. Oxford University Press; New York.

4 Bhanojirao VV (1991). Human development report 1990: review and assessment. *World Development*, **19**(10):1451–60.

5 United Nations Development Programme (UNDP) (2006). Human development report 2006. UNDP (cited 2009 June 8).1–422. Available from: http://hdr.undp.org/en/reports/global/hdr2006/.

6 Boyle P, Autier P, Bartelink H, et al (2003). European code against cancer and scientific justification: third version (2003). *Ann Oncol*, **14**(7):973–1005.

7 Pietinen P, Lahti-Koski M, Vartiainen E, & Puska P (2001). Nutrition and cardiovascular disease in Finland since the early 1970s: a success story. *J Nutr Health Aging*, **5**(3):150–54.

8 Srinath RK & Katan MB (2004). Diet, nutrition and the prevention of hypertension and cardiovascular diseases. *Public Health Nutr*, **7**(1A):167–86.

9 Zatonski WA & Willett W (2005). Changes in dietary fat and declining coronary heart disease in Poland: population-based study. *BMJ*, **331**(7510):187–88.

10 Vartiainen E, Jousilahti P, Alfthan G, Sundvall J, Pietinen P, & Puska P (2000). Cardiovascular risk factor changes in Finland, 1972–1997. *Int J Epidemiol*, **29**(1):49–56.

11 Jemal A, Thun MJ, Ries LA, et al (2008). Annual report to the nation on the status of cancer, 1975–2005, featuring trends in lung cancer, tobacco use, and tobacco control. *J Natl Cancer Inst*, **100**(23):1672–94.

12 Menotti A, Lanti M, Kromhout D, et al (2007). Forty-year coronary mortality trends and changes in major risk factors in the first 10 years of follow-up in the seven countries study. *Eur J Epidemiol*, **22**(11):747–54.

13 Kabir Z, Connolly GN, Clancy L, Jemal A, & Koh HK (2007). Reduced lung cancer deaths attributable to decreased tobacco use in Massachusetts. *Cancer Causes Control*, **18**(8):833–38.

14 Tucker WT, Ferson S, Finkel AM, & Slavin D (2008). Strategies for risk communication: evolution, evidence, experience. Proceedings of a symposium sponsored by the Society for Risk Analysis and the National Science Foundation. May 15–17, 2006. Montauk, New York. *Ann N Y Acad Sci*, **1128**:1–137.

15 Jemal A, Thun MJ, Ries LA, et al (2008). Annual report to the nation on the status of cancer, 1975–2005, featuring trends in lung cancer, tobacco use, and tobacco control. *J Natl Cancer Inst*, **100**(23):1672–94.

16 Steliarova-Foucher E, Stiller C, Kaatsch P, et al (2004). Geographical patterns and time trends of cancer incidence and survival among children and adolescents in Europe since the 1970s (the ACCIS project): an epidemiological study. *Lancet*, **364**(9451):2097–2105.

17 Sinha G (2007). United Kingdom becomes the cancer clinical trials recruitment capital of the world. *J Natl Cancer Inst*, **99**(6):420–22.

18 Morris E, Haward RA, Gilthorpe MS, Craigs C, & Forman D (2006). The impact of the Calman-Hine report on the processes and outcomes of care for Yorkshire's colorectal cancer patients. *Br J Cancer*, **95**(8):979–985.

19 Barr VJ, Robinson S, Marin-Link B, et al (2003). The expanded Chronic Care Model: an integration of concepts and strategies from population health promotion and the Chronic Care Model. *Hosp Q*, **7**(1):73–82.

20 Pollack LA, Greer GE, Rowland JH, et al (2005). Cancer survivorship: a new challenge in comprehensive cancer control. *Cancer Causes Control*, **16**(Suppl 1):51–59.

21 Harries AD, Makombe SD, Schouten EJ, Ben-Smith A, & Jahn A (2008). Different delivery models for antiretroviral therapy in sub-Saharan Africa in the context of 'universal access'. *Trans R Soc Trop Med Hyg*, **102**(4):310–11.

22 World Health Organization, International Agency for Research on Cancer (IARC) (2008). World Cancer Report 2008. IARC (cited 2009 July 2).1–524. Available from: http://www.iarc.fr/en/publications/pdfs-online/wcr/2008/index.php.

23 International Union Against Cancer (UICC) (2009). World Cancer Declaration 2008. UICC (cited 2009 June 26):1–2. Available from: http://www.uicc.org/templates/uicc/pdf/wcd2008/wcden09low.pdf.

24 World Health Organization (WHO) (2005). Preventing chronic diseases: a vital investment: WHO global report. WHO (cited 2009 Mar. 19).1–182. Available from: http://www.who.int/chp/chronic_disease_report/full_report.pdf.

25 World Health Organization (WHO), International Union Against Cancer (UICC) (2005). Global action against cancer – Updated version. WHO (cited 2009 Mar. 19). (2nd). 1–24] Available from: http://www.who.int/cancer/media/GlobalActionCancerEnglfull.pdf

26 World Health Organization (WHO), Commission on Social Determinants of Health. Closing the gap in a generation: health equity through action on the social determinants of health (2008). Final Report of the Commission on Social Determinants of Health. WHO (cited 2009 Apr. 2);1–247. Available from: http://whqlibdoc.who.int/publications/2008/9789241563703_eng.pdf

27 World Health Organization (WHO) (2009). WHO Framework Convention on Tobacco Control (FCTC). WHO FCTC (cited 2009 June 8). Available from: http://www.who.int/fctc/en/.

28 World Health Organization (WHO) (2008). The world health report 2008: primary health care now more than ever. WHO 2008 (cited 2009 Apr. 2). 1–119. Available from: http://www.who.int/whr/2008/whr08_en.pdf.

29 World Health Organization (WHO) (2004). Global strategy on diet, physical activity and health. WHO (cited 2009 July 2). 1–18. Available from: http://www.who.int/dietphysicalactivity/strategy/eb11344/strategy_english_web.pdf.

30 World Cancer Research Fund (WCRF) (2007), American Institute for Cancer Research (AICR). Food, nutrition, physical activity, and the prevention of cancer: a global perspective. WCRF/AICR (cited 2009 July 2). 1–517. Available from: http://www.dietandcancerreport.org.

31 World Cancer Research Fund (WCRF), American Institute for Cancer Research (AICR) (2009). Policy and action for cancer prevention. Food, nutrition, and physical activity: a global perspective. WCRF/AICR (cited 2009 Apr. 8). 1–188].Available from: http://www.dietandcancerreport.org/.

32 International Atomic Energy Authority (IAEA) (2008). Building partnerships to fight the cancer epidemic: Programme of Action for Cancer Therapy (PACT). IAEA. 1–24. Available from: http://cancer.iaea.org/documents/PACT_2008_Small.pdf.

33 Mackay J, Jemal A, Lee NC, & Parkin DM (2006). The cancer atlas. American Cancer Society (ACS) (cited 2009 July 2). 1–128. Available from: http://www.cancer.org/docroot/AA/content/AA_2_5_9x_Cancer_Atlas.asp.

34 Sloan FA & Gelbrand H (eds) (2007). Institute of Medicine. *Cancer control opportunities in low- and middle-income countries.* The National Academies Press, Washington, DC. (cited 2009 July 2). 1–325.

35 Curado MP, Edwards B, Shin HR, et al (2007). Cancer incidence in five continents, Vol. IX. International Agency for Research on Cancer (IARC) (IX). 1–896. Available from: http://www-dep.iarc.fr/CI5_IX_frame.htm.

36 Coleman MP, Quaresma M, Berrino F, et al (2008). Cancer survival in five continents: a worldwide population-based study (CONCORD). *Lancet Oncol*, **9**(8):730–56.

37 Berrino F, De AR, Sant M, et al (2007). Survival for eight major cancers and all cancers combined for European adults diagnosed in 1995–99: results of the EUROCARE-4 study. *Lancet Oncol*, **8**(9):773–83.

38 Boyle P, Autier P, Bartelink H, et al (2003). European code against cancer and scientific justification: 3rd version (2003). *Ann Oncol*, **14**(7):973–1005.

39 Steliarova-Foucher E, Stiller C, Kaatsch P, et al (2004). Geographical patterns and time trends of cancer incidence and survival among children and adolescents in Europe since the 1970s (the ACCIS project): an epidemiological study. *Lancet*, **364**(9451):2097–2105.

Index

Locators for headings which also have subheadings refer to general aspects of the topic
Locators in **bold** refer to major content
Locators in *italic* refer to figures/tables